PHALDEEPIKA

(Bhavartha Bodhini)

PHALDEEPIKA

(Bhavartha Bodhini)

English Translation

PANDIT GOPESH KUMAR OJHA
PANDIT ASHUTOSH OJHA

MOTILAL BANARSIDASS PUBLISHERS
PRIVATE LIMITED • DELHI

Reprint: Delhi, 2012
First English Edition: Delhi, 2008

ISBN: 978-81-208-3340-1 (Cloth)
ISBN: 978-81-208-3341-8 (Paper)

MOTILAL BANARSIDASS
41 U.A. Bungalow Road, Jawahar Nagar, Delhi 110 007
8 Mahalaxmi Chamber, 22 Bhulabhai Desai Road, Mumbai 400 026
203 Royapettah High Road, Mylapore, Chennai 600 004
236, 9th Main III Block, Jayanagar, Bangalore 560 011
Sanas Plaza, 1302 Baji Rao Road, Pune 411 002
8 Camac Street, Kolkata 700 017
Ashok Rajpath, Patna 800 004
Chowk, Varanasi 221 001

Printed in India
By Jainendra Prakash Jain at Shri Jainendra Press,
A-44, Naraina Phase-I, New Delhi 110 028
and Published by Narendra Prakash Jain for
Motilal Banarsidass Publishers Private Limited,
Bungalow Road, Delhi 110 007

CONTENTS

PREFACE

॥ ओम श्री परमात्मने नमः ॥

Om Shri Paramatmane Namah

The first of the three sounds 'अ' constituting the sacred Syllable vkse contains the symbol of Vishnu, the second one 'ऊ' that of Maheshwar and the third one 'म' symbolises Brahma. All the three Brahma, Vishnu and Mahesh are in the Pranava. This is the beginning, the end, and the middle.

अकारो विष्णुरुद्दिष्ट उकारस्तु महेश्ववर।
मकारस्तु स्मृतो ब्रह्मा प्रणवस्तुत्रयात्मक:॥

This is a holy exclamation at the beginning and end of reading of the Vedas or prior to the commencement of a prayer, mantra or scared work.

The घोष - The resounding sound which occurs when ओम is uttered, in itself, is the sound of assent, respectful affirmation, removal or warding off of all evils and every obstacle. This is the 'AKASH' Tatwa and it is similar to the sound of a good 'conch-shell'. It is ruled by the Planet Jupiter and the sound helps not only in the rectifying the hearing problems but in all matters connected to the Vata disorders particularly the troubles caused by the entities living in the 4th dimensions.

Constant thinking of 'Pranav' releases the energy in body. The kindling of the Kundalini from its sleeping state, and then it starts to move upwards and passes through the various Chakras resulting in the evolvement and attainment of Maya by endowing one with the Ashta Siddhis and Nava Niddhis and then the ultimate Moksha, the freedom from the cycle of life and death.

Depending upon the right and capability of a person the worship is done as the Saguna - Nirguna Bheda as well as 'Abheda'.

The second school of thought 'Prakrit Paropasna' which is known more as 'अजपा - जपा' that is the साधना of अभेद or अद्वैत सिद्धान्त। In the 'Tantrasara' the subject matter is described as :-

"One which is completed through the inhaling* and exhaling of breath, which is not uttered as Japa but still is a Japa, that is called the Ajapajap". The 'Kumbhak (stopping of Breath) in between the two is the ardhachandra (ँ) and it brings to consciousness the process of breathing.

This element which comprises the two letters 'ह' (Ha) and 'स' (Sa) and the ardhachandra (ँ) is the Kalpa Vriksha, the Mahamantra of Shri Vidya. This is visible and takes form during the meditation of Ardha- Narishwar Shiva in the form of Guru.

उद्यद्भानुस्पुरिततडिदाकारमर्धाम्बिके ।
पाशाभीती वरदपरशूं संदधानं कराब्जैः ॥
दिव्याकल्पैर्नवमणिमयैः शोभितं विश्वमूलं ।
सौम्याग्नेयं वपुरवतु नश्चन्द्रचूडं त्रिनेत्रम् ॥

जिनका आकार उदयकाल के सूर्य एवं चमकती हुई बिजली के समान दीप्तिमान है, जो अपनी चारों भुजाओं में क्रमशः पाश, अभयमुद्रा, वरमुद्रा और परशु धारण किये हुये हैं, दिव्य मणिमय सिंहासन पर विराजमान हैं और विश्व के मूल कारण हैं- ऐसे सौम्य (शान्त) एवं आग्नेय उग्र अथवा अग्नीशोम - स्वरूप त्रिनेत्रधारी चन्द्रचूड़ भगवान अर्धनारीश्र्वर हमारी रक्षा करें।

One whose formation is like illumination of the Rising Sun and Lightening; one who holds in his four arms - Pasha and Parshu and shows the Abhaya Mudra and Vara Mudra, respectively. Who is

---

*In the Dakshina Murti Samhita, it is written that -

It starts from birth and continues till death i.e. why प्राण Pran is Hansa. This is Atmaswaroopa. This prana is 21600 times. Everyone subconsciously does this Japa but as soon as he becomes conscious of the Shwas - Prashaws - all his Chakras open up leading the Atma to Paramatama.

enthroned on a throne embedded with unparalleled (दिव्य) lustrous Gems and is the Universal (root) cause of the Universe - Such a peaceful as well as Ugra (fiery looking) or Agnishowm (अग्निशोभ) with three eyes - Chandra Chuda (with the Crescent Moon on his forehead). The Supreme Power, Bhagwan Ardha Narishwar - half Iswar and the other half in the Female form, the Almighty God protect us. (त्राहिमाम् त्राहिमाम् त्राहिमाम्)।

This is the book about which to write or say anything is like showing candle to the Rising Sun. Many learned scholars had commented and translated this book, originally in Sanskrit, into various languages prevailing in India. This well known book Phaldeepika was created in the 12th Century by Mantreshwar* who was the greatest of all the Astrologers of his time. He took up the Astrological Principles prevailing and propagated by great sages like Maharishi Parashar, Gemini and many more.

A few decades ago this book was only available in the local languages prevailing in the South India and was not available to the vast majority of the Hindi speaking people in the North India. Then the learned Pandit Gopesh Kumar Ojha commented and translated it, 50 years ago, in the Devnagri Script (Hindi language) for the benefit of the Hindi - knowing persons.

Now I, his son Pandit Ashutosh Ojha have the opportunity to present it in the present set-up to the English speaking people. The 225 Principles of the "Bhavarth Ratnakar" which was earlier in the Hindi Edition are also present in this English work. From our side we have given some more examples and illustrations which were not in the Hindi Version so that the book in itself is complete.

The present book Bhavartha Bodhini Phaldeepika was in the 12th/ 13th Century written by Mantreshwar. Mantreswar was a Siddha Purush an evolved soul. He was a well read person and was successful in Tantra-Shastra as such he was called Mantreshwar with the Blessings of the lords of the Mantras. Pandit Gopesh Kumar Ojha was a scholar of Sanskrit, English, Persian and many other Indian languages. He came from a traditional family of the learned Pandits

*See Introduction.

who were the Gurus of the Maharajas of Alwar (Rajasthan) in India. Many years ago he thought of writing the not so far available 'Phaldeepika' to the Hindi knowing people which was available either in Sanskrit or in some other languages prevailing in South India. Some part of the original was in coded language just like a hint in solving a puzzle so Panditji thought of enriching the translation with his deep knowledge of the subject matter and presenting it for us in a simple and easy to understand manner. Bhavarthabodini Phaldeepika is one out of many other books like Jataka Parijata, Jataka Deshmang Chandrika etc. which he translated and gave his lucid commentary upon.

We have now brought out this present English Edition so that Astrology lovers in the West and those who are proficient in the English language can take advantage of the so far secret Principles of Vedic Astrology enshrined in Mantreshwar's Phaldeepika. Astrologers know that the Karma of a person in the past lives has resulted in the present birth. We are here to bear the brunt or to enjoy the effects of stars. Still the God Almighty has given to us a Will to improve or tarnish our destiny. We refer here to the Chapter 26, Sloka No. 50 of Phaldeepika itself.

अहिंसकस्य दान्तस्य धर्मार्जितधस्यच।
सर्वदा नियमस्थस्य सदा सानुग्रहा ग्रहा:॥

One who does not want others to be killed, has control on his senses (behaviour and mind) and earns his living in a righteous manner, always follows the rules and principles laid down in the scriptures, the planets are always pleased with him i.e. are always favourable to him.

(Phaldeepika, Sloka No. 50, Chapter 26)

Here we would like to quote the horoscope of Shri Ravana. He was Pandit of the Pandits. The most handsome, intelligent and eligible person and a victorious King, who not only conquered the Planets but defeated Lord Indra, the King of Gods. He used the planets as steps to climb to his throne.

Horoscope of Ravana

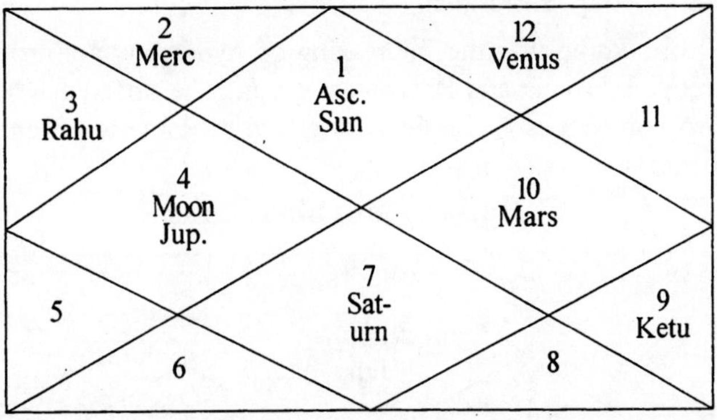

He had the blessings of lord Shiva. He was the person who could never be defeated, surrounded by good counsellors and was a Brahmin of the highest class, son of Rishi Visravas and Kaikasi and grandson of Pulastya, with such a powerful horoscope which was no less than that of Shri Rama.

He strayed from the path of religion and wanted Sita for himself. Sita the wife of Lord Rama had everything desirable in a woman but then Ravana's own wife Mandodari was no less.

The idea got imbibed in his mind that he should get Sita because whoever will marry her will be the king emperor. She was a beautiful woman endowed with all the qualities desirable in a woman - all the characteristics of a Padmini.

Exalted Saturn in the 7th house gave Ravana a faithful, good looking wife. Exalted Mars in the 10th house made him conquer the world, the Moon and Jupiter in the 4th house in Cancer gave him the throne of Shri Lanka, the city of gold.

But then the full aspect of Saturn and Mars on the first house and on his Sun (exalted) gave him the idea, the desire to possess Sita. No sooner he left the path of morality, religion and ethics, he become arrogant and his stars lost the luster and power. They become incapable to help him. He kicked his brother out and the significator of brother Mars became weak. Vibhishan brought about his fall and death. He would not listen to older people of his court, nor to his wife and his exalted Saturn lost the power and the strength to protect him.

His Atma his soul became weak and got coloured so ultimately he was killed by Shri Rama.

Lord Rama was the future king of Ayodhya - a warrior. The horoscope of Rama and Ravana are given. The difference between the two horoscopes is that the Rising sign of Rama was Cancer and that of Ravana was Aries.

Horoscope of Shri Rama

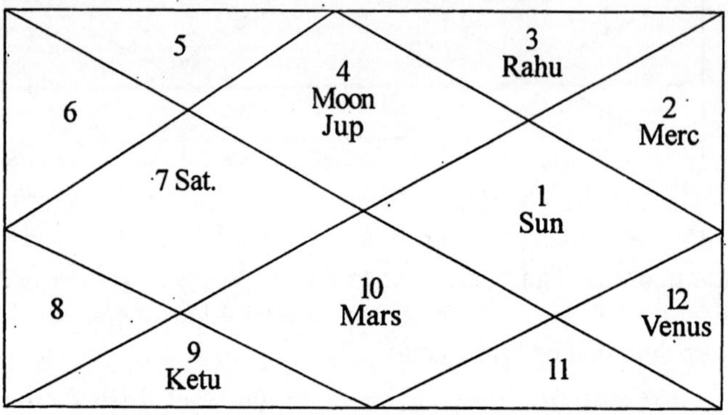

No doubt Rama was the Incarnation of Lord Vishnu but Ravana had the blessing of Lord Shiva. Why was Ravana defeated? The reason is not far to seek. He went astray from the path of religion and as soon as he abducted Sita his downfall started.

Exalted Sun in the first house endowed Ravana with luster, courage, anger and pride. 'Pride has a fall' and this applied to Shri Ravana.

City of gold, palatial buildings existed. A faithful and loving wife too was there to comfort him. The question is raised why did he lose to Rama? The answer is clear in bold letters. Ravana due to his actions brought about his own doom.

History indicates that Duryodhan threw his lustful eyes on Draupadi and so he got destroyed together with all the family and friends. Helen was abducted and Troy was burnt- Every time it happens but we do not learn from it.

Their beauty became a curse not only for themselves but for those too who laid their eyes on them. That is the way the Maya operates.

The purpose of indicating this is that many times people meet Astrologers and put up these questions why their horoscope is not showing good effect? The reason is that when we do certain deeds in life which weaken the 'Karakas', the Significators, then how can the planets show good effects? If you want your horoscope to show good then be on the path of religion. Do not do such things the loss of which will cause mental anguish to others. Every action bounces back.

Turning out his brother – reduced the effect of his Mars. Not listening to his wife and advisers dulled his Venus, Moon and Saturn and going through the established norms he kidnapped the wife of Rama.

On the other hand Ram never did anything against the established principles.

Just because his father desired him to leave - he did and so he improved his Sun - Love and support of his brother Lakshman strengthened his Mars; Respect for spiritual and religious people improved his Jupiter and Saturn - Therefore with almost parallel horoscopes Rama triumphed and Ravana did not and the victor is always worshipped.

Rama could not strike him in the Chest (the heart) as his Jupiter and Moon were protecting him so he sent the arrow to his naval and his source of all energy (supposed to have nectar in his naval) dried out then his heads were cut by the blast of arrows.

Many person with the Economic securities, forget the line of demarcation forget the moral principles of life they earn their wealth without any adherence to how they do it money is their God and then other evil creep in. They cast their lustful looks left and right and cause problems not only to others but for themselves. They do not take lesson from History.

When Ravana could not accomplish his desires because it was against the structure of the society of that time then how can a frail person like us attain it. Even if for a moment we gain then against all odds it is a temporary gain and ends in mental anguish.

They go to Astrologers and Babajis and want their help by using Vashikaran and what not. Their stars by their Karmas has already lost their hue and luster and how can they achieve anything.

By one action all good effects of planets are washed out and by one deed - good deed even debilitated planets show effects like exalted planets.

All this is written out for the learned reader to emphasize that Astrology is great, mathematical interpretations are fine but unless we follow the path of religion and keep the significators of different planets happy - good results will not come from a horoscope.

I wish that readers will enjoy this version of the Bhavartha Bodhini Phaldeepika and in case of any doubts or clarifications will solve it themselves or get back to us.

धर्मेण हन्यते व्याधि धर्मेण हन्यते ग्रहा:।
धर्मेण हन्यते शत्रु यतो धर्मास्ततो जय:॥

Ashutosh Ojha
1952/Sector - 4,
Gurgaon (Haryana)- 122001,India
E mail: aojha @vsnl.com
(91-124-2306168)

INTRODUCTION

वन्दे वन्दारूमन्दारमिन्दु भूषण नन्दनम् ।
अमन्दानन्दसन्दोह बन्धुरं सिन्धुराननम् ॥

The present unique classical treatise has come into being for the first time for the benefit of the Hindi[1] knowing population on account of the infinite grace of the Supreme Power of God Head.

Earlier this work was available only in the South Indian languages in the litho form. The original Sanskrit text in 'Dev Nagri' format was published approximately 40 years ago[2] from Calcutta and its commentary and notes were subsequently available in Tamil, Telgu, Kannada, Malyalam, Gujrati, English etc. yet its Hindi* version did not exist.

The present commentary highlights the meaning and substance of the Sanskrit text. It also elaborates the meanings of the twelve houses in a horoscope. Besides this we have added 450 yogas of the (Bhavarath Ratnakar[3] Shri Ramanuja in the Hindi Version; so the title of 'Bhavartha Bodhini Phaldeepika' is an appropriate and most befitting title for the book.

Shri Mantreshwar in his younger days was known as Markundeya Bhattardi. He was born in Southern India, in a Namboodari Brahmin family. One opinion is that his birthplace was 'Shaveeti' in the Tamil province. Another opinion is that his birthplace is Kerala. He was a worshipper of "Goddess Sukantala". There are differences about his birth period as well. Some learned

---

[1]National Language in India

[2]Interpreting part of Yogas (combination)

[3]Written in the year 1969.

persons are of the opinion that his birth was in the 13th century A.D. and yet others are of the opinion that it was the 16th century A.D.

For intensive learning he travelled to 'Bhadrikashram' in the Himachal Pradesh and also lived in Mithila (Bihar) to gain the proximity of the learned scholars for quite a long time. He was a grand scholar of Nayaya, Vedanta etc., the six philosophies. He was constantly engaged in the rigorous rites of fasting, japas and yagyas and succeeded in mastering and attaining the proximity of the Presiding Deities of the mantras. His name then became 'Mantreshwar'. He discarded his mortal body through 'yoga' at the age of the One hundred and fifty years.

Due to the study of various types of learning and rigorous practices, his knowledge of Astrology was intense and unlimited and therefore the readers will come across such practical and unparalleled interpretations in 'Phaldeepika' that they will get enchanted. 'Phaldeepika' is a mature creation of Astrology. Together with the commentary, the original slokas has also been included so that the kind hearted Sanskrit knowing readers could also enjoy the beauty of original poetry enunciated by Mantreshwar. It is of no use to praise the grandeur, benefits and substance of this treatise as the present book is in itself in front of the readers.

We expect that the officials will include this interpretive part of the unparalleled book in the list of recommended books for the purpose of proficiency and various types of examinations related to the learning and mastery of Astrology. The learned readers are requested to provide and suggest improvements for the next printings at the address given below:

'Saravali States'

यदुपचित मन्य जन्मनि शुभाशुभं कर्मणः पक्तिम्।
व्यञ्जयति शास्त्र मेतत्तमसि द्रव्याणि दीप इव।।

Astrology throws light like a lamp illuminates the goods kept in darkness, i.e. the results of the good and bad 'karma' that one has done in his previous birth. 'Jyotish Kalpadrum' has three divisions viz' 'Samhita'; 'Siddhanta' and 'Hora'. The interpretations of birth charts and horary charts fall under 'Hora'. 'Phaldeepika' was created to indicate the results of the past 'Karma'.

Sd: G.K. Ojha
Vijaya Dashmi Vikram Samvat 2026
93 Daryaganj, Delhi [1952 / Sector-4
Gurgaon, Haryana]
e-mail: aojha@vsnl.com

[The above is the literal translation in English of the Introduction written by the learned Pandit Gopesh Kumar Ojha, M.A., LL.B. whose knowledge has no parallel.

1

Rashibheda
Mangala Charan (Analysis of Signs)

One who dresses in white, has the luster of the Moon, is Glory and Happiness incarnate, has four arms (The Lord Almighty), meditate on to Him for eliminating all obstacles.

शुक्लाम्बरधरं देवं शशिवर्णं चतुर्भुजम्।
प्रसन्नवदनं ध्यायेत्सर्वविघ्नोपशान्तये॥

सन्दर्शनं वितनुते पितृदेवनृणां
मासाब्दवासरदलैरथ ऊर्ध्वगं यत्।
सव्यं क्वचित्क्वचिदुपैत्यपसव्यमेकं
ज्योतिः परं दिशतु वस्त्वमितां श्रियं नः ॥१॥

वाग्देवीं कुलदेवतां मम गुरून् कालत्रयज्ञानदान्
सूर्यादींश्च नवग्रहान् गणपतिं भक्त्या प्रणमयेश्वरम्।
संक्षिप्यात्रिपराशरादिकथितान् मन्त्रेश्वरो दैवविद्ऽ
वक्ष्येऽहं फलदीपिकां सुविमलां ज्योतिर्विदां प्रीतये॥२॥

The Supreme Illumination (Sun God), who to the Gods in the Sky, for half of the year (six months): to the departed forefathers for half the month (one fortnight): and to the human beings for half a day/night, all together, blesses with his appearance; who at times moves *via* the left (in the Northern Hemisphere) and then to the right (*via* the Southern Latitude) bestows, infinite (unlimited) prosperity (wealth, luxuries, good fortunes and beauty etc.)

The Gods are supposed to reside at the 'Dhruva'[1] Loka. At that place the night and day each, are of six months duration. The departed forefathers reside in the Chandra Loka (Moon). The Sun lights up the Moon for half the month (the bright half), the dark half belongs to the departed forefathers. The Earth, the abode of human beings, receives light for half of the day and night (i.e., twelve hours). All the above three have been stated in the prayers above. The Goddess of speech (Saraswati), the family God, and the giver of knowledge (of the past, present and future), my Gurus, as well as to Sun,[2] Moon, Mars, Mercury, Jupiter, Venus, Saturn, Rahu, Ketu - these nine planets, to Shri Ganeshji and to Ishwar (Bhagwan Shankar), I pay my obeisançe with respect and then I, Mantreshwar, present for the enjoyment of Astrologers, with frankness and simplicity the present scripture (Predictive Astrology) spoken, by the learned Maharishi Atri, Maharishi Parashar etc.

पदाभाद्यैर्यन्त्रैर्जननसमयोऽत्र प्रथमतो
विशेषाद्विज्ञेयः सह विघटिकाभिस्त्वथ तदा।
गतैदृक्तुल्यत्वं गणितकरणैः खेचरगतिं
विदित्वा तद्भावं बलमपि फलं तैः कथयतु॥३॥

First of all, the child's birth time should be recorded correctly and accurately with the use of various yantras mentioned in Astrology. The Ghatis, Palas, and Vipalas should be recorded expertly (It is very simple these days with the use of a watch). Calculation of the planetary position with the help of Astronomy, as to its sign, degree, minutes and seconds should be done.

If different positions are indicated from various ephemeris then the ephemeris which gives the exact location where the planets are actually visible, should be taken to be accurate [The present day Lahiri's

---

[1]The Pole Star

[2]The traditional system which still prevails is that before any writing or yagyas or auspicious events are undertaken, we invoke the blessings of different Gods, Gurus, the nine planets etc. to make the passage of completion smooth and without obstacles. Only after using different mantras we proceed with the main work.

Ephemeris and Raphael's Ephemeris are quite good]. Planetary longitude, cusps of houses, strength of planets and houses should be calculated and then predictions should be undertaken.

शिरोवक्त्रोरोहृज्जठरकटिवस्तिप्रजनन-
स्थलान्यूरूजान्वोर्युगलमिति जंघे पदयुगम्।
विलग्नात्कालाङ्गन्यलिझषकुलीरान्तिममिदं
भसन्धिर्विख्याता सकलभवनान्तानपि परे ॥४॥

The entire horoscope should be equated with that of the build up of the 'Kala Purusha', and then from the first house (Bhava, sign) consideration for head; from the second that of face; from the third Chest; from the fourth heart; from the fifth stomach; from the sixth waist; from the seventh 'Basti' (the lower part, if the portion between Naval and organ is divided in two parts), from the eight house private part, from the ninth thighs, from the tenth - the knees; from the eleventh shin, and the twelfth the feet, should be considered. If benefics are placed or aspect a house or if the Lord of that house is endowed with strength then the portion of the body which is indicated by that house is well developed, proportionate and beautiful to look at. If the lord of a house is weak or if the house is teneted or aspected by malefic then the part indicated by that house is thin, weak looking and disease may afflict that portion.

The ending portion (degree) of Cancer, Scorpio as well as Pisces is called the Joint (Sandhi in Sanskrit). Some Sages think that whenever two signs meet is called the joint *i.e.*, Rashi Sandhi.

अरण्ये केदारे शयनभवने श्वभ्रसलिले
गिरौ पाथः सस्यान्वितभुवि विशां धाम्नि सुषिरे।
जनाधीशस्थाने सजलविपिने धाम्नि विचरत्
कुलाले कीलाले वसतिरुदिता मेषभवनात् ॥५॥

We mention the places indicated by Aries, Taurus etc. - the twelve signs respectively.

(1) Forest (2) Agricultural land full of water (3) The Bed room (4) The Creeks, split space (Cracks) full of water (5) The hills

(6) The land full of grains and water (7) The abode of a businessman (Vaisya) (8) A hole (9) The ruler (King or a high official like Collector) (10) A flooded forest (11) A place of pottery makers and (12) Water.

In a horoscope or in a horary chart whichever sign is considered then in prediction, help should be taken from the above mentioned places indicated by that sign.

[Example: Suppose a question is asked as to where the lost article can be located. If in the answer the planet indicated Gemini (the 3rd sign) then inference should be drawn that the article lost or misplaced is in the bedroom]

भौमः शुक्रबुधेन्दुसूर्यशशिजाः शुक्रारजीवार्कजाः
मन्दो देवगुरुः क्रमेण कथिता मेषादिराशीश्वराः।
सूर्यादुच्चगृहाः क्रियो वृषमृगस्त्रीकर्किमीनास्तुला
दिक्त्र्यंशैर्मनुयुक्तिथीषुभनखांशैस्तेऽस्तनीचाः क्रमात् ॥६॥

Aries and Scorpio are ruled by Mars; Taurus and Libra by Venus; Gemini and Virgo by Mercury; Sagittarius and Pisces by Jupiter; Capricorn and Aquarius by Saturn; Leo ruled by Sun and the lord of Cancer is Moon.

Now in the chart below we have given the exaltation sign, sign of debilitation, the highest degrees where a planet is exalted or debilitated

Chart of Exaltation / Debilitation

Planet	Exalted Sign	Highest Degree of Exaltation	Debilitated Sign	Maximum Debilitation
Sun	Aries	10°	Libra	10°
Moon	Taurus	3°	Scorpio	3°
Mars	Capricorn	28°	Cancer	28°
Mercury	Virgo	15°	Pisces	15°
Jupiter	Cancer	5°	Capricorn	5°
Venus	Pisces	27°	Virgo	27°
Saturn	Libra	20°	Aries	20°

For example Jupiter when in the 5th degree in Cancer is in its maximum exaltation and after it reaches the meridian, it starts to descend; in Capricorn in 5 degrees it is debilitated to the maximum extent and after that it starts to get stronger *i.e.*, the debilitated effect is gradually getting reduced.

सिंहोक्षाजवधूहयाङ्गवणिजः कुंभस्त्रिकोणा रवेः
झेन्द्वोस्तूच्चलवान्नखोड्विनशरैर्दिग्भूतकृत्यंशकैः।
चापाद्यर्धवधूनृयुग्घटातुला मर्त्याश्च कीटोऽलिभं
त्वाप्याः कर्किमृगापरार्द्धशफराः शेषाश्चतुष्पादकाः ॥७॥

For some planets, the signs which are there own or exalted signs are also their Moola - Trikona signs as well. How can we distinguish as to where a planet is in own sign or in exalted sign or in its Moola - Trikona ? Which is the portion of the Moola - Trikona ? It is explained in the Table below :

Table of Moola Trikona

Planet	Sign	Moola-Trikona	Remaining portion
Sun	Leo	0° to 20°	Balance own sign
Moon	Taurus	3° to 30°	First 3 exalted to
Mars	Aries	0° to 12°	Balance own sign
Mercury*	Virgo	16° to 20°	20 to 30 Own sign 1 to 15 exaltation
Jupiter	Sagittarius	0° to 10°	Balance own sign
Venus	Libra	0° to 5°	Balance own sign
Saturn	Aquarius	0° to 20°	Balance own sign

Now we divide the signs into four sections *viz.*, Manushya, Keeta, Jalachar and Chatushpada.

*Mercury in Virgo is exalted in between 0 degree to 15 degree; from 16th degree to 20th degree; it is Moola - Trikona; and from 20th degree to 30th degree it is in own sign.

Manushya (human)	Chatushpada (four legged)	Keeta (worms)	Jalachar (entities residing in water)
Gemini	Aries	Scorpio	Cancer
Virgo	Taurus		Capricorn (second half)
Libra	Leo		Pisces
Sagittarius (first half)	Sagittarius (second half)		
Aquarius	Capricorn (first half)		

गोकर्क्यश्व्यजनक्रभान्यथ नृयुड्मीनौ परे राशय-
स्ते पृष्ठोभयकोदयाः समिथुनाः पृष्ठोदयाश्चैन्दवाः।
सौराः शेषगृहा क्रमेण कथिता रात्रिद्युसंज्ञा क्रमा-
दूर्ध्वाध:समवक्रभानि तु पुनस्तीक्ष्णांशुमुक्ताद् गृहात्॥८॥

Now we give below as to which signs rise from the front and which signs rise from the back (hind) first. Some signs rise from both sides.

Aries	From the back (hind) first	Libra	Front first
Taurus	Hind	Scorpio	Front first
Gemini	From both ways	Sagittarius	Hind first
Cancer	Hind first	Capricorn	Hind first
Leo	Front first	Aquarius	Front first
Virgo	Front first	Pisces	From both ways

Some people are of the view that the sign rising from the Front first are better and the sign rising 'hind first' are malefic. Planets posited in the signs rising front first, show their effect from the beginning itself (*i.e.* in the beginning of the periodic influences as well as in the earlier years of life). Planets in the hind first - rising show effect in the end. Those in the end. Those in the signs rising both ways, during the middle portion.

Now we give below the signs that are strong during the day[3] and also those which are strong at night.

Signs strong during the day - 5[4], 6, 7, 8, 11, 12

Signs strong during the night - 1, 2, 3, 4, 9, 10.

Sun has special power on signs which are stronger by day.

Moon has special power on signs which are stronger by night.

Start counting from the sign which Sun has already traversed.

These are in order called as 'Urdha', 'Adha', 'Sama', 'Vakra'. For example if Sun has crossed Virgo and has entered into Libra, then count from Virgo to Leo. These signs will respectively be known as 'Urdha', 'Adha', 'Sama', 'Vakra', 'Urdha', 'Adha', 'Sama', 'Vakra', 'Urdha', 'Adha', 'Sama' and 'Vakra'.

मेषादाह चरं स्थिराख्यमुभयं द्वारं बहिर्गर्भभं
धातुर्मूलमितीह जीव उदितं क्रूरं च सौम्यं विदुः ।
मेषाद्याः कथितास्त्रिकोणसहिताः प्रागादिनाथाः क्रमा–
दोजर्क्षं समभं पुमांश्च युवतिर्वामाङ्गमस्तादिकम् ॥९ ॥

Now we indicate some other features and characteristics of signs:-

Table or Chart of Features and Characteristics of Signs

Aries	Moveable	On the gate (threshold)	Metals	Odd	Malefic	East
Taurus	Fixed	Outside	Farm products	Even	Benefic	South
Gemini	Dual	Inside	Living beings	Odd	Malefic	West
Cancer	Movable	On the gate	Metals	Even	Benefic	North
Leo	Fixed	Outside products	Farm	Odd	Malefic	East
Virgo	Dual	Inside	Livings beings	Even	Benefic	South

[3]Sunrise to Sunset is day and Sunset to Sunrise is night

[4]'5' stands for Leo,'6' for Virgo and so on.

Libra	Movable	On the gate	Metals	Odd	Malefic	West
Scorpio	Fixed	Outside	Farm products	Even	Benefic	North
Sagitta-rius	Dual	Inside	Living beings	Odd	Malefic	East
Capri-corn	Movable	On the gate	Metals	Even	Benefic	South
Aqua rius	Fixed	Outside	Farm products	Odd	Malefic	West
Pisces	Dual	Inside	Living beings	Even	Benefic	North

We give below the Sanskrit names which depict the meaning and sense as well. We also give the English words that they indicate chart (movable) *i.e.* in which the work is done faster. If one starts travelling when a movable sign is rising then he returns at an early date.

Isthira (fixed) work done in these signs is long lasting. Entering into a house for living in a fixed sign, indicates living in that place for many years.

The first half of 'Ubhaya' (dual) shows the effect of fixed. The second half shows that of a movable sign. Because it shows both types of effect so it is called a dual sign.

'Dwar' means the gate *i.e.* the 'threshold'. 'bahi' means 'outside' and 'Garbha' stands for inside.

'Dhatu' (metals) include all types of metals, gold, silver, copper, iron etc.

'Moola' (the origin) stands for trees, fruits, corns, grains, farm products etc.

"Jeeva' (living beings) - one who has life - sons, grandsons etc.

Suppose a planet indicates 'Gains'? Then the question is what type of Gains? The sign that a planet is posited in will indicate the nature of the gains (or losses) - if that be of metals, roots or living beings. Malefics becomes more malefic in odd signs but in even signs, they show less evil.

In what manner that planets will show their effect should be decided after taking the nature as well as the placement and other important things mentioned in the book.

'Visham' means 'Una' or 'ojas', (or luster) 'Sama' means 'Pura' (perfect, soft). If more planets are placed in 'Visham' sign then the person is endowed with active elements. He will have courage, ability to take initiative etc. to a great extent. In 'sama sign', the nature is soft, beautiful, tolerant etc.

All the signs 1, 3, 5, 7, 9 and 11 are hard but comparatively 3, 7 and 9 are less hard (*i.e.* soft)

It is so because the lords of these signs are natural benefic. Similarly 2, 4, 6, 8, 10 and 12 are benefic (mild) still 2, 4, 6 and 12 are specially more benefic (mild) as the lords of these signs are also natural benefic.

The purpose of indicating the 'direction' (Disha) of a planet is that the placement of a 'karaka' *i.e.* , significator in a sign points out to the direction (of that sign) in which it will be fruitful. For example if in a horoscope, the lord of the first, ninth and tenth houses are in Scorpio then the indication is that the fortunes will come to him in the North (from his birth place)

लग्नं होरा कल्यदेहोदयाख्यं रूपं शीर्षं वर्तमानं च जन्म।
वित्तं विद्या स्वान्नपानानि भुक्तिं दक्षाक्ष्यास्यं पत्रिका वाक्कुटुम्बम् ॥१० ॥

दुश्चिक्योरो दक्षकर्णं च सेनां धैर्यं विक्रमं भ्रातरं च
गेहं क्षेत्रं मातुलं भागिनेयं बन्धुं मित्रं वाहनं च ॥११ ॥

राज्यं गोमहिषसुगन्धवस्त्रभूषाः पातालं हिबुकसुखाम्बुसेतुनाद्यः ।
राजाङ्कं सचिवकरात्मधीभविष्ययज्ज्ञानासून् सुतजठरश्रुतिस्मृतीश्च ॥१२ ॥

ऋणास्त्रचोरक्षतरोगशत्रून् ज्ञात्याजिदुष्कृत्यघभीत्यवज्ञाः ।
जामित्रचित्तोत्थमदास्तकामान् द्यूनाध्वलोकान् पतिमार्गभर्याः ॥१३ ॥

माङ्गल्यरन्ध्रमलिनाधिपराभवायुः
क्लेशापवादमरणाशुचिविघ्नदासान्।
आचार्यदैवपितृन् शुभपूर्वभाग्य-
पूजातपःसुकृतपौत्रजपार्यवंशान्॥१४॥

व्यापारास्पदमानकर्मजयसत्कीर्तिं ऋतुं जीवनं
व्योमाचारगुणप्रवृत्तिगमनान्याज्ञां च मेषूरणम्।
लाभायागमनाप्तिसिद्धिविभवान् प्राप्तिं भवं श्लाध्यतां
ज्येष्ठभ्रातरमन्यकर्णसरसान् सन्तोषमाकर्णनम्॥१५॥

दुःखांघ्रिवामनयनक्षयसूचकान्त्य-
दारिद्र्यपापशयनव्ययरिःफबन्धान्।
भावाह्वया निगदिताः क्रमशोऽथ लीन-
स्थानं त्रिषड्व्ययपराभवराशिनाम॥१६॥

There are twelve houses in a birth chart. Each house is called by more than one name. The different names of various houses are given below which indicate the matters that fall under the respective house.

First House

Lagna (Ascendant); Hora; kalaya; (Sunrise *i.e.*, beginning); Udaya (the beginning); Roopa (appearance), head, the present (present period); Janma (Birth) - all these are considered from the first house.

Second House

Wealth, education, ownership (control on wealth); eatables food, right eye, face, letters, speech, family - these are the (translation of the) names of second house. *i.e.*, consider these matters from the second house.

Third House

Chest, right ear, army, courage (valour), power and brothers (sisters) are considered from the third house. It is also called 'Dushchikya'.

Fourth House

Home (residence), Agriculture, maternal uncles, nephews, relatives, friends, vehicles, mother, cows-buffaloes (herds), scents, clothiers, ornaments and happiness are considered from the fourth house. Water, river, bridges are also considered from this house. This house is also called "Hibuk'.

Fifth House

King's Royal Seal (Insignia); Minister, Tax, Atma (Soul), wisdom, knowledge of the future, life (longevity), children, stomach, Shruti (Veda), Smriti (manusmriti *etc.*), all these should be considered from the fifth house. Shruti-Smriti means knowledge of scripture - so all types of spiritual knowledge should be considered from the fifth house.

Sixth House

Debts, Arms (weapons), thief, injury, disease, enemies, caste (relatives who keep a feeling of enmity), war, Bad acts, sins, fear, insults etc., should be judged from the sixth house.

Seventh House

The desires of heart (lust), pride, road, public, husband, wife etc. should be considered from the seventh house. At Sunset ('Asta'), Sun is in the seventh house so this house is also given the name 'Asta'.

Eighth House

Conjugal Bliss (Longevity of the husband), Chidra (hole), mental sickness - anxiety, insult or defeat, Longevity, sorrow, scandal, death, obstacles, Ashuchi (impurity due to death etc. known as 'Sutak'), slaves are considered from the 8th house. Private parts (anus) falls under the Eighth house. Mars in the Eighth at times causes piles, fistula etc.

Ninth House

Teacher (Guru), God (family deity), father, Prayers, previous birth (good deeds etc.), grand son, high family are considered from the ninth house. In South India father is considered from the ninth house but in other parts of India from the tenth house.

Tenth House

Business, status, respect, career, victory, fame yagya (fire sacrifice), livelihood, interest in work, manners (good or bad), departure, Authority (boss), good traits, sky etc. are considered from the tenth house. This is also called 'Meshurana' or the place of giving directions (orders).

Eleventh House

Gains, income, receipts, incoming of persons, realisation (siddhis), Riches (wealth-luxuries), welfare, praise, older brother or older sister, left ear, softness (glaze), good news etc. are to be considered from the eleventh house.

Twelfth House

Grief, feet, left eye, enjoyment, backbiters, end (last results), poverty, sins, sleep (sleeping on a bad intimate relationship), expenses, imprisonment etc. should be considered from the twelfth house. The twelfth house is also known as 'Vaya' or 'Rifa'

दुःस्थानमष्टमरिपुव्ययभवमाहुः सुस्थानमन्यभवनं शुभदं प्रदिष्टम्।
प्राहुर्विलग्नदशसप्तचतुर्थभानि केन्द्रं हि कण्टकचतुष्टयनामयुक्तम् ॥१७॥

The 6th, 8th and 12th houses are called 'Dusthan'. The meaning of this Sanskrit word is 'bad places'. The other houses *viz*., 1, 2, 3, 4, 5, 7th, 9th, 10th and 11th are called 'Shubha' - benefic houses. The 1st, 4th, 7th and 10th are known as Angles the other names for these in Sanskrit are 'Kendra' or 'Kantaka' or 'Chatushtaya'.

पणफरमिति केन्द्रादूर्ध्वमापोक्लिमन्तत्-
परमथ चतुरस्रं नैधनं बन्धुभं च।
अथ समुपचयानि व्योमशौर्यारिलाभा
नवमसुतभयुग्मं स्यात् त्रिकोणं प्रशस्त ॥१८॥

The second, fifth, eighth and eleventh are known as 'panaphar' meaning succeedent house. The third, sixth, ninth and twelfth are called 'Apoklim' and are Cadent houses. The third, sixth, tenth and eleventh are known as 'Upachaya'.

The fifth and ninth are known as 'Trikona' - Trine in English. Trines are excellent houses. Benefic planets in Trines show even more benefic results. The lords of the Trines also give benefic results in their major* or minor periods.

* See chapter dealing with Periods of Planets

2

Graha Bheda Planetary Characteristics

In the beginning of this Chapter first of all, we indicate as to what should be judged from a planet. What materials does a planet signify? In the first Chapter we had explained as to what should be decided from different houses (Bhava) if this principle is taken to be universal, then the lords of the houses should also indicate the same things and matters which fall under their respective signs.

For example, if the 6th house indicate enemies, then the lord of the 6th should also indicate enemies. This speciality has come to the planet due to the ownership of the house. But what are its basic characteristics? Suppose that in ten horoscopes Sun rules ten different houses. Then Sun will show the results of first house, if it rules the first, of the second house if it rules the second-all this is true but what are the natural traits of Sun-its assets, accomplishments, power to confer, etc.

All these things and what the planets signify, have been discussed in the Slokas below-

ताम्रं स्वर्णं पितृशुभफलं चात्मसौख्यप्रतापं
धैर्यं शौर्यं समितिविजयं राजसेवां प्रकाशम्।
शैवं कार्यं वनगिरिगतिं होमकार्यप्रवृत्तिं
देवस्थानं कथयतु बुधस्तैक्ष्ण्यमुत्साहमर्कात्॥१॥

मातुः स्वस्ति मनःप्रसादमुदधिस्नानं सितं चामरं
छत्रं सुव्यजनं फलानि मृदुलं पुष्पाणि सस्यं कृषिम्।
कीर्तिं मौक्तिककांस्यरौप्यमधुरक्षीरादिवस्त्राम्बुगो-

योषाप्तिं सुखभोजनं तनुसुखं रूपं वदेच्चन्द्रतः ॥२॥
स्त्वं भूफलितं सहोदरगुणं क्रौर्यं रणं साहसं
विद्वेषं च महानसाग्निकनकज्ञात्यस्त्रचोरत्रिपून्।
उत्साहं परकामिनीरतिमसत्योक्तिं महीजाद्वदे-
द्वीर्यं चित्तसमुन्नतिं च कलुषं सेनाधिपत्यं क्षतम्॥३॥

पाण्डित्यं सुवचः कलानिपुणतां विद्वत्स्तुति मातुलं
वाक्यचातुर्यपासनादिपटुतां विद्यासु युक्तिं मतिम्।
यज्ञं वैष्णवकर्म सत्यवचनं शुक्तिं विहारस्थलं
शिल्पं बान्ध्यवयौवराज्यसुहृदस्तद्भागिनेयं बुधात्॥४॥

ज्ञानं सद्गुणमात्मजं च सचिवं स्वाचारमाचार्यकं
माहात्म्यं श्रुतिशास्त्रधीस्मृतिमतिं सर्वोन्नतिं सद्गतिम्।
देवब्राह्मणभक्तिमध्वरतपःश्रद्धाश्च कोशस्थलं
वैदुष्यं विजितेन्द्रियं धवसुखं संमानमीड्याद्दयाम्॥५॥

संपद्वाहनवस्त्रभूषणनिधिद्रव्याणि तौर्यत्रिकं
भार्यासौख्यसुगन्धपुष्पमदनव्यापारशय्यालयान्।
श्रीमत्त्वं कवितासुखं बहुवधूसङ्ग विलासं मदं
साचिव्यं सरसोक्तिमाह भृगुजादुद्वाहमर्मोत्सवम्॥६॥

आयुष्यं मरणं भयं पतितां दुःखावमानामयान्
दारिद्र्यं भृतकापवादकलुषाण्याशौचनिन्द्यापदः।
स्थैर्यं नीचजनाश्रयं च महिषं तन्द्रीमृणं चायसं
दासत्वं कृषिसाधनं रविसुतात्कारगृहं बन्धनम्॥७॥

Sun

Copper, gold, father, benefic results (own betterment), patience valour, success in war, Atma (Soul), happiness, fame and status,

Government - job, strength, light, work and worship related to Sun, travels in forest and hills, inclination in Hawna (Yagya)- fire sacrifice, temples (and places of worship), penetrating, enthusiasm, etc. should be judged from Sun by a wiseman *i.e.* Sun is the significator of the above mentioned matters.

Moon

Welfare of mother, inner contentment, bathing in the sea, white flag or white material and white fan (made of white hair used to fan gods and kings with), umbrella, beautiful fans and royal insignia, fruits, flowers, soft material, agriculture, grains, fame, pearl, silver, Kansa (material out of which gongs are made), milk, sweet materials, clothes, water, cow, gain of woman, in take of food with happiness, looks (beauty)-all these should be judged from the Moon. Moon signifies these things.

Mars

Now we take up what Mars represents? Satwa (physical and mental strength). Things which come out of the bowels of earth, brother-sisters (and relationship with them), cruelty, courage, war, enmity, fire in kitchen, gold, kinsmen, arms, thief, enemies, enthusiasm, interest in the wife of others, lies, semen (strength, courage) mental receptivity and joyful attitude, generosity, courage or high qualities, sinful or indecent activities, injury, commanders (high position in army) etc. falls under Mars.

Mercury

What matters are influenced by Mercury or say as to what is ruled by Mercury? Learning, excellent power of speech, art, expertness, praise by learned people, maternal uncle, cleverness in speech, expertness in prayers, intellectual capacity in acquiring education (to be intelligent is one thing and to use intelligent in acquiring education is another).

Yagya, religious rites related to Lord Vishnu, truthful speech, in mother of pearls, place of entertainment, sculpture (and expertness in sculpture), relative, Yuvraj (the prince next to the throne), friends nephew, niece etc.- all these should be considered from Mercury.

Jupiter

Now we mention the matters which come under Jupiter: Knowledge (wisdom), good qualities, Son (male child), Minister (kings, minister), good behaviour and manners, or one's own character and work, teaching or initiating, important soul (high class innerself) knowledge of Vedas (Shruti) and Smiriti, rise for all, moksha (enlightenment after death), worship of Gods and Brahmins, Yagya, Tapasya, respect for others, treasure, expertness in learning, control on senses, honour, kindness etc., should be judged from Jupiter. If a woman's horoscope is under consideration then her husband's longevity and conjugal bliss should be judged from Jupiter.

Venus

Prosperity, vehicles, clothes, ornaments, Nidhi (treasure sure or wealth secreted under the earth), inclination and attainment in dancing, music, instrumental music etc. fragrance, flowers, satisfaction and relationship (husband wife), bed and business related to the above things, richness, prosperity, contentment, poetry, enjoyment, position as a minister, softness, marriage and other religions good deeds, celebrations etc. are judged from Venus. In the horoscope of a male, happiness from wife (women) should also be considered from Venus. The happiness from one's own wife as well from other women. As it has been mentioned in Sloka No. 5 that Jupiter is the significator of husband, similarity in Sloka No. 7 it is mentioned that Venus is the significator of wife.

The permanent significator of different planets which have been mentioned in Phal Deepika, they have great importance in interpreting birth charts. Those Astrologer who do not consider these significators they commit many mistakes. One person showed his horoscope to us. The rising sign was Aquarius. The periodic influence was of Venus and the age of the person was 22 years. When the native was supposed to enter in his 24th year then he was entering into the Mahadasha i.e. the major period of Sun. Many Astrologers have predicted that as Sun is the lord of the 7th house, which in this was case Leo, so the native will be married when he will be in the period of Sun as the lord of the 7th causes marriage or partnership. But our opinion was that as Venus is the significator of wife and women so we suggested that in the

Mahadasha of Venus he will be married and our predictions came true. The purpose of stating this is that we should not get into a wrong judgement only because of the Lordship of a planet of a certain house but should also put weigtage on the significator.

We should not only concentrate and predict according to the lordship but we should also take the significator, signified by a planet. If Jupiter is the ruler of any house and if it is placed in a good house and the native is passing through the minor period of Jupiter, then even at a young age the person so born, will have a child or he will be blessed with happiness from children. If Venus is well placed then even in young age it gives relationship and happiness from women. Longevity, death, fear, falling down from a high place or to lose one's status, to be an outcast, insult, sickness, sorrow, poverty, defame, sins, labour, impurity, back biting or bad name, calamities, impurity of the mind and to be engaged in sinful and bad activities, impurity due to the death of someone, steadiness, to live under the patronage of low people - Buffalo, laziness, fatigue, debts, things made out of iron, service, slavery or working for other imprisonment, getting arrested, farm equipments. All these should be considered from Saturn.

पित्तास्थिसारोऽल्पकचश्च रक्तश्यामाकृतिर् स्यान्मधुपिंङ्गलाक्षः ।
कौसुम्भवासश्चतुरस्रदेहः शूरः प्रचण्डः पृथुबाहुरर्कः ॥८ ॥

स्थूलो युवा च स्थविरः कृशः सितः कान्तेक्षणश्चासितसूक्ष्ममूर्धजः ।
रक्तैकसारो मृदुवाक् सितांशुको गौरः शशी वातकफात्मको मृदुः ॥९ ॥

मध्ये कृशः कुञ्चितदीप्तकेशः क्रूरेक्षणः पैत्तिक उग्रबुद्धिः ।
रक्ताम्बरो रक्ततनुर्महीजश्चण्डोऽत्युदारस्तरुणोऽतिमज्जः ॥१० ॥

दूर्वालताश्यामतनुस्त्रिधातुमिश्रः सिरावन्मधुरोक्तियुक्तः ।
रक्तायताक्षो हरितांशुकस्त्वक्सारो बुधो हास्यरुचिः समाङ्गः ॥११ ॥

पीतद्युतिः पिङ्गकचेक्षणः स्यात् पीनोन्नतोराश्च बृहच्छरीरः ।
कफात्मकः श्रेष्ठमतिः सुरेड्यः सिंहाब्जनादश्च वसुप्रधानः ॥१२ ॥

चित्राम्बराकुञ्चितकृष्णकेशः स्थूलाङ्गदेहश्च कफानिलात्मा।
दूर्वाङ्कुराभः कमनो विशालनेत्रो भृगुः साधितशुक्लवृद्धि ॥१३॥

पङ्गुर्निम्नविलोचनः कृशतनुर्दीर्घः सिरालोऽलसः
कृष्णाङ्गः पवनात्मकोऽतिपिशुनः स्नाय्वात्मको निर्घृणः।
मूर्खः स्थूलनखद्विजः परुषरोमाङ्गोऽशुचिस्तामसो
रौद्रः क्रोधपरो जरापरिणतः कृष्णाम्बरो भास्करिः ॥१४॥

Now we talk about the appearance and attributes of planets.

What is the purpose of this? If there is a planet in the ascendant then the native's virtues, temperament and behaviour will be according to the planet so placed.

One who has Mars in the 1st house, will have courage, ability to fight, sudden temper and heat. It also depends upon is in which sign Mars is in the ascendant. The position of Mars in different signs will give different results to some extent. If Mars is strong then the person will be brave and will be a commander and will fight. If Mars is weak or is associated with malefic then a person can only fight like a eunuch.

If there is no planet in the first house then the native's appearance will be like the lord of the ascendant.* His temperaments, his attributes, prakriti etc. will be like the ascendant lord. It is therefore necessary to understand the appearance, the behaviour, the temperament of various planets.

---

*We have noted that the Navansha of the ascendant and the ruler of the Navansha also controls the basic temperament and prakriti of a person. If for example– Cancer rises and Leo is the Navansha then at times the native will behave like– a Leo ascendant person, although the ascendant here is Cancer. At other times he will be more like a Cancerian. We should take both these things into account. The planet which aspects the ascendant also brings its effect on the person. The native will take the nature and dosha generated by these planet.

For example– Sun causes imbalance of the pitta. Saturn causes imbalance of wind this is the reason that we should understand the temper, virtues, good qualities or ill effect that come under the planets.

Now we give below different matters, virtues, temper etc. of planets.

Sun

Sun has control on pitta. The bones are strong. The hair on the head are less (or curly). The appearance is reddish black like deep red, the eyes are like- honey coloured. A little bit of brown and redness, square buildup, long arms and is dressed in red. By temper Sun is brave (full of courage) and violent.

Moon

Moon has heavy and big appearance (plump). On one side he is young, and on the other side he is mature. The body is white and weak.

Moon is said to be big and also thin. It looks that according to 'Pakshabal' the bright half and dark half, the appearance changes. Hair on the head are little and black. The eyes are very beautiful. The main thing of prime importance is the blood i.e. Moon has control on the circulation of blood. The voice is sweet. He is very fair in complexion and dresses in white. Moon is soft by nature and by appearance. Out of the three doshas it has control on phlegm and wind i.e. Moon in its periodic influences gives disease related to the imbalance or wind and phlegm or it could be vata or cough disorder.

Mars

Mars is thin in the middle that is his waist is thin. The hair is wavy and bright. There is penetration in his looks. By nature is violent and quick in temper, has control on pitta. He is dressed in red and the body has reduce. By nature is hot but is also very generous. It has control on the substance inside bones (bone marrow) in the body. Thus if Mars is strong then the bone marrow is also strong. If Mars

---

*If Saturn is in the 4th house in any horoscope then it will have full aspect on the 1st house. The aspect of Saturn is not always bad and from the 4th house aspecting the 1st house, it will make the native very wise and impart wisdom from the childhood and the person will start to behave in a mature manner. He will also understand the psychology of others. However the 4th house is also related to old age. Saturn alone in the 4th house causes a very lonely old age full of problems.

is weak then the majja will weak. Mars* is of young age (youth) i.e. if in the horoscope of a person, a strong Mars is posited in the ascendant then even at the age of 50 years, he will have the appearance of a 30 year old young man.

Mercury

Now we talk of the appearance and nature of Mercury

The view of Mercury is like new grass. It has the three doshas-vata, pitta and phelgm i.e. if Mercury is under malefic influences or does not show good effect then it can cause disease connected to the three doshas during it major or minor periods. It is full of nerves i.e. Mercury has control on the nervous system in the body. If Mercury is afflicted then possibility of disorder of the nervous system is possible. By nature it is fond of speaking sweet and appealing words. His body is symmetrical and well formed. The body is proportionate.

Mercury likes humour i.e. the sense of humour is well developed. Those man or women who have Mercury and Moon together they have a tremendous sense of humour. All the time they say things to make other people smile and laugh. The manner Mars has control on the majja. Mercury rules the skin. The topmost level of the skin. If Mercury is good skin is good. If Mercury is afflicted by malefic, the possibility of disease connected with skin may happen. The eyes of Mercury are long and he is dressed in green. This is a general description of Mercury.

Jupiter

Jupiter is yellow in colour but the eyes and hair on the head are a little bit brown. The chest is well formed and high, and the body is big. It rules the phlegm. In Ayurveda the appearance of people with cough prakriti that have been mentioned will also be in a person in whose horoscope Jupiter is strong and placed in the 1st house or is the ruler of the Navansha of the ascendant. The person so born will be big in build and will have the appearance of Jupiter. When Jupiter is strong then it makes a person very intelligent. We see intellectual abilities from Mercury as well as from Jupiter. When intellectual abilities

*Homoglobin problems are caused by Mars.

are considered from both then what will be the logic? Mercury gives ability to comprehend quickly any subject, and to remember it very fast. But Jupiter gives an analytical and logical mind, the will power is very strong. Good ideas, good virtues are the characteristic of Jupiter that is why Jupiter is called the Guru of the gods. The speech or the sound when a Jupiter person speaks is like that of a lion or like conch shell - very deep. It is a planet which indicate wealth. It gives wealth. If Jupiter is good in a chart then a person will be wealthy. When in transit Jupiter is a favourably situated then it endows one with wealth. If Jupiter in the birth chart is afflicted by malefic or is associated with malefic then wealth is destroyed. All these things are indicated in a Sanskrit word, which is Vasupradhan.*

Venus

Now we speak of the appearance and attributes of Venus

Dressed in multi coloured clothes. The hair are wavy and black. The body and the parts of the body are heavy. It has control on the phelgm and the vata. The hue of the body is like bright like the seeds of grass.

For Mercury the hue of the body given is like blades of the grass because it is more green and for Venus it is the seeds of the grass because it look white and bright in appearance. Venus is very beautiful that means one who has Venus in the first house or has a strong Venus in a horoscope, that person will be beautiful in appearance. The eyes are big and it has control on semen. Semen is called Shukra in Sanskrit. This is why Venus is the ruler of semen. If Venus is in the 8th house then it given disease connected with semen.

Saturn

Now we speak of the appearance of Saturn

Saturn is lame and particularly if Saturn is in the 12th house then

---

*In many books– Vasupradhan is indicated that means importance of wealth. But in many other books the Sanskrit word is Vasupradhan. Vasa is the fat in the body. So one who has more fat in the body and is fat in appearance.

it causes disease connected with legs. Many times people suffer from polio and they get injury in the feet. The eyes are deep set, in Sanskrit the word- 'Nimna Vilochan' which has two meanings. One is deep set the other meaning is that those who always look downwards. The body is big (big frame) but thin. That means the bones are big. The nerves are too many. By nature is lazy. The colour is dark. It has control on the vata. By temper he is hard hearted and a back biter. He is a fool. The teeth and nails are thick. The body parts and down are hard. He is impure. To look at he is frightening and by nature angry. He is dressed in black and old in age. It has specific omens of 'Tamogunas'.

शैवं धाम बहि:प्रकाशकमरुद्देशो रवे: पूर्वदिक्
दुर्गास्थानवधूजलौषधिमधुस्थानं विधोर्वायुदिक्।
चोरम्लेंच्छकृशानुयुद्धभुवि दिग्याम्या कुजस्योदिता
विद्वद्विष्णुसभाविहारगणकस्थनान्युदीचीं विदु: ॥१५॥

कोशाश्वत्थसुरद्विजातिनिलयस्त्वैशानदिग्गीष्पते-
र्वेश्यावीथ्यवरोधनृत्तशयनस्थानं भृगोरग्निदिक्।
नीचश्रेण्यशुचिस्थलं वरुणदिक्छास्तु: शनेरालयों
वल्मीकाहितमोबिलान्यहिशिखिस्थानानि दिग्रक्षस: ॥१६॥

After talking about the seven planets, their appearance and traits, we talk about the gods, the directions and special abodes of planets.

Temple of Shiva– Open spaces, where there is more light, Desert area and the Eastern direction, fall under Sun. What is the purpose of telling all this? The answer is that if some thing is lost and Sun is placed in the 1st house in Horary Chart, then we can tell where the lost thing can be located. If Sun is strong in a horoscope then we say that the native's fortunes will rise when he moves in the Eastern direction from his birth place. In political astrology Sun when afflicted by malefic can cause problems in Maru country or it can be concluded that there will be war and uprising. These matters are indicated just by infinitesimal manner in the Slokas. In horoscope or in Horary Charts, we should use our logical decisions in arriving at conclusion.

Now we go to state what comes under Moon. The temples of goddess Durga. The room where women or more then one women live. The place where there is water, medicines are grown or made, honey and wine. Moon rules the North West places and directions.

Now we talk about Mars

Mars- Mars has control on the lands where fighting takes place, where there is fire, the place where thieves and muslims and bad people live. Mars has control on these matters. The direction of Mars is South.

Now we come to Mercury

Mercury has control on the place where the temple of lord Vishnu, on the places where learned people gather, the place of celebrations and entertainment where mathematician and astrologers sit. Mercury rules the North.

Now we come to Jupiter

Jupiter has jurisdiction where treasures, the pipal tree, the place where Brahmins and gods live, all these places are controlled by Jupiter. The direction of Jupiter is North East.

Venus

Venus has jurisdiction on houses where prostitutes and dancers live where women wear veils, bed-rooms, the place of dancing. Venus rules the South East.

Saturn

Saturn has ruling on the persons of the low caste, where the temple of Sastha– (Sastha has been mentioned as a God). Unholy places, impure places, they all came under Saturn. Saturn rules the West.

Now we talk of Rahu and Ketu

Valmeetk- the place where termites gather and make mounds in forests. Where snakes live or holes where their is darkness. Rahu and

Ketu rules the South West. Rahu is the North Node of Moon and the Ketu is the South node of Moon.

Now we come to Sloka No. 17 to Sloka No. 20

शैवो भिषडनृपतिरध्वरकृत्प्रधानी
व्याघ्रो मृगो दिनपतेः किल चक्रवाकः
शास्ताङ्गनारजककर्षकतोयगाः स्यु-
रिन्दोः शशश्च हरिणश्च बकश्चकोरः ॥१७॥

भौमो महानसगतायुधभृत्सुवर्ण-
काराजकुक्कुटशिवाकपिगृध्रचोराः ।
गोपज्ञशिल्पगणकोत्तमविष्णुदासा-
स्तार्क्ष्यः किकी दिविशु कौ शशिजो बडालः ॥१८॥

दैवज्ञमन्त्रिगुरुविप्रयतीशमुख्याः
पारावतः सुरगुरोस्तुरगश्च हंसः ।
गानी धनी विटवणिङ्नटततन्तुवाय-
वेश्यामयूरमहिषाश्च भृगोः शुको गौः ॥१९॥

तैलक्रयी भृतकनीचकिरातकाय-
स्काराश्च दन्तिकरटाश्च पिकाः शनेः स्युः ।
बौद्धाहितुण्डिकखराजवृकोष्ट्रसर्प-
ध्वान्तादयो मशकमत्कुणकृम्युलूकाः ॥२०॥

When we understand the matters ruled by different planets, only then we can predict correctly. Therefore we should know as to what comes under which planet. This is mentioned below in details—

Sun

Worshiper of Shiva, Vaidya which is Ayurvedic doctors, king, one who performs yagya or fire sacrifice, ministers, tiger, deer, chakor (a bird).

Moon

Under Moon the worshipper of Shastha, women, (any women) washerman, farmer, animals residing in water, rabbit, deer, cranes and chakor.

Mars

Any work connected with kitchen or where work connected with fire takes place and one who uses weapons, goldsmith, Ram, cock and hen, jackal, monkey, vulture and thief.

Mercury

Learned person one who is engaged in sculpture, excellent Accountant or Astrologer, worshipper of Vishnu, Garud, (Eagle) Chatak (a bird), Parrot and Cat come under Mercury.

Jupiter

Under Jupiter– Astrologer, Minister, Guru, Brahmins, Sanyasi*, main administrator or chief of a household, pigeon, horses, swans.

Venus

Engaged in singing or singer, wealthy persons, business community, lustful people. Weaver, prostitutes, peacock, cow, buffalow, parrots and gymnasts.

Saturn

Those engaged in the business of buying and selling of oil, servants, low type of people, hunters, ironsmith, elephant, crow and cuckoo.

Rahu and Ketu

Buddhists, snake charmers or those engaged in catching snakes, donkey, Ram, sheep, camel, snakes, mosquitoes, bug of all types, insects, termites, owl. Places where there is always darkness.

---

*Many commentators has translated the Slokas as the main– Sanyasi. But we do not agree with this. It has two meanings. One is Sanyasi i.e. an Ascetic and the second one is the main person i.e. the main administrator (or leader).

In order to understand the different type of animals, matters, profession, clothes and places mentioned above, it will require a big space to explain them in details. But we will just give one example– so that people reading the book can understands. Suppose in a horoscope Venus is strong and its periodic influence is about to commence, then the things which have been mentioned for Venus like people or material etc. will give benefit. But out of so many things from which things he will benefit? For that logic should be used. Suppose a person is a villager and he lives in a village and engaged in farming. Then it is possible that he might benefit from the business connected with cow, grains etc. If this person lives in a big metropolitan city like Bombay and is a director making films or producing films, then if he engages prostitutes or women actors and starts to make new movies then he will gain much. Similarly these planetary things should be considered after taking into account the person and his background.

सौम्यः समाऽर्कजसितावहितौ खरांशो-
रिन्दोर्हितौ रविबुधावपरे समाः स्युः।
भौमस्य मन्दभृगुजौ तु समौ रिपुर्ज्ञः
सौम्यस्य शीतगुररिः सुहृदौ सितार्कौ ॥२१॥

सूरेद्विषौ कविबुधौ रविजः समः स्या-
न्मध्यौ कवेर्गुरुकुजौ सुहृदौ शनिज्ञौ।
जीवः समः सितविदौ रविजस्य मित्रे
ज्ञेया अनुक्तखचरास्तु तदन्यथा स्युः ॥२२॥

In these Slokas it has been mentioned as to which planets are friends of a planet. Which planets are enemies and what other planets are neutral i.e. neither enemy nor friend. In astrology a planet which is neither a friend nor an enemy is called Sama i.e. neutral. These are the natural friends, enemies and neutrals. We illustrate them in a tabular form.

Table of Natural Friends, Neutrals, Enemies

Planet	Friend	Neutral	Enemies
Sun	-Moon, Mars, Jupiter	-Mercury	-Venus, Saturn
Moon	-Sun, Mercury	-Mars, Jupiter, Venus, Saturn	----------
Mars	-Sun, Moon, Jupiter	-Venus, Saturn	-Mercury
Mercury	-Sun, Venus Saturn.	-Mars, Jupiter,	-Moon
Jupiter	-Sun, Moon, Mars	-Saturn	-Mercury, Venus
Venus	-Mercury, Saturn	-Mars, Jupiter.	-Sun, Moon
Saturn	-Mercury, Venus.	-Jupiter	-Sun, Moon, Mars

This is the table of the natural friendship of planets. By temperament which planet is friend of which and which planet is enemy. In the coming Slokaṣ we will explain how to decide it in a horoscope as to which planets are friends or which planets are enemies.

अन्योन्यं त्रिसुखस्वखान्त्यभवगास्तकालमित्राण्मयमी
तन्नैसर्गिकमप्यवेक्ष्य कथयेत्तस्यातिमित्राहितान्।
शौर्याज्ञे रविजो गुरुर्गुरुसुतौ भौमश्चतुर्थाष्टमौ
पूर्णं पश्यति सप्तमं च सकलास्तेष्वंघ्रिवृद्ध्या क्रमात्॥२३॥

After stating above the natural friendship of planets. We come to the temporary friendships. Look to the planet about which we have to consider friends and enemies. Planets placed in the 2nd, 3rd, 4th, 10th, 11th and 12th houses from it are friends and those which are in same sign where the planet in question is placed i.e. in the 1st house, or in the 5th , 6th, 7th, 8th and 9th house are enemies. Here either a planet is a friend or an enemy. This is for the temporary friendships. After looking into both the natural and temporary friendships we would decide if planets are friends or neutral or enemy.

1. Those planets which are friends both ways i.e natural and temporary are called great friend.
2. Those planet which are enemy both ways or called great enemies.
3. Those planet which are friend from one method and enemy from the other, they are called Neutrals.
4. If a planet is friend in one place and neutral in the other manner then he will be called a friend.
5. A planet enemy in one place and neutral in the second, then he will be a enemy.

In a horoscope we should make a chart indicating friendship and enmity between planets. The question is what is the purpose of all this? The answer is that when a planet is in the house of a great friend or friend then it gives benefic results. Even if it is a malefic planet it does not show bad results as otherwise it would show. A planet in the house of an enemy or in the house of a great enemy does not bestow good effect. If it is a benefic then its benefic effect is reduced and a malefic will give real bad results.

Aspect of planet is given below

Planet	Full aspect	three fourth aspect	half aspect (50%)	25% (one fourth)
Sun	7	4-8	5th and 9th houses.	3-10
Moon	7	4-8	5th, 9th houses.	3-10
Mars	4-7-8	–	5th, 9th houses.	3-10
Mercury	7	4-8	5th, 9th houses.	3-10
Jupiter	5-7-9	4-8	------	3-10
Venus	7	4-8	5th, 9th houses.	3-10
Saturn	3-10-7	4-8	5th, 9th houses.	---

Which planet aspect which house has been indicated in the chart above.

Sun aspects the 7th house will full aspect and on the 4th and 8th has 75% aspect. On the 5th and 9th it has 50% and on the 3rd and

10th it has 25%. Similar things has been described in the table above for other planets.

सूर्यादिरयनं क्षणो दिनमृतुर्मासश्च पक्षः शर-
द्विप्रौ शुक्रगुरु रविक्षितिसुतौ चन्द्रौ बुधोऽन्त्यः शानिः।
प्राहुः सत्त्वरजस्तमांसि शशिगुर्वर्काः कविज्ञौ परे
ग्रीष्मदर्ककुजौ शशी शशिसुतो जीवः शनिर्भार्गवः ॥२४॥

We have spoken about the appearance and some symptoms of planets above, and some of these are given below-

1. For how long (duration of time) a planet rules and what is its caste? Whether it is Sathoguni, Rajoguni or Tamoguni. Which seasons are rules by them? These will be clear from the Table below-

Planet	Kaal (i.e. duration of time)	Caste (which is Jaati)	Gunas (I) (Attributes)	Season (Ritu)
Sun	Half a year	Kshatriya	सात्विक	Summer
Moon[1]	Two Ghatikas (one)ghaties = 24 minutes)	Vaisya	सात्विक	Rainy Season
Mars	One day	Kshatriya	तामसिक	Summer
Mercury	Two months	Sudra	राजसिक	Sarad
Jupiter	One month	Brahmin	सात्विक	Hemant
Venus	15 days	Brahmin	सात्विक	Basant (Spring)
Saturn	1 year	Malecha (Shilpkar)	तामसिक	Shishir (winter)

तातम्बे रविभार्गवौ दिवि निशि प्राभाकरीन्दू स्मृतौ
तद्व्यस्तेन पितृव्यमातृभगिनीसंज्ञौ तदा तत्क्रमात्।

[1]Many astrologers and books have mentioned Moon as Brahmin, Mercury as Vaishya.

वामाक्षीन्दुरिनोऽन्यदक्षि कथितो भौमः कनिष्ठानुजो
जीवो ज्येष्ठसहोदरः शशिसुतो दत्तात्मजः संज्ञितः ॥२५॥

Now we discuss as to what matters should be decided from which planets—

Sun–If the birth is during the day time then Sun is the significator of father. If the birth is at night then Sun signifies Uncle from the father's side. It has special control on the right eye.

Moon- If the birth is at night then Moon represents mother and if the birth is during the day time then Moon represents the mother's sister i.e. Aunt. On the body it has control on the left eye.

Mars- Mars is significator of younger brothers.

Mercury- Has control on adopted sons.

Jupiter- Signifies older brothers.

Venus- If the birth is during the day time then it signifies mother. If at night then from it mother's sister should be considered.

Saturn- If the birth is during the day time then father's brothers (Uncle) should be considered from it and if the birth is at night then father should be considered from Saturn i.e Saturn will be the significator of father.

देहो देही हिमरुचिरिनस्त्विन्द्रियाण्यारपूर्वा
आदित्यद्विड्गुलिकशिखिनस्तस्य पीडाकराः स्युः ।
गन्धः सौम्यो भृगुजशशिनौ द्वौ रसौ सूर्यभौमौ
रूपौ शब्दो गुरुरथ परे स्पर्शसंज्ञाः प्रदिष्टाः ॥२६॥

From every planet many things are considered. Here we talk of some more subject as to what matter falls under which planet.

1. Sun - is the Atma (Soul)
2. Moon - is the Body and
3. Mars, Mercury, Jupiter, Venus and Saturn the five planets have control on the five senses.

The Sun and Mars they are the rulers of luster, (tej) and eye sight. The power to see. Moon and Venus have special control on Rasa like- liquids as these two are the rulers of water.

Mercury rules the power to smell because it has more element of earth.

Jupiter is endowed with the Akasha Tathwa, 'Ether', so has control on the power of hearing.

Saturn, Rahu and Ketu are the rulers of Vayu- the wind (Air) and so touch comes under it.

What is the purpose of all this? The purpose is that if Jupiter is afflicted in a horoscope then the native can be deaf. He will be listen less.

Rahu, Gullika and Ketu are enemies of Sun. So they cause mental anguish and problems to the soul.

Body comes under Moon and Rahu, Gullik and Ketu being enemies of Moon as well so they cause physical discomfort and disease.

क्षीणेन्द्वर्ककुजाहिकेतुरविजाः पापाः सपापश्च वित्
क्लीवाः केतुबुधार्कजाः शशितमःशु क्राः स्त्रियोऽन्ये नराः ।
रुद्राम्बागुहविष्णुधातृकमलाकालाह्यजा देवताः
सूर्यादग्निजलाग्निभूमिख पयोवाय्वात्मकाः स्युर्ग्रहाः ॥२७॥

Weak Moon- that means the waning Moon,

Sun, Mars, Rahu, Ketu and Saturn are malefic. If Mercury is placed with a malefic then it also become a Pappi a malefic; If Mercury is posited with a benefic planet then it becomes a benefic. We have talked above of the waning Moon, Sun etc. The manner we have written the name of the planet, in the same manner they should be considered more and more malefic. Like in the ascending order Mars is more malefic then Sun, Rahu is much more malefic then Mars, Ketu is more then Rahu and the Saturn is the most malefic.

This look to be the purpose of the creator of this Book. According to the opinion of some people the malefic are only Mars, Saturn, Rahu and Ketu. Sun* is cruel but not a Pappi. Does not harm. Mercury

---

*Sun destroys the house it is in. In the 5th gives problems to children; in the 7th to spouse– and operates as a malefic.

and Moon by nature are benefic. Mercury, Ketu and Saturn are eunuch. Moon, Rahu and Venus are female planets. Sun, Mars and Jupiter are male planets.

The element of Sun is fire and the lord presiding is Rudra. Rudra is another name of lord Shiva.

Moon rules water and the presiding deity of Moon is Goddess Amba (Parvati).

Mars presides over fire. The element is fire and the god here is Kartik Swami. The element of Mercury is earth and its presiding deity is God Vishnu. Jupiter's element is Aakash (Ether) and the presiding deity is lord Brahma. The element of Venus is water and the deity is Lakshmi. The tatwa of Saturn is Vayu and the presiding god is Yama.

The presiding deity of Rahu is 'Sheshnag' and that of Ketu is Brahma. Rahu and Ketu are not planet in reality. They are just shadow planets (like a place) so there element does not exist. They show effect like Saturn, so their element can be taken as Vayu. The purpose of talking about the presiding deity of planets is that whichever planet is associated with the 9th or the 5th house, the natural affinity of the native will be towards the god ruling them.

We refer to a monthly magazine Kalyan– Year–28, No. 4. In our article– "Bhagwat Bhakti and the 9th Planets". If a person is suffering during a planet's major or minor period then worshipping the gods presiding on that planet will give immediate relief and the negative effect will subside immediately.

गोधूमं तण्डुलं वै तिलचणककुलुत्थाढकश्याममुद्गा
निष्पावा माष अर्केन्द्वसितगुरुशिखिक्रूरविद्भृग्वहीनाम्।
भोगिनार्क्यारजीवज्ञशशिशिखिसितेष्वम्बराख्यं कलिङ्गङ्
सौराष्ट्रवन्तिसिन्धूनसुमगधयवनान्पर्वतान्कीकटांश्च ॥२८॥

मणिक्यं तरणेः सुधार्यममलं मुक्ताफलं शीतगो-
र्माहेयस्य च विद्रुमं मरकतं सौम्यस्य गारुत्मतम्।
देवेड्यस्य च पुष्परागमसुरामात्यस्य वज्रं शने-
नीलं निर्मलमन्ययोश्च गदिते गोमेधवैदूर्यके ॥२९॥

Now we talk which planet has effect on what type of grain and what are the country or provinces on which they have special control. We write this in a tabulation form.

Sun	Wheat	Kaling	Ruby
Moon	Rice	Yavan	White Pearl
Mars	Lentils	Avanti	Coral
Mercury	Klygreen	Maghad	Emerald
Jupiter	Gram	Sindhu	Yellow Sapphire
Venus	Black Moong	Keekat	Diamond
Saturn	Sesame	Saurashtra	Blue Sapphire
Rahu	Klyblack	Ambar	Gomeda
Ketu	Kulthi	Parvat	Cat's eye.

India is a big country. In which part of the country the native's rise will come? In order to decide it look to the strongest planet in the birth chart. See which part of the country it rules. A persons rise will come, if he moves to that place or does some type of work connected with that place. A planet which is weak or afflicted then in the country or place ruled by that planet, rise will not come.

The only use of the grains on which a planet has control or jurisdiction is that when a planet is not so good and is showing bad effects by transit or due to its periods then that grain on which the planet has control should be donated. Easting the grains indicated by planets which are strong will bring much better effects.

ताम्रं कांस्यं धातुताम्रंत्रपु स्यात् स्वर्णं रौप्यं चायसं भास्करादेः।
वस्त्रं तत्तद्वर्णयुक्तं विशेषाज्जीर्णं मन्दस्याग्निदग्धं कुजस्य ॥३० ॥

भानोः कटुर्भूमिसुतस्य तिक्तं लावण्यमिन्दोरथ चन्द्रजस्य।
मिश्रीकृतं यन्मधुरं गुरोस्तु शुक्रस्य चाम्लं च शनेः कषायः ॥३१ ॥

Now we speak of the metals, clothes, taste viz., sour, sweet etc. on which a planet has control. In a tabulation from we write it:

Planet	Metals	Clothes or garments	Taste
Sun	Copper	-Kesaria- (sort of orange).	Bitter
Moon	'Cansa' is a mixed metal Copper and Brass	White	Salted
Mars	Copper	-Red- (burned Red)	Spicy
Mercury	Sisa (lead)	-Green	Mixed
Jupiter	Gold	-Yellow	Sweet
Venus	Silver	-White or spotted.	Sour
Saturn	Iron	-Black -(old, well) used).	Pungent.

The special thing is that from Mars we should understand a burnt cloth. A cloth which has been burnt and from Saturn old tattered cloth. The taste indicated by Sun is bitter and that of Mars is tikta or sharp. In the Indian system six types of tastes have been mentioned. Sweet, Bitter, Ambla, Tikta, Kasaila and Salted. These six are under the control of six planets. Mercury has mixed Ras like– sort of mixture.

भास्वग्दीष्पतिचन्द्रजक्षितिभुवां स्याद्दक्षिणे लाञ्छनं
शेषाणामितरत्र तिग्मकिरणात्कट्यां शिरःपृष्ठयोः ।
कक्षेंऽसे वदने च सक्थिचरणे चिह्नं वयांस्यर्कतो
नेमे नाथ तटं नखं नग सनि ज्ञानाढ्य नग्नाटनम् ॥३२ ॥

We talk of the marks that planets give on the body and the age of planet on which they have special control. We write this in four columns given below:

Planet	Side of Body	Place	Age
Sun	Right side	On the hips or waist	50 years
Moon	Left side	Head	70 years
Mars	Right side	Back	16 years
Mercury	Right side	Flanks	20 years
Jupiter	Right side	Shoulders	30 years
Venus	Left side	Face	7 years
Saturn	Left side	Legs	100 years

That means Saturn controls very old people. The age of Rahu is also mentioned as 100 years. Where the age has been mentioned as 100 years there instead of taking as actually 100 it should be taken as a very old age. When the question arises in the Horary Chart about theft etc. then in prediction it should be mentioned the signs, birth mark are on this part of the body. The part which is indicated by a planet. The age of thief can also be judged from the age mentioned for the planet. All these can help in arriving at conclusion.

नीलद्युतिर्दीर्घतनुः कुवर्णः पामी सपाषण्डमतः सहिक्कः।
असत्यवादी कपटी च राहुः कुष्ठी परान्निन्दति बुद्धिहीनः ॥३३॥

रक्तोग्रदृष्टिर्विषवागुदग्रदेहः सशस्त्रः पतितश्च केतुः
धूम्रद्युतिर्धूमप एव नित्यं व्रणाङ्किताङ्गश्च कृशो नृशंसः ॥३४॥

सीसं च जीर्वसवसनं तमसस्तु केतो-
मृद्भजनं विविधचित्रपटं प्रदिष्टम्।
मित्राणि विच्छनिसितास्तमसोर्द्वयोस्तु
भौमः समो निगदितो रिपवश्च शेषाः ॥३५॥

Now we give some special attributes of Rahu and Ketu.

The body of Rahu is big, blue colour, by caste is malecha* i.e. low caste. In the body has ezema or skin disease, is not religious and indulges in showiness – confidence trickster. It has hicoughs, tells lies, is cunning, suffers from disease, has low mental I.Q. and always indulges in talking ill of others and backbiting.

Ketu's eyes are red and piercing. There is poison in his speech. High body, always bears arms. The colour of his body is like smoke, and he is always engaged in smoking, drugs etc. On his body there are spot marks of wounds, physically is thin. But by nature he is cruel and always indulges in causing anguish and hurt to others. By caste is low. What is the purpose of mentioning these symptoms? The answer is that if some one has Ketu, which is the South node of Moon, in the 2nd house, then he always speaks harsh and sarcastic remarks. If in the minor period of Rahu a person suffers, then we can say that due to the backbiting of other people, he suffered. When many symptoms and characteristic are indicated then influence should be drawn by considering all the factors and then the predictions will be correct. This is the opinion of astrologers. When many characteristic are indicated about a planet, then Astrologers use logic and experience to predict.

The Metal of Rahu is lead and it has control on tattered clothes. What happens when a person is passing through the period of Rahu? The this person by habit keeps himself unkempt, may not take a wash for many days, may grow his beard and dresses in dirty and tattered clothes. The pot of Ketu is made of earth (earthern pots) and has spotted clothes. The friends of Rahu and Ketu are, Mercury, Venus and Saturn. Mars is neither a friend nor an enemy so neutral. Sun, Moon and Jupiter are enemies of Rahu and Ketu.

मूढोऽपि नीचरिपुगोऽष्टमषड्व्ययस्थो
दुस्थः स्मृतो भवति सुस्थ इतीतरः स्यात् ॥

If a planet is combust, is debilitated in a sign, or is debilitated in Navansha, is posited in **the sign of an enemy** or is placed in the 6th, 8th and 12th houses from the ascendant, then it is a 'Dustha' (placed in a bad house). If it is in any other place then ones mentioned above, then it called 'Sustha' like placed in a good house.

चन्द्रे व्ययायतनुषट्सुतकामसंस्थे
तोयाभिवृद्धिमिह शंसति वृद्धिकार्ये ॥३६ ॥

If there is a question regarding or related to water[1] and if Moon

---

*The word is used in Sanskrit to indicate 'Yavana' people of non-Aryan races, and those who are dirty and badly dressed.

[1]What comes under water? To build a Dam or to dig up a well or reservoir. What is Asta? Asta is in English combust. When a planet is so close to Sun that due to the rays of the Sun it is not visible then it is called combust. Moon when 12 degrees away from Sun i.e. when Moon on either side is 12 degree or less from Sun, then it is combust. This is possible during Amawasya and on the first day of the New Moon (bright half).

is in the 1st, 5th, 6th, 7th, 11th or 12th house then the water will increase. This should be predicted from the chart.

Mars is combust within 17 degrees, Mercury when direct then within 14 degree, if Mercury is retrograde then upto 12 degree is combust. Jupiter is combust within 11 degree, Venus if direct then upto 10 degree but if Venus is retrograde it is combust upto 8 degree. Saturn is combust on either side of Sun within 15 degree, whether preceding or following Sun. This is all in the footnote.

अन्तः सारसमुन्नतद्रुररुणो वल्ली सितेन्दू स्मृतौ
गुल्मः केतुरहिश्च कण्टकनगौ भौमार्कजौ कीर्तितौ।
वागीधः सफलोऽफलः शशिसुतः क्षीरप्रसूनद्रमौ
शुकेन्दू विधुरोषधिः शनिरसारागश्च सालद्रुमः ॥३७॥

Which planet has control on what type of trees has been given below–

1. Those trees which are tall and
 strong and hard– Sun has control on them.
2. Climbers Valli etc. are controlled by Moon and Venus.
3. Uneven portion and Bushes are controlled by Rahu and Ketu.
4. The trees which has thorns are controlled and comes under Saturn and Mars.
5. The trees which have fruits are under the section of Jupiter.
6. The trees which have no fruits come under Mercury.
7. Those trees which are full of flowers or one which have lot of juice or which eject milk, they come under Venus and Moon.
8. Ayurvedic medicinal plants and herbs come under Moon.
9. Those trees which do not have much juice, are weak and old then Saturn has control them.
10. Rahu has control on the trees of Saal, Eucalyptus etc.

According to another opinion Jupiter has control on trees which give fruits, the tree which have more flowers come under Venus and those trees which have lot of leaves come under Mercury. Generally all tress have leafs and flowers and fruits but we have to look for the main thing in that tree. In the trees which give fruits is Jackfruit, Mouloshree is very nice tree where flowers are of main importance and Ashok trees where leaves are the main thing.

3

Divisions of a Horoscope

क्षत्रत्रिभागनवभागदशांशहोरात्रिंशांशसप्तलवषष्टिलवाः कलांशाः।
ते द्वादशांशसहिता दशवर्गसंज्ञा वर्गोत्तमो निजनिजे भवने नवांश ॥१॥

दशांशषष्ट्यंशकलांशहीनास्ते सप्तवर्गाश्च विसप्तमांशाः।
षड्वर्गसंज्ञास्त्वथ राशिभावतुल्यं नवांशस्य फलं हि केचित् ॥२॥

क्षेत्रेषु पूर्णमुदितं फलमन्यवर्गे-
ष्वर्द्धं कलादशमषष्टिलवेषु पादम्।
बालः कुमारतरुणौ प्रवया मृतःषड्
भाग क्रमाद्युजि विपर्ययमित्यवस्थाः ॥३॥

क्षेत्रस्यार्द्ध हि होरा त्वयुजि रविसुधांश्वोः समे व्यस्तमेतद्
द्रेष्काणेशास्त्रिभागैस्तनुसुतशुभपा द्वादशांशस्तु लग्नात्।
भौमार्कीड्यज्ञशुक्राः शिशुजसमलवा ह्योजभे युग्मभे तद्-
व्यस्तं त्रिशांशनाथाः क्रियमकरतुलाः कर्कटाद्या नवांशाः ॥४॥

यज्ञं रत्न जनं धनं नय पटं रूपं शुकं चेटिना
नागं योग खगं बलं भग शिला धूलिर्नवं प्रस्वनम्।
लाभं विश्व दिवं कुशं रम धमं षष्ट्यंशकाश्चौजभे
क्रूराख्या समभे विपर्ययमिदं शेषास्तु सौम्याह्वयाः ॥५॥

स्वात् सप्तांशदशांशकौ तु विषमे युग्मे तु कामाच्छुभात्

स्वादीशाश्च कलांशपा विधिहरीशार्काः समर्क्षेऽन्यथा।
ख्यातैः कोणयुतैस्त्रिकोणभवनस्वर्क्षोच्चकेन्द्रोत्तमै-
वर्गाः सप्त दश त्रयोदशमिता वर्गाः प्रदिष्टाः परैः ।।६।।

In the 1st Chapater we have introduced different houses.

In the 2nd Chapter the planets were introduced and now in the 3rd Chapter, we are presenting the Vargas in the Horoscope. Varg means- Parts - Divisions. If one sign is supposed to be one and we divide it into two equal parts then half the part is called Hora. If the same is divided into three equal divisions then every part is called Dreshkana or Decanet. Similarly the sign of 30 degree is divided in 5 parts, 7 parts, 9 parts, 10 parts, 12 parts, 16 parts, 60 parts and these divisions are called the Vargas. Why do we do these divisions? These divisions are for measuring the strength of planets in mathematical manner. The table of the 10 parts are given below as they are ten so we called them Dash Vargas.

Table

1.	One part-	Each sign-	30 degree
2.	Two parts	Hora	15 degree
3.	Three parts	Dreshkana	10 degree
4.	Five parts	Trinshansha*	5,7, or 8 degree
5.	Seven parts	Saptumansha	4°-17'-8'
6.	Nine parts	Navansha	3°-20'
7.	Ten parts	Dashmansha	3 degree
8.	Twelve parts	Dwadashansha	2°-30'
9.	Sixteen parts	Shodashansha	1-16'-52'
10.	Sixty parts	Shastansha	0°-30'

If we take only the 6 parts viz. sign, Hora, Decanet, Navansha, Dwadashansha and Trinshansh then it is called the 'Shad Vargas'. The six divisions.

All Trinshansha are not equal. In Trinshansh some parts are of 5

* Some part is of 5 degree, some of 7 degree and some is of 8 degree. All Trinshansha are not equal.

Hora Chakra

Aries	Taurus	Gemini	Cancer	Leo	Virgo	Libra	Scorpio	Sagittarius	Capricorn	Aqarius	Pisces	Sign	
Sun	Moon	Sun	Moon	Sun	Moon	Sun	Moon	Sun	Moon	Sun	Moon	Degree	15
Moon	Sun	Moon	Sun	Moon	Sun	Moon	Sun	Moon	Sun	Moon	Sun	Degree	30

Decanet Chakra

Aries	Taurus	Gemini	Cancer	Leo	Virgo	Libra	Scorpio	Sagittarius	Capricorn	Aqarius	Pisces	Sign
1	2	3	4	5	6	7	8	9	10	11	12	1 to 10°
5	6	7	8	9	10	11	12	1	2	3	4	11 to 20°
9	10	11	12	1	2	3	4	5	6	7	8	21 to 30°

Saptamansha Chakra

	Aries	Taurus	Gemini	Cancer	Leo	Virgo	Libra	Scorpio	Sagittarius	Capricorn	Aqarius	Pisces	Degree
I Part	1	8	3	10	5	12	7	2	9	4	11	6	4-17-8
II Part	2	9	4	11	6	1	8	3	10	5	12	7	8-34-17
III Part	3	10	5	12	7	2	9	4	11	6	1	8	12-51-26
IV Part	4	11	6	1	8	3	10	5	12	7	2	9	17-8-34
V Part	5	12	7	2	9	4	11	6	1	8	3	10	21-25-42
VI Part	6	1	8	3	10	5	12	7	2	9	4	11	25-42-51
VII Part	7	2	9	4	11	6	1	8	3	10	5	12	30-0-0

degrees, some are of 7 degrees, and some of 8 degrees. If we also consider the Saptamansh, the 7th part together with the Shad Vargas then we call it "Sapta Varga". The 10 Vargas that we have given above when we consider them, then it is called Dash Vargas consideration.

We now give below the tables of the 10 Vargas as a ready reckoner. This will clarify as to which sign owns what degree, minutes and seconds.

First of all is the Hora Table. The decanet Table, then the Saptamansha table. This is page, 56.

If we divide the 30 degrees of a sign by Seven then we get 4 degrees, 17 minutes, 8 second and 34. However from practical angle we take it to be as 4 degrees, 17 minutes and 8th seconds. The last portion 34 is left out because these divisions of planet is done only until the seconds. In the Hora of Parasar the seven parts are respectively called as– Chaar, Cheer, Dadhi, Aajya, Ikchu Ras, Madya, Sudha Jal. Chaar stands for Salted liquid. Cheer for the Sea or Kheer, Dadhi is the Curd or Yogurt. Aajya, Ikchu Ras, Madya and pure water. The Sanskrit names are used because at times it is difficult to find a word which gives an exact meaning.

Navansha Chakra

Part	Aries	Taurus	Gemini	Cancer	Leo	Virgo	Libra	Scorpio	Sagittarius	Capricorn	Aqarius	Pisces	Degree
I	1	10	7	4	1	10	7	4	1	10	7	4	3-20
II	2	11	8	5	2	11	8	5	2	11	8	5	6-40
III	3	12	9	6	3	12	9	6	3	12	9	6	10-00
IV	4	1	10	7	4	1	10	7	4	1	10	7	13-20
V	5	2	11	8	5	2	11	8	5	2	11	8	16-40
VI	6	3	12	9	6	3	12	9	6	3	12	9	20-00
VII	7	4	1	10	7	4	1	10	7	4	1	10	23-20
VIII	8	5	2	11	8	5	2	11	8	5	2	11	26-40
IX	9	6	3	12	9	6	3	12	9	6	3	12	30-00

After the Navansha Table we give the Dashmansha Chakra, Dwadashansha Chakra and then the Sodashansha Chakra.

Dashmansha Chakra

Aries	Taurus	Gemini	Cancer	Leo	Virgo	Libra	Scorpio	Sagittarius	Capricorn	Aqarius	Pisces	Degree
1	10	3	12	5	2	7	4	9	6	11	8	3
2	11	4	1	6	3	8	5	10	7	12	9	6
3	12	5	2	7	4	9	6	11	8	1	10	9
4	1	6	3	8	5	10	7	12	9	2	11	12
5	2	7	4	9	6	11	8	1	10	3	12	15

6	3	8	5	10	7	12	9	2	11	4	1	18
7	4	9	6	11	8	1	10	3	12	5	2	21
8	5	10	7	12	10	2	11	4	1	6	3	24
9	6	11	8	1	11	3	12	5	2	7	4	27
10	7	12	9	2	12	4	1	6	3	8	5	30

Dwadansha Chakra

Aries	Taurus	Gemini	Cancer	Leo	Virgo	Libra	Scorpio	Sagittarius	Capricorn	Aqarius	Pisces	Uto Deg. Min.
1	2	3	4	5	6	7	8	9	10	11	12	2-30
2	3	4	5	6	7	8	9	10	11	12	1	5-00
3	4	5	6	7	8	9	10	11	12	1	2	7-30
4	5	6	7	8	9	10	11	12	1	2	3	10-00
5	6	7	8	9	10	11	12	1	2	3	4	12-30
6	7	8	9	10	11	12	1	2	3	4	5	15-00
7	8	9	10	11	12	1	2	3	4	5	6	17-30
8	9	10	11	12	1	2	3	4	5	6	7	20-00
9	10	11	12	1	2	3	4	5	6	7	8	22-30
10	11	12	1	2	3	4	5	6	7	8	9	25-00
11	12	1	2	3	4	5	6	7	8	9	10	27-30
12	1	2	3	4	5	6	7	8	9	10	11	30-00

Shodashansha Chakra

Aries	Taurus	Gemini	Cancer	Leo	Virgo	Libra	Scorpio	Sagittarius	Capricorn	Aqarius	Pisces	D-M-S
1	5	9	1	5	9	1	5	9	1	5	9	1-52-30
2	6	10	2	6	10	2	6	10	2	6	10	3-45-00
3	7	11	3	7	11	3	7	11	3	7	11	5-37-30
4	8	12	4	8	12	4	8	12	4	8	12	7-30-00
5	9	1	5	9	1	5	9	1	5	9	1	9-22-30
6	10	2	6	10	2	6	10	2	6	10	2	11-15-00
7	11	3	7	11	3	7	11	3	7	11	3	13-7-30
8	12	4	8	12	4	8	12	4	8	12	4	15-00-00
9	1	5	9	1	5	9	1	5	9	1	5	16-52-30
10	2	6	10	2	6	10	2	6	10	2	6	18-45-00
11	3	7	11	3	7	11	3	7	11	3	7	20-37-30
12	4	8	12	4	8	12	4	8	12	4	8	22-30-00
1	5	9	1	5	9	1	5	9	1	5	9	24-22-30
2	6	10	2	6	10	2	6	10	2	6	10	16-25-00
3	7	11	3	7	11	3	7	11	3	7	11	28-7-30

Shodashansha

In the 6 odd sign viz. Aries, Gemini, Leo, Libra, Sagittarius, Aquarius, the lords of the 16 divisons are respectively.

(1) Brahma

(2) Vishnu

(3) Har–Har Stands for lord Shiva.

(4) Sun

(5) Brahma

(6) Vishnu

(7) Har

(8) Sun

(9) Brahma

(10) Vishnu

(11) Har

(12) Sun

(13) Brahma

(14) Vishnu

(15) Har

(16) Surya

In the even signs i.e. Taurus, Cancer, Virgo, Scorpio, Capricorn and Pisces. The lord of the 16 divisons are presided over by –

(1) Sun

(2) Har

(3) Vishnu

(4) Brahma

(5) Sun

(6) Har

(7) Vishnu

(8) Brahma

(9) Sun

(10) Har

(11) Vishnu

(12) Brahma

(13) Sun

(14) Har

(15) Vishnu

(16) Brahma

Trinsansh means 30 divisions. But actually the system prevails that one sign of 30 degree is divided into 5 parts. In the odd signs. Aries, Gemini, Leo Libra, Sagittarius and Aquarius.

The. 1st part is from 0 degree to 5 degree.

The 2nd part is from 6 degree to 10 degree.

The 3rd from 11 degree to 18 degree.

The 4th from 19 degree to 25 degree and

The 5th from 26 degree to 30 degree.

In the even signs which is– Taurus, Cancer, Virgo, Scorpio, Capricorn and Pisces.

The 1st part or the 1st division is until 5 degree.

The 2nd from 6 degree to 12 degree.

The 3rd from 13 degree to 20 degree.

The 4th from 21 degree to 25 degree and

The 5th from 26 degree to 30 degree.

The table of the trinsansh are given below which will make if clear as to how many degrees are assigned to different division.

Trinshansha Chakra

Division	Aries	Taurus	Gemini	Cancer	Leo	Virgo	Libra	Scorpio	Sagittarius	Capricorn	Aqarius	Pisces
I	1	2	1	2	1	2	1	2	1	2	1	2
II	11	6	11	6	11	6	11	6	11	6	11	6
III	9	12	9	12	9	12	9	12	9	12	9	12
IV	3	10	3	10	3	10	3	10	3	10	3	10
V	7	8	7	8	7	8	7	8	7	8	7	8

Trinsansh- In the Trinsansh in odd signs.

In the 1st part up to 5 degree.

In the 2nd part up to10 degree.

In the 3rd part up to 18 degree.

In the 4th part up to 25 degree.

In the 5th part up to 30 degree.

Trinshansh - The even signs-

In the 1st part up to 5 degree.

In the 2nd part up to 12 degree.

In the 3rd part up to 20 degree.

In the 4th part up to 25 degree.

In the 5th part up to 30 degree.

Shasthiansha- Every sign has 30 degree and if we divide each degree by 2 then we get 60 parts and all the signs will be divided in 60 parts of half a degree each.

In the odd signs– The Aries, Gemini, Leo, Libra, Sagittarius and Aquarius.

1, 2, 8, 9, 10, 11, 12, 15, 16, 30, 31, 32, 33, 34, 35, 39, 40, 42, 43, 44, 48, 51, 52 and 59 are malefic. The remaining are benefic.

In the even sign which are– Taurus, Cancer, Virgo, Scorpio, Capricorn and Pisces.

The 3, 4, 5, 6, 7, 13, 14, 17, 18, 19, 20, 21, 22, 23, 24, 25, 26, 27, 28, 29 and then 36, 37, 38, 41, 45, 46, 47, 49, 50, 53, 54, 55, 56, 57 and 60th are malefic the remaining are benefic.

These are the 10 Vargas. If we have to consider the malefic and benefic effect of a planet then see if the planet is placed in its exalted or in its own sign or in sign of a friend etc. in the sign, Hora, Dreshkana etc. or in the sign of an enemy, or in the sign of a great enemy etc. If they are in good divisions like exalted, own sign, or in the sign of friend then they are good. If they are not so placed viz., in the sign of enemy or great enemy or are debilitated etc. in the 10 Varga then the effect will be bad . However all the divisions (Vargas) are not of equal importance. If we assign importance to the sign of 16 points then

Hora, Decanet, 7th division, 9th division, 12th division and trinsansh will get 50% i.e. 8 points. According to opinion of others, the Navansha should also be assigned the same 100% importance as we give to the sign. The remaining three divisions viz. Dashmansh– 10th, Sodashansh– 16th Sashtiansh– 60th, should be assigned 25% i. e. 4 points of importance. Our own view is that the sign and Navansha should be given the same importance. If sign is the body, Navansha is the heart of the horoscope. If body is weak and the heart is strong. The person can live long. But if the body is strong and the heart is weak then danger and ill health can come any time.

If a planet is in the same sign and same Navansha then its called Vargottam.

For example– If Moon is in Aries in two degrees then Moon will be in the sign of Aries and also in the Aries Navansha which is the 9th division of Aries, So it will be Vargottam. Vargottam means in an excellent division. The Vargottam planets are supposed to be very strong as if they are in their own sign. Besides these there is another characteristic of the planets – these are Bal, Kumar, Yuva, Prodha and Vridha. In the odd signs i.e. in Aries, Gemini, Leo, Libra, Sagittarius and Aquarius.

Until 6 degree the planets are in their Bal Avashta like– very very young.

Until 12 degree they are Kumar Avastha. Kumar means young age.

Until 18 degree Yuva which is youth.

Upto the 24 degree mature i.e. prodha and

the last 6 degree the planet is supposed to be lifeless. In Taurus, Cancer, Virgo, Scorpio, Capricorn and Pisces the counting is in the reverse manner from 0 degree to 6 degree is lifeless. Then till 12 degree – Prodha– that's mature old. Upto 18 degree young. Upto to 24 degree very good and the last 6 degree a child (kumar).

In order to measure the strength of any planet, we should see if a planet is in an angle or in a trine, if it is in own sign, is in Mool Trikoan sign, is exalted or Vargottam where is it situated? Then we should consider the 7 Vargas or 10 Vargas. Many people look if a planet is in the house of a friend or in its own sign or is exalted and so they considered the 13 vargas.

वर्गान्योजयतु त्रयोदश सुहृत्स्वर्क्षोच्चभेषु क्रमाद्-
द्विस्त्रिः पञ्च चतुर्नवाद्रिवसुषट्संख्यासु वर्गैक्यतः ।
प्राहुश्चोत्तमपारिजातकथितौ सिंहासनं गोपुरं
चेत्यैरावतदेवलोकसुरलोकांशंश्च पारावतम् ॥७ ॥

In the 13 Vargas the things to be considered are if a planet is exalted, in the house of a friend, or in its own sign. If it is in own sign in two divisions then it is called that the planet is in "Parijatansh". If it is in three benefic Vargas then is called in "Uttam Ansh". If, in four Vargas, it is in benefic then is called in "Gopuransh". In five good Vargas it is called in 'Singhasansha', when in six benefic Vargas then it is called "Paravatansh". In Seven good Vargas it is called "Devlokansha". If in eight benefic Vargas then it is called Surlokansh and if in nine benefic division then it is called Aairavathansh.

The more the number of benefic Vargas a planet is in, so much better is its strength. One commentator has illustrated it that suppose Jupiter in a horoscope, is 8 sign, 1 degree, 25 minute and 1 second then Jupiter is in its Moola Trikona Rashi, own Decanet, own Sapthamansh, own Seven Parts, own Dwadashansh, own Dashmansh and own Sodhasansh. So the 6 divisions are its own and therefore Jupiter is in 'Parvatansh'. The effects of Parvathansh, Gopuransh etc. are given in the coming Slokas.

आर्यानल्पगुणार्थसौख्यविभवान्यः पारिजातांशकः
स्वाचार विनयान्वितं च निपुणं यद्युत्तमांशे स्थितः ।
खेटो गोपुरभागगः शुभमतिं स्वक्षेत्रगो मन्दिरं
यः सिंहासनगो नृपेन्द्रदयितं भूपालतुल्यं नरम् ॥८ ॥

श्रेष्ठाश्वद्विपवाहनादि विभवं पारावताधिष्ठितः
सत्कीर्तिं यदि देवलोकसहितो भूमण्डलाधीश्वरम् ।
वन्द्यं भूपतिभिः सुरेन्द्रसदृशं त्वैरावतांशास्थितः
सद्भाग्यं धनधान्यपुत्रसहितं भूपं विदध्याद् ग्रहः ॥९ ॥

यद्वर्गेष्वखिलेषु मृत्युबलेष्वत्राथ वक्ष्ये क्रमा-
न्नाशं दुःखमनर्थतां च विसुखं बन्धुप्रियं तद्वरम्।
भूप्रेष्टं धनिनं नृपं नृपवरं वर्गे बलिष्ठेऽखिले
वर्धिष्णु सुखिनं नृपं गदमृती बालाद्यवस्थाफलम्॥१०॥

We have stated earlier as to what names have been given to the planets according to the number of benefic Vargas they occupy.

Now we give the results when planets are in different 'Ansha'.

1. Parijatansh– If a planet is in Parijatansh then the native is endowed with many good qualities, rich, happy and gets honour.
2. If a planet is in Uttamansh then it makes one good in behaviour according to his family traditions, clever, humble and well liked by other people. He walks on trodden path of his forefathers.
3. When a planet is in Gopuransh then his thinking is pure. He has happiness from cows, agricultural lands, wealth and his own houses.
4. When a planet is in 'Singhansh' then the person is close to the Ruler and well liked by the ruler. He may be equal to a ruler or may become a ruling person. This interpretation should be drawn according to the circumstances.
5. When a planet is in a 'Paravatansha' then the native attains the best elephants, horses, vehicles and endowed with all type of riches.
6. When a planet is in Devlokansh then the native gets fame. He is the owner of lots of lands a King or a Governor etc.
7. When a planet is in Airavatansh then the native is equal in luxuries to King of Gods Indra. Many kings are under him.
8. When a planet is in 'Surlokansh' then the effect is similar to one mentioned above. The person will be endowed with wealth, prosperity, good fortunes, happiness from sons and will be a ruler of rulers. The good effects that has been mentioned above are when planets are in benefic divisions. Varga means division. So at places we used division or Vargas. It is the same thing.

The point to be noted over here is that the general effect has been given as to what can happen. We should draw the inference that when a planet is in more benefic Vargas then it will show that much more happiness and is capable to show better effects.

No one becomes a king. If only one planet is good and no one becomes a poor person or loses every thing if a planet is weak or has no strength. It is not possible that either all the planets are good or all the planets are bad. We should use logic in arriving at conclusions by measuring the strength of all planets. Now we describe as to what effects are shown by planets when they are weak.

The effect of all these should be taken in the essence and not in a literal manner. We have discussed the effect of planet when they are strong in the above Slokas.

If a planet has no strength in all the Dash Vargas then it causes death or sufferings equal to death.

If it is weak in Nine Vargas then it causes destruction and losses.

If a planet is weak in 8 Vargas then it give deep sorrow.

If weak in the Seven it causes calamities.

In Six it destroys happiness.

Now if a planet is strong in five and weak in five then it makes a person dear and close to the relatives. If it is strong in Six Vargas and weak in four then he is the leader of his kinsmen. If it is strong in Seven and weak in three then he gets happiness from the kings. If strong in Eight then he is rich and strong in Nine he is a king and it is strong in all Ten Vargas then he will be an Emperor.

These days we do not have kings and emperors and all that. So the interpretation should be that the stronger a planet is in the Vargas so much better results it will show.

Now we take the effect of planet according to their Avasthas. Avasthas means– age. If a planet is Bal– means child or is Kumar like– young or mature or Vridha etc.

When a planet is in child stage then it enables the native to attain prosperity.

If in the Kumar Avastha, the planet endows one with happiness.

If in the Youth (Yuva) it makes the native a king i.e. he rises in life.

When the planet is in much mature stage in the Prodhvastha it gives sickness and disease.

In Vridha Avastha, old age, it can cause death or sufferings equal to death.

Here also we should not take the literal meaning, but we should take the sense. We should draw practical inference from this i.e. if in Bala Stage it gives ascending rise. In the Kumaravastha it gives much better results. In the Yuvavastha it gives the strongest results. In the Prodhavastha the native is not capable to do any good . He is engaged in bad deeds and in the Vridhavastha it gives very bad results.

षड् वर्गेषु शुभग्रहाधिकगुणै:* श्रीमांश्चिरं जीवति
क्रुरांशे बहुले विलग्नभवने दीनोऽल्पजीव: शठ: ।
तन्नाथा बलिनो नृपोऽस्त्यथ नवांशेशो दृगाणेश्वरो
लग्नेश: क्रमश: सुखी नृपसम: क्षीणोपतिर्भाग्यवान् ॥११ ॥

If benefic planets are strong in the Shadvarga, the six division, then the native will be rich and long lived. As we observe the Six Vargas of planets in the same manner, we should also measure the strength of the Ascendant in the Vargas. We take the sign, degree,

---

In one Sanskrit Text of Phaldeepika Sloka No. 13 and 14 are not given which show the appearance of Dreshkana. In another copy of a Sanskrit Text in the beginning the 1st Decanet of Leo the appearance is mentioned as Vulture faced (13 Sloka lines 3-4). Similarly the Leo 1st Decanet is called Chatuspadh four legged in Sloka No. 14 line 1-2). It looks like there is some type of misprint in the Sanskrit Text.

What is the meaning of the words used in the Decanet table? We mention them now.

Ayudh	-	Weapon or one who bears them
Chatushpada	-	Four Legged
Kolanan	-	Pig faced.
Gridhasya	-	Vulture faced
Pash	-	Net
Pakshi	-	Bird
Sarpa	-	Snake
Nigad	-	One who is chained.

minutes and second rising at birth. We observe if the rising degrees, minutes etc. are placed in the division of its own lord or in the divisions of benefic planets. If the rising degrees of the ascendant falls in malefic Shadvargas then the native will be short-lived, poor and will be a person of a bad character. However if the degrees and the lords of the Vargas are strong then the native will attain a very high status in life.

If the Navansha of the lord of ascendant is strong then also the native is happy. If the Dreshkana of the ascendant is strong then the person so born will attain a position equal to that of a king. If the lord of the ascendant is strong in itself then the native will be the ruler of the Earth and fortunate in life.

ओजे क्रूरेऽर्कहोरां गतवति बलवान् क्रूरवृत्तिर्धनाढ्यो
युग्मे चान्द्रीं शुभेषु द्युतिविनयवचोहृद्यसौभाग्ययुक्तः ।
व्यस्तेऽत्र मिश्रे समफलमुदितं लग्नचन्द्रौ बलिष्ठो
तन्नाथौ द्वौ च तद्वद्यदि भवति चिरंजीव्यदुःखी यशस्वीं ॥१२॥

In the horoscope of a person if malefic are placed in Aries, Gemini, Leo, Libra, Sagittarius and Aquarius and are in the Hora of Sun, i.e. in the 1st 15 degrees then the native so born will be cruel by nature. They have courage and wealth. However if it is the other way round like in the horoscope the benefic planets are in Taurus, Cancer, Virgo, Scorpio, Capricorn and Pisces and they are in the Hora of Moon i.e. in the first 15 degrees, then they are full of grace, luster,

---

	First	Second	Third
Movable sign (Aries, Cancer, Libra, Capricorn).	Benefic	Neutral	Malefic
Fixed sign (Taurus, Leo, Scorpio, Aquarius)	Malefic	Benefic	Neutral
Dual sign (Gemini, Virgo, Sagittarius, Pisces)	Malefic	Neutral	Benefic

The above results should be used after verifying if the sign rising is movable, fixed or dual as well as which decanet first, second or third is ascending.

humble and they speak softly, they have power to draw people towards them and are fortunate in life. The conditions which have been given above if they are different (reverse) then the results are also different. If the conditions are mixed then the result should also be interpreted as mixed. In the horoscope if the ascendant and Moon both are strong and the lords of the ascendant and Moon sign also have full strength then the native is long lived, happy and well known.

सिंहाजाश्वितुलानृयुग्मभवनेष्वन्त्या हयाजादिमाः
मध्यौ स्त्रीयमयोरिहायुधभृतः पाशोलिमध्यो भवेत्।
नक्राद्यो निगलो मृगेन्द्रघटयोराद्यो वणिड्मःध्यमो
गृध्रास्यो वृषभान्तिमश्च विहगः कर्क्यादि कोलाननम्॥१३॥

कौर्प्याद्यः कर्कटान्त्यो भषचरममहिश्चाजगोमध्यसिंहा-
द्यलयन्त्यं स्याच्चतुष्पादिह फलमधनक्रूरनिन्द्या दरिन्द्राः।
द्वन्द्वर्क्षे स्युर्दृगाणैरधमसमशुभान्यस्थिरे चोत्क्रमेण
प्राहुस्तज्ज्ञाः स्थिरर्क्षेष्वशुभशुभसमान्येव लग्ने फलानि॥१४॥

In this Slokas the appearance of the Decanet are given. The following are the Decanets:

Sign	I Decent	II Decent	III Decent
Aries	Weapon	Four Legged	Weapon
Taurus	-	Four Legged	Bird
Gemini	-	Weapon	Weapon
Cancer	Pig-faced	-	Snake
Leo	Vulture faced four legged	-	Weapon
Virgo	-	Weapon	-
Libra	-	Vulture faced	-
Scorpio	Snake	Net	Weapon
Sagittarius	Weapon	-	Four Legged
Capricorn	Chained	-	Weapon
Aquarius	Vulture faced	-	-
Pisces	-	-	Snake

द्रक्काणेशे स्ववर्गे शुभखगसहिते स्वोच्चमित्रर्क्षगे वा
तद्वत्त्रिंशांशनाथे बलवति यदि चेद् द्वादशांशाधिपे वा।
होरानाथे तथा चेन्निखिलगुणगणो नित्यशुद्धप्रवीणो
दीर्घायुः स्याद्दयावान् सुतधनसहितः कीर्तिमान्नजभोगः ॥१५॥

If the dreshkana of the Ascendant is in exalted divisions, own division, or in the division of a friend posited with benefic and the Ascendant-Hora, Ascendant– Trinshansha and Ascendant–Dwadashansha are also in their respective exalted, own or in the division of friends, with benefic then that person is endowed with many qualities. He is long lived, kind, pure, famous, intelligent equal to kings and enjoys life like a king. He has happiness from sons and has wealth.

मन्दिस्थराशिपतिसङ्गतसुत्रिकोणं
तस्यांशराशिपतिसंयुतमंशकोणम्।
लग्नं वदन्ति गुलिकांशकराशिकोणं
तद्वद्विधौ बलयुते शनिनैव विद्यात्॥१६॥

Observe where Mandi is placed and where the lord of the sign of Mandi is placed. So first we observe the sign of Mandi and then we have to observe sign occupied by the dispositer of Mandi.

The native's ascendant falls in trine to these sign i.e. in the 5th and 9th signs from these signs mentioned above or in the 5th– 9th from the Navansha which Mandi occupies or look to the 5th and 9th from the Navansha lord occupied by Mandi or the 5th-9th from the Navansha occupied by Gulik. Here we use these methods for rectifying the ascendant. But before we use these principles these are given for people who are new in the field of Astrology. These rules are given again for their benefit. In the movable signs the 1st, 2nd and 3rd Decanet are benefic, neutral and bad respectively. In fixed signs the 1st Decanet is malefic, the middle one benefic and the last one i.e. the 3rd one is neutral. In dual signs the 1st Decanet is bad, the 2nd one is neutral, the 3rd one is benefic. The movable, fixed dual, signs are also mentioned here. The above result should be mentioned after taking into consideration which Decanet is rising. How to arrive at the conclusion as to which is the rising sign. This is done when there is a doubt about birth time or if the birth time is at the border line. The things which should be considered are:

1. The sign occupied by Mandi.
2. The dispositer of the Mandi.
3. The Navansha of Mandi or the lord of the Navansha occupied by Mandi.
4. The Navansha occupied by gulik.

कुर्यादात्मसुहृद्दृशाणगशशी कल्याणरूपं गुणं
श्रेयांस्युत्तमवर्गजस्त्वपरगस्तन्नाथजातान् गुणान।
स्वत्रिंशांशगता ग्रहा विदधते तत्कारकत्वोदितं
तत्रैकोऽपि सुहृद्ग्रहेक्षितयुतः स्वोच्चेऽर्थयुक्तं नृपम् ॥१७॥

If Moon is in own Decanet or in the decanet of a friend then the person so born will be handsome and will be endowed with good qualities. If the Moon attains Uttam Vargas then also the native is very fortunate. If it is better in more divisions then so much the better. The ordinary rule is that Moon takes away the good or bad qualities of the sign if occupies. Moon is the Mann. The emotions and whichever sign it occupies a persons emotional bent changes, according to that sign.

Which planet indicates what type of strength has been mentioned above. If we have to observe how a planet will show the effect of the matters if signifies then we should see in which Trinshansha the planet is placed. The best effect comes when the Trinshansha is ruled by the planet itself. If the Trinshansha is ruled by a friend then the result is medium and if the Trinshansha is ruled by an enemy then the results

---

Although gulik and Mandi are one thing yet some people take them as separate due to confusion. The ascendant will be the 5th or 9th from the four which have been mentioned above it. The manner which have been prescribed by using Mandi as the base for arriving at the rising sign in the same manner if Moon is strong then Moon should be used and then we should decide the ascendant.

are bad. If the lord of the Trinshansha are malefic, great enemies then the result is the worst. Even if one planet is in own sign, or in exalted sign, and it is placed with a planet which is a friend or is aspected by it, then the native will have good fortunes, wealth, high position and status. The other opinion is that only an exalted planet or one in own sign in Trinshansha will show this effect.*

स्वोच्चे प्रदीप्तः सुखितस्त्रिकोणे स्वस्थः स्वगेहे मुदितः सुहृद्भे।
शान्तस्तु सौम्यग्रहवर्गयुक्तः शक्तो मतोऽसौ स्फुटरश्मिजालः ॥१८॥

ग्रहाभिभूतः स निपीडितः स्यात् खलस्तु पापग्रहवर्गयातः।
सुदुःखितः शत्रुगृहे ग्रहेन्द्रो नीचेऽतिभीतो विकलोऽस्तयातः ॥१९॥

पूर्णं प्रदीप्ता विकलास्तु शून्यं मध्येऽनुपाताच्च शुभं क्रमेण।
अनुक्रमेणाशुभमेव कुर्युं र्नामानुरूपाणि फलानि तेषाम् ॥२०॥

Different names which themselves depict the condition and efficacy of a planet are given in these slokas. According to the strength of the planet if it is in the exalted sign, the Moola Trikona, in own sign, or in the house of a friend etc. When a planet is in its exalted sign, it is called 'Pradipth'. Pradipth means– shining with luster lighted. When it is in Mool Trikoan, it is called Sukhit i.e. the planet is happy. When it is in own sign it is called Swastha which means in good health. When in the sign of friend, it is called Mudit – means happy, smiling contented. When it is in the division of benefic planets and is also conjoined with a benefic then the planet is called– Shanta - *i.e.* peaceful. When a planet is visible in the sky that means away from the Sun and is shining, is not combust then the planet is called 'Shakta' that means full of strength and capable of showing good results.

---

*If the sign, decanate, Navansha, all the three of a planet are in their own or exalted divisions, then it is said to be in the 'Uttam' 'Varga'. Some astrologers are of the view that if a planet is in any three, out of the ten Vargas, in own or exalted divisions it is in the 'Uttam Varga'. This opinion is considered to be a weak opinion.

When a planet is combust then it shows negative results. It is so weak that it is not capable to do any good, is not able to show any good results. A combust planet is called Vikala.

If a planet is not Shakta then it is Vikala, which is the reverse of Shakta. When a planet is lost in a war then is called – Nepeedith.* That means it has no strength and is a malefic. When any planet is in the divisions of malefic then it is called Khal. When a planet is in the house of an enemy, then it is called 'completely unhappy' i.e. Poorna Dukhi and when it is in the debilitated sign it is called 'Atibheath' which means extremely afraid. These words depicts the meaning itself in Sanskrit language– Pradipth, Sukhit, Swastha, Mudit, Shanta, Shakta, Nipidith, Khal, Sudukith, Shakta and Vikala etc. These 11 conditions are called the Avasthas. They show the results according to their names.

In the first 6th Avasthas a planet gives benefic results. What will be the percentage of the benefic results? This has been explained according to the system of currency prevailing in India. In the old times before 1962 the Rupee had 16 Annas. Like a Rupee had 16 Divisions. When a planet is exalted then it gets 16 out of 16 benefic resutls.

In the Sukhit it has 14 out of 16; In Own sign it gets 12 out of 16. In the sign of a friend it gets 10 out of 16, and in the Shanta

---

Which planet is called a defeated planet?

The answer to this question is that-

a. When two planets are in the same sign, degree, minutes– then they are side to be engaged in war with each other.

b. The three balas viz. (i) Sthanbala (ii) Dikbala (iii) Kalabala should be calculated out of the Shadbalas (six type of strength) which includes the above mentioned 3 balas and also (iv) Ayanbala (v) Chestabala (vi) Naisargikbalas.

c. Add the first 3 balas only in order to arrive at the 'Yudhbala'.

d. Subtract the one with lesser strength (bala) from the one which has more strength.

e. The remainder should be divided by the Bimba Parimana (the area inside the circumstances) of the two planets.

Avastha it gets 8 out of 16, and in the Sakta Avastha it get 6 out of 16. In Nipeedith Awastha 6 out of 16 malefic. In Khal Awastha 8 out of 16 ill effects. In Sudukhit Awastha it has negative effect which is 10 out of 16 . In debilitated sign it shows 12 out of 16 bad and in Vikala Awastha that means combust the negative is 100%, 16 out of 16.

When a planet is in good Awastha then the results are very good in its major and minor periodic influences. When planets are in bad Avasthas then the results are malefic in their periods.

---

f. Add the quotient to the (Yudhbala) (three balas) of the planet in the North direction and subtract the quotient from the planet in the South direction.

g. The planet in the North is the victorious one and the after one in the South is the defeated one. The planetary Bimba Parimana are as follows-

Planet	**Bimba Parimana**
Mars	9.4 Seconds
Mercury	6.6 Seconds
Jupiter	190.4 Seconds
Venus	16.6 Seconds
Saturn	158.0 Seconds

4

Graha Bala (Planetary Strength)

How to calculate the strength of Planets and houses has been dealt with in this chapter. It is necessary to state the opinion of the other teachers of Astrology before coming to the opinion of Mantreshwar Maharaj.

Those who know how to calculate the six types of strength (shadbala), for them it is easy to understand the meaning of the Slokas in 'Phaldeepika'. But those of us who are not acquainted with the shadbalas, should read the details given below:

'Shadbala' - The Sanskrit word means six type of strengths and these six types of strength of planets is a unique feature of Vedic Astrology (Indian Astrology)

SHADBALA INCLUDES

(a) Sthana bala (Strength of Placement)

(b) Dig bala (Directional strength)

(c) Kala bala (Strength of Time)

(d) Chesta bala (Strength due to the Movement)

(e) Naisargik bala (Natural Strength), and

(f) Drik bala (Strength of Aspect)

Now we will explain each of the above one by one.

Sthana bala

1. Uchchabala - Strength due to exaltation. When a planet is posited in the degree of its highest* exaltation then it is allotted 1 roopa (=60 points) of strength. If the planets is in exact degree of its

debilitation then it gets 0 i.e. nothing at all. If it is some where in between the exaltation and the debilitation point then the strength is calculated by the rule of three. This is called Uchchabala.

2. If a planet is in its Moola - Trikona sign (see ch. I) then it get 45 points; in its own sign the planets is allotted 30 points; if it is in the sign of a great friend then 22.5 points; in the sign of a friend, it gets 15 points; In a neutral sign (i.e. where the lord is neither a friend nor an enemy), it gets 7.5 points; in the sign belonging to an enemy - 3.75 points; and in the sign of a great enemy, the planets gets the lowest just 1.875 points.

3. If a planet is in own Hora then it gets 30 points, in the hora of a great friend then 22.5 points, in a friend, hora 15 points in neutral hora 7.5 points, in a enemy hora 3.75 points and in a great enemies hora 1.875 points.

4. If a planet is in its own decanate then 30 points, in a great friend's 22.5 points, in the decanate of a friend 15 points, in a neutral decanate 7.5 points, in an enemy's 3.75 points and in the decanate of a great enemy then 1.875 points.

5. In the Saptamansha a planet is allotted 30, 22.5, 15, 7.5, 3.75

---

*The exact degree in which a planet is exalted in a sign is, its highest point of exaltation and the exact degree in which a planet is debilitated in a sign is called its highest debilitation point.

N.B. (1) Money is counted in the units of Rupees, Anna, Paisa (Pound, Shilling etc.). Stock of grains are weighted (with) in Kilograms, grams (or seer, chatank) just as in one rupee there are one hundred paisa (new) in the same manner one 'Roopa' has, sixty units called 'Shashtaansha' or 60 points. If it is difficult to express the strength of a planet in full one 'rupa' then it is expressed in a fraction viz., 30 points, 22.5 points etc.

N.B. (2) Suppose Sun is in the decanate of Jupiter and Juipter is a great friend of Sun then the Sun will be allotted 22.5 points of strength. This is as per "Shripati Padhdhti)". Some leanred persons while doing the commentary on 'Keshavi Jataka' has written that (I) If Sun is in the drekana of Jupiter and (ii) Jupiter is also in the division of a great friend then Sun will get 22.5 points. We side with the opinion of Shripati Padhdhati. We don't agree with the commentators of 'Keshvi Jataka'.

and 1.875 according as it is placed in own, great friend, friend, neutral, enemy and great enemies sign respectively.

6. In the navansha a planet is allotted 30, 22.5, 15, 7.5, 3.75 and 1.875 according as it is in own, great friend, friend, neutral, enemy and great enemies sign respectively.
7. In the Dwadshansha (12th part) a planet is allotted 30, 22.5, 15, 7.5, 3.75 and 1.875 according as it is in its own, great friend, friend, neutral, enemy and great enemy's sign respectively.
8. In Trinshansha a planet is allotted 30, 22.5, 15, 7.5, 3.75 and 1.875 marks according as it is in its own, great friend, friend, neutral enemy and great enemy's sign respectively.
9. (a) Sun, Mars, Mercury, Jupiter and Saturn - out of the five, whichever are in odd signs (Aries, Gemini, Leo, Libra, Sagittarius and Aquarius) get 15 points each..

   (b) Moon and Venus, out of these two those who which are in even signs (Taurus, cancer, Virgo, Scorpio, Capricorn and Pisces) get 15 points each.

(10) (a) The same method of allotment is done if in the Navansha - Sun, Mars, Mercury, Jupiter and Saturn are in odd signs 0 then the one in odd sign gets 15 points.

   (b) Out of the Moon and Venus whichever is in an even Navansha - also get 15 points each.

11. The planet in angular position get 60 points (=1 roopa); the one in succeedent a house gets 30 points; and those in cadent house get 15 points.
12. (a) Out of Sun, Mars or Jupiter whichever is in the first decanate of any sign gets 15 points. In other decanates they get no points (i.e. 0)

   (b) Out of Mercury and Saturn whichever is in the second decanate gets 15 points. In other decanates none.

   (c) Out of Moon and Venus whichever is in the 3rd decanate gets 15 points. In other decanate (i.e. in the 1st or 2nd) they get 0.

The sum total of the above 12 types of strength is known as the

'Sthana Bala' i.e. (I) the exaltation strength, (ii) to (viii) the Saptavarga bala, (ix) odd signs bala (x) odd Navansha bala (xi) Angular position bala, and (xii) the decanate bala.

Dik bala (Directional Strength)

Dikbala, Dishabala or directional strength is one and the same.

(a) Sun and Mars - Out of these two whichever is on the cusp of the 10th house gets 1 Roop (= 60 points). If these are on the cusp of the 4th house then they get 0 point. Other positions are calculated by the rule of three (proportionate allotments).

(b) Out of Moon and Venus whichever is one the cusp of 4th house gets 1 Roop (= 60 points). On the 10th cusp they get 0 point.

(c) Mercury and Jupiter on the cusp of I house (rising degree) get 1 Roop (= 60 points). On the cusp of the 7th house they get 0 point.

(d) If Saturn is in the 7th house then 1 Roop is allotted to it and if it is on the cusp of Ascendant then 0 point.

The table below gives a quick idea as to the points allotted to Planets*.

Planet	10th Cusp	7th Cusp	4th Cusp	1st Cusp
Sun Mars	1 roop	---	0 points	---
Moon Venus	0 points	---	1 roopa	---
Mercury Jupiter	---	0	---	1 roopa
Saturn	---	1	---	0

Kala bala

This is the sum total of the nine types of strength. These are mentioned below:

1. (a) Sun, Jupiter and Vensus - each one of them at noon gets 1 Roopa (= 60 points). Exactly at mid night they get 0. At any other time in between the strength should be calculated proportionately.

(b) Moon, Mars and Saturn - each one of them get 1 Roopa (= 60 points) at mid night. Exactly at Noon they get 0. Any other time, proportionate strength should be allotted.

(c) Mercury always gets 1 Roopa all through out the 24 hours.

2. (a) When Sun and Moon are exactly 180 degrees from each other then benefic planets are allotted 1 roopa. When Sun and Moon are exactly in the same degree then the benefic planets get 0 points. Proportionate strength is allotted if these are anywhere from 0° to 180°.

Moon, Mercury, Jupiter and Venus are benefic planets. 'Keshavi Jataka' mentions that Mercury with malefics should be considered as malefic. But some other Pandits state that Mercury is always a benefic planet.

(b) When Sun and Moon both of them are in the same degree, the malefic planets get full 1 roopa (= 60 points). However the malefic planets get 0 point when Sun and Moon are exactly opposite to each other (180 degree apart). The in between strength should be calculated by the rule of three when Sun and Moon are separated from each other by other than 0° or 180 degree.

Sun, Mars and Saturn are malefic. This bala (strength), is called 'the Paksha bala' (i.e. Krishna Paksha - the dark half and Shukla Paksha - the bright half)

(c) The Paksha Bala of Moon should be doubled.

3. (a) If the birth is during the daytime then the duration of the day (i.e. between Sun Rise and Sun Set) is divided by 3.

If the birth time falls in the I part then Mercury, in the II part then Sun, and in the III part then Saturn will be allotted 1 roopa (= 60 points) respectively.

(b) If the birth is at night, then the time between Sunset to Surise, should be divided by 3.

If the time of birth falls in the I part then Moon gets 1 roopa, in the II part then Venus gets 1 roopa, and in the III part then Mars will get 1 roopa (= 60 points).

(c) Irrespective of the time of birth (the birth can be at any time of the day and night), Jupiter always gets 1 roopa (= 60 points).

4. Since the Earth came into being, one year or 360 days (30 days in each month), we should calculated up to the birthday as to what was the day of the week on the first day of that year. The lord of that day will be the lord of the year.

   Whichever planet is the year lord that planet will be allotted 15 points.

5. Similarly beginning with the universe (30 days to each month) count up to the month of birth. The lord of the day, which falls on the first day of that month, will get 30 points.

6. The lord of the day on which the birth took place gets 45 points.

7. The planet which is the ruler of the Hora in which the birth took place will get 1 roopa (= 60 points) [see page 98 - 101, of 'Anka Vidya']

Ayan Bala

8. The planet in the North latitude from the center line in the sky has North (Kranti) and when in the South then it has the South (Kranti). Exactly on the meridian (center line) it has zero kranti.

   (a) Sun, Mars, Jupiter, Venus get 1 roopa on 24 degree North Kranti and 0 bala in the 24 degree of South Kranti. In between bala should be proportionately calculated.

   (b) Moon and Saturn get 1 roopa of strength on the 24 degree of South Kranti and on 214° North Kranti they get 0 bala. Proportionate calculated should be done to get the bala in between.

   (c) The Special feature about Mercury is that if its Kranti is zero then it gets 30 points of bala. If it proceeds from zero Kranti to 24° North Kranti then its bala keeps on increasing till 1 roopa. Its bala also keeps on increasing.

   (d) Even if it moves towards the 24° South Kranti - So the

---

N.B. As Moon does not gct any point due to retrogression (Chesha bala) because it is always in direct motion so Moon gets twice of the Paksha bala.

bala of Mercury increases all the time immaterial of its movement towards the South or North. Proportionate bala should be allotted for the other positions between 0° and 24°.

(e) Sun's* Ayan bala should be doubled.

Yudh Bala

9. This is the ninth Bala under the Kala Bala. In any two out of the five planets Mars, Mercury, Jupiter, Venus and Saturn are in the same sign, degree and minute, then it is inferred that they are in war with each other. To calculate Yudhbala please refer to Shripati Paddhiti, Keshvi Paddhiti or Parashar Horoshastra. Here it has not been explained as it would require a lengthy space. Some details have already been given in the note on page 71.

The nine types of balas (strength) given above fall under kala bala (These Sanskrit names are as follows:)

(1) Natoanta Bala or Day - Night Bala

(2) Paksha Bala (dark half / bright half)

(3) Tribhag Bala (Three Divisions)

(4) Abda Bala

(5) Mase Bala (Month Bala)

(6) Var Bala (Day of week bala)

---

1. From the beginning of the Universe till the date of birth how many years (360 days each), and how many months (30 days each) has elapsed - to calculated these please see 'Surya Siddhanta' - I chapter Slokas 45 to 51.

Another opinion is that it is not necessary to do these intensive calculations. The lord of the first week day in the Vikram Samvat in which the birth took place will be the year lord. Similarly the Lord of the first week day of the month is the lord of the month.

*Sun is always in direct motion, it never is retrograde so it does not get and chesta or retrogression bala. Therefore its Ayanbala is doubled up.

Rarely, Mars, Mercury, Jupiter, Venus, Saturn out of these five two of them are in the same sign, degree and minutes, only then it is required to calculate 'YudhBala'.

(7) Hora Bala

(8) Ayan Bala

(9) Yudh Bala

Some persons take the first seven under the Kala Bala and 8th and 9th balas are treated separately.

Chesta Bala (Strength due to movement)

Now we explain the term "Chest Bala'. Sun and Moon are always direct in motion. They are never retrograde. The remaining Mars, Mercury, Jupiter, Venus and Saturn are at times direct and at other times retrograde in motion. Due to their motion, they get bala and this bala is called Chesta Bala.

In order to calculate Chesta bala, an exhaustive mathematical methods are employed for knowing the centre of motion, slow speed etc. So it has not been explained here in detail. We are however mentioning some broad method to know the strength.

(a) When a planet is retrograde it gets 1 roopa (= 60 points).

(b) Anuvakra (or Riju motion) then it is allotted 30 points.

(c) If it is Vikal then 15 points.

(d) Samagam motion then 30 points.

(e) Slow in motion (motion is on the increase but less than average slow motion) in direct motion then 15 points.

(f) Comparatively slow in motion (but less than average motion) and the planet is direct in motion then 7.5 points.

(g) faster in motion (direct motion is going down but more than average motion) then 45 points.

(h) Comparatively faster (direct motion is increasing and more than average motion) then 30 points are allotted.

This is a rough and ready method. For exact calculation, proceed with mathematical manner.

Natural Strength (Naisargik Bala)

Which planet has how much of strength by nature is called the Natural Strength. This is fixed and never changes.

The following is the strength of planets:

Sun	60.00 Points
Moon	51.43 Points
Venus	42.85 Points
Jupiter	34.28 Points
Mercury	25.70 Points
Mars	17.14 Points
Saturn	8.57 Points

Drik Bala (Drishti Bala) Viz. The strength of Aspect

When planets receive aspect from benefic planets then it is called Shubha Drishti.

In order to calculate the aspect strength, we should know the distance between the planet and then mathematically calculate the strength*.

Note

1. Sun, Moon, Mercury, Venus, get 0 on a planet which is away from them by:

	Strength	Aspect Distance
	0	30°
on	0.25	60°
on	0.75	90°
on	0.50	120°
on	0	150°
on	1	180°
on	0.75	210°
on	0.25	170°
on	0	300°

In between strength of aspect should be proportionately calculated.

The aspect of Mars, Jupiter, Saturn are as follows:

On	Mars	Jupiter	Saturn
30°	0	0	0
60°	0.25	0.25	1
90°	1	0.75	0.75
120°	0.50	1	0.50
150°	0	0	0
180°	1	1	1
210°	1	0.75	0.75
240°	0.50	1	0.50
270°	0.25	0.25	1
300°	0	0	0

The aspect in between should be calculated by the rule of three.

If a planet has the aspect of malefic then it is called Papa Drishta. These aspects are also calculated in the manner described above. Most books of Astrology give a table of Aspects.

If benefic aspects are more, then from these, subtract the malefic aspect. The remainder should be then subtracted from the total of Sthanbala, Kalabala etc. Now the balance is called the total of six types of strength i.e. 'Shadbala Pinda'.

How to calculate the strength of planets has been discussed to some extent so far; now we proceed to show as to the manner of calculating the 'Bhavabala'.

Bhava Bala (Strength of Houses)

The total of 3 types of strength is added together to calculate the Bhavabala.

1. Bhaveshbala - The strength of the Lord of the house.
2. Bhava Dikbala- Strength due to the placement of the house.
3. Shubha Drishtibala- Strength due to the benefic/malefic aspects on the house.

The lord of the house is called 'Bhavesh'. Calculating the strength of a planet has been mentioned above.

Bhava Dikbala

a. Gemini, Virgo, Libra, Aquarius and the first half of Sagittarius are two legged signs and if they are in the Ascendent then they get 1 roopa (=60 points). In the 7th house they get 0- point. In other houses their strength is calculated proportionately.

b. The second half of Aries, Taurus, Leo, Sagittarius and the first half of Capricorn are four legged signs and if they fall in the 10th house then 1 roopa is allotted to them. In the 4th house they get 0 and in other house the strength is calculated proportionately.

c. Cancer and Scorpio are 'Keet' signs. In the 7th house they get 1 roopa. In the 1st they get 0 point. In other houses the strength is calculated by the rule of three.

d. Pisces and the second half of the Capricorn are water signs. In the 4th house they get 1 roopa in the 10th they get 0 point. In other house the strength is calculated proportionately.

Strength of the Aspect

If benefic aspect on a house is more then deduct the malefic aspect from it and the remainder should be added to the total of the strength of the lord of the house and the Dikbala of the house. The Sum total of the these will be the Bhavabala.

If the malefic aspect is more then subtract the benefic aspect. The remainder should be again deducted from the total that we get from adding together the strength of the lord* of the house and Bhava Dikbala. This is the Bhava Dikbala.

To calculate the malefic and benefic aspect - on a house is a matter which needs a detailed process and this should be learned from any book dealing with Astrological calculationing (Jatak Paddhatis). (1).

---

*The planet which is the ruler of the house.

1. How to calculate the six balas and bhava balas, please refer to (a) Keshavi Jataka (b) Shripati Paddhati and (c) Jataka Paddhati by Vatashreni Bhudev.

We have given above some what of an outline about the planetary strength and the Bhava (house) strength. In the fourth chapter of Phal Deepika, Mantreshwar has elaborated the above subject. Now we give below the literal translation of the Slokas of Phal Deepika :

वीर्यं षड्विधमाह कालजबलं चेष्टाबलं स्वोच्चजं
दिग्वीर्यं त्वयनोद्भवं दिविषदां स्थानोद्भवं च क्रमात्
निश्यारेन्दुसिताः परे दिवि सदा ज्ञः शुक्लपक्षे शुभाः
कृष्णेऽन्ये च निजाब्दमासदिनहोरास्वङघ्रिवृद्ध्या क्रमात् ॥१ ॥

1. The strength of a planet is of six types. These are Kala Bala, Chestabala, Uchchabala, Dikbala, Ayanbala and Sthanbala.

Mars, Moon and Venus are strong at night- Other planets are strong during the day time. Mercury is deemed strong around the clock– during day and night all the time. During the waxing Moon, benefic planets are strong– the remaining planets are strong during the waning Moon.

'Abda' ruler has one fourth strength. The lord of the month get half the strength out of 1 roopa. The lord of the week day gets 3 by 4 (three out of 4) strength. The planet whose Hora is at birth get one full roopa.

राकाचन्द्रस्य चेष्टाबलमुदगयने भास्वतो वक्रगानां
युद्धे चोदक्स्थितानां स्फुटबहुलरुचां स्वोच्चवीर्यं स्वतुङ्गे ।
दिग्वीर्यं खेऽर्कभौमौ सुहृयदि शशिसितौ विद्गुरू लग्नगौ चे-
न्मन्देऽस्ते याम्यमार्गे बुधशनिशशिनोऽन्येऽयनाख्ये परस्मिन् ॥२ ॥

Moon gets full Chestabala (full strength) on full Moon day. The remaining planets when retrograde gets chestabala. In the war between planets one who is not combust and is in the North, is the victorious one. When a planet is in the degree of its highest exaltation then it should deemed to be in its full exalted state.

Now we tell about - Dikbala (Directional strength) Sun and Mars are strong in the 10th house. Moon and Venus are strong in the 4th house. Mercury and Jupiter are strong in the first house and Saturn is strong in the 7th house.

Now we tell of the Ayan Bala. Saturn, Mercury and Moon are strong in South Ayan. The remaining planets are strong in the North Ayan.

स्वोच्चस्वर्क्षसुहृद्गृहेषु बलिनः षट्सु स्ववर्गेषु वा
प्रोक्तं स्थानबलं चतुष्टयमुखात्वपूर्णार्द्धपादाः क्रमात्
मध्याद्यन्तकषण्डमर्त्यवनिताः खेटा बलिष्ठाः क्रमात्
मन्दारज्ञगुरूशनोब्जरवयो नैजे बले वर्द्धनाः ॥३॥

The strength (bala) a planet gets by being in its exalted, own or in the sign of a friend or being placed in the six Vargas, that is called the Sthanbala.

If a planet is in an angel then it gets 1 roopa, in the succedent house half a roopa and in cadent house then it get one fourth roopa.

Neutral planets in the middle of a sign (from 1 degree to 20 degree), male planets in the first part (from 1 degree to 10 degree) and female planets in the last part (from 21 degree to 30 degree) are strong.

In natural strength, Saturn, Mars, Mercury, Jupiter, Venus, Moon and Sun are stronger in the ascending order i.e. Mars is stronger than Saturn, Mercury is stronger than Mars and so on.

वक्रं गतो रुचिररश्मिसमहपूर्णो
नीचारिभांशसहितोऽपि भवेत्स खेटः
वीर्यान्वितस्तुहिनरश्मिरिवोच्चमित्र-
स्वक्षेत्रगोऽपि विबलो हतदीधितिश्चेत् ॥४॥

Even if a planet is debilitated in sign or Navansha, but if it is retrograde and is bright in its own rays i.e. not combust, then it is taken as a strong planet.

Even if a planet is exalted or in own sign or in the sign of a friend, like Moon, but its rays are dead due to the effect of being combust then it is deemed to be weak. The meaning of this is that

---

*Ayan- the path of planet via the North and South of the equator.

even if Moon is placed in Taurus or Cancer but it is the Moon of Amavasya (Sun-Moon are in the same degree then it is weak). On the other hand a debilitated Moon (in Scorpio) if it is a full Moon as well then it is strong. The same principle applies to other planets.

तुङ्गस्था बलिनोऽखिलाश्च शशिनः श्लाघ्यं हि पक्षोद्भवं
भानोर्दिग्बलमाह वक्रगमने ताराग्रहाणां बलम्।
कर्क्य क्षाजघटालिगोहिरबलान्त्योक्षाश्विपाश्चात्यगः
केतुस्तत्परिवेषधन्वसु बली चेन्द्वर्कयोगो निशि ॥५ ॥

All planets if exalted are strong. Special importance should be given to the fortnight of the Moon (bright half and dark half). Sun's directional strength is of main importance as well as the retrograde strength of other planets.

Rahu (North Node of Moon), in Cancer, Taurus, Aries, Aquarius and Scorpio and Ketu (South Node of Moon) in Pisces, Virgo, Taurus and in the second half of Sagittarius are strong and in Parivesh and Indrachap are also strong at night if Sun and Moon are placed in one sign. (Sun and Moon are conjoined).

रूपं मानुषभेऽलिभेऽङ्घ्रिपरेष्वर्द्ध बलं स्यात्तनोः
तुल्यं स्वामिबलेन चोपचयगे नाथेऽतिवीर्योत्कटम्।
स्वामीड्यज्ञयुतेक्षिते कवियुते चान्यैरयुक्तेक्षिते
शर्वर्यांत्रिशि राशयोऽहनि परे वीर्यान्विताः कीर्तिताः ॥६ ॥

If any Manushya Rashi is in the Ascendant then it gets 1 Roopa. If Scorpio is in the first house then one by fourth roopa and for other signs one half of a roopa. Ascendant gets the same strength as is the strength of its lord..

If the lord of the Ascendant is placed in Upachya, then Lagna is deemed to be very strong. If Venus is in the Ascendant or is teneted by its lord Mercury or Jupiter or is receiving full aspect from its lord Mercury or Jupiter and is not aspected by or teneted by other planets then also it is taken to be very strong. The essence of this is that the placement of Venus is of importance but not that much importance is given to its aspect but on the other hand the aspect and placement of

Mercury or Jupiter if these are the rulers of the Ascendant then both of these are of prime importance and endows the Ascendant with strength.

The signs which are strong during the day are strong and those strong at night are strong at night.

स्वोच्चे पूर्णं स्वत्रिकोणे त्रिपादं स्वक्षेत्रऽर्द्धं मित्रभे पादमव।
द्विट्क्षेत्रेऽल्पं नीचगेऽस्तं गतेऽपि क्षेत्रं वीर्यं निष्फलं स्याद् ग्रहानाम्॥७॥

If a planet is exalted then it gets 1 roopa, in its Mooltrikona three by four roopa; in own sign half and in the sign of a friend then one by four. In an enemy sign a planet gets very little bala and if debilitated or combust then if does not get any bala i.e. 0.

केन्द्रे ग्रहाणामुदितं बलं यत्सुखे नभस्यस्तगृहे निलग्ने।
उपर्युपर्युक्तपदक्रमेण बलाभिवृद्धिं हि विकल्पयन्ति॥८॥

Out of the four angles, which angle has what bala is given now. In the Ascendant full strength i.e. 1 roopa, in the 7th, three by four; in the 10th one by two (half); and in the fourth one by four (*i.e.* a quarter).

Now what importance should be attached to which aspect is given below:

श्रेष्ठति सा सप्तमदृष्टिरेव सर्वत्र वाच्या न तथाऽन्यदृष्टिः।
योगादिषु न्यूनफलप्रेदति विशेषदृष्टिर्न तु कैश्चिदुक्ता॥९॥

All the time the 7th house aspect is the best. Other aspects viz. the 5th and 9th are not that effective. However some learned Astrologers are of the opinion that where 'Yoga' is considered then the 5th-9th aspect of Jupiter; 4th-8th aspect of Mars; and the 3rd-10th aspect of Saturn, are capable to show full effect of an aspect.

Planetary friendship and enmity are of two types i.e. natural and temporal. Now we elaborate as to what and how much importance should be given to them.

नैसर्गिकं शत्रुसुहृत्त्वमेव भवेत्प्रामाणं फलकारि सम्यक्।
तात्कालिकं कार्यवशेन वाच्यं तच्छत्रुमित्रत्वमनित्यमेव॥१०॥

Natural friendship or natural enmity etc. of planets show the main results. Temporal friendship/enmity is due when work* realisation is considered. This is not permanent.

(The planets which are natural enemies– Show bad results in the major period of one and the minor period of the other. The enemy of the Ascendant or whichever house is to be considered, the enemy of the lord of that house spoils the house during its major and minor periods all these should be considered).

निःशेषदोषहरणे शुभवर्द्धने च
वार्यं गुरोरधिकमस्त्यखिलग्रहेभ्यः ।
तद्वीर्ययपाददलशक्तिभृतौ ज्ञशुक्रौ
चान्द्रं बलं तु निखिलग्रहवीर्यबीजम् ॥११ ॥

Jupiter is endowed with powers to reduce the negative effects of all types. It is the most efficacious planet to increase good results. Whatever is the capacity of Jupiter, the benefic effect of Venus is half of that,. and Mercury's benefic effect is even half of that of Venus. However the strength of Moon is the root (Moola) of the effectiveness of all planets.

Chandra Kriya etc.

Now we speak of (a) Chandra Kriya (b) Chandra Avastha and (c) Chandravela. How to calculate them and what is their effect in prediction. The above three should be considered in a nativity, in a horary chart as well as in Muhurta (finding an auspicious date and time). Chandra Kriya are 60 in all. Chandra Avastha are 12 and Chandravela-36.

जन्मर्क्षविघटी नीतैर्ज्ञानाङ्कैर्नयैर्भजेत् ।
लब्धाश्चन्द्रक्रियावस्थावेलाख्यास्तत्फलं क्रमात् ॥१२ ॥

---

*In the original Sanskrit Sloka the word 'Karyavash' i.e. due to work i.e. if a work will be done or not. 'Phaldeepika' is a treatise dealing with a nativity at birth and not with the horary charts. Still in order to observe if a work will be realised or not, temporal relationship should be looked into in horary Astrology.

Consider the constellation (of Moon) at birth, or in horary chart or at the time of a Muhurta-

(1) The number of Ghatis and Palas which has passed should be reduced to Palas. Then divide this by 60-Whatever is the quotient has been written in the Slokas 13 to 15. This is Chandra Kriya.

(2) Consider the constellation which has already been traversed by Moon at the time of Muhurta or horary chart convert it into Palas and then divide by 300. The quotient is the Chandra Avastha. The interpretation of all these are given in Sloka No. 16 below.

(3) Convert the Ghatis and Palas elapsed from birth, horary question, or Muhurta, into Palas, then divide this by 100. The resultant quotient is the Chandravela. The effect of every Chandravela has been given in the Slokas # 17 to Slokas # 19 which follows.

Chandra Kriya Effects

स्थानाद्भ्रष्टस्तपस्वी परयुवतिरतो द्यूतकृद्धस्तिमुख्या-
रूढः सिंहासनस्थो नरपतिररिहा दण्डनेता गुणी च।
निष्प्राणश्छिन्नमूर्द्धा क्षतकरचरणो बन्धनस्थो विनष्टो
राजा वेदानधीते स्वपिति सुचरितः संस्मृतो धर्मकर्ता॥१३॥

संद्रश्यो निधिसंगतः श्रुतकुलो वयाख्यापरः शत्रुहा
रोगी शत्रुजितः स्वदेशचलितो भृत्यो विनष्टार्थकः।
अस्थानी च सुमन्त्रकः परमहीभर्ता सभार्यो गज-
त्रस्तः संयुगभतिमानतिभयो लीनोन्नदाताग्निगः॥१४॥

क्षुद्र्बाधासहितोऽन्नमत्ति विचरन्मांसानोऽस्त्रक्षतः
सोद्वाहो धृतकन्दुको विहरति द्यूतैर्नृपो दुःखितः।
शय्यास्थो रिपुसेवितश्च ससुहृद्योगी च भार्यान्वितो
मिष्टाशी च पयः पिबन् सुकृतकृत् स्वस्थस्तथास्ते सुखम्॥१५।

If quotient is.......

1. Displaced (from position/residence)
2. Hard working
3. Engaged in other's women
4. Gambler
5. Riding on the main elephant
6. Sitting on the throne
7. King
8. Destroyer of enemies
9. Commander-in-Chief or high Official in Army
10. Endowed with many qualities
11. Lifeless (dead)
12. One whose head is cut
13. One injured in hand and feet
14. Imprisoned (Kidnapped)
15. Venistha
16. King
17. Recitor of Vedas
18. Sleeping
19. Good character
20. Engaged in deeds as per the religious rules
21. From Aristocratic family
22. Recipient of treasure
23. Famous or from the family of scholars
24. Commentator
25. Annihilator of enemies
26. Patient
27. Defeated by enemies
28. One who has left his country
29. Servant

30. One whose wealth is destroyed
31. Person in the court
32. Good Minister or adviser
33. Landlord of others lands
34. With wife
35. One who has been frightened by elephant
36. Coward
37. Extremely frightened persons
38. Person in hiding
39. One who gives corns to others
40. In the Fire (placed in fire)
41. Hungry
42. Engaged in eating corn
43. Likes to travel
44. Meat eater
45. Wounded from a weapon
46. Married
47. One who has a ball in the hand
48. Gambler
49. King
50. Unhappy
51. Lying on a cot
52. Who is served by enemies
53. Together with friend
54. Yogi
55. With wife
56. One eating sweets
57. One who drinks milk
58. One who does good deeds
59. Healthy
60. Happy

Chandra Awastha Phala

आत्मस्थानात्प्रवासो महितनृपहितो दासता प्राणहानि-
भूपालत्वं स्ववंशोचित्तगुणनिरतो रोग आस्थानवत्त्वम्।
भीतिः क्षुद्बाधितत्वं युवतिपरिणयो रम्यशय्यानुषक्ति
र्मृष्टाशित्वं च गीता इति नियमवशात्सद्भिरिन्दोरवस्था ॥१६॥

1. One who is out of his house
2. Benevolent of a great king
3. Death due to Slavery
4. Kingdom (Rajatwa)
5. Endowed with good qualities of his family
6. Disease
7. Present in the Court
8. Fear
9. Distress due to hunger
10. Marriage with a girl
11. Desire to rest in a beautiful couch (bed)
12. One who eats excellent food.

मूर्द्धामयो मुदितता चजनं सुखस्थो
नेत्रामयः सुखितता वनिताविहारः।
उग्रज्वरः कनकभूषणमश्रुमोक्षः
क्ष्वेला नं निधुवनं जठरस्य रोगः ॥१७॥

क्रीडा जले हसनचित्रविलेखने च
क्रोधश्च नृत्तकरणं घृतभुक्तिनिद्रे।
दानक्रिया दशनरुक् कलहः प्रयाण-
मुन्मत्तता च सलिलाप्लवनं विरोधः ॥१८॥

स्वेच्छारनानं क्षुद्भयं शास्त्रालाभं स्वैर गोष्ठी योधनं पुण्यकर्म।

पापा चार: क्रूरकर्मा प्रहर्ष प्राज्ञैरेवं चन्द्रवेला प्रदिष्टा ॥१९॥

The effects of Chandravelas are as follows-

1. Headache
2. Happiness
3. To perform Yagya
4. Happy or sitting comfortably
5. Eye disease
6. To be happy
7. Engaged in playful activities with women
8. High fever
9. Gold Ornaments
10. With shedding tears
11. Consume poison
12. Intimate relationship
13. Disease of Stomach
14. Play in water, laughing, painting
15. Anger
16. Dancing
17. Eating Ghee (purified butter)
18. Sleeping
19. Donating
20. Disease of Teeth
21. Quarrel
22. Travelling
23. Mental imbalance (due to drinking or madness)
24. To swim in water
25. Opposition
26. To bathe due to one's own desire
27. Hunger
28. Fear
29. To Study (Scripture)
30. One who does whatever he wants to do

31. Get together with friends
32. To be engaged in warfare
33. Good activities
34. Sinful activities
35. One who does cruel acts
36. Extreme happiness.

To observe Chandra Kriya one constellation is divided into 60 parts. The measurement of one constellation is 13 degree and 20 minutes. When this is divided by 60 then every part comes to be of 13' 20" (13 minutes 20 seconds).

Table of Chandra Kriya

	D-M-Sec.		D-M-Sec.		D-m-Sec.
1.	0-13-20	21.	4-40-0	41.	9-6-40
2.	0-26-40	22.	4-53-20	42.	9-20-0
3.	0-40-0	23.	5-6-40	43.	9-33-20
4.	0-53-2	24.	5-20-0	44.	9-46-40
5.	1-6-40	25.	5-33-20	45.	10-0-0
6.	1-20-0	26.	5-46-40	46.	10-13-20
7.	1-33-20	27.	6-0-0	47.	10-26-40
8.	1-46-40	28.	6-13-20	48.	10-40-0
9.	2-0-0	29.	6-26-40	49.	10-53-20
10.	2-13-20	30.	6-40-0	50.	11-6-40
11.	2-26-40	31.	6-53-20	51.	11-20-0
12.	2-40-0	32.	7-6-40	52.	11-33-20
13.	2-53-20	33.	7-20-0	53.	11-46-40
14.	3-6-40	34.	7-33-20	54.	12-0-0
15.	3-20-0	35.	7-46-40	55.	12-13-20
16.	3-33-20	36.	8-0-0	56.	12-26-40
17.	3-46-40	37.	8-13-20	57.	12-40-0
18.	4-0-0	38.	8-26-40	58.	12-53-20
19.	4-13-20	39.	8-40-0	59.	13-6-40
20.	4-26-40	40.	8-53-20	60.	13-20-0

For example if the longitude of Moon is 11ˢ-20⁰-37'-21", and as the span of Revati constellation is from 11ˢ-16'-40'-0", to 12ˢ-0⁰-0'-0", so we write.

Longitude of Moon	11ˢ-20⁰-37'-21"
Beginning of Revati	11ˢ-16'-40'-0"
Revati traversed by Moon	3⁰-57'-21"

Now look to the table above and we find that 3-46-40 indicates that the 17th part is completed. The 18th position finishes at 4-0-0. Therefore as 17th part being completed, the effect of Chandra Kriya of 17th part shows. One who teaches Vedas', will apply in this instance. One who teaches Vedas i.e. the native will be learned.

To know about the 'Chandra Avastha' one constellation of 13⁰-20' is divided by 12 and each part here will be of 1⁰-6'-40".

Table of Chandra Awastha

	D-M-Sec.		D-M-Sec.		D-M-Sec.
1.	1-6-40	5.	5-33-20	9.	10-0-0
2.	2-13-20	6.	6-40-0	10.	11-6-40
3.	3-20.0	7.	7-46-40	11.	12-13-20
4.	4-26-40	8.	8-46-40	12.	13-20-0

For example the traversed Revati constellation (as shown above) is 3⁰-57'-21'. In the above table part 3 is completed at 3⁰-20'-0'. The 4th part runs with 4⁰-26'-40". So the completed part 3 will be the Chandra Awastha.

The result of this is shown as death due to slavery, i.e. making effort in doing work for others (in service can cause death). The reduction in stamina, physical and mental, in service, can be deducted.

In order to get 'Chandravela' one constellation of 13⁰-20' when divided by 36, gives each part of 0⁰-22'-13" and 20 Prativikala.

Table of Chandravela

	D-M-Sec.		D-M-Sec.		D-M-Sec.
1.	0-22-13-20	13.	4-48-53-20	25.	9-15-33-20
2.	0-46-26-40	14.	5-11-6-40	26.	9-37-46-40
3.	1-6-40-0	15.	5-33-20-0	27.	10-0-0-0
4.	1-28-53-20	16.	5-55-33-20	28.	10-22-13-20
5.	1-51-6-40	17.	6-17-46-40	29.	10-44-26-40
6.	2-13-20-0	18.	6-40-0-0	30.	11-6-40-0
7.	2-35-33-20	19.	7-2-13-20	31.	11-28-53-20
8.	2-57-46-40	20.	7-24-26-40	32.	11-51-6-40
9.	3-20-0-0	21.	7-46-40-0	33.	12-13-20-0
10.	3-42-13-20	22.	8-8-53-20	34.	12-35-33-20
11.	4-4-26-40	23.	8-31-6-40	35.	12-57-46-40
12.	4-26-40-0	24.	8-53-20-0	36.	13-20-00-00

For example the Revati constellation has been traversed 3^0-57'-21" (see examples above). The 10th part in the Chandravela Table shows 3-42-13-20 as the ending. The 11th part shows the ending as 4-4-26-40. This is more than the distance covered in Revati. So, the finished 10th part is applicable here. The result of this is given as one who is shedding tears i.e. such native will be unhappy.

जातके च मूहूर्ते च प्रश्ने चन्द्रक्रियादशः ।
सम्यक् फलप्रदास्तस्माद्विशेषेण विचिन्तयेत् ॥२० ॥

In the birth chart, Muhurta and Horary Astrology, the effect of Chandra Kriya, Chandra Avastha etc. are very much true– So these should be specially considered.

पक्षोद्भवं हिमकरस्य विशेष्शमाहुः
स्थानोद्भवं तु बलमप्यधिक्रं परेषाम् ।
तत्संप्रयुक्तमितरैरधिकाधिकं स्या-
दन्यानि तेन सदृशानि बहूनि ते स्युः ॥२१ ॥

Much significance is attached to the Pakshebala of Moon (Bright half/dark half). In the case of rest of the planets special importance should be given to the Sthanabala.

Generally due to the sum total of all six types of strength, the strength of one planet compared to other increases much. This is so because some planets are strong in one or two types of balas whereas others may be strong in others. All these should be considered thoroughly.

Bala Pinda

सार्द्धानि षशतीक्ष्णकरो बलीयान् चन्द्रस्तु षशपञ्च वसुन्धराज:
सप्तेन्दुसूनो रविवद्गुरोस्तु सार्द्धानि पञ्चाथ सितो बली स्यात्॥२२॥

Now we speak as to at least how many roopa a planet should get to be called strong.

If Sun gets 6.5 roopa, Moon 6 roopa, and Mars 5 roopa then these are considered strong. Similarly if Mercury gets 7 roopas, Jupiter 6.5 and Venus 5.5. roopas then they are called strong.

Note:

How to calculate extra territorial planets like 'Dhoom', 'Vyatipata' etc.

1. Add 4 signs, 13 degrees, 20 minutes to the longitude of Sun. The resultant sign, degree etc. will be 'DHOOM'.
2. Deduct 'Dhoom' from 12 signs 0 degree, 0 minute- The balance is 'Vyatipata'.
3. Add six signs to the sign, degree minute of 'Vyatipata, then we get 'Parivesh.'.
4. Subtract 'Parivesh' from 12 signs-Degree, minutes the residue is called 'Indrachap'.

For example if the longitude of Sun at birth as:

	Sign	-	Degree	-	Minutes	-	Secs.
1. Sun	7	-	26	-	11	-	38
Add +	4	-	13	-	20		

Dhoom is (0)	12	- 9	- 31	- 38
	12	- 0	- 0	- 0
2. -	0	- 9	- 31	- 38
Vyatipata is	11	- 20	- 28	- 22
3.	11	- 20	- 28	- 22
+	6	- 0	- 0	- 0
Parivesh is	5	- 20	- 28	- 22
	12	- 0	- 0	- 0
4. -	5	- 20	- 28	- 22
Indrachap is	6	- 9	- 31	- 38

मन्दस्तु पंञ्चैव हि षड्बलानां संयोग एवापरथान्यथा स्युः ।
एवं ग्रहाणां स्वबलाबलानि विचिन्त्य सम्यक्कयेत्फलानि॥२३ ॥

If Saturn gets even 5.5. roopa balas then it is called strong. If the total of Shadbala of any planet is less than that mentioned above, then it is considered weak. This way the strength of planets should be elaborately considered and then prediction should be done.

We have explained as how much roopa a planet should get in the total of Shadbala to be considered strong. Now we talk about the system discussed in other books.

1. Sthana
2. Dik
3. Chesta
4. Kala and
5. Ayan

Out of five types of strength, how much a planet should get to be considered strong? The natural strength of planet has not been mentioned because the natural strength of planets is the same in every horoscope.

Table of Balas for Planets– which make them strong

Planet	Sthana	Dik	Chesta	Kala	Ayan	Total
Sun	2-45	0-35	0-50	1-52	0-30	6-32
Moon	2-13	0-50	0-30	1-40	0-40	5-53
Mars	1-36	0-30	0-40	1-07	0-20	4-13
Mercury	2-45	0-35	0-50	1-52	0-30	6-32
Jupiter	2-45	0-35	0-50	1-52	0-30	6-32
Venus	2-13	0-50	0-30	1-40	0-40	5-53
Saturn	1-36	0-30	0-40	1-07	0-20	4-13

One roopa has 60 points. Here the doubt comes that in Sloka No. 22 it has been stated that the total of six balas of Sun when 6.5 then it is considered strong and here only where the total of five types of strength is 6 Roopa 32 points - it is strong. The answer to this is that it is similar to the fact that in an examination the total per cent of pass marks should be 33 per cent in aggregate but in each paper 40 per cent is required to pass it.

Now we speak of the strength of a house:

लग्नादिकानामधिपस्य पिण्डे रूपान्विते तद्बलपिण्डमाहुः ।
गृहस्य यस्यां दिशादिग्बलं स्यात्तद्भाववीर्य सहितस्य दृष्ट्या ॥२४॥

If we have to find the strength* of a house then we should add

(a) Bhava Dikbala

(b) Bhava Drikbala and

(c) The strength of the lord of the house.

This will give us the Bhava Bala (the strength of the house).

---

*One commentator has written that we should add one roopa to the bala of the lord of the house to gets its strength.

If the house is teneted by its lord, Jupiter, Venus or Mercury or aspected by its lord, Jupiter or Mercury then that bala should also be added (see Sloka No. 6).

The purpose of finding the strength of a house is that if a house is strong then benefic results related to that house will be felt. If a house is weak then benefic results will be less and malefic results will be more.

5

Career

The name of this chapter is 'Career" *i.e.* Where and What type of work one should undertake for livelihood (to acquire wealth).

Generally many people while consulting astrologers ask as to the most suitable profession for them to earn a decent income. This is the subject matter of this chapter.

अर्थाप्ति कथयेद्विलग्नशशिनोः प्राबल्यतः खेचरैः
कर्मस्थैः पितृमातृशात्रवसुहृद्भ्रात्रादिभिः स्त्रीधनात्।
भृत्यद्वा दिननाथलग्नशशिनां मध्ये बलीयांस्ततः
कर्मेशस्थनवांशराशिपवशाद्वृत्तिं जगुस्तद्विदः ॥१॥

Which is the planet that helps one to acquire wealth? Before proceeding further, let me point out that in a horoscope we have to consider each and all aspects. For example, if the earning capacity is limited, or prosperity is not indicated in the birth chart, then a person may rise in life, but will not be able to earn his living. He may earn fame, prestige and honour, but wealth will not be there. The tenth house and the planets posited therein from the Ascendent or Moon, whichever is stronger, will give the source of wealth. If Sun is in the 10th house then the native will benefit from his father.

If Moon is there, then benefit comes from mother.

If Mars is there, then he will gain through enemies. By defeating his enemies he will win wealth.

If it is Mercury, then benefit comes through friends.

If it is Jupiter then from brothers.

If it is Venus, then from women..

If it is Saturn, then benefit comes from servants.

We have indicated above the relatives through whom the native is likely to benefit. When these books were written, then the sources of revenue were limited. But these days, they have increased, and we should interpret according to the background of the present industrial developments, import-exports etc. We should not only consider benefit from father, but also from all those things which are indicated by Sun. Benefits accrue from one or more sources indicated.

Similarly, we should understand from the Moon and other planets. For example, if Moon is placed in 10th house from the Ascendant then the person will benefit through white materials, silver, liquids, and from such things which come out of the sea. He will benefit from Pearls, and if he does business with overseas countries, exports/ imports, and particularly of such materials which are used by the masses. similarly we should consider the various sources of benefit from other planets.

We have spoken so far only about the planet in the 10th from the rising sign or Moon. Now we discuss another principle.

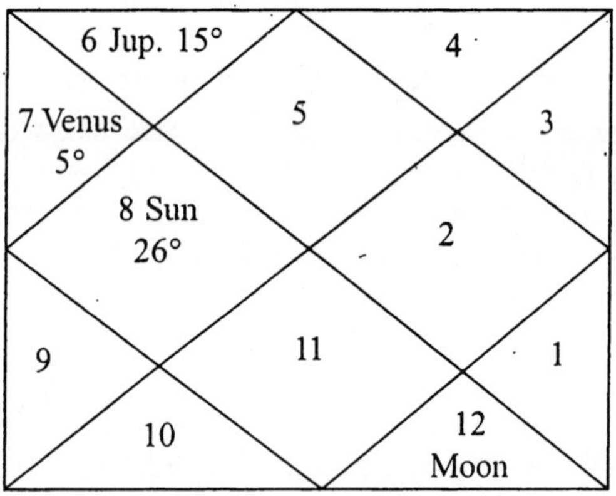

Consider as to which is the strongest out of the rising sign, Sun and Moon and then examine the tenth sign from it. The lord of the Navansha in which the lord of the 10th sign from the strongest is placed, will indicate the sources of revenue. For example, we give above a horoscope with Leo rising, Sun is in Scorpio in the 4th house, Moon in 8th house in Pisces.

Out of these we find that the Ascendant is the strongest then the 10th house from Ascendant is owned by Venus and Venus is in the Navansha of Mars, say 5 degree in Libra, then Mars will indicate the type of work that the native should take up in order to do better in life. If Sun is the strongest, then the 10th house from Sun is Leo and being in the 26th degree falls in Aquarius Navansha which is ruled by Saturn so the work will be related to the matter and products which fall under Saturn. The native will also benefit from people who have the nature, characteristics, physical buildup etc. of Saturn and are engaged in the related work falling under Saturn.

If Moon is the strongest, then we should consider the 10th house from it, which is Sagittarius, Jupiter is the lord of Sagittarius and it is posited in Virgo in the 15 degree, i.e. it is in Taurus Navansha. The lord of this Navansha is Venus, so we should indicate that the native will benefit from people who have the nature, appearance and characteristics of Venus, i.e. refined, balanced body, attractive personality and amicable disposition. Secondly, he should deal in things which come under Venus. For example, jewellery, ornaments, silk, perfumes, ivory, paintings, film industry, film line, photography etc. He will also benefit from people engaged in this type of work.

We have mentioned above that whichever is the strongest out of the Ascendant, Sun. and Moon, then the Navansha occupied by the lord of the 10th from that sign should be considered as the nature of acquisition of wealth. The question arises if only the strongest should be considered? The answer is no.

Some astrologers are of the opinion that we should consider all the three. At times, we find that the source of revenue is not continuous. At one period of life one person is engaged in one business, then he changes his business altogether. This is indicated according to the periodic influences or the transit one is passing through. For example, if it is the periodic influence of Moon, he would benefit from liquids, white things, etc. If it is through Sun, then he will benefit through his own efforts, father, people in better position etc. during Rahu's periodic influence, a person definitely changes or relocates to a new place. He is likely to benefit from import and export, from foreigners and foreign countries. During Venus's periodic influence the natural inclination runs towards nice things, fine arts, and other things which are soft, lustrous, and attractive. Whether he will benefit much will be indicated by the strength of these planets in the birth chart. It is a very complicated thing, but with knowledge and practice one will arrive at the right conclusion.

फलद्रुमैर्मन्त्रजपेश्च शाठ्यद्द्यूतानृतैः कंबलभेषजाद्यैः।
धातुक्रियाद्वा क्षितिपालपूज्याज्जीवत्यसौ पङ्कजवल्लभांशे ॥२॥

जलोद्भवानां क्रयविक्रयेण कृषिक्रियागोमहिषीसमुत्थैः।
तीर्थाटनाद्वा वनिताश्रयाद्वा निशाकरांशे वसनक्रयाद्वा ॥३॥

भौमांशके धातुरणप्रहारैर्महानसाद्भू मिवशात्सुवर्णात्।
परोपतापायुधसाहसैर्वा म्लेच्छाश्रयात्सूचकचोरवृत्या ॥४॥

काव्यागमैर्लेखकलिप्युपायैर्ज्योतिर्गणज्ञानवशाद्बुधांशे।
परार्थवेदाध्ययनाज्जपाञ्च पुरोहितव्याजवशात्प्रवृत्तिः ॥५॥

जीवांशके भूसुरदेवतानां समाश्रयाद्भू मिपतिप्रसादात्।
पुराणशास्त्रागमनीतिमार्गाद्धर्मोपदेशेन कुसीदवृत्या ॥६॥

स्त्रीसंश्रयाद्गोमहिषीगजाश्वैस्तौर्यत्रिकैर्वा रजतैश्च गन्धैः।
क्षीरराद्यलङ्कारपटीपटाद्यैः शुक्रांशकेऽमात्यगुणैः कवित्वात् ॥७॥

शन्यंशके मूलफलैः श्रमेण प्रेष्यैः खलैर्नीचधनैः कुधान्यैः।
भारोद्यहात्कुत्सितमार्गवृत्या शिल्पादिभिर्दारुमयैर्वधाद्यैः ॥८॥

We have mentioned above the lord of Navansha of the sign occupied by the 10th lord from the Sun, Moon and Ascendant. Now we give below the matter and sources, which come under different planets.

Sun : Fruits and fruit trees, mantra, religious prayers and japa, cleverness, treachery, mischief, gambling, speculation, lying, blankets, wool, woollen clothers, medicine, chemicals used in medicines, chemistry, metals, work for important person, kings, or government service.

Moon : Things which come out of the sea and water (Pearls, Corals, Sea food), overseas work, import and export, shipping, agriculture, milk, from cows and buffaloes, milk products, cheese, yogurt, butter, etc., travelling to holy places with the patronage of a woman, or through textile – sale and purchase of textiles.

Mars : If Mars is the lord of the Navansha, then the following will indicate the sources of revenue : metals (like iron, copper, and work connected with it, electricity, radio) fighting - physically as well as legal cases, war, army, dacoity, military service, work connected with gold - manufacturing of gold ornaments, etc., Cooking, working in hotels and restaurant, from other after causing them injury from weapons anguish, firearms, courage, through the patronage of Muslims, Intelligence Department or as an informer, and from theft. Infact, Mars indicates wealth because the person is aggressive and takes initiatives to earn wealth.

Mercury : If Mercury is the planet indicating work then one benefits through poetry, scriptures, as a writer (where reading and writing is involved) through commission, cleverness, brokerage and trading, astrology and other occult sciences, due to his learning, teaching reciting of Vedas and from other religious books, working as a priest.

Looking to the present times, a person benefits from journalism, newspaper, through Railways, communications, working in Embassies, grains, tourism, etc. all these come under Mercury.

Jupiter : The following matters fall under Jupiter: Brahmins, living in temples and holy places or under their patronage or due to the benevolence of kings, Puranas (holy texts), education, Veda's (teaching of it), from the path of truth and not through unfair means, preaching of religion -- all these are the sources of income. Jupiter also indicates income from interest. Those people who have interest as to the main source of income do have a very strong Jupiter in their birth charts. The banks mortgage companies and financial institutions also come under Jupiter.

Venus : Venus indicates benefit though women or patronage of women (even if it is one's spouse, or prostitute, queen, actress -- anyone), cows, buffaloes, elephants (ivory); horses etc. through music, musical instruments, dancing -- singing, silver, scented rings, silk and refined textiles, ornaments, poetry, by becoming an adviser to a minister, a king or an influential women; movies, milk - milk products, photography, luxury goods, perfumes cosmetics etc. also come under Venus. We have found that people with strong Venus in the second house earn money by working in banks or financial institutions.

Saturn : If Saturn indicates the source of wealth then benefit comes from Vegetables which grow under the earth like potatoes, sweet potatoes, etc., physical work (like labourers, helpers etc.), service under others or employ others bad-characters or through the wealth of bad people, through bribes and money acquired from illegal and underhand means*, working as touts or agents for prostitutes; through coarse grains. Saturn gives wealth through hard labour and persistence. If the person is not educated then he will work as a labourer or a farm labourer, if he is educated then he will sit in a chair and work throughout the day. It also gives wealth through wood, wooden furniture, etc.

अंशेशे बलवत्ययत्नधनसंप्राप्तिं बलोनेंशपे।
स्वल्पं प्रोक्तफलं भवेदुदयतः कर्मर्क्षदेशे फलम्।
अंशस्योक्तदिशं वदेत्पतियुते दृष्टे स्वदेशे फलं
सत्यन्यैः परदेशजं तदधिपस्यांशे स्वदेशे स्थिरे॥९॥

When the lord of the Navansha, about which we have discussed in the preceding slokas, wealth is strong, then acquired easily that is with less efforts more money comes. But if the lord of the Navansha is weak, then the amount of earnings is very little.

Now we will discuss the country and the direction from which the wealth will come.

---

*Bribes accepted by magistrates from culprits or by jail superintendent from prisoner is a bad source of income.

(1) Whichever sign falls in the 10th house that sign will indicate the country and the direction from which money is earned.

Or

(2) The lord of the Navansha in which the lord of the 10th house is posited will indicate the country and the direction from where money will be earned.

For example, in the horoscope gives earlier, Leo rises and it is strong, and then the 10th sign from it is Taurus. The native will benefit from countries which come under Taurus and the direction indicated by it. In second case Venus rules Taurus, and it is in the Scorpio Navansha, then the native will benefit from countries which fall under Scorpio, and the direction indicated by Scorpio. However, one thing should be kept in mind. If the lord of the sign or the Navansha through which we are getting the indication is posited therein or aspects it, then the native will earn wealth in his own country. If the lord of the 10th is posited in a fixed Navansha, then also the native earns in his own country. However the two signs viz., the 10th sign, or the Navansha occupied by the lord of the 10th sign, are tenanted by or aspected by other planets and not the lord threof, then the native will do better in other countries and not in his own country. He lives in a foreign country, or he will travel to foreign countries in order to earn his livings. In some astrological books it is mentioned that if the lord of the 9th house is in a movable sign, then the native benefits in other countries (overseas). If it is in a fixed sign, then he will have rise in life in his own country, and if it is in a dual sign, then the native will earn at times from foreign countries and at other times he will make money in his own country.

(The direction indicated by different signs and planets, please see Chapter 2.).

N.B. (i) Planets in the first house or (ii) planets which aspect the 10th house will indicate the method of earnings.

6

Yogadhyay — Combination and Placement of Planets

रुचकभद्रकहंसकमालवाः
सशशका इति पञ्च च कीर्तिकाः ।
स्वभवनोच्चगतेषु चतुष्टये
क्षितिसुतादिषु तान् क्रमशे वदेत् ॥१ ॥

In this chapter we will discuss many yogas. The relationship if any between the lords of two houses and the placement of planets in particular positions which will endow the native with some type of special power and strength.

First of all we shall take up the five yogas which are called the 'Pancha Mahapurush' Yogas (five special Yogas). These are based on the five planets viz., Mars, Mercury, Jupiter, Venus and Saturn.

If Mars is in Aries, Scorpio or Capricorn and is posited in an angle (1, 4, 7 or 10th house) from Ascendant then it is called 'Ruchak' Yoga.

If Mercury is posited in an angular position and occupies Gemini or Virgo, then it is called 'Bhadra' Yoga.

If Jupiter is in an angular position and occupies Cancer, Sagittarius, or Pisces, then it is called 'Hamsa' Yoga.

If Venus is posited in Taurus, Libra, or Pisces, and is in an angular position, then it is called 'Malavya' Yoga.

If Saturn is posited in an angle in Libra, Capricorn, or Aquarius then it is called 'Sasa' Yoga.

दीर्घास्यो बहुसाहसाप्तविभवः शूरोऽरिहन्तां बल
गर्विष्ठो रुचके प्रतीतगुणवान् सेनापतिर्जित्वरः ।
आयुष्मान् सकुशाग्रद्धिरमलो विद्वज्जनश्लाघितो
भूपो भद्रकयोगजोऽतिविभवश्चास्थानकोलाहलः ॥२ ॥

हंसे सद्भिरभिष्टुतः क्षितिपतिः शङ्खाब्जमत्स्याङ्कशै-
श्चिह्नैः पादकराङ्कितः शुभवपुर्मुष्टान्नभुग्धार्मिकः ।
पुष्टाङ्गो धृतमान्धनी सुतवधूभाग्यान्वितो वर्धनो
मालव्ये सुखभुक्सुवाहनयशा विद्वान्प्रसन्नेन्द्रियः ॥३ ॥

शस्तः सर्वजनैः सुभृत्यबलवान् ग्रामाधिपो वा नृपो
दुर्वृत्तः शशयोगजोंऽन्यवनितावित्तान्वितः सौख्यान् ।
लग्नेन्द्वोरपि योगपञ्चकमिदं साम्राज्यसिद्धिप्रदं
तेष्वेकादिषु भाग्यवान् नृपसमो राजा नृपेन्द्राऽधिकः ॥४ ॥

If one or more of the above five yogas are present in a nativity then what will be the physical appearance or fortunes of a person, has been given below:

If a person is born in Ruchak yoga, then he will have a large face, and he will earn wealth on account of his courage. He will be strong and brave. He will annihilate his enemies and is proud. He will be a general in the army and will maintain his dignity. (It is likely that the person will occupy a high position of power in the political sphere). He will be famous on account of his capabilities. He will have fame and will be well known. He will achieve success in whatever work he undertakes.

If a person is born in Bhadra Yoga, then he has a piercing intelligence, pure, would like to dress well, will maintain a neat and clean appearance. Learned people will praise him. He is very good and clever in speech. This type of person will be very fortunate and will possess all types of luxuries. He will be a king, or equal to a king.

One who is born in Hamsa Yoga, has the signs of conch-shells, lotus, fish, and trident in his hands and feet, he is very charming, good looking, and peaceful in appearance. He likes to eat good and nice food, and good people praise him.

If a person is born in Malavya Yoga, then he has patience and is strong in built. He has well-developed parts of his body. He loves rich food. He is learned, has happy appearance. He is not easily disturbed. He is blessed with women and sons. He will rise in life towards good fortunes and success. His fame is spread throughout the world. He will own or will enjoy luxurious cars and residence.

If someone is born in Sasa Yoga then he is very influential. He is the head of a village, or head of a Sect. He is strong and many good people work under him. "Good" here stands for capable. People born in Sasa yoga, are praised by others. However his character is not good. He is interested in other women, but he is wealthy and happy.

We have given above five yogas, which take effect due to Mars, Mercury, Jupiter, Venus and Saturn. If any one of them occupies its sign of exaltation or own sign, which falls in an angle in the horoscope, then one of the five yogas mentioned above is formed. The 1st, 4th, 7th, and 10th houses are angles. We must also keep in mind that we should consider these yogas not only from the Ascendant, but also from Moon. If a Planet occupies an angular position from Moon, and is powerful in its own sign, or in its sign of exaltation, then it will endow the native with wealth, prosperity, success and fame. We should therefore consider the angular position from the rising sign, as well as from the Moon sign. If one planet create yoga then it will make the native fortunate. If two planets create two of the above five yogas then the native will be equal to a king.

If three planets create three different yogas, then the person so born is a king. If four planets are in such powerful position, then the person concerned will be King of Kings. If five planets are causing all the five yogas, Ruchak, Bhadra, Hamsa, Malavya and Sasa then he occupies the highest position in life. These five yogas cannot be simultaneously present in a horoscope if we consider only from the Rising Sign. If we consider just from the Moon sign then also is not possible because Mercury and Venus can not occupy angular position as well as be in their sign of exaltation or own sign, only from the

Moon, or only from the rising sign. Therefore we have to consider all the five yogas both from Moon and from the rising sign.

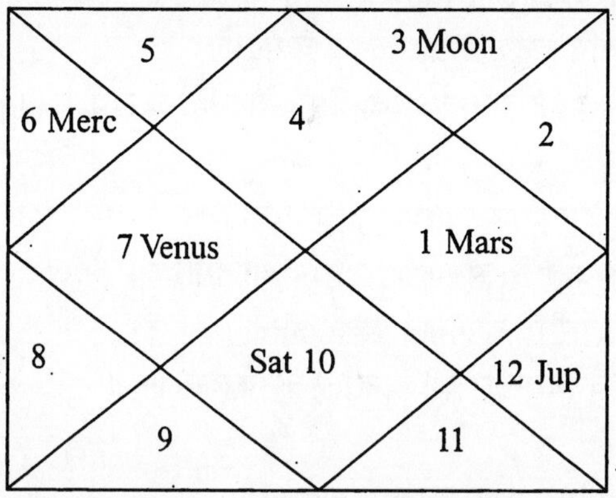

Consider a horoscope with Cancer rising, Venus in Libra in the 4th house, Saturn in Capricorn in the 7th house, Mars in Aries in the 10th house, Mercury in Virgo in the 3rd house, Moon in Gemini in the 12th house. When we consider from the rising sign, then in this chart, Venus is causing Malavya Yoga, Mars is causing Ruchak Yoga, and Saturn is causing Sasa Yoga. If we consider from Moon also then Mercury is creating Bhadra Yoga. If Jupiter is also in Pisces, then there will be Hamsa Yoga also, so all the five yogas will be present.

In almost all-old textbooks of astrology, which are famous for hundreds of years, they have given these five Mahapurusha Yogas. However in a book, called Mansagari it has been pointed out that at times these five Mahapurusha Yogas are cancelled. If the planet, which is creating the Mahapurusha Yoga conjoins with Sun or Moon, then the yoga is cancelled.

The native will not be a king but when he passes through the periodic influence of such a planet then he will enjoy only certain good results. He will have wealth but his wealth will not be so much as king's possess he will have courage, but not of a very extraordinary type. The intensity is reduced. This is called cancellation of the Panchamahapurusha Yoga. (If a planet is combust then the effects will be bad instead of good).

विधोस्तु सुनफानधुरुधुराः स्वारिः फोभय-
स्थितैर्विरविभिर्ग्रहैरितरथा तु केमद्रुमः ॥
हिमत्विषि चतुष्टये ग्रहयुतेऽथ केमद्रुमो
न हीति कथितोऽथवा हिमकराद्ग्रहैः केन्द्रगैः ॥५॥

स्वयमधिगतवित्तः पार्थिवस्तत्समो वा
भवति हि सुनफायां धीधनख्यातिमांश्च
प्रभुरगदशरीरः शीलवान् ख्यातकीर्ति-
र्विषयसुखसुवेषो वनर्तृतश्चानफायाम् ॥६॥

उत्पन्नभोगसुखभाग्यधनवाहनाढ्य-
स्त्यागान्वितो धुरुधुराप्रभवः संभृत्यः ।
केमद्रुमे मलिनदुःखितनोचनिःस्वाः
प्रेष्याः खलाश्च नृपतेरपि वंशजाताः ॥७॥

Now we give another four yogas. We consider these four yogas from the sign occupied by Moon in the birth chart. Wherever we refer to planets, we consider only Mars, Mercury, Jupiter, Venus and Saturn. We do not consider Sun in this yoga.

(1) If any planet occupies the 12th house from Moon, and there is no planet in the second from Moon, then it is called Anpha Yoga.

(2) If there are no planets in the 12th house from Moon, and a planet occupies the second house from Moon, then it is called sunpha yoga.

(3) If both the 2nd and the 12th houses from Moon have planets, then it is called Durdhara Yoga.

(4) If there is no planet either in the 2nd or 12th from Moon, then it is called Kemudrum Yoga.

Some astrologers are of the view that if one of the following takes place, then the Kemudrum Yoga will not show effect.

(1) If a planet is posited in the same sign with Moon.

(2) If a planet occupies an angular position from the rising sign.

(3) If a planet occupies the 4th or 10th house from Moon.

Famous astrologers like Mantreshwar insists that Kemudrum Yoga is there if there is no planet on either side of Moon i.e. in the 2nd and 12th from Moon. He does not adhere to the view that it is cancelled.

The results of Kemudrum yoga is not good. If Kemudrum Yoga is there, then the person will be unhappy in life. He will be uncomely. He will be poor. He works for others, and never rises in life. Kemudrum Yoga has been endowed with so much bad results that even if a person is born in a royal family, then the above mentioned things will apply to his life. We like to direct the attention of the learned readers that we should not draw conclusion from only one yoga but should consider all other factors.

Now we shall tell the effects of these 3 yogas we have referred above viz., Anpha, Sunpha, and Durdhara.

(1) A person who is born in Sunpha Yoga becomes a king or equal to a king. He is intelligent, wealthy, and he will become famous.

(2) One who is born in Anpha Yoga is pleasant to look at, has a good character and behaviour. He has material prosperity and pleasures. He is well satisfied and happy by temperament. He dresses well and keeps good health. He gets respect in society.

(3) A person who is born in Durdhara Yoga is ready to sacrifice everything for the benefit for others. He is happy and wealthy. He will never lack vehicles. He has material prosperity, and he enjoys it.

हित्वेन्दुं शुभसिवेवास्युभयचर्याख्या: स्वरि:फोभय-
स्थानस्थै: सवितु: शुभै: स्युरशुभैस्ते पपसंज्ञा: स्मृता: ।
सत्पार्श्वे शुभकर्तरीत्युदयभे पापैस्तु पापाह्वयो
लग्नाद्वित्तगतै: शुभैस्तु सुशुभो योगो पापेक्षितै: ॥८ ॥

In the yogas above, if any planet (with the exception of Sun) is either in the 2nd, 12th or on both (2nd and 12th) places from the Moon, then a Yoga takes place.

Now we are going to tell that if any other planet except the

Moon, is either in the 2nd or 12th or in 2nd and 12th (both) places from Sun then the following yogas are formed:

(1) If Mars, Mercury, Jupiter, Venus, and Saturn, either of them, or more than one, are in the 2nd house from Sun, then the yoga such formed is called Subhavesi Yoga.

(2) If Mars, Mercury, Jupiter, Venus, or Saturn is in the 12th from sun, then it is called Subhavesi Yoga.

(3) If out of these 5 planets, one or more is in the 12th and 2nd, i.e. on either side of the house in which sun is posited, then the yoga such formed is called UBAHYACHARI Yoga. "Ubahyachari ", a Sanskrit worked, means " on both sides Of Whom " that is the sign in which Sun is posited. The yoga will not take place if the planets are on either side of sun but not in the same sign. It is necessary that they should be in the sign proceeding and following the sign in which Sun is posited. In this yoga we do not consider Moon. We do not take Rahu and Ketu also. We do not consider Uranus, Neptune, and Pluto, but only the 5 planets Mars, Mercury, Jupiter, Venus, and Saturn. These 3 yogas and other yogas we have given above are given in many books of astrology however according to Maharaj Mantreshwar, if benefic form this Subhavesi, subgavasi, and Ubahyachari, then it will show good results. But if malefic are in such position and are causing these yogas, then instead of Subha Yogas they will be called Papavasi and Papaubahyachari. 'Papa means it will show bad effects or restrict the good effects.

We should also consider these yogas from the Rising sign i.e. if there are on either side (the 2nd and 12th). Of the rising sign, then it will also create a yoga. If there are malefic in the sign proceeding and the sign following the rising sign, then it is called Papakartari, but if there are benefic on either side of the rising sign, then it is called Subha-Kartari. If there are benefic in the 2nd house from the rising sign and no malefic aspect it then it is called susubha Yoga. We should remember that if there are benefic in the 2nd house from the Ascendant, it is a good yoga. If there is no planet in the 2nd house from the Lagna and there is one or more planet in the 12th house from the rising sign, then it is not considered any yoga, because the 12th house is considered to be inauspicious.

जातः स्यात् सुभगः सुखी गुणनिधिर्धीरो नृपो धार्मिको
विख्यातः सकलप्रियोऽतिसुभगो दाता महीशप्रियः
चार्वङ्ग प्रियवाक्यप्रपञ्चरसिको वाग्मी यशस्वी धनी
विद्यादत्र सुवेसिवास्युभयचर्याख्येषु पादक्रमात् ॥९ ॥

A person who is born in Subhavesi Yoga will be handsome, happy, endowed with many good qualities, patience and perseverance, religious, and he will rule many people. A person who is born in Subhavesi Yoga will be very good looking, will be a giver, will be a favourite of the king and will occupy a high post in the government and he will be famous. He will be loved by all. A person who is born in Subhayachari Yoga will be a good orator; will win in debates and competitions. He will be sweet tongued. He will be learned, wealthy and famous. All parts of his body are attractive, and he will please everyone.

अन्याययाज्जननिन्दको हतरुचिर्हीनप्रियो दुर्जनो
मायावी परनिन्दकः खलयुतो दुर्वृत्तशास्त्राधिकः ।
लोके सयादपकीर्तिदुःखितमना विद्यार्थभाग्यैश्च्युतो
जातश्चाशु भवेसिवास्युभयचर्याख्येषु पादक्रमात् ॥१० ॥

A person who is born in Papavesi loves to talk ill of others. He will find fault with everyone. He is dull, will not be attractive. He is bad by nature and keeps the company of low people.

A person who is born in Asubhavasi will also be a person who will find faults with others. He is a confidence trickster and cheats others. He is a Friend of rogues. He indulges in sinful activities and will try to substantiate his sinful activities by reciting the scriptures and painting out and explaining all his bad conducts in a logical manner.

A person who is born in Asubhaubhayachari Yoga is devoid of education and learning, fortunes and wealth. He is always unhappy and gets public censure.

जैवातृको विभरोगरिपुः सुखी स्या–
दाढ्यः श्रिया च शुभकर्तरियोगजातः ।

निःस्वोऽशु चिर्विसुखदारसुतोऽङ्गहीनः
स्यात्पापकर्तारिभवोऽचिरमायुरेति ॥११ ॥

A person who is born in Subhakartari Yoga will be longlived, wealthy, happy and prosperity of all types. He will not suffer from disease and enemies.

But a person who is born in Papakartari Yoga is poor, impure, sinful unhappy, and loses some portion of his body. He is short-lived. He is devoid of wife and children. In short, Subhakartari shows good results, and Papakartari shows negative effects. It does not mean that all these results will take place fully. We must consider the essence of all these yogas. We have to draw our conclusion from experience and learning as to how much to take from one yoga, how much from the other, how much from the third one. Generally speaking, the effect of these yogas will manifest throughout life, but much more so when a person passes through the periodic influences of a planet which is creating any of the yoga. For example, if Venus is in the 2nd house from Sun and a person passes through the periodic influence of Venus, then it will indicate good results. Or, if Venus is in the 2nd house from the rising sign, then also during the periodic influence of Venus, the person will be very good in speech. He will have much wealth, he will have happiness, and he will have happiness from women, and he will get benefit through their advice. So the good effects which are indicated by Venus will get intensified due to this particular placement. His health will be good and he will live in nice surroundings.

A subhavasi and Papavasi is one and the same thing.

आचारवान् धर्ममतिः प्रसन्नः
सौभाग्यवान् पार्थिवमाननीयः ।
मृदुस्वभावः स्मितभाषणश्च
धनी भवेच्चामलयोगजातः ॥१२ ॥

There is another yoga which is called Amla Yoga, but how is it formed has not been mentioned so far. A person who is born in Amla Yoga is very religious and interested in religious activities; he will be happy by temperament; he will be blessed with good fortunes. He will receive honour from kings. He will speak softly and will be cheerful. He will be wealthy.

सुशभेशुभर्कतर्यां वेस्यादौ सुनभादिवत्।
शुभैः क्रमात्फलं ज्ञेयं विपरीतमसद्ग्रहैः ॥१३॥

Whatever results have been indicated for Sunpha, Anpha, etc., should also be considered for Susubha, Subha Kartari and Subhavesi, *i.e.* Subhvesi and Susubha will indicate the results of Sunpha, and Subhavasi will give results similar to Anpha Yoga. Subhaubhyachari will give the same results as Durdhara. If planets are in the (a) 2nd house (b) in the 3rd house (c) in the 2nd and 3rd house from sun-then benefic results are indicated. If malefic create the yogas then we must draw the opposite conclusions. However if malefic are either in their exaltation sign, or in their own house, and are strong, with directional strength, then they will show mixed results.

In a similar manner, if benefic are well placed, then they will enhance the good results. If they are not so well placed, then mixed effect will ensue.

ओजेश्वर्केन्दुलग्नान्यजनि दिवि पुमांश्चेन्महाभाग्ययोगः
स्त्रीणान्तद्व्यत्ययेस्याच्छशिनि सुरगुरोः केन्द्रगे केसरीति।
जीवान्त्याष्टारिसंस्थे शशिनि तु शकटः केन्द्रेगे नास्ति लग्ना-
च्चन्द्रे केन्द्रादिगेऽर्कादधमसवरिष्ठाख्ययोगाः प्रसिद्धाः ॥१४॥

(A) In the horoscope of a man, if the following four yogas take place, then it is known as Mahabhagya Yoga:

(1) If the native is born during the daytime (between sunrise and before sunset)

(2) If the rising sign is an odd sign.

(3) If sun is in an odd sign.

(4) If moon is also in an odd sign.

In the case of a woman, it is the reverse; i.e.:

(1) If she is born during the night time (between sunset and sunrise).

(2) Her Rising sign falls in an even sign.

(3) Moon is also in an even sign.

(4) Sun is also in an even sign.

When these four conditions are fulfilled in the horoscope of a girl, then she is said to be born in Mahabhagya Yoga.

Now we tell of other yogas, which will take place in the case of anyone, whether a man or a woman.

(B) If Jupiter is in an angular position from Moon, then it is called Kesari Yoga. In many textbooks the same yoga is called Gajkesari Yoga, i.e. the person born in this yoga possesses the strength of a lion and the intelligence of an elephant, so he will do well in life.

If Moon is in the 6th, 8th or 12th houses from Jupiter, then it is called Sakat Yoga. However if Moon occupies an angular position from the Ascendant then the Sakat Yoga will not take place.

If Moon occupies a Kendra position from Sun, then it is called Adham Yoga.

If Moon is in the 2nd, 5th, 8th, or 11th from sun. Then it is called Sama Yoga.

If Moon occupies the 3rd, 6th, 9th or 12th from Sun, then it is called Varishta Yoga.

Now we give the results of these different yogas:

महाभाग्ये जातः सकलनयनानन्दजनको
वदान्यो विख्यातः क्षितिपतिरशीत्यायुरमलः ।
वधूनां योगेऽस्मिन् सति धनसुमाङ्गल्यसहिता
चिरं पुत्रैः पौत्रैः शुभमुपगता सा सुचरिता ॥१५ ॥

The person who is born in Mahabhagya Yoga pleases the eyes of everyone, generous, famous, pure in character owns lands and properties, and prosperous like a king. Those women who have this Mahabhagya Yoga have good character, their husband live for long time and they are wealthy. They have happiness from husband, sons, and grand sons for a long time. They will leave this body before their husband, and will never suffer widowhood.

केसरीव रिपुवर्गनिहन्ता प्रौढवाक् सदसि राजसवृत्तिः ।
दीर्घजीव्यत्तियशाः पटुबुद्धिस्तेजसा जयति केसरियोगे ॥१६ ॥

Now we tell the results of Kesari Yoga. A person who is born in Kesari Yoga destroys his enemy, annihilates his enemies like a lion. In the society of educated and learned people he will have full control and convincing abilities due to his speech, He will discuss every subject with authority and seriousness. He enjoys life and occupies a high post. He is respected. He is always a leader due to his inner strength.

क्वचित्क्वचिद्भाग्यपरिच्युतः सन् पुनः पुनः सर्वमुपैति भाग्यम् ।
लोकेऽप्रसिद्धोऽपरिहार्यमन्तः शल्यं प्रपन्नः शकटेऽतिदुःखी ॥१७ ॥

A person who is born in Sakat Yoga is unhappy. He has acute suffering in his heart so much so that it will always prick him like a thorn. He will not get fame will lead an ordinary life. At times, he will rise very high in life and at other times, he will fall to the bottom. That is why it is said that like a wheel his fortunes go up and down constantly.

Horoscope of Pandit Nehru, born 14.11.1989

At 41 Ghatis and 38 palas

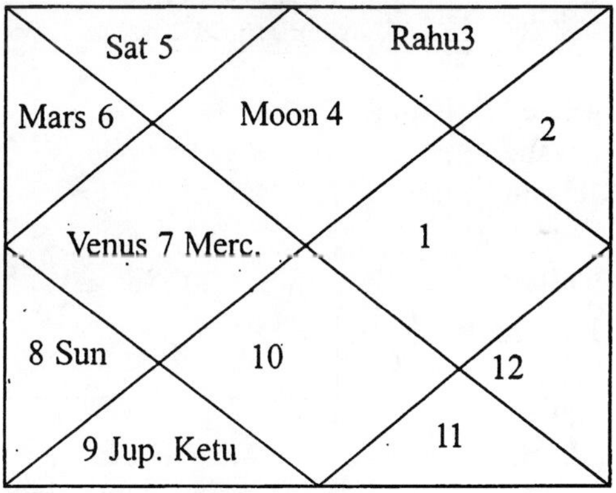

If Moon is in the first house as in the horoscope (given above) which has Cancer in the Ascendant with Moon in it. Jupiter is in the 6th house. As Moon is in the 8th from Jupiter so it should cause Sakat Yoga but because Moon occupies an angular position, so this Sakat Yoga will not take place. This person became Prime minister of his country (India).

In many old books it is also written that if benefic occupy the 3rd, 6th, 10th, and 11th houses from Moon, then it is called Vasuman Yoga.

If benefic occupy the 3rd, 6th, 10th and 11th houses from Ascendant then it is called Ativasuman Yoga.

If benefic occupy the 6th, 7th and 8th houses from Moon then it is a very good yoga.

The main purpose of telling this is that some yogas give mixed results.

If benefic, like Moon and Jupiter, which are causing the yoga are both very strong, or in their own houses, then the yoga will show good results (see the horoscope given above).

Now we are going to tell the effects of Adham, Sama, and Varishta Yoga.

Horoscope of Sh. J.N.Vyas

Born – Samvat 1955 Magh Mase, Krishna Pakshe, Navami, Saturday, Ishtum 12 Ghatis 48 Palas.

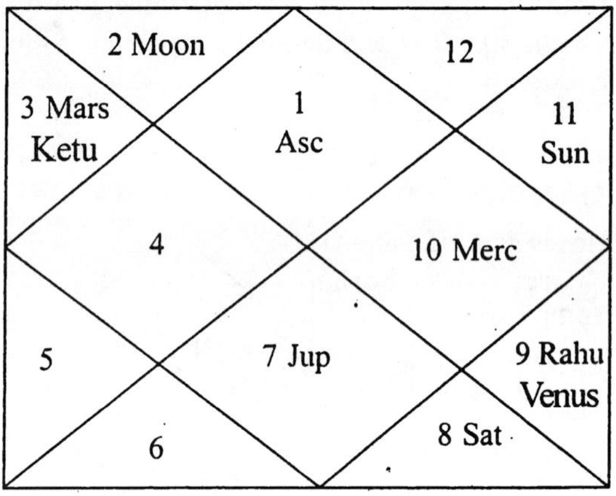

(1) If a native is born in Adham Yoga, then he has very little of fame, happiness, wealth, vehicles, immovable property, knowledge, intelligence, humbleness, expertness, education and generosity.

कष्टमध्यमवराह्वययोगे द्रव्यवाहनयशः सुखसंपत्।
ज्ञानधीविनयनैगुणविद्यात्यागभोगजफलान्यपि तद्वत् ॥१८ ॥

(2) If a person is born in Sama Yoga, then he has happiness up to

fifty per cent of all those things, which we have mentioned for Adham Yoga.

(3) If a person is born in Varishta Yoga, then he enjoys wealth, happiness, knowledge, intelligence and fame. He is very expert and humble. He is generous and educated. He will enjoy the maximum good results and will be endowed with good qualities.

चन्द्राद्वा वसुमांस्तथोपचयगैर्लग्नात्समस्तैः शुभै-
श्चन्द्राव्द्योम्न्यमलाह्वयः शुभखगैर्योगो विलग्नादपि।
जन्मेशे सहिते विलग्नपतिना केन्द्रेऽधिमित्रर्क्षगे
लग्नं पश्चति कश्चिदत्र बलवान्योगो भवेत्पुष्कलः ॥१९॥

तिष्ठेयु स्वगृहे सदा वसुमति द्रव्याण्यनल्पान्यपि
क्ष्मेशः स्यादमले धनी सुतयशः संपद्युतो नीतिमन्।
श्रीमान् पुष्कलयोगजो नृपवरैः संमानितो विश्रुतः
स्वाकल्पाम्बरभूषितः शुभवचाः सर्वोत्तमः स्यात्प्रभुः ॥२०॥

The effects of Vasuman, Amla, and Pshkal Yogas:

(1) If all the benefic occupy the 3rd, 6th, 10th and 11th houses from the Rising Sign (it does not matter if they are in one or more houses), then the yoga such formed is called Vasuman.

(2) If all the benefic planets occupy the Upachaya houses, that is the 3rd, 6th, 10th and 11th from Moon, then it is also known as Vasuman Yoga.

(3) If benefic occupy the 10th house from the Ascendant or the Moon, then it is called Amla Yoga.

(4) If the lord of the rising sign and the lord of the sign occupied by Moon are placed together in an angle from the Rising sign which is also the house of a great friend, and a strong planet aspects the ascendant, then the yoga so formed is called Pushkal Yoga.

The effects of these yogas are given below:

(1) If a person is born in Vasuman Yoga then he will always live in his own house and will be wealthy. In the good old days, it was

considered troublesome to go to foreign countries, and far away places in order to earn one's living, and it was always supposed that one who lives in his own house is the happiest.

(2) One who is born in Amla Yoga is the owner of lands, wealthy and he is very discreet, knows what is good and bad. He is blessed with sons, fame and prosperity.

(3) If a person is born in Pushkal Yoga, then he is honoured by the kings. He is wealthy and famous. He is fond of good dress and ornaments. He speaks auspicious words. He is the owner of many persons and occupies a high position.

सर्वे पञ्चसु षट्सु शुभा मालाश्च पङ्क्त्या स्थिता
यद्येवं मृतिषड्व्ययादिषु गृहेष्वत्राशु भाख्याः स्मृताः ।
स्वर्क्षोच्चे यदि कोणकण्टकयुतौ भाग्येशशुक्रावुभौ
यक्ष्म्याख्योऽथ तथाविधे हिमकरे गौरीति जीवेक्षिते ॥२१ ॥

जनाधिकारी क्षितिपालशस्तो भोगी प्रदाता परकार्यकर्त्ता।
बन्धुप्रियः सत्सुतदारयुक्तों धीरः सुमालाह्वययोगजातः ॥२२ ॥

कुमार्गयुक्तोऽशुभमालिकाख्ये दुःखी परेषां वधकृत् कृतघ्नः ।
स्यात्कातरी भूसुरभक्तिहीनो लोकाभिशप्तः कलहप्रियः स्यात् ॥२३ ॥

नित्यं गङ्गलशीलया वनितया क्रीडत्यरोगी धनी
तेजस्वी स्वजनान् सुरक्षित महालक्ष्मीप्रसादालयः ।
श्रेष्ठान्दोलिकया प्रयाति तुरगस्तम्बेरमध्यासितो
लोकान्नदकरो महीपतिवरो दाता च लक्ष्मीभवः ॥२४ ॥

सुन्दरगात्रः श्लाघितगोत्र पार्थिवमित्रः सद्गुणपुत्रः ।
पङ्कजवक्त्रः संस्तुतजैत्रो राजति गौरीयोगसमुत्थः ॥२५ ॥

Now we are going to tell the effects of four other yogas viz., Subhamala, Asubhamala, Lakshmi and Gauri.

(1) If all the planets are respectively in the 5th, 6th, and 7th house and none of these houses is vacant, then it is called Subhamala yoga.

(2) Starting from the 6th, 8th, or 12th, if all the planets occupy the 5th, 6th, and 7th houses respectively, then it is termed as Asubhamala Yoga.

(3) If the lord of the 9th house and Venus occupy own or exalted signs, and are simultaneously posited in an angle or trine from the rising sign, then it is termed as Lakshmi Yoga.

(1st, 4th, 7th, and 10th houses are called angles; 5th and 9th are known as trine).

(4) If Moon is either in Cancer or Taurus and is posited in an angle or trine from the rising sign, and is also aspected by Jupiter, then it is called Gauri Yoga.

One who is born in Sumala or Subhamala yoga is the ruler of many persons, enjoys life. He gives donations and is generous. He is loved and respected by his kinsmen. He has good sons and wives and is endowed with much patience. He is honoured and praised by the kings. He will always oblige others by doing good deeds and helping them.

(5) One who is born in Asubyhamala or Asubhamalika Yoga kills others, will never feel obliged to others, quarrelsome, and always follows the path of evils. He is a coward and draws in public censure. He does not respect the Brahmins and elderly people. He is full of sorrow and unhappiness.

(6) One who is born in Lakshmi Yoga enjoys the company of a good-tempered woman. He is powerful. He is capable of protecting his kinsmen and is wealthy. He has good health. He possesses horse, elephants, vehicles, and gives happiness to all. He is famous for his generous nature, and owns much property. This Lakshmi Yoga is considered to be good raja yoga.

(7) If a person is born in Gauri yoga, then his body is very attractive. He is a friend of the king. He is endowed with good qualities and has many sons. He overcomes his enemies. He will be praised. Every one will praise his ancestors. His face is like a lotus, good looking and attractive. In short, this yoga is also considered to be very good.

Now we tell the effects of Saraswati Yoga.

शुक्रवाक्पतिसुधाकरात्मजैः केन्द्रकोणसहितैर्द्वितीयगैः ।
स्वोच्चमित्रभवनेषु वाक्पतौ वीर्यगे सति सरस्वतीरिता ॥२६ ॥

धीमं न्नाटकगद्यपद्यगपानालङ्कारशास्त्रेश्वयं
निष्णतः कविताप्रबन्धरचनाशास्त्रार्थपारंगत ।
कीर्त्याक्रान्तजगत्त्रयोऽतिधनिको दारात्मजैरन्वितः
स्यात् सारस्वतयोगजो नृपवरैः संपूजितो भाग्यवान् ॥२७ ॥

If Mercury, Jupiter, Venus are in angular or trikon position or in the 2nd house and Jupiter occupies its own sign, or the sign of a friend, or is exalted, then it is termed as Saraswati Yoga.

Swami Karpatriji
Maharaj born
11.08.1907
Pratapgarh (U.P.)

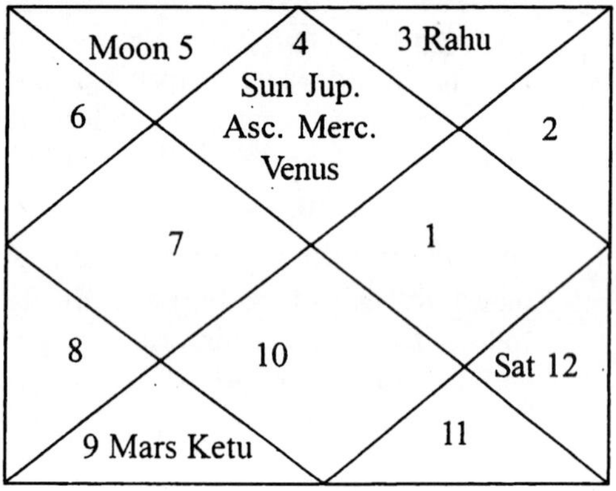

The horoscope of Swami Karpatriji Maharaj (given above) has Cancer rising with Sun, Jupiter, Venus and Mercury in the 1st house (he renounced everything and even refused the seat of Sankaracharya). He was born on 11th August 1907. In this horoscope Venus and Mercury and Jupiter are in angular position in the 1st house. Simultaneously, Jupiter is exalted, so Saraswati Yoga is formed. He was a very learned person, and because of powerful Jupiter this Saraswati Yoga is very powerful in his horoscope.

A person who has Saraswarti yoga is very intelligent, endowed with dramatics, writing capacity, and all types of learning. He is strong in mathematics and a scholar. He is fond of writing poetry, his fame spreads throughout the world. He is very wealthy. Such a person has happiness from wife and sons, until he turns to sanyas. These persons are honoured and worshipped by kings. They are very fortunate (infact when a person acquires wisdom and realisation comes to him then he will go beyond material things and will seek spiritual heights). In the above horoscope, due to powerful Jupiter and Mercury, he had purity of mind. Sun is also there and so four planets together caused Sanyas yoga.

लग्नधींश्वरभास्करामृतकरा: केन्द्रत्रिकोणाश्रिता:
स्वोच्चस्वर्क्षसुहृद्गृहानुपगता: श्रीकण्ठयोगो भवेत्।
तद्वद्भार्गवभाग्यनाथशशिजा: श्रीनाथयोगस्तथा
वागींशात्मपसूर्यजा यदि तदा वैरिञ्चियोगस्तत: ॥२८

रुद्राक्षाभरणो विभूतिधवलच्छायो महात्मा शिवं
ध्यायत्यात्मनि सन्ततं सुनियम: शैवव्रते दीक्षित:।
साधूनामुपकारक: परमतेष्वेव नसूयो भवेत्
तेजस्वीं शिवपूजया प्रमुदित: श्रीकण्ठयोगोद्भव: ॥२९॥
लक्ष्मीवान् सरसोक्तिचाटुनिपुणो नारायणङ्काङ्कित:
तन्नामाङ्कितहृद्यपद्यमनिशं संकीर्तयन् सज्जने:।
तद्भक्तापचितौ प्रसन्नवदन: सत्पुत्रदारान्वित:
सर्वेषां नयनप्रियोऽतिसुभग: श्रीनाथयोगोद्भव: ॥३०॥

ब्रह्मज्ञानपरायणो बहुमतिर्वेदप्रधानो गुणी
हृष्टो वैदिकमार्गतो न चलति प्रख्यातशिष्यव्रज:।
सौम्योक्तिर्बहुवित्तदारतनय: सद्ब्रह्मतेजोज्वलन्दी-
र्घायुर्क्जितेन्द्रीयो नतनृपो वैरिञ्चियोगोद्भव: ॥३१॥

Now we give below 3 other yogas:

(1) Shrikantha Yoga.

(2) Shri Natha Yoga.

(3) Viranchi Yoga.

Vishnu is known as Sri Natha. 'Shri' is Lakshmi, 'Natha' is Husband of Lakshmi. Siva is known as Shri Kantha. Brahma is known as Viranchi. These 3 yogas are termed according to the names of Brahma, Vishnu and Mahesh (Siva).

(1) Shrikantha Yoga: If lord of the rising sign, sun and moon are posited in their own sign, or in the house of a friend or in their exalted signs and are simultaneously in an angle or trine from the Ascendant, then it is called Shrikantha Yoga.

(2) If Mercury, Venus and lord of the ninth house are exalted or in own signs, or posited in the house of a friend and simultaneously occupy an angle or trine from the Ascendant then it is called Shrikantha Yoga.

(3) If Lord of the 5th house, Jupiter, and Saturn are exalted, or in own sign, or in the house of a friend and simultaneously occupy an angle or trine position then it is called Viranchi Yoga.

(1) One who is born in Shrikantha Yoga is one who is fond of wearing Rudraksha. Rudraksha is a fruit whose beads are used for Japa. The Saivites (the followers of lord Siva) do their japa on these beads. They decorate their body with ashes, he has a great soul. His body is lustrous. He is a worshipper of Lord Sankara, very religious and he follows the principles of good behaviour and character vigorously. He is a Saivite. He looks after the religious and saintly people. He is not jealous of those people whose follow other religious principles. He devotes all his time, energy and mind to the worship of lord Sankara. He is powerful. All these good traits are found in the native who is born in Shrikantha Yoga.

Note: The three planets, which are causing the yoga, are exalted, then the best results will come. If they are in their own sign or in the house of a friend, then the effect is a little less. When we consider these yogas, then we must consider the physical possibilities, whether all the planets mentioned above could be exalted simultaneously or not. Generally, they will be mixed. Some planets will be exalted, and some will be in the house of a friend or in own sign. We must consider the basic strength of planets, which form the different yogas in order to measure the intensity of their effect.

(2) One who is born in Shrinatha Yoga is very wealthy, always speaks sweet and endearing words. His speech, writings, and letters – all have softness and are very pleasing. He is an expert in pleasing other on account of his soft and endearing words. He is endowed with the signs of conch shells, chakra etc. of Narayana, i.e. his palms and feet possess these markings. He recites poetry in praise of Him and always does sankiratna. The worshippers of Vishnu are very much respected and treated extremely well by these people. People born in Shrinatha Yoga are extremely good looking and pleasing to the eyes. These natives are endowed with good sons and wife.

(3) One who is born in Viranchi Yoga is extremely intelligent, follows the religious principles of Vedas, is endowed with Brahmagyan and gifted with all types of knowledge. His is always happy and will never leave the religious path, which is mentioned in the Vedas.

Many famous people are his disciples he speaks well of others. He will be endowed with wealth, sons, and wife and will have happiness from them. His face is lustrous and shining due to deep knowledge. He is long lived and has full control over his senses even kings pay homage to him.

अन्योन्यं भवनस्थयोर्हिहगयोर्लग्नादिरिःफान्तकं
भावाधीश्वरयोः क्रमेण कथिताः षट्षष्टियोगा जनैः ।
त्रिंशद्दैन्यमुदीरितं व्ययरिपुच्छिद्रदिनाथोत्थिता-
स्त्वष्टौ शौर्यपतेः खला निगदिताः शेषा महाख्याः स्मृताः ॥३२ ॥

मूर्खः स्यादपवादको दुरितकृन्नित्यं सपत्नार्दितः
क्रूरोक्तिः किलदैन्यजश्चलमतिर्विच्छिन्नकार्योद्यमः ।

उद्वृत्तश्च खले कदाचिदखलं भाग्यं लभेताखिलं
सौम्योक्तिश्च कदाचिदेवमशुभं दारिद्र्यदुःखादिकम् ॥३३॥

श्रीकटाक्षनिलयः प्रभुराढ्यश्चित्रवस्त्रकनकाभरणश्च।
पार्थिववाप्तबहुमानसमाज्ञो यानवित्तसुतावांश्च महाख्ये ॥३४॥

We give below 66 other yogas, which are formed on account of exchange of houses between the Lords of two different houses. Out of these sixty-six yogas, twenty-eight are termed as Maha Yogas, and they show good results. One who is born in the Maha Yoga is wealthy and is blessed by goddess Lakshmi. He is the ruler of many. He dresses himself in soft and good clothes and decorates himself with ornaments. He is honoured by kings and government and occupies a high position of responsibility. He has happiness from sons and enjoys wealth and vehicles. The Maha yoga is formed under the following conditions:

(1) Lord of the 1st and lord of the 2nd exchange their house. For example, Lord of the 2nd is placed in the 1st house and the Lord of the 1st goes to the 2nd house. (2) An exchange between 4th and 1st. (3) An exchange between 1st and 5th. (4) An exchange between 7th and 1st. (5) Exchange between 9th and Ascendant. (6) Exchange between 1st and 10th. (7) Exchange between 1st and 11th. (8) 2nd and 4th. (9) 2nd and 5th. (10) 2nd and 7th. (11) 2nd and 9th. (12) 2nd and 10th. (13) 2nd and 11th. (14) 4th and 5th. (15) 4th and 7th. (16) 4th and 9th. (17) 4th and 10th. (18) 4th and 11th. (19) 5th and 7th. (20) 5th and 9th. (21) 5th and 10th. (22) 5th and 11th. (23) 7th and 9th. (24) 7th and 10th. (25) 7th and 11th. (26) 9th and 10th.

This exchange between the lord of the 9th and 10th is also called a raja yoga.

(27) 9th and 11th. (28) 10th and 11th.

Now we tell the other 38 yogas which are not considered to be auspicious. These yogas are divided further in two parts. There are 8 yogas, which are called Khala yoga, and the rest of the 30 are called Dainya Yoga.

One who is born in Dainya Yoga is a fool himself but is always engaged in disapproving and backbiting others. He indulges in bad deeds and suffers through his enemies, he uses sarcastic and insulting speech and is fickle-minded. Whatever work he undertakes will meet with obstacles. These thirty Dainya yogas are formed when there is an exchange between the lords of the following houses:

> 12th and 1st ; 12th and 2nd. ; 12th and 3rd;12th and 4th.;12th and 5th.;12th and 6th.;12th and 7th; 12th and 8th; 12th and 9th.; 12th and 10.12^{th} and 11th.
>
> 8th and 1st. 8th and 2nd. 8th and 3rd. 8th and 4th.8th and 5th.8th and 6th.8th and 7th. 8th and 9th. 8th and 10th. 8th and 11th.
>
> 6th and 1st. 6th and 2nd. 6th and 3rd. 6th and 4th. 6th and 5th. 6th and 7th. 6th and 9th. 6th and 10th. 6th and 11th.

The readers will notice that any association of the lord of the 6th, 8th or 12th house with the lord of any other house results in Dainya Yoga. Out of these 30, the Lord of the 8th is considered to be the most inauspicious. In fact if the lord of the 8th or the lord of the 11th comes in contact with other planets then this association spoil that planet, even the best of Raj yogas are nullified.

Now we give the eight Khala Yogas, which are formed if there is an exchange between the following:

> (1) 3rd and 1st : 3rd and 2nd : 3rd and 4th : 3rd and 5th : 3rd and 7th : 3rd and 9th: 3rd and 10th : 3rd and 11th :

These 8 yogas also give bad results. 'Khala' is a Sanskrit word, which indicates bad character. One is born in Khala Yoga is fickle minded. At times he follows the good path, and at other times he is on the other side of the fence. Sometimes he is endowed with good fortune, at other times he loses everything and as such poor and unhappy. At times he has good speech, but often he uses the most sarcastic and bad remarks. His temperament, fortunes, happiness fluctuates between good and bad. In short, the effect is not good and steadiness is missing in his life.

Subsequently Mantreshwar Maharaj discuss some yogas which are formed when the lord of the 6th is placed in the 8th or 12th house; or the lord of the 8th is placed in the 6th or 12th, or the lord of the 12th is placed in the 6th or 8th house. These yogas are called Harsha Yoga, Saral yoga and Vimal yoga respectively. The purpose of telling is that in the next yoga exchange is not mentioned, only the placement is mentioned. For example, if it is a complete exchange, like lord of the 6th in the 8th then Dainya yoga will be formed. But if only the lord of the 6th goes to the 8th house and the lord of 8th occupies any other house but not the 6th then it will be called Harsha Yoga. We will discuss it further at the appropriate places.

In an old Sanskrit text Uttarkalamrit of Kalidas an exchange between the lords of the 6th , 8th or 12th house is supposed to give auspicious results, This view is exactly opposite to the view expressed in Phaldeepika.

(i) If lord of 8th house is in the 6th or 12th.

(ii) Lord of the 6th is in the 8th or 12th.

(iii) Lord of the 12th is in 6th or 8th.

(iv) Lord of these three houses aspect each other or exchange houses.

(v) They should not be placed with or aspected by the lords of other houses.

Then such a person will be an Emperor endowed with prosperity of all types. This is called reverse Raja Yoga.

There have been different textbooks, which are considered authoritative on astrology. They have been written hundreds of years ago. But at certain places they have interpreted the results in different manner. Actual knowledge and results will come only from experience and with the blessings of the Guru. In Uttarkalamrit the association between the lords of the 6th and 8th and 12th will be fruitful only when these are mutually connected and are not connected with the lords of other houses. This is the most essential rule that they should not be connected with others.

Reference to Uttarakalamrit has been given to authenticate that great Astrologers also have differences in their views. Now we come back to the main subject. Mutual exchange between the lords of two benefic places, create Mahayogas. Certain yogas are illustrated by example horoscopes.

In the horoscope of Mrs. Indira Gandhi born on 19 November

1917 at 41 Ghatis 52 Plalas and 23 Vipalas at Allahabad, we find that —

Mrs. Indira Gandhi

Asc. 3-27°-13'
Sun 7-4°-8'
Moon 9-5°-37'
Mars 4-13°-23'
Merc. 7-13°-15'
Jup. 1-15°-1'
Venus 8-21°-0'
Sat.3-21°-47'
Rahu 8-10°-33'
Ketu 2-10°-33'

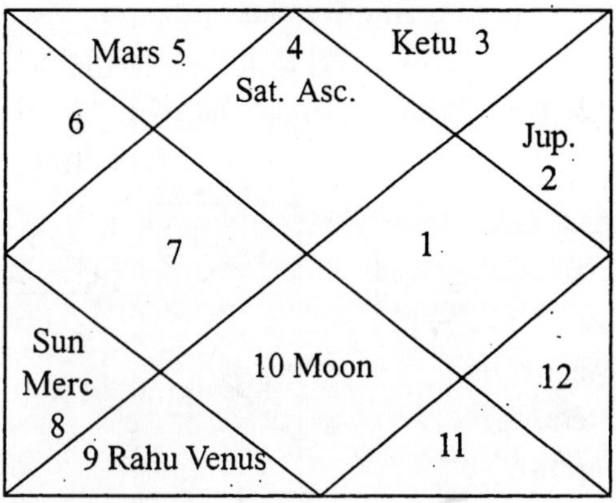

(1) An exchange between 1st and 7th.

(2) An exchange between 2nd and 5th are two Maha yogas.

However

(3) an exchange between 6th and 11th is Dainya Yoga.

In the horoscope of Queen Elizabeth II, born on 21 April 1926 at London —

Queen Elizabeth II

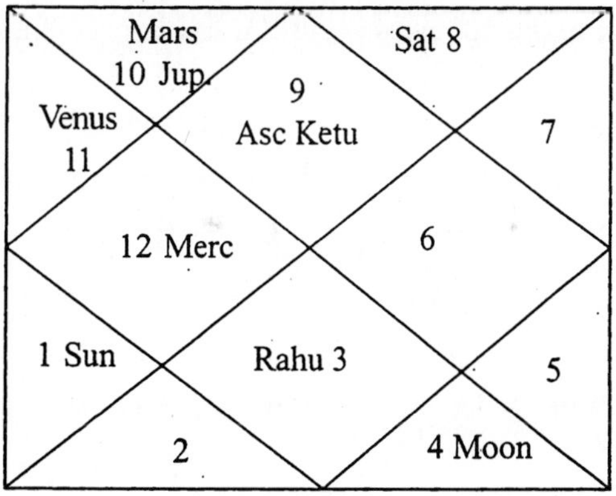

(1) An exchange between 2nd and 12th is a Dainya yoga.

(2) However Sun and Mars are exalted, Moon is in its own sign and so are powerful. The birth being in a royal family so she became a queen. However due to Dainya Yoga her kingdom will shrink.

In the horoscope of H.E. Robert Nixon, born on 9th January 1912, 9.30 p.m. P.S.T. at California (Long. 117.51 West; lat. 33.47 North)

H.E. Robert Nixon

Asc. 4-23°-33'-26'
Sun 8-26°-45'-48'
Moon 9-27°-26'
Mars 8-7°-7'
Merc. 8-7°-24'
Jup. 8-9°-6'
Venus 10-11°-43'
Sat.1-4°-40'
Rahu 11-14°-8'
Ketu 5-14°-8'

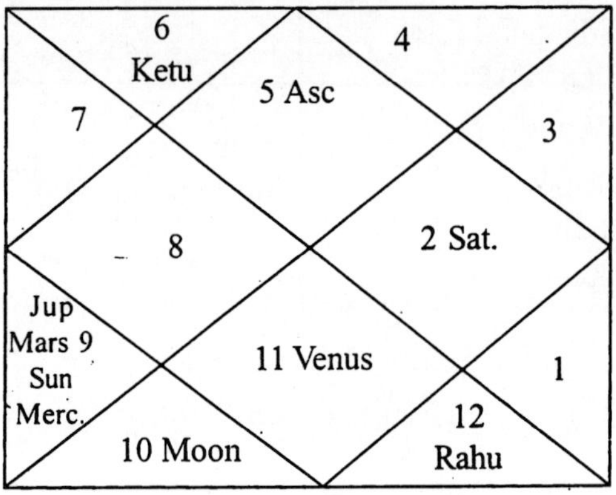

(1) An exchange between the lords of the 7th and 10th is a Maha yoga.

(2) The placement of Sun, Mars, Mercury and Jupiter in one house is also raja yoga. It is also a Sanyas yoga.

(3) Saturn in the 10th house causes a fall in position, a set back in power.

The horoscope is given to indicate an example of Maha yoga.

In the horoscope of Late Pandit Mahamopadhyaya Shri Shiv Kumar Shastri , born in the year Vikram Samvat 1904 (Indian Calendar)

Pandit Mahamopadhyaya Shri Shiv Kumar Shastri

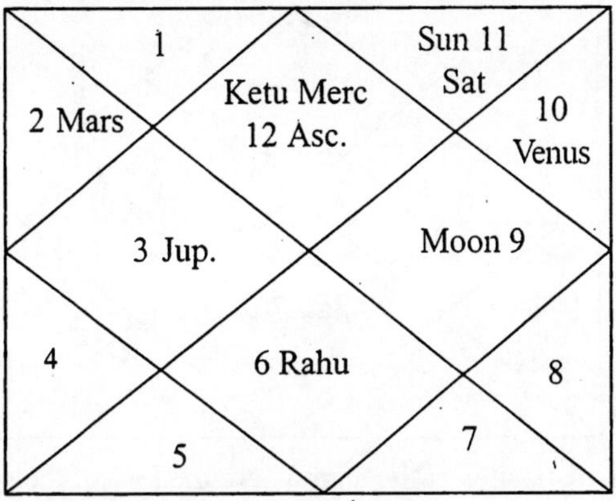

(1) An exchange between the lords of the 1st and 4th causes Maha yoga.

लग्नाधिपाप्तभपतिस्थिरतराशिनाथः
स्वोच्चस्वभेषु यदि कोणचतुष्टयस्थः ।
योगःस काहल इति प्रथितोऽथत्तद्वत्
लग्नाधिपाप्तभपतिर्यदि पर्वताख्यः ॥३५ ॥

वर्द्धिष्णुरार्यः सुमतिः प्रसन्नः क्षेमङ्करः काहलजो नृमान्यः
स्थिरार्थसौख्यः स्थिरकार्यकर्त्ता क्षितीश्वरः पर्वतयोगजातः ॥३६ ॥

(i) The lord of the sign (say X) in which the lord of the Ascendant is placed.

(ii) Now observe the lord of the sign (say Y) in which X is placed.

(iii) Now if Y is exalted or in its own house which is also an angle or trine, then Kahal yoga is formed.

In the horoscope given below the lord of the Ascendant is in the sign of Sun – which is placed in the sign of Saturn - which in its place is exalted in the7th house – so Kahal yoga is formed.

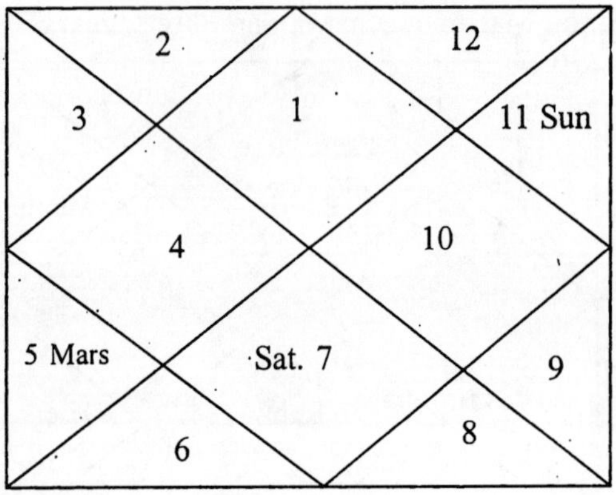

In short the dispositer of the sign where the lord of the sign occupied by the rising sign is placed, if it is in its own sign or sign of exaltation and side by side which is also an angle and trine then Kahal yoga is formed.

One who is born in Kahal yoga is endowed with purity, intelligence, and intelligence of the highest order, happiness and will do good to others. He will be honoured and respected by the masses.

In the horoscope of Sir Ashutosh Mukerjee born on 29th June 1864 –

(1) The lord of Ascendant is in Aries; the lord of Aries is Mars, which is in its own sign but because Mars is neither in an angle or trine so Kahal yoga is not formed.

Sir Ashutosh Mukerjee

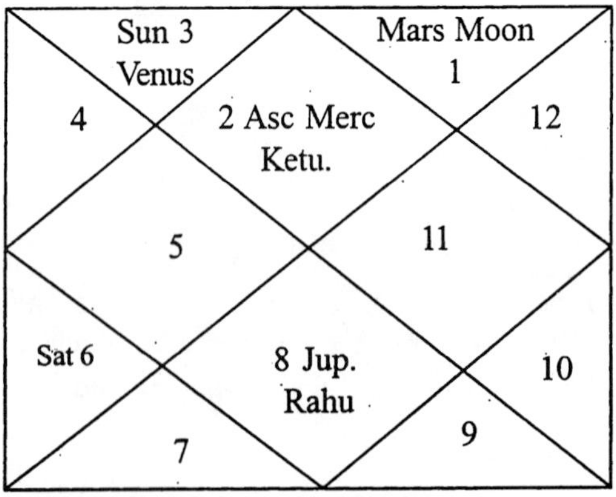

The native was born on 27 – 10-1908 –

Mr. Shah

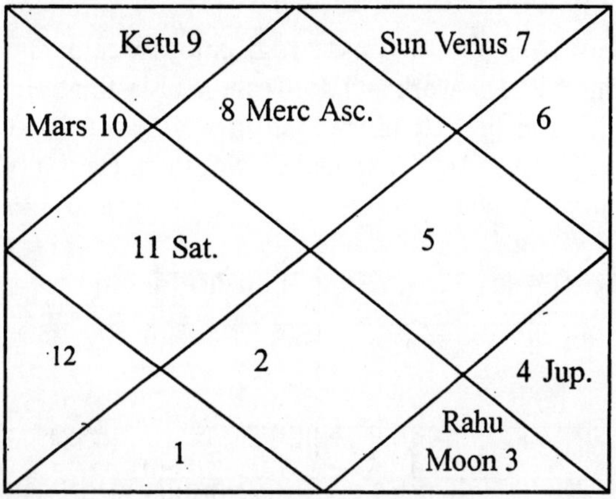

(1) The lord of the Ascendant Mars is in the house of Saturn, which is also in its own sign and also in an angle so Kahal yoga is formed.

Parvat Yoga

Look for the lord of the sign (say A) in which the lord of the Ascendant is placed. If this lord (a) is in its sign of exaltation or own house which also falls in an angle or trine then Parvat Yoga is formed.

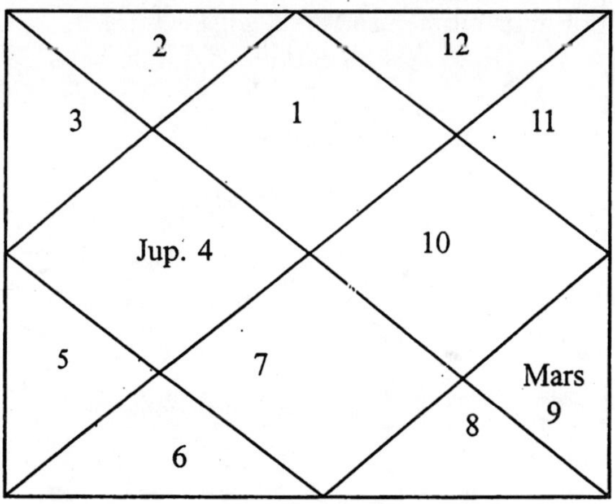

In the horoscope given just above Mars (the lord of Ascendant) is in the house of Jupiter, which is exalted in the 4th house - so Parvat Yoga is also formed.

One who is born in Parvat yoga enjoys wealth and happiness throughout life. His work and deeds are long lasting. He occupies a high position in life. He is engaged in work related to charity viz. Builds temples, gardens, orphanages, wells etc. He is a ruler (a high position in the Government).

धर्मकर्मभवनाधिपती द्वौ संयुतौ महितभावगतौ चेत्।
राजयोग इति तद्वदिह स्यात् केन्द्रकोणयुतिर्यति शङ्खः ॥३७॥

भेरीशङ्खप्रणादैर्धृ तमृदुपटिकाजातवृत्तातपत्रो
हस्त्यश्वान्दोलिकाद्यैः सह मगधकृतप्रस्तुतिर्भूमिपालः।
नानारूपोपहारस्फुरितकरयुतैः प्रार्थितः सज्जनैः स्या-
द्राजा स्याक्छङ्खयोगे बहुवरवनिताभोगसम्पत्तिपूर्णः ॥३८॥

In the horoscope of Mr. Shah also the lord of the Ascendant Mars is in Capricorn and the lord of the Saturn is in own sign in an angle so Parvat yoga is present.

In the horoscope of Morarji Desai the lord of the Ascendant is posited in Capricorn. The lord of Capricorn is Saturn and it is exalted in the 5th house (in a trine), so Parvat yoga is formed.

Shri Morarji Desai was born on 29 February 1896. In his horoscope–

Morarji Desai

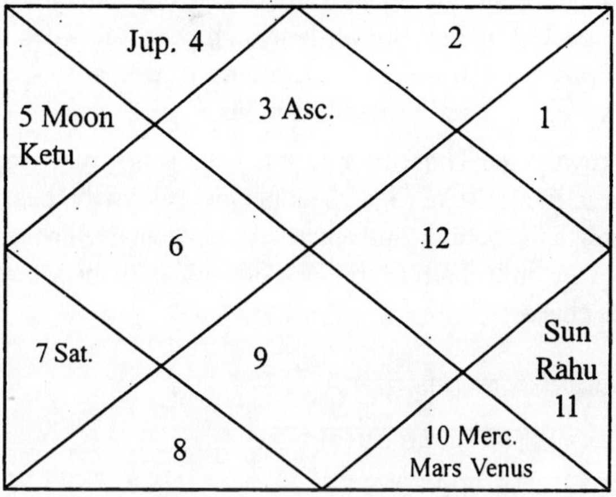

(1) The lord of Ascendant is in the house of Saturn and Saturn is exalted in the 5th house – so Parvat yoga is formed.

(2) In this horoscope an exchange between the lords of 5th and 8th houses constitutes Dainya yoga – so time and again he fell from his high positions.

   (1) If lord of the 9th and 10th are placed together in a benefic house, then it is called a Rajyoga (ups and down in life).

   (2) If lord of an angle (1, 4, 7 or 10) is placed with the lord of a trine, (5th and 9th) in a benefic sign then it is called a Shankha yoga.

One who is born in Rajyoga is a king or equal to a king when he travels with Emblems of royalty then musicians and good people walk with him with bands and music. He occupies a very good position and is followed by a army of horses, elephants, and chariots. People sing his praises and present him with different kinds of gifts. He enjoys the best of women and is endowed with wealth.

Rajyoga is a Sanskrit word means yoga to be a king. In the good old days kings used to keep many women and they were endowed with all types of luxuries. During the present time this Rajyoga should be interpreted that the native will be wealthy and attain a high position. Very few people these days will walk with bands and music of their own free-will or use horses and elephants in big cities. We should interpret that they will have luxurious cars, will live in nice places and will be respected on account of their high position. They enjoy life and are happy. When we say 'enjoyment' it means 'material bliss', which is different from spiritual happiness.

Sankhya yoga: Those born in this yoga gets praise from others. This yoga is like a Raja Yoga. The person enjoys the best when he passes through the periodic influences of the planets, which are creating Raj Yoga in the birth chart. (Periodic influences of planets are discussed in another chapter).

संख्यायोगाः सप्तसप्तर्क्षसंस्थै-
रेकापायाद्वल्लकीदामाशम्।
केदाराख्यः शूलयोगो युगं च
गोलश्चान्यान् पूर्वमुक्तान्विहाय ॥३९

वीणयोगो नृत्तगीतप्रियोऽर्थी
दाम्नि त्यागीभूपतिश्चोपकारी।
पाशे भोगी सार्थसच्छीलबन्धुः
केदारख्ये श्रीकृषिक्षेत्रयुक्तः ॥४० ॥

शूले हिंस्रः क्रोधशीलो दरिद्रः
पाषण्डी स्याद् द्रव्यहीनो युगाख्ये।
निस्वः पापी म्लेच्छयुक्तः कुशिल्पीं
गोले जातश्चालसोऽपायुरेव ॥४१ ॥

(1) If Sun, Moon* etc., the 7 planets are in different signs, then it is called Vallaki yoga. The same yoga is also known as the VinaYoga. One who is born in this Vina yoga is an expert in dancing and music. He is wealthy.

---

* In the Yogas mentioned here only five planets and the Luminaries are to be considered. Rahu and Ketu are not taken in account.

(2) If all the 7 planets are placed in 6 signs in any order, then it is called Dama Yoga. One who is born in Dama Yoga wants to oblige and look after others like a king but he himself is a detached person.

(3) When all the 7 planets - - Sun, Moon, Mars, Mercury, Jupiter, Venus and Saturn are spread out in five signs only, then it is called Pasha Yoga. The person born in this yoga enjoys life, is wealthy, well behaved, and has many relatives and kinsmen.

(4) If the seven planets are placed only in four signs only, then it is called Kedar Yoga. A person born in Kedar yoga has much agricultural lands, farms and wealth.

(5) If all the 7 planets are spread out in 3 signs only, then it is called Shool Yoga. A person born in Shool yoga is cruel, poor and bad tempered.

(6) If the 7 planets are posited in two signs then it is called Yuga Yoga. This person is a trickster and without wealth.

(7) If all the planets are in one sign then is called Gola yoga. One who is born in this yoga is lazy, short–lived, poor, lives with low class of people and is engaged in sinful activities. He is dull in every work.

सौम्यैरिन्दोर्द्यूनषड्रन्ध्रसंस्थैस्तद्वल्लग्नात्संस्थितैर्वाधियोगः ।

नेता मन्त्री भूपतिः स्यात्क्रमेण ख्यातः श्रीमान्दीर्घजीवी मनस्वी ॥

अधियोगभवो नरेश्वरः स्थिरसंपद्बहुबन्धुपोषकः ।

अमुना रिपवः पराजिताश्चिरमायुर्लभते प्रसिद्धताम् ॥४३ ॥

(1) If benefic occupy the 6th, 7th and 8th houses from the Moon, then it is called Adhi Yoga.

(2) Even if benefic occupy the 6th 7th and 8th houses from Ascendant, then it is also termed as Adhi Yoga. If the three benefic, Mercury, Jupiter and Venus are endowed with full strength then the person is a Ruler (a king). If these planet are of medium strength, then the native acts as an advisor to big people, or is a minister to a king. If these three planets are endowed with very little strength

even then the good effect prevails but the person is only a leader of men.

One who is born in Adhi Yoga is wealthy. He has long life and is proud. He has immovable property, rules over others and Lakshmi never deserts him. He looks after his kinsmen. He is successful over his enemies and is famous.

According to the opinion of some, if the 6th, 7th and 8th houses from moon have Mercury, Jupiter and Venus, and if none of these houses are empty then and only then Adhi Yoga is formed. However according to other Astrologers even if all the 3 planets are together in one house out of the 6th, 7th and 8th houses or are separately placed in two or more houses then also the Adhi Yoga is formed.

भावैः सौम्ययुतेक्षितैस्तदधिपैः सुस्थानगैर्भास्वरैः
स्वोच्चस्वर्क्षगतैर्विलग्नभवनाद्योगाः क्रमाद्द्वादश।
संज्ञाश्चामरधेनुशौर्यजलधिच्छत्रास्त्रक मासुरा–
भाग्यख्यातिसुपारिजातमुसलास्तज्ज्ञैर्यथा कीर्तिताः ॥४४॥

प्रत्यहं ब्रजति वृद्धिमुदग्रां शुक्लचन्द्र इव शोभनशीलः।
कीर्तिमान् जनपतिश्चिरजीवी श्रीनिधिर्भवति चामरजातः: ॥४५॥

सान्नपान्नविभवोऽखिलविद्यापुष्कलोधिककुटम्बविभूतिः।
हेमरत्नधनधान्यसमृद्धो राजराज इव राजति धेनौ॥४६॥

कीर्तिमद्भिरनुजैरभिष्टुतो लालितो महितविक्रमयुक्तः।
शौर्यजी भवति राम इवासौ राजकार्यनिरतोऽतियशस्वी॥४७

गोंसंपद्धनधान्यशोभिसदनं बन्धुपूर्णं वर–
स्त्रीरत्नाम्बरभूषणानि महितस्थानं च सर्वोत्तमम्।
प्राप्नोत्युम्बुधियोगजः स्थिरसुखो हस्त्यश्वयानादिगो
राजेड्यो द्विजदेवकार्यनिरतः कूपप्रपाकृत्पथि॥४८॥

सुसंसारसौभाग्यसन्तानलक्ष्मी
निवासो यशस्वी सुभाषी मनीषी।
अमात्यो मीशस्य पूज्यो धनाढ्यः
स्फुरत्तीक्ष्णबुद्धिर्भवेच्छत्रयोगो ॥४९ ॥

शत्रून् बलिष्ठान् बलवन्निगृह्य क्रूरप्रवृत्त्या सहितोऽभिमानी।
व्रणाङ्किताङ्गश्च विवादकारी स्यादस्त्रयोगे दृढगात्रयुक्तः ॥५० ॥

परदारपराङ्मुखो भवेद्वरदारात्मजबन्धुसंश्रितः।
जनकादधिकः शुभैर्गुणैर्महनीयां श्रियमेति कामजः ॥५१ ॥

हन्त्यन्यकार्य पिशुनः स्वकार्यपरो दरिद्रश्च दुराग्रही स्यात्।
स्वयंकृतानर्थपरार्तः कुकर्मकृच्चासुरयोगजातः ॥५२ ॥

चञ्चच्चामरवाद्यघोषनिबिडामान्दोलिकां शाश्वतीं
लक्ष्मीं प्राप्य महाजनैः मृतनतिः स्याद्धर्ममार्गे स्थितः
प्रीणात्येष पितृन् सुरान्द्विजगणांस्तत्तत्प्रियैः पूजनैः
स्वाचारः स्वकुलोद्वहः सुहृदय स्याद्भाग्ययोगोद्भवः ॥५३ ॥
सत्क्रियां सकललोकसंमतामाचरन्नवति सज्जनान्नृपः।
पुत्रमित्रधनदारभाग्यवान् ख्यातिजो भवति लोकविश्रुत ॥५४ ॥

नित्यमङ्गलयुतः पृथिवीशः संचितार्थनिचयः सुकुटुम्बी।
सत्कथाश्रवणभक्तिरभिज्ञो पारिजातजननः शिवतातिः ॥५५ ॥

कृच्छ्रलब्धधनवान परिभूतो लोलसंपदुचितव्ययशीलः।
स्वर्गमेव लभऽन्तेत्यदशायां जाल्मको मुसलजश्चपलश्च ॥५६ ॥

(1) If benefic aspect or are posited in the Ascendant, and the lord of the Ascendant is not combust and is in its own sign or sign of exaltation, then it is called Chamar Yoga. One who is born in

Chamar Yoga attains increasing prosperity in life, like a waxing Moon. He is good-looking and gentle, like the moon. He is wealthy, famous, long lived, and is a ruler of men.

(2) If benefic aspect or occupy the 2nd house, and the lord of the 2nd house is not combust and is in its own sign or sign of exaltation and is placed in a good house, then it is called Dhenu Yoga.

One who is born in Dhenu Yoga possesses good wealth, jewels, and is like a king. He is rich and very successful in financial control (treasurer like Kuber). From the second house we judge education, family, the type of food and drink one is fond of. If the lord of the 2nd house is strong then such a person will get good food, good things to drink, will be educated, will have a large family, etc. In south India education is also considered from the 2nd house, as well. In fact, 2nd house is the house of speech, lips, and mouth, tongue. Generally it is thought that one who is educated will have good speech and voice. Or one, who has knowledge, speaks well – these are inter-related matters.

(3) If benefic aspect or are posited in the 3rd house, and the lord of the 3rd is not combust, occupies its own sign, or sign of exaltation, and is placed in a good house then it is called Shorya Yoga. A person who is born in Shorya Yoga is full of valour, very courageous and his younger brothers rise to great heights in life and worship him. From the third house we judge younger brothers/sisters, valour, etc. and the person with this configuration has happiness from this source, Such a person himself is famous, and occupies a high position in the Government. Mantreswar Maharaj says that "he is full of courage and valour like Rama".

(4) If benefic occupy or aspect the 4th house and the lord of the 4th is in its own sign, or in its sign of exaltation, is not combust and occupies a good house, then it is known as Ambudhi or Jaladhi Yoga. Ambudhi or Jaladhi is the name for the sea. One who is born in this yoga possesses all types of cattle, corns and wealth in sufficient quantity he owns good houses and lives in a good place. He has many relatives and happiness from them. He has a good wife, jewels, clothes, and ornaments, etc. He also attains

an honourable position in life. He is happy throughout. He owns vehicles, elephants, horses etc. and receives honour from Kings. Such a person is engaged in the worship of Brahmins and (gods), and has a strong religious aptitude of mind. He will get hospitals and places of worship constructed. In short fourth house is the house of happiness, and one who is born with strong 4th house, enjoys happiness, and vehicles and all things which are considered from it. If he deals in real estate or construction activities, building materials, agriculture etc. he will benefit much.

(5) If benefic occupy or aspect the 5th house and the lord of the 5th is in its exaltation or own sign, is not combust, is placed well, then it is called Chatra Yoga. One who is born in Chatra Yoga has all type of fortunes. He is wealthy, famous, intelligent, and speaks well. He has a keen intellect. He will be good in research. He becomes a Minister to a king. He receives honour from the government or kings. He has good children. From the 5th house we consider children knowledge, education, etc. and one who has a strong 5th house has plenty of the things which fall under the 5th house.

(6) If the lord of the 6th house is in its own sign or sign of exaltation, is not combust, is placed well, and benefic occupy or aspect the 6th house, then it is called Astra Yoga. In general 6th house is considered to be inauspicious, but if the lord of the 6th is placed in the 6th itself then it will be good because it is in its own sign. Generally astrologers say that if malefic occupy the 6th house it is good, because 6th house is the house of enemies and disease and Mars, Saturn, or North Node of Moon will destroy enemies, and disease. It is also well known that malefic in the 3rd, 6th and 11th are considered good, and the same thing applies here. The Mantreshwar Maharaj says that, "we get happiness from a house whose lord is very strong". If benefic aspect or occupy a house, then they intensify the good effect of that house. There is a difference of opinion here that we must emphasize. If benefic occupy the 6th house then it is good, and according to other astrologers if malefic occupy the 6th house, then it is good.

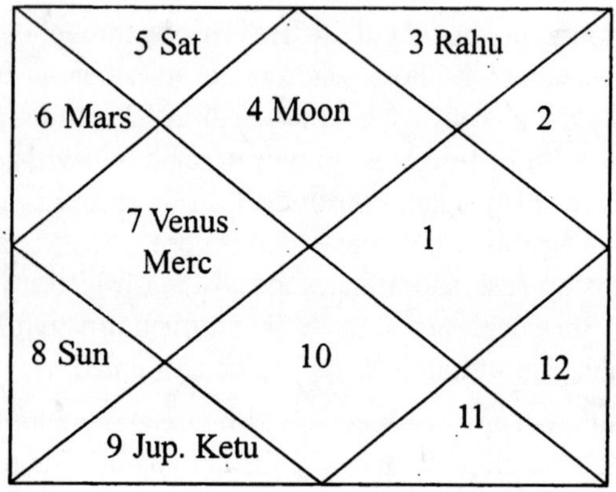

In horoscope given above Jupiter and Ketu are in the 6th house; Saturn aspect it only 50 per cent, Mars aspect is full and Venus and Mercury aspect is 25 per cent. Due to both good and bad aspects and due to the placement of a malefic Ketu and a benefic Jupiter – the Astra Yoga will not show full effect. However the lord of the 6th house is strong and placed in its own sign so we think that Astra yoga is present. This is a controversial matter.

According to Mantreshwar

Those who are born in Astra Yoga annihilates even the strongest of their enemies due to their strength. They are proud and cruel. They have strong arms and muscles, but they have marks of injury on the body. They are argumentative by nature.

(7) If benefic occupy or aspect the 7th house and the lord of the 7th is well placed in its own sign or in its exaltation, is not combust, then it is called Kama Yoga. One who is born in Kama Yoga is not interested in extra-marital relationship at all. He gets a very good wife, children and happiness from relatives. Such a person acquires much wealth on account of his capabilities and he rises to better heights much above those attained by his father.

(8) If benefic occupy or aspect the 8th house and the lord of the 8th house occupies its own sign or exalted sign, is not combust, and is posited in a good House then it is called Asur Yoga. The interpretation of this yoga is not good. The native is engaged in bad deeds, is poor, intolerant, a backbiter, and indulges in spoiling

the works of others. Due to the results of his bad acts, such a person has sorrow and losses.

(9) If benefic occupy or aspect the 9th house, the lord of the 9th house, is not combust* occupies a benefic house is placed in its own sign or sign of exaltation then it is known as Bhagya Yoga. A musical band and emblems of royalty accompanies such a person when he goes out in a palanquin. These things were taken to be a sign of extreme prosperity and authority a few decades ago. He is always wealthy. Highly placed persons respect him. He worships his parents, elderly people, Brahmins and Gods. He increases the good name and fame of his family. He is pure and gentle. If benefic are placed in the 9th house then the native is good at heart or if malefic are placed in it then he is cruel and does bad deeds. The same should also be interpreted if benefic or malefic aspect the 9th house.

(10) If benefic occupy or aspect the 10th house; the lord of the 10th house, occupies a benefic house (any house except the 6th, 8th or 12th house), is posited in its own sign or exalted sign; is not combust, then the yoga so formed is termed as Khyati Yoga. One who is born in Khyati Yoga does good deeds and everyone shower praises on him. He becomes a king and protects his people. He attains fame. He has wife, sons, friends and wealth. He is fortunate.

(11) If benefic occupy or aspect the eleventh house and the lord of the eleventh is posited in a benefic house, is not combust and is in its own sign or exalted sign then Suparijata Yoga is formed. One who is born in this yoga belongs to a good family (famous family), accumulates wealth and thus becomes rich. He is engaged in religious and auspicious deeds constantly. He is learned and does good to others.

(12) If benefic aspect or occupy the 12th house and the lord of 12th house is posited in a benefic house, is not combust, occupies its

---

*In the slokas given between # 44 to # 56 this should be remembered that the lord of the house which is being considered should not be combust. Planets lose their good effect and become weak in the rays of sun and weak planets do not show good effects.

own sign or sign of exaltation then it is known as Musal Yoga. One who is born in Musal Yoga earns wealth with great difficulties. His prosperity is not stable. He spends money freely but only in essential things. Others (enemies) suppress him. He is changeable in disposition and a fool but he gets liberation in the end.

We have shown above the twelve yogas which will be formed if benefic occupy or aspect different houses from Ascendant to the 12th house. If side by side the lord of the respective house is not combust, occupies a benefic house and is also in its own sign or sign of exaltation.

दुःस्थैर्भावगृहेश्वरैरशुभसंयुक्तेक्षितैर्वा क्रमा-
द्भावैः स्युस्त्ववयोगनिःस्वमृतयः प्रोक्ताः कुहूः पामरः ।
हर्षो दुष्कृतिरित्यथापि सरलो निर्भाग्यदुर्योगकौ
योगा द्वादश ते दरिद्रविमले प्रोक्ता विपश्चिज्जनैः ॥५७॥

अप्रसिद्धिरतिदुःसहदैन्यं स्वल्पमायुरवमानमसद्भिः ।
संयुतः कुचरितः कुतनुः स्याच्चञ्चलस्थितिरिहाप्यवयोगे ॥५८॥

सुवचनशून्यो विफलकुटुम्बः कुजनसमाजः कुदशनचक्षुः ।
मतिसुतविद्याविभवविहीनो रिपुहृतवित्तः प्रभवति निस्वे ॥५९॥

अपरिभूतः सहजविहीनो
मनसि विलज्जो हतबलवित्तः ।
अनुचितकर्मश्रमपरिखिन्नो
विकृतिगुणः स्यादिति मृतियोगे ॥६०॥

मातृवाहनसुहृत्सुखभूषाबन्धुभिर्विरहितः स्थितिशून्यः ।
स्थानमाश्रितमनेन हतं स्यात् कुस्त्रियामभिरतः कुहुयोगे ॥६१॥

दुःखजीव्यनृतवागविवेकी वञ्चको मृतसुतोऽप्यनपत्यः।
नास्तिकोऽल्पकुजनं भजतेऽसौ घस्मरो भवति पामरयोगे ॥६२॥

सुखभोगभाग्यदृढगात्रसंयुतो
निहताहितो भवति पापभरुकः।
प्रथितप्रधानजनवल्लभो धन-
द्युतिमित्रकीर्तिसुतवांश्च हर्षजः ॥६३॥

स्वपत्नीवियोगं परस्त्रीरतीच्छा
दुरालोकमध्वानसंचारवृतिः
प्रेमहादिगुह्यार्तिमुर्वीशपीडां
वदेद्दुष्कृतौ बन्धुधिक्कारशोकम् ॥६४॥

दीर्घायुष्मान् दृढतिरभयः श्रीमान्विद्यासुतधनसहितः।
सिद्धारम्भो जितरिपुरमलो विख्याताख्यः प्रभवति सरले ॥६५॥

पित्रार्जितक्षेत्रगृहादिनाशकृत्
साधून् गुरून्निदति धर्मवर्जितः।
प्रत्नातिजीर्णम्बरधृच्च दुर्गतो
निर्भाग्ययोगे बहुदुःखभाजनम् ॥६६॥

शरीरप्रयासैः कृतं कर्म यत्तत्
व्रजेन्निफलत्वं जनेषु।
जनद्रोहकारी स्वकुक्षिंभरिः स्यात्

अजस्रं प्रवासी व दुर्योगजात: ॥६७॥
ऋणग्रस्त उग्रो दरिद्राग्रगण्यो
भवेत्र्करोगी च सौभ्रात्रहीन: ।
अकार्यप्रवृत्तो रसाभासवादी
परप्रेष्यक: स्याद्दरिद्राख्ययोगे ॥६८॥

किञ्चिद्व्ययो भूरिधनाभिवृद्धिं
प्रयात्ययं सर्वजनानुकूल्यम् ।
सुखी स्वतन्त्रो महनीयवृत्ति
र्गुणै: प्रतीतो विमलोद्भव: स्यात् ॥६९॥

These next 12 yogas indicate the results if the lords of different houses are posited in a bad house. There is no such house as a 'bad house', but still the 6th, 8th and 12th houses are inauspicious. These 12 yogas are also according to the lords of the 12 houses and that house is occupied by or receives aspect of malefic. The following two conditions should be fulfilled:

(1) Malefic occupy or aspect a particular house.

(2) The lord of the house should be posited in the 6th 8th or 12th.

Note: If the lord of the house is also aspected or conjoins with malefic then further bad effects will take place.

(1) If 1st house has malefic or malefic aspect it and the lord thereof goes to the 6th, 8th or 12th, then it is known as Avayoga. One who is born in Avayoga has a changeable disposition verging on to fickle mindedness. He moves about with bad characters. Neither his health not his character is good. He does not live long, and leads an ordinary life. He is very poor, and is insulted by others.

Mantreshwar Maharaj has written very nicely and emphasized that when the Ascendant and its lord are strong, then the entire horoscope improves. If the rising sign and the lord of the rising sign are weak, then the horoscope will not show any good effect at all. We agree with this view due to our experience. For example, if the ascendant and its lord are weak, then the receptive capacity of a person is reduced. He may have wealth, but he will not be able to enjoy. Due to some disease or the other, he will not be able to acquire knowledge, he will not get a job, he will not be able to eat i.e. he will be restricted in everything.

(2) If lord of the 2nd house is posited in the 6th, 8th, or 12th or if malefic aspect or are placed with the lord of the second house and is also aspected or occupied by malefic then it is called Niswa Yoga. It means one who does not possess anything and is poor. He has bad teeth and defect in eyes. He does not speak good words. He has a limited family i.e. if he has a wife then there are no children or no sons. He does not have good association. His wealth is taken over by his enemies.

In short the native lacks all the things indicated by the second house.

(3) If the lord of the 3rd house is posited in the 6th, 8th or 12th house and the 3rd house and its lord are aspected by or associated with malefic then it is called Mriti Yoga. One who is born in this yoga is defeated by his enemies, engaged in underhand deeds, passes through mental anguish and is devoid of honour. He loses his wealth and courage. He receives no happiness through his brothers (sisters). He has no control on his mind and takes emotional decisions and then repents at leisure.

(4) If the lord of the fourth house is posited in the 6th, 8th or 12th house and malefic conjoins with or aspect the 4th house or its lord then it is known as Kuhu yoga. One who is born in Kuhu yoga does not get happiness from mother, vehicles, friends, ornaments and relatives. The fourth house is the house of happiness and old age. If this house is afflicted then the native is devoid of happiness and his old age is troublesome. He does not get peace anywhere and such things happen which compel him to leave his residence and wander about from place to place. He is not welcome anywhere. He indulges in clandestine affairs with worthless women.

In short the native suffers on account of the matters indicated by the fourth house. Women are not judged from it but the native indulges in sinful activities with worthless women and it is the beginning of unhappiness.

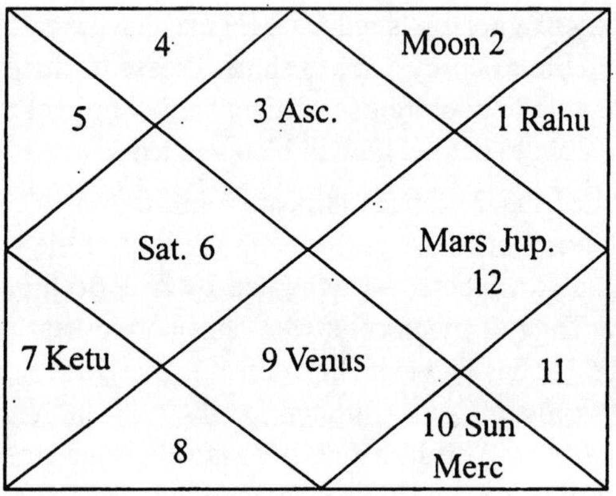

Mantreshwar Maharaj has ignored this point but we have found that if Saturn is posited in the 4th house and the lord thereof is also afflicted then the native's old age is very unhappy and it is spent in poverty and problems. In the horoscope given above Saturn is in the 4th house afflicted by the full aspect of Mars and the lord of the 4th house is also in the 8th house with Sun a malefic). The native enjoyed life in the middle portion but his old age was very unhappy and difficult.

(5) If the lord of 5th house or the 5th house is afflicted or receive aspect of malefic then Pamar Yoga is formed. One who has this Pamar Yoga in his horoscope spends life unhappily. He indulges in lies and is a cheat. He does not beget children or the children do not survive long. If by chance they live then they are a source of problems. His children hate him. He does not believe in God and his circle of friends is people from low class. He loves to eat constantly.

(6) If the 6th house is occupied or aspected by malefic and the lord of the 6th house is posited in the 6th, 8th or 12th house then it is called Harsha Yoga. Such a person is fortunate, endowed with strong body, happy, and afraid of sins, overcomes his enemies and enjoys life. He is famous and favoured by highly placed persons. He has happiness from sons, wealth and friends. His face is lustrous and he gets respect in life *.

(7) If the lord of the 7th house or 7th house is afflicted or aspected by

malefic and the lord of 7th is also posited in the 6th, 8th or 12th house then the yoga so formed is called Dushkriti Yoga. Such a person suffers from all types of ills - indicated by the 7th house viz., separation from wife – due to divorce or her death, involvement with other married women leading to unhappiness, tiring journeys, insults from relatives (and partners) which causes mental anguish, troubles through government (and rulers). If the 7th house and the lord of the 7th house are both spoiled then urinary or kidney troubles.

(8) If the lord of the 8th house is posited in the 6th, 8th or 12th house and the 8th house is afflicted by malefic then it is called Saral Yoga. One who is born in this yoga is long lived, strong minded, fearless, wealthy and famous. He overcomes his enemies and endowed with education, sons and success in his career (works). Mantreshwar Maharaj says that the lord of the 8th in the 6th, 8th or 12th is like an enemy who has fallen in a pit and so unable to cause any harm. According to some opinion the Saral Yoga takes place if the 8th house is not teneted or aspected by other malefic because in such case the good effects of the house owned by them is spoilt and side by side they will spoil the 8th house and thus reduce longevity or may cause chronic sickness. However Saturn (if posited in the 8th house) increases longevity but it gives long and lingering diseases in old age. Mars is extremely bad in the 8th house. It causes urinary troubles, piles, fistulas etc. and also accidents. In the case of girls it destroys their conjugal happiness (by widowhood or otherwise). Ketu is also bad in the 8th house and causes urinary troubles, prostrate lands, injuries etc. We have illustrated all this to point out that if the eighth house is teneted by malefic then Saral Yoga is not formed.

(9) If the lord of the 9th house is posited in the 6th, 8th or 12th house and malefic afflict or aspect it and the 9th house is also occupied or aspected by malefic then it is called Nirbhagya yoga. One who is born in it has sorrow, dresses in old and shabby looking clothes. The 9th house is the house of religion and such a person speaks ill of Gurus, saints and gods. Whatever property he inherits from his ancestors is destroyed.

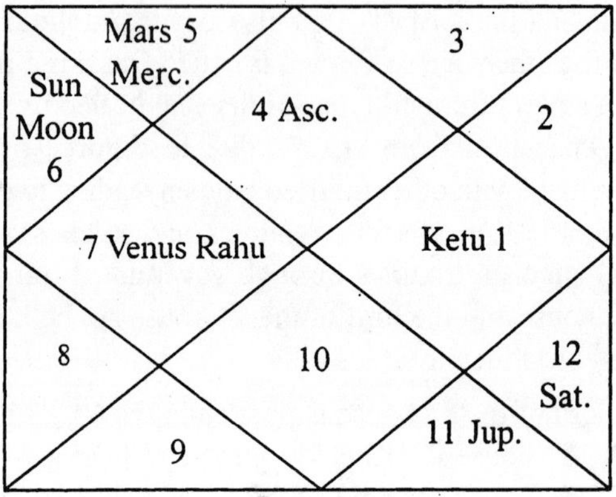

'In this horoscope the lord of the 9th is in the 8th house and Saturn a malefic is posited in the 9th house; the 9th house is also aspected by Mars and Sun. The lord of the 9th Jupiter is also aspected by Mars. This is an illustration of Nirbhagya yoga. However as Jupiter and Saturn: Sun and Mercury have exchanged places and Sun and Moon are together so wealth and prosperity is indicated.

Side by side Jupiter the lord of the 6th is in the 8th house and the 6th house receives full aspect of Saturn - so Harsha Yoga also takes place.

Thirdly an exchange between the lord of the 8th and 9th creates a Dainya yoga.

Fourthly an exchange between the lord of the 2nd and 3rd (i.e. Sun and Mercury) creates a Khala yoga.

Fifthly Venus is in its own house in an angle (4th house) - so Malavya yoga is also formed.

Sixthly Moon is in the 8th house from Jupiter so Shakat yoga also takes place.

In any horoscope all the yogas should be synthesized and then conclusions should be arrived at.

(10) If malefic occupy or aspect the 10th house, and the lord of the 10th house is also posited in the 6th, 8th ,or 12th house and is also aspected by or conjoins with malefic then it is known as Duryoga.

One who has this yoga in his horoscope fails in his work even when he puts in all efforts. All his efforts go waste and he lives away from his birthplace (in other cities and countries) i.e. away from his wife and children. He is not respected by others. He is jealous of others and is only engaged in looking after his earnings.

(11) If the lord of the 11th house is posited in the 6th, 8th or 12th. We have earlier mentioned that If the lord of any house is posited in the 6th, 8th or 12th house and the concerned house is also teneted or aspected by malefic only then a certain yoga will take place – this is the opinion of one school. However Mantreshwar Maharaj – the real authority on Astrology points out that if the lord of a house is posited in the 6th, 8th or 12th house and the concerned house and its lord both are aspected by or associate with malefic then the various yogas will be fully effective.

However there are exceptions. If a house is spoilt due to the placement of malefic in the 11th house then it should cause Daridra yoga (yoga for poverty). But Astrologers differ here. Because in "Saravali" an old Sanskrit text it is written that all planets increase the efficacy of the 11th house i.e. endow one with wealth and fortunes. So if the lord of the 11th house is in the 6th, 8th or 12th houses then it is Daridra yoga. If planets are posited in the 11th house then they will cancel the effect of Daridra yoga.

One who is born in Daridra yoga owes money to others, is poor, suffers from diseases of the ears, devoid of good brothers, engages in bad deeds, speaks lies and uses bad words, sorrowful and works for others.

(12) If the lord of the 12th house is placed in the 6th, 8th or 12th house and is also aspected by or conjoins with malefic then the yoga is called 'Vimal'. The native who has Vimal yoga is careful while spending money i.e. he spends less and accumulates wealth. He is happy, independent and famous for his capabilities. He does good deeds, which are liked by everyone.

In the twelve yogas given above, two things have been emphasized-

(1) The lord of the house should occupy the 6th, 8th or 12th house.

(2) The house should be teneted or aspected by malefic. If the lord of a particular is also afflicted due to the association or aspect of malefic then the resultant effect would be worst.

Some astrologers have pointed out that if the lords of some houses are posited in the 6th, 8th or 12th house and the house in question is also occupied or aspected by malefic then the yogas take place. The second opinion is that the lord of that particular house in question should also be afflicted.

In fact the following five factors destroy the good effects of a house –

(1) If the lord of a house is placed in the 6th, 8th or 12th house (trik).

(2) If the lord is placed with a malefic.

(3) If the lord of a house receives the aspect of a malefic.

(4) If the house is teneted by malefic.

(5) If the house is aspected by malefic.

The more the number of factors present; the more negative effects related to that house will ensue.

These factors have been pointed out in connection with the above yogas. There are five other factors, which restricts the good effect of a house.

(a) If the house in question is hemmed in between malefic.

(b) If the lord of a house is hemmed in between malefic.

(c) If the significators of a house are afflicted.

(d) If the lord of a house is combust.

(e) If the significator of a particular matter is combust.

छिंद्रारिव्ययनायका: प्रबलगा:केन्दन्त्रिकोणाश्रिता:
लग्नव्योमचतुर्थभाग्यपतय: षड्रन्ध्ररि:फस्थिता:
निर्वीर्या विगतप्रभा यदि तदा दुर्योग एव स्मृत-
स्तद्व्यस्ते सति योगवान्धनपतिर्भूप: सुखी धार्मिक: ॥७० ॥

If the lord of the 6th, 8th or 12th are strong and occupy an angle (1, 4, 7, 10) or trine (5, 9) and the lords of that angle is devoid of strength or combust and placed in the 6th, 8th or 12th house then it is called 'Duryoga'. This is a bad yoga.

If it is the reverse i.e. The 6th, 8th, 12th lords are devoid of strength and placed in the 6th, 8th or 12th house and the lords of angles are well placed in good houses, are full of strength, are not combust then the native will be rich. He will be prosperous like a king, happy and religious.

The purpose of mentioning is that the lords of the 6th, 8th and 12th are not good houses and their lords should be comparatively weak. The 1st, 4th, 7th, and 10th are good houses and their lords should be strong, endowed with all types of strength. If the dose of poison is weak and less in quantity and the nectar is more and strong. - so much the better.

7

Raj Yoga

त्र्याद्यैः खेटैः स्वोच्चगैः केन्द्रसंस्थैः स्वर्क्षस्थैर्वा भूपतिः स्यात्प्रसिद्धः।
पञ्चाद्यैस्तैरन्यवंशप्रसूतोऽप्युर्वीनाथो वारणाश्वौघयुक्तः॥१॥

If three or more planets are in angles and are exalted or posited in their own signs, then the native will become king who will be well known. If five or more planets occupy angular positions and are exalted or occupy their own signs then the native irrespective of his family status, becomes the owner of this Earth (an Emperor). He has herds of horses and elephants i.e. he is a very prosperous king.

It is necessary the planets should be in angles, otherwise the yoga does not operate in full.

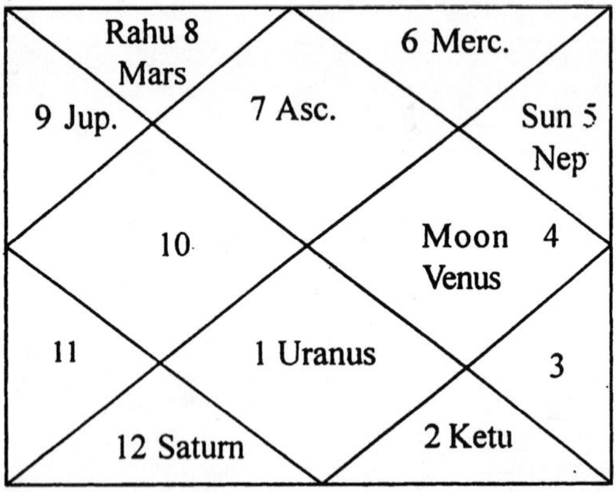

Look at the above horoscope. The native of the above horoscope was born on 2nd September 1937, In this horoscope Sun, Moon, Mars, and Jupiter are in their own signs and Mercury is exalted. The native was born in a very good family but the raja yoga did not operate because no planet except Moon is in an angular position.

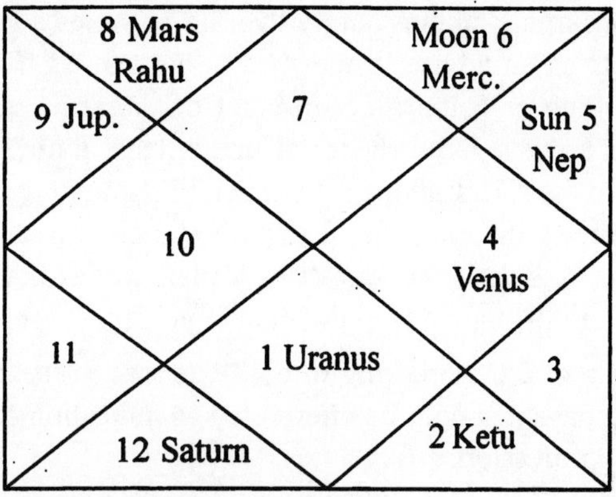

A second examples is also given:

भूपाः स्युर्नृपवंशजास्तु यदि दुर्योगे न जातास्तथा
ह्यन्तर्धिर्नहि चेत्करादि्दनकराज्जाताः स्फुरन्त्येत ते।
त्र्याद्यैः केन्द्रगतैः स्वभोच्चसहितैर्भूपोद्भवाः पार्थिवाः
मर्त्यास्त्वन्यकुलोद्भवाः क्षितिपेस्तुल्याः कदाचिन्नृपाःङ्करङ्क

The native was born on 6th September 1937. The horoscope above has four planets in their own signs. However as no planet, which is in its own sign, is in an angle so he was a sanyasi. This person is a Sanyasi with a large following. He was able to collect money to get a fabulous temple constructed. The raja Yoga did not show full effect. However due to Mercury and Jupiter in angles from the Moon sign, he is well respected.

If one is born in a royal family and there is (i) no bad yogas. (ii) No combust planets in the horoscope then he will definitely be a king. If three or more than three planets are in angles and are also posited in the exalted or own signs then one who is born in a royal family will definitely be a king. (He supersedes his brothers and becomes a ruler). If the birth is in an ordinary family then with the above yoga the native will be prosperous like a king and in exceptional cases may become a king.

Note : In any interpretation the background of a person should be considered. It is also mentioned in Astrology that if one, with raja yoga, is born in a Brahmin family then he becomes a Minister to a king (or acts as an adviser); one who is born in a Shatriya family becomes a king or commander-in-chief of the army due to a raja yoga, and in a vaisya family he is rich enough that at times he extends loans even to the rulers. If one is born in a Shudra family then he will be a favourite of the king and in exceptional circumstances acquire power. Side by side if the karaka of a planet does not get a good treatment from the native then the raja yogas fail to operate.

The use of the work king in old texts was in the context of a ruler. These days it should be interpreted as indication of success in politics and profession.

यद्येकोऽपि विराजितांशुनिकरः सुस्थानगो वक्रगो
नीचस्थोऽपि करोति भूपसदृशं द्वौ वा त्रयो वा ग्रहाः ।
एवं चेज्जनयन्ति भूपतिममी शस्तांशराशिस्थिता
स्तद्वच्चेद्बहवो नृपं समकुटच्छत्रोल्लसच्चामरम् ॥३॥

If Even one planet is placed in a good house (except 6th, 8th or 12th house) and is retrograde (even if it is debilitated) but not combust*, then the native is prosperous like a king. The planet should have full brightness. If two or three planets are so placed in a nativity then it makes one a king. If many planets are so placed and are also in benefic signs and benefic navansha then it ushers in a prosperous kind endowed with all the signs of royalty (crown, umbrella, chawar etc.). In our opinion this yoga should be specially considered in the case of persons born in royal family.

द्वौ वा त्र्याद्या दिग्बलयुक्ता यदि जातः
क्ष्माभृद्वंशे भूमिपतिः स्याज्जयशीलः ।

---

*Combust: Any planet which comes within fifteen degrees of Sun is combust. It is not visible and its effect is neutralized. Mercury does not lose its effect due to combustion because it is always within 28 degrees of Sun but for clarity of thinking it should better be as far away as possible. When a planet is with in Eight minute of Sun then it shows very powerful and positive effect. When a planet is away from Sun then it looks very bright and visible such a planet is strong.

हित्वा मन्दं पञ्जखगा दिग्बलयुक्ता-
श्वत्वारो वा भूपतिरन्यान्वयजोऽपि ॥४॥

If one is born in a royal family and two or more planets are endowed with directional strength in his nativity then he becomes a king and is victorious at all places. Sun and Mars on the cusp of the 10th house; Mercury and Jupiter on the cusp of the 1st house; Moon and Venus on the cusp of the 4th house; and Saturn on the cusp of the 7th house has full directional strength.

If, except Saturn, out of the remaining six planets, five planets or even four have full directional strength then the native, irrespective of his status at birth, becomes a king.

गणोत्तमे लग्ननवांशकोद्गमे निशाकरश्चापि गणोत्तमेऽपि वा।
चतुर्ग्रहैश्चन्द्रविवर्नितैस्तदा निरीक्षतः स्यादधमोद्भवो नृपः ॥५॥

If the Ascendant and Moon are both Vargottam i.e. in the same sign and same navansha, and the Ascendant is aspected by four other planets except the Moon then the native will be a king, even if he is born in a low family.

Horoscope

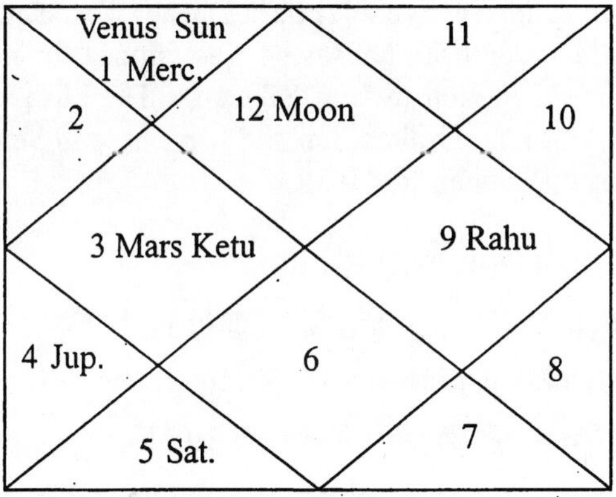

Navansha

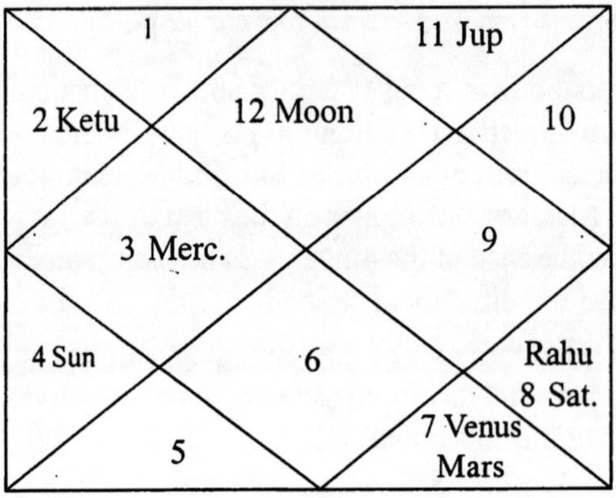

The horoscope of Shri Ravindra Nath Tagore. Given above has Pisces Ascendant both in the nativity and in the Navansha chart. Moon is also in Pisces in both the charts - so one condition that the ascendant and Moon should be vargttom is fulfilled. Jupiter (the lord of the Ascendant) aspects the Ascendant with full aspect. In order that the yoga is fruitful, four Planets should aspect the Ascendant which is not the case here so the yoga does not exist in this chart. However only though a part of the yoga is there, this endowed him with long life, honour, recognition and (noble prize). Due to an exchange between the lords of the 1st and 5th houses he was famous for his writings and educational institution (Shanti Niketan). (The birth was on 7th May 1861, at 4.02 a.m. Exalted Sun and Mercury and Venus in own sign in the Navansha chart, did help.

विलग्नेश: केन्द्र यदि तपसि वर्गोत्तमगत:
स्वतुङ्गे स्वर्क्षे वा गुरुपतिरपि स्याद्यपि तथा।
गजस्कन्धे कार्तस्वरकृतविमानेऽतिसुषमे।
सुखीसीनं भूपं जनयति लसच्चामरयुगम्॥६॥

If the lord of the Ascendant is vargottam and is posited in the 1st, 4th, 7th, 9th, or 10th house and side by side the lord of the 9th house is also vargottam in its own sign or sign of exaltation and is also posited in an angular position (*1, 4, 7 or 10) or in the 9th house itself, then the native will be an extremely prosperous king who rides a throne of gold placed on the shoulders of an elephant and is accompanied by other signs of royalty.

निषादमपि पार्थिवं जनयतीन्दुरुच्चस्वभ-
स्थितग्रहनिरीक्षतो धवलकाम्तिजालोज्ज्वलः ।
विहाय तनुभं कलास्फुरितपूर्णकान्तिः शशी
चतुष्टयगता नृपं जनयति द्विपाश्वान्वितम् ॥७ ॥

Two other rajayogas are given below:

(a) If in a nativity Moon, endowed with strength during the bright half receives full aspect of a planet from its own sign or sign of exaltation then the native even if born in a family of slaves, will be a king.

(b) If 'Full Moon' occupies any angle but not the ascendant i.e., 4th, 7th or 10th house then the native will be a king. He will possess herds of horses and elephants.

Our opinion is that in this yoga if Moon is in the 4th house then Sun will be in the 10th house (because on full Moon, Sun and Moon are opposite to each other) and so both of them will be endowed with full directional strength and therefore very powerful. Side by side the 4th house indicates vehicles, horses, elephants, etc. so the native will own a number of these. In other houses (7th and 10th) the effect will be modified.

अश्विन्यामुदयगतो भृगुर्ग्रहेन्द्रै-
र्दृष्टश्चेज्जनयति भूपतिं जितारिम् ।
नीचार्योर्गृहमपहाय वित्तसंस्थो
लग्नेशः सह कविना बली च भूपम् ॥८ ॥

Two other raja yogas based on Venus are given below:

(a) If Venus is in the constellation of Ashwini (i.e. from 0 degree to 13 degrees 20 minutes in Aries) and is posited in the Ascendant and is simultaneously aspected by three planets then the native will be a strong king who is victorious over his enemies.

In the above case Sun and Mercury cannot aspect Venus because they are always near it. The remaining planets are Mars, Saturn, Jupiter and Moon. The best position would be as shown in the horoscope below:

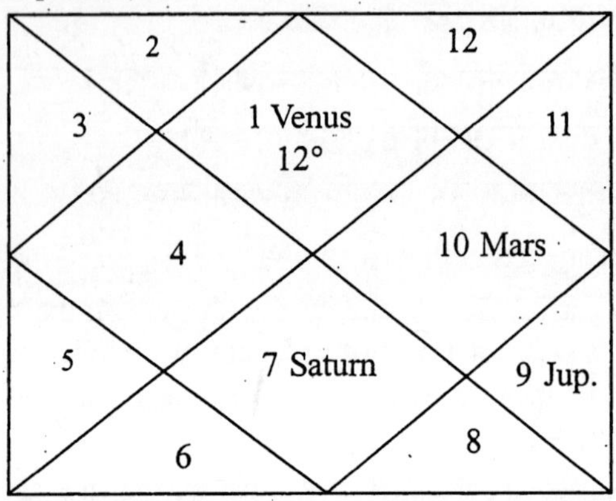

Here Saturn and Mars are both exalted and Jupiter is in its own sign. Saturn and Mars also possess full directional strength.

(b) If the lord of the first house is strong and is posited along with Venus in the second house (this sign should neither be the sign of debilitation nor owned by an enemy - of the lord of the Ascendant or Venus), then the native will be a king.

भौमश्चेदजहरिचापलग्नसंस्थः
पृथ्वीशं कलयति मित्रखेटदृष्टः ।
कर्मेशो नवमगतश्च भाग्यनाथो
मध्यस्थो भवति नृपो जनैः प्रशस्तः ॥९ ॥

The next two raja yogas are very powerful:

(a) If Mars is posited in Aries, Leo or Sagittarius in the first house and friendly planet aspects it then the native will be a king.

(b) If there is an exchange of houses between the lords of the 9th and 10th, then the native will be a king and others will praise him, i.e. it is very powerful raja yoga.

चापार्द्धे भगवान् सहस्रकिरणस्त्रैव ताराधिपो
लग्ने भानुसुतेऽतिवीर्यसहितः स्वोच्चे च भूनन्दनः ।

यद्येवं भवति क्षितेरधिपतिः संश्रुत्य दूरं भयात्
त्रस्ता एव नमन्ति तस्य रिपवो दग्धाः प्रतापग्निना ॥१०॥

If sun is in the first half of Sagittarius (from 0 degree to 15 degrees), Moon is also in Sagittarius, Saturn* is in the Ascendant and Mars is exalted then the native is a King full of courage and valorous. Due to fear his enemies pay their obeisance to him from a distance.

सुधामृणालोपमविम्बशोभितः शशी नवांशे नलिनीप्रियस्य
यदि क्षितीशो बहुहस्तिपूर्णः शुभाश्च केन्द्रेषु न पापयुक्ताः ॥११॥

If white Moon of full disc like nectar on a day preceding or succeeding full Moon is in Leo navansha and benefic planets (who are not conjoined with malefic), are in angles then the native is a king who owns a fleet of elephants.

नीचारिवर्गरहितैर्विहगैस्त्रिभिस्तु
स्वांशोपगैर्बलयुतैः शुभदृष्टिजुष्टैः
गोक्षीरशाङ्खधवलोमृगलाञ्छनश्च
स्याद्यस्य जन्मनि स भूमिपतिर्जितारिः ॥१२॥

If Moon is lustrous like cow's milk or a conch shell (i.e. a waxing Moon from the 8th day onwards) and three other planets (i.e. four in all including Moon) are strong in their vargas. They should not be in the signs and vargas of enemies or debilitation and benefic planets aspect them, then the native is the owner of lands viz., a king. He is victorious over his enemies".

कुमुदगहनबन्धुं श्रेष्ठमंशं प्रपन्नं
यदि बलसमुपेतः पश्यति व्योमचारी।
उदयभवनसंस्थः पापसंज्ञो न चैवं

---

*Saturn : Saturn is deemed to be very powerful in Libra, Pisces, Sagittarius, Capricorn and Aquarius particularly in the Ascendant.

According to the opinion of some astrologers, the moon should be in the Ascendant.

भवति मनुजनाथः सार्वभौमः सुदेहः ॥१३॥

If there is no malefic in the Ascendant and Moon[Ω] is in its highest varga i.e., in its own sign, own navansha and own decanet and Moon is also aspected by a strong planet then the native is handsome (very attractive in physical appearance) and a king who owns much lands.

जीवो बुधो भृगुसुतोऽथ निशाकरो वा
धर्मे विशुद्धतनवः स्फुटरश्मिजालाः ।
मित्रैर्निरीक्षितयुता यदि सूतिकाले
कुर्वन्ति देवसदृशं नृपतिं महान्तम् ॥१४॥

Jupiter, Mercury, Venus or Moon - if they are not combust and has no malefic influences, occupy the 9th house^ from the Ascendant and simultaneously conjoined with or receive aspect from benefic then the native is a great king he is equated to a god by his subjects.

Note : When a planet does not occupy the sign and navansha of malefic or an enemy, does not conjoin with or afflicted by malefic and is aspects by malefic, then it is said to be devoid of malefic influence and is called a planet with a 'pure body'. A planet which is in exalted, own or benefic vargas is 'Pure'. The causes, which make it malefic, are considered its negative points.

शुक्रेड्यौ सवितुः शिशुस्तिमियुगे स्वोच्चे च पूर्णः शशी
दृष्टीस्तीव्रविलोचनेन दिनकृन्मेषोदयेऽसौ नृपः ।
सेनायाश्चलनेन रेणुपटलैर्यस्य प्रविष्टे रवा-
वस्तभ्रान्तिसमाकुला कमलिनी संकोचमागच्छति ॥१५॥

[Ω]Subramaniam Shastri's opinion is that a planet who is in three vargas (which are owned by his great friends is called to be in highest varga. Other famous astrologers are of the view that when a planet is in its own sign, navansha and decanet only then he is in its highest vargas.

^In the original sloka the word 'Dharam" has been used and as religion falls under the 9th house so the house of religion is the 9th the Ascendant.

If

(1) Venus, Jupiter and Saturn are in Pisces;

(2) Full Moon is in its sign of exaltation;

(3) Sun receives aspect from Mars

and (4) the ascendant is Aries; then the native will be a great king that so much dust is raised when his army marches that an image of evening is created and the lotus flower closes its petals - (thinking that the night is approaching.)

If the above four conditions are fulfilled then we have a horoscope of the following configuration:

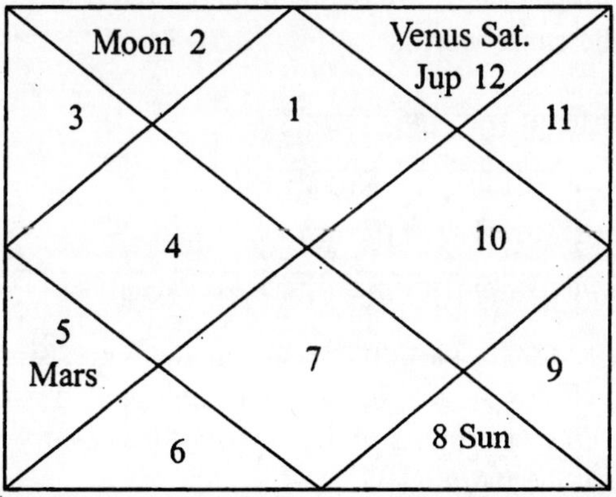

Mars should be either in Aries, Taurus or Leo and then and only then, it can aspect sun. If it is in Aries then 'Ruchak yoga' is also created which is good in itself. If it is in Leo then an exchange of houses between Mars and Sun takes place and it is a Dainya yoga and does not give good results. If Mars is in Taurus then it is with Moon and endows the native with tremendous courage, wealth and property.

The main thing here is that Venus cannot be in Pisces if Sun is in Scorpio, because Venus cannot go beyond 48 degrees from Sun. So this yoga cannot take place unless one condition is relaxed and the Moon instead of exalted in sign is substituted with exalted in Navansha or if we amend that full moon is in its own sign, instead of in its sign of exaltation then the yoga is possible.

नीचारिस्थैर्भवभवनगैः षष्ठदुश्चिक्यगैर्वा।
सौम्यैः स्वोच्चं परमुपगतैर्निर्मलैः केन्द्रगैर्वा।
आज्ञां याते शिशिरकिरणे कर्कटस्थे निशाया-
मेकच्छत्रं त्रिभुवनमिदं यस्य स क्षत्रियेशः ॥१६॥

(a) If the birth is at the night.

(b) Moon is in Cancer in the 10th house.

(c) Debilitated planets or planets who are posited in the signs of enemies occupy the 3rd, 6th, 11th houses or all the benefic in their highest degree of exaltation are in angular positions and no benefic planet is combust, then the native is an Emperor who rules the entire world.

वर्गोत्तमे हिमकरः सकलः स्थितोंऽशे
कुर्यान्महीपतिमपूर्वयशोऽभिरामम्।
यस्याश्वबृन्दखुरघातरजोऽभिभूतो
भानु प्रभातशशिनोऽनुकरोति रूपम् ॥१७॥

If full Moon is vargottam (i.e. in the same sign and same navansha) then this singla yoga makes one a powerful king that the dust thrown up by the hoofs of the horses of his cavalry reduces Sun to an image of the morning Moon.

कन्द्रगौ यदि च जीवशशाङ्कौ
यस्य जन्मनि च भार्गवदृष्टौ।
भूपतिर्भवति सोऽतुलकीर्ति
र्नीचगो यदि न कश्चिदिह स्यात् ॥१८॥

(a) If at the time of birth Jupiter and Moon are in angles and receive aspect of Venus; (b) no planet is debilitated, then the native is a king whose fame lasts forever.

जलचरराशिनवांशक इन्दुस्तनुभवने शुभदस्वकवर्गे।
अशुभकरः खलु कण्टकहीनो भवति नृपो बहुवारणनाथः ॥१९॥

If moon occupies a watery sign and navansha and is placed in the first house in its own Vargas or in the varga of benefic planets and there is no malefic planets in angles, then the native will be a king who will possess an army of elephants.

शुक्रो जीवनिरीक्षितो वितनुते भूपोद्भवं भूपति
देवेड्यो मृगभं विहाय तनुगो मत्तेभयुक्तं नृपम्।
केन्द्रे जन्मपतिर्बलाधिकयुत:* कुर्याद्धरित्रीपतिं
दृष्टे वाक्पतिना बुधे दधति दृथ्वीशाश्च तच्छासनम् ॥२० ॥

We are giving four yogas - they are all separate from one another:

(a) if a person is born is a royal family and Venus receives and aspect of Jupiter then the native will be a king.

(b) If Jupiter is in the 1st house in any sign except Capricorn, then this an excellent raja yoga.

(c) The lord of the Ascendant* is strong and occupies an angle then it is a powerful yoga.

(d) If Mercury receive an aspect from Jupiter then kings follow the advice of such a person. It is an indication that the native with such configuration is intelligent and practical.

We would clarify here that Jupiter aspects the 5th, 7th and 9th house from it and when Mercury occupies the 5th and 9th house (or is conjoined with) from Jupiter it will give good results and makes one practical and intelligent. However if Mercury is in the 7th house from Jupiter, then the advice and decisions of such a person are not practical. His purity of intellect and helping attitude is all their but his decisions not only in his own case but also for others lack depth.

एकोप्युच्चक्षेत्रगो मित्रदृष्ट:
कूर्याद्भूपं मित्रयोगाद्धनाढ्यम्।
स्वांशे सूर्ये स्वर्क्षगश्चन्द्रमा-
श्चेद्देशाधीशं साश्वनागं विधत्ते ॥२१ ॥

---

*The Sanskrit word mentions - 'Janmapati' which could apply either to the lord of the Ascendant or to the lord of the Moon sign.

(a) If even one planet occupies its sign of exaltation and receive aspect from planets, which are his friends, then the person so born will be a king. If such an exalted planet conjoins with a friendly planet then the native is rich.

(b) If Sun is in its own navansha and Moon occupies Cancer then it is excellent raja yoga. Sun should be strong by sign and Moon should also be strong in the Navansha i.e. the Signs and navansha both in a horoscope then the full horoscope improves.

मीने पूर्णज्योतिषि मित्रग्रहदृष्टे चन्द्र
लोकानन्दकरः स्यान्नृपमुख्यः।
पूर्णज्योतिः स्वोच्चगतश्चेत्तुहिनांशु-
स्त्यागाधिक्यं सज्जनशस्तं जगदीशम्॥२२॥

(a) If Moon is illuminated in full (full Moon) occupies Pisces and receives aspect from a friendly planet then it is strong raja yoga.

(b) A full Moon in Taurus at birth ushers in a generous person who is highly praised by good people. It is good raja yoga.

चन्द्रेऽधिमित्रांशगते सुदृष्टे शुक्रेण लक्ष्मीसहितो नृपः स्यात्
तथा स्थिते वासवमन्त्रिदुष्टे पूर्णां धरित्री परिपालयेत्सः॥२३॥

(a) If Moon is in the navansha of a great friend and receives aspect from Venus, then not only the native gets wealth but it is strong raja yoga as well.

(b) If in the yoga mentioned above, Jupiter aspects Moon as well, then the native will be a king*

पापास्त्रिशत्रुभवगा यदि जन्मनाथ-
ल्लग्नाद्धने कुजबुधौ हिबुकेऽर्कशुक्रौ।

*According to Varahmihir if the birth is during the daytime and Moon is in its own or great friend's navansha and is also receive aspect of Jupiter then it is a raja yoga. If the birth is during the night and Moon, who is in its own or great friend's navansha receives aspect of Venus then much prosperity comes.

कर्मायलग्नसहिताः कुजमन्दजीवा-
स्तज्ज्ञा वदन्ति चतुरस्त्विह राजयोगान् ॥२४॥

Another four raja yogas are mentioned below:

(a) If malefic occupy the 3rd, 6th, and 11th houses from the lord of the Ascendant.

(b) Mars and Mercury occupy the second house from the Ascendant.

(c) Sun and Venus are in the 4th houses from Ascendant.

(d) Mars in the 10th, Jupiter in the 1st and Saturn in the 11th house.

All these are excellent raja yogas.

According to many people the position in (a) should be counted from the lord of the sign occupied by Moon.

In the yoga above Mars in 10th and Jupiter in the first house are endowed with full directional strength and Saturn in the 11th house is powerful so this is a better inference from the Sanskrit text.

लाभेशधर्मेशधनेश्वराणामेकोऽपि चन्द्रग्रहकेन्द्रवर्ती।
स्वपुत्रलाभाधिपतिर्गुरुश्चेदखण्डसाम्राज्यपतित्वमेति ॥२५॥

If anyone out of the (a) lord of second, ninth or eleventh house occupies an angular position from Moon and (b) Jupiter owns one out of the 2nd, 5th or 11th house, then it is strong raja yoga.

Neechbhanga Raja Yoga

नीचस्थितो जन्मनि यो ग्रहः स्यात्तद्राशिनाथोऽपि तदुच्चनाथः।
स चन्द्रलग्नाद्यपि केन्द्रवर्ती राजा भवेद्धार्मिकचक्रवर्ती ॥२६॥

If any planet occupies its sign of debilitation then it is considered a weak planet, which will show evil effects. However at times such a debilitated planet shows excellent results - i.e. the effect of debilitation is not only cancelled but also good results ensue. The question is when does it happen?

We give the conditions, which lead to cancellation of the negative effects:

(1) If the lord of the sign in which a planet is debilitated occupies an angle from the Moon, and (2) the planet who is exalted in that sign should also be in an angle from Moon then it is a neechbhanga raj yoga and the results are extremely good. In the Sanskrit Sloka the word 'Uchchanath" can have two meanings-

For example Saturn is debilitated in Aries which is the exaltation sign of Sun - so both Sun and Mars should be in angles from Moon.

The second opinion is that Saturn is exalted in Libra, which is owned by Venus, and so if Saturn has to lose its debilitation effects then Mars and Venus should occupy angular positions from Moon. In our opinion the second interpretation looks more authentic.

To make it more clear we give below :

(a) If Sun is debilitated then Venus and Mars.

(b) If Moon is debilitated then Mars and Venus.

(c) If Mars is debilitated then Saturn.

(d) If Mercury is debilitated then Jupiter and Mercury.

(e) If Jupiter is debilitated then Saturn and Moon.

(f) If Venus is debilitated then Mercury and Jupiter.

(g) If Saturn is debilitated then Mars and Venus should occupy angular positions from Moon.

Only if both the conditions (1) and (2) are present then the neechabhanga Raja yoga is take place.

(2) We give below another yoga for the neechabhanga raja yoga to take place.

One commentator is of the opinion that:-

(i) The lord of the sign in which the planet is debilitated should occupy an angular position from the Ascendant.

Or

(ii) The lord of the sign in which the planet is debilitated should be in an angle from Moon.

Or

(iii) The lord of the exaltation sign of the debilitated planet should occupy an angle from the Ascendant.

Or

(iv) The lord of the exaltation sign of the planet which is debilitated should be in an angle from the Moon.

If any of he above condition is fulfilled then the neechbhanga raja yoga will be effective.

We do not adhere to this view because in the original Slokas the word "APP' that means both the lord of he sign in which the planet is debilitated and also the lord of the exaltation sign of the planet which is debilitated, should occupy an angular position from the Moon.

The Sanskrit text 'Chandralagna" clearly indicates that it should be from the Moon (and not the Ascendant).

A third opinion is of the view that the lord of the sign in which a planet is debilitated or the lord of the exaltation sign of the planet, which is debilitated, should occupy an angular position from the debilitated planet.

यद्येको नीचगतस्तद्राश्यधिपस्तदुच्चपः केन्द्रे ।
यस्य स तु चक्रवर्ती समस्तभूपालवन्द्यांघ्रिः ॥२७॥

The lord of the sign in which a planet is debilitated and the lord of the exaltation sign of the debilitated planet should be in angular position from each other. Then it is also a neechbhanga Raja Yoga.

यस्मिन्राशौ वर्तते खेचरस्तद्राशीशेन प्रेक्षितश्चेत्स खेटः ।
क्षोणीपालं कीर्तिमन्तं विदध्यात् सुस्थानश्चेत्किंपुनः पार्थिवेन्द्रः ॥२८॥

The Lord of the sign in which a planet is debilitated, should fully aspect the debilitated planet. Then it is another instance of neechabhanga raja yoga. However if this debilitated planet occupies the 6, 8, or 12th house then it would not be powerful raja yoga. In good houses the raja yoga will be strong.

नीचे तिष्ठति यस्तदाश्रितगृहाधीशो विलग्नाद्यदा
चन्द्राद्वा यदि नीचगस्य विहगस्योच्चर्क्षनाथोऽथवा।
केन्द्रे तिष्ठति चेत्पूर्णविभवः स्याच्चक्रवर्ती नृपो
धर्मिष्ठोऽन्यमहीशवन्दितपदस्तेजोयशोभाग्यवान् ॥२९ ॥

It a planet is in its debilitated sign then (a) The lord of that sign or (b) the lord of the sign in which the debilitated planet is exalted, either of them are in angular position from the Ascendant or the Moon, then Neechbhanga Raja Yoga takes place.

नीचे यस्तस्य नीचोच्चभेशौ द्वावेक एव वा
केन्द्रस्थश्चेच्चक्रवर्ती भूपः स्याद्भूपवन्दितः ॥३० ॥

If a planet is posited in its sign of debilitation and the lord of this sign as well as the lord of the sign where the planet is exalted - anyone or both are in an angle from the Ascendant then the neechbhanga raja yoga takes place.

Note 1: In the slokas from 26 to 30, many neechbhanga raja yogas are repeated.

Note 2: If we consider all the conditions then by permutation and combinations most of the debilitated planets will create Neechbhanga Raja yogas. So proper judgement is headed.

Note 3: Sloka 27 can be interpreted in another manners i.e., If a planet is debilitated then the lord of the sign where the debilitated planet gets exalted, should be in an angular position then Neechbhanga raja yoga takes place. For example if Sun is debilitated (in Libra) in a chart, then the lord of the sign is Venus. Venus is exalted in Pisces. The ruler of Pisces is Jupiter, So if, Jupiter is posited in an angle then it is a 'Neechbhanga Raja yoga'.

[The Sanskrit word 'Neecha' mean 'Debilitated' 'Bhanga' means 'annulled' and Raja yoga is the combination (yoga) for becoming a King (Raja).]

8

Bhavashraya Phal (Effects of Planets in Houses)

In this chapter the effects of the placement of Sun, Moon, Mars, etc. in different houses are discussed:

लग्नेऽर्केऽल्पकचः क्रियालसतमः क्रोधी प्रचण्डोन्नतो
मानी लोचनरूक्षकः कृशतनुः शूरोऽक्षमो निर्घृणः।
स्फोटाक्षः शशिभे क्रिये सतिमिरः सिंहे निशान्धः पुमान्
दारिद्र्योपहतो विनष्टतनयो जातस्तुलायां भवेत्ङ्क१ङ्क

विगतविद्याविनयवित्तं स्खलितवाचं धनगतः
सबलशौर्यश्रियमुदारं स्वजनशत्रुं सहजगः।
जनयतीमं सुहृदि सूर्यो विसुखबन्धुक्षितिसुहृद्
भवनमुक्तं नृपतिसेवा जनकसंपद्व्ययकरम्ङ्क२ङ्क

सुखधनायुस्तनयहीनं सुमतिमात्मन्यटविगं
प्रथितमुर्वीपतिमरिस्थः सुगुणसंपद्विजयगम्।
नृपविरुद्धं कुतनुमस्तेऽध्वगमदारं ह्यवमतं
हतधनायुः सुहृदमर्को विगतदृष्टिं निधनगःङ्क३ङ्क

विजनकोऽर्के ससुतबन्धुस्तपसि देवद्विजमनाः
ससुतयानस्तुतिमतिश्रीबलयशाः खे क्षितिपतिः।
भवगतेऽर्के बहुधनायुर्विगतशोको जनपतिः
पितुरमित्रं विकलनेत्रो विधनपुत्रो व्ययगतेङ्क४ङ्क

Sun in Various Houses:

If Sun is in the first house at the time of birth, the native has little hair (on the head), is lazy, hot tempered, violent, tall, proud, courageous, cruel and for giing).

His hairs are dry. If Sun is in Cancer (in the Ascendant), the native will have distinct and prominent eyes. When Sun is in Aries then the native has prominent eyes. When Sun is in Aries then the native suffers from eye-disease (at times blindness). When the Sun is in Leo then the native is night – blind. When the Sun is in Libra then many bad effects occur – the native is poor and his sons are destroyed.

When Sun is in the second house then the native is devoid of education, gentleness and wealth; his voice is defective (stammering or similar type of defective).

When Sun is in the third house the native is strong, a fighter, rich and generous but has enmity with relatives.

When Sun is in the 4th house the native is devoid of happiness, relatives, friends, and property. He does not possess a house (or problems always arise in connection with property matters). These things are considered from the 4th house and the placement of a malefic cause bad effects. The native squanders his inherited property. He works in the government service.

If Sun is in the 5th house then the native is devoid of happiness, wealth, longevity and sons. He has a limited family and at times the eldest child (son in particular) is destroyed or problems occur through him. The native is however intelligent and loves to walk in forest. It is a good placement for publications. (At times it restricts birth of a child till 30th year).

Sun in the 6th house makes the native prosperous like a king, famous, wealthy, and victorious and he is gifted with good qualities.

Sun in the 7th house gives deformity in body (unbalanced - not proportionate). Such a person works in opposition to the government. He roams about and is insulted. Sun here destroys happiness from wife (at times the wife is proud, hot tempered) - the rapport is missing.

Sun in the 8th, the wealth is lost, the native is short lived, his friends forsakes him or are destroyed; causes trouble in the eyesight - particularly the right eye – sight.

Sun in the 9th house limits happiness from father (the father dies in early age). Some people consider father from the 9th house and so Sun in the 9th house is not good for father. The native has happiness from children and relatives (It delays birth of grand children). Such a person worships Gods and Brahmins.

Sun in the 10 house gives a abundance of vehicles and children. The native is intelligent, wealthy, and strong and is famous. Other people shower praises on him and he is prosperous like a king. Sun has full directional strength here and it is extremely good for rise in life.

Sun in the 11th house endows on with wealth and long life. He is happy (has no sorrow). He rules over others. Sun here gives very good friends who are well up either in the political or financial world.

Sun in the 12th house cause enmity with father. The native suffers, from disease in the eyes (loss of eyesight – particularly the left eye. The native is devoid of wealth and sons. We have found that Sun here restricts the rise of a person till 22nd year. The second part of life is prosperous.

सिते चन्द्रे लग्ने दृढतनुरदभ्रायुरभयो
बलिष्ठो लक्ष्मीवान् भवति विपरीतं क्षयगते।
धनाढ्योऽन्तर्वाणिर्विषयसुखवान् वाचि विकल:
सहोत्थे सभ्रातृप्रमदबलशौर्योऽतिकृपण: ॥५॥

सुखी भोगी त्यागी सुहृदि ससुहृद्वाहनयशा:
सुपुत्रो मेधावी मृदुगतिरमात्य: सुतगते।
क्षतेऽल्पायुश्चन्द्रेऽमतिरुदररोगी परिभवी
स्मरे दृष्टे: सौम्यो वरयुवतिकान्तोऽतिसुभग: ॥६॥

मृतौ रोग्यल्पायुस्तपसि शुभधर्मात्मसुतवान्
जयी सिद्धारम्भो नभसि शुभकृत्सत्प्रियकर:।

मनस्वी बह्वायुर्धनतनयभृत्यैः सह भवे
व्यये द्वेष्यो दुःखी शशिनि परिभूतोऽलसतमः ॥७॥

Moon in different houses:

When the waxing Moon (Moon in the bright half) occupies the Ascendent then the native is courageous, strong built, brave, wealthy and long lived. But if the Moon is waxing (dark half) then it indicates the reverse effects.

Moon in the second house makes on soft of speech, pleasure loving and wealthy. However he has emotional speech (excitable manner of speech).

Moon in the third confirms happiness from brothers. Such a person is proud, strong, and brave but is a miser.

Moon in the 4th house makes the native happy, one who enjoys life, spends money freely, endowed with good friends, vehicles and property. He is well known.

Moon in the 5th house gives good walk, intelligence, and good sons. Such a person is Minister to a king. In Libra, Moon gives two sons.

Moon in the 6th house reduces longevity and intelligence. The native suffer from the disease of the stomach. He is defeated or insulted.

Moon in the 7th house makes one good looking and gentle. He has a good wife and he has conjugal happiness.

Moon in the 8th house makes the native sick and short lived.

However if no planet aspect the Moon in the 8th house then the native has long life.

Moon in the 9th house makes one pure, religious and he will be blessed with sons.

Moon in the 10th house, the native is victorious. He gets early success in whatever work he attends to, such a person does good deeds and obliges gentle person.

Moon in the 11th house makes one proud, long-lived, and wealthy and he has sons. He possesses many servants.

Moon in the 12th house shows bad effects. The native is lazy, unhappy and is insulted by others. He is hated by other people.

Note: Moon in the 6th, 8th and 12th houses causes sickness in early life (up to four years of age).

Mars in different houses

Mars in the Ascendent makes one cruel and very courageous. The person suffers from injury on the body (face and forehead in particular). He is short lived.

The native is argumentative.

Mars in the second house makes on ugly in looks or he is not good in speech. He is devoid of education, wealth and associates with bad characters (at times he uses cutting remarks and creates enemies all round).

Mars in the third house endows one with good qualities, wealth, happiness and courage. Such a person never gets defeated by others. However he does not get happiness from younger brothers.

If Mars is in the 4th house then the native lacks good friends, happiness, vehicles and property. He does not get happiness from mother (has strained relationship). The 4th house indicates the things mentioned above and Mars here reduces happiness from these sources.

Mars in the 5th house diminishes happiness from sons (children). The children are adamant and strong willed and a source of unhappiness the native in not intelligent and is a backbiter. Mars here does give success in teaching and management of educational institutions.

Mars in the 6th house makes one wealthy, famous, victorious over enemies, and prosperous like a king. He is lustful.

Mars* in the 7th house makes on engage in bad deeds, suffers from disease, fond of walking. His wife dies (i.e. he does not get happiness from wife).

The position of Mars is bad for the second child. Mars in the 7th house makes one strongly mangalik and the native should marry a mangalik woman then the negative effects are cancelled.

Mars, Saturn, the North Node of Moon (Rahu), the South Node

of Moon (Ketu) and Sun are natural malefics. The 7th house is the house of wife (or husband), the fourth house is the house of mother and vehicles the first house is mental happiness and self; the 12th house indicates pleasures of the bad – happiness from wife and other women.

The placement of malefics destroys happiness in marriage either by destroying the wife of making her sick or by constant differences in life with her. The sum total of it is to limit conjugal happiness.

In order to arrive at solid conclusion the horoscope should be examined from the Ascendent, the Moon (taking the sign in which the Moon is placed as the first house) and Venus. Venus is also considered because it rules conjugal happiness and it is the significator of wife (or women).

In the case of women consider the Ascendent, moon and Mars (instead of Venus). Mars is considered because it is related to the conjugal pleasure in the life of a woman. According to the opinion of some astrologers Sun and Jupiter should also be taken into account. For example Sun and Saturn or Sun and Mars together are bad for the husband.

Mars in the 8th house is also not good. Such a person is sickly, devoid of wealth, short lived and other people talk against him. (The native overspends money and suffers from urinary troubles).

Mars in the 9th house makes one hated by others even if he is a lose to the king. He does not get happiness from father. The native causes pains and sufferings to others. (He changes his religion and goes to extremes. He invites public ensure because of his religious views and because of his habit of championing controversial issues.

Mars in the 10th house makes one cruel, generous in giving to others (donations), like a king, ambitious and he is praised by highly placed persons. (He is good in organizing – however he is a hard taskmaster and drives others).

Mars in the 11th house makes one wealthy, happy gentle, courageous. He does not have any sorrow in his life (However he suffers through the elder brother or does not get happiness from him).

Mars in the 12th house makes one a backbiter, cruel, without wife and he is irreligious. He suffers diseases of the eyes. (Mars in this position makes the native, accident prone, he has secret enemies who bring about his downfall, he is imprisoned and loses property and wealth through law).

Mercury in different houses:

Mercury in the first house makes one learned; sweet tempered, good in speech and long lived. (In the Ascendant it endows one with quick perception and subtle wit.

In Aries, Leo and Sagittarius quick in anger, good in dramatics, skilful in mathematics. Endowed with fanciful ideas. In Taurus and Capricorn, the native is crafty, malicious, opinionative, fond of food. In Gemini, malicious, opinionative, fond of wit, orator, doctor, scholar, scientific mind. In Scorpio crafty, good in chemist, not to be trusted. In Cancer and Pisces - a shallow mind – a chatter box and possess a very high opinion of his abilities. Not to be depended upon.

Mercury in the second house makes one intelligent, fond of poetry, soft of speech and he eats sweet food. He earns money through his intelligence (Teaching, writing, brokerage or commission, interpreter or as a messenger).

Mercury in the third house makes one brave but he has longevity is average (medium around 64 years. he works hard and even then does not get wealthy. He has good brothers and sisters.

Mercury in the 4th house makes one learned. He praises others by using only good words in order to receive advantage from them. He has friends, wealth, lands and property. He enjoys them and lives happily.

Mercury in the 5th house makes one intelligent. He gets fame and happiness due to his learning and intelligence. He has many children. (In Gemini, Leo and Virgo it does not give happiness form children or destroys them; in Cancer, Scorpio and Pisces, the children will be deformed or insane more so if Mercury is related to Mars and Saturn, inspite the mind to risky ventures - speculation).

Mercury in the 6th house makes one lazy, cruel in speech, victorious over enemies but such a person loses his temper if opposed.

He is argumentative. (He is cheated by his servants - if Mars associates then he is robbed and even injured by the servants and people working under him. If Mercury owns the first house and is placed in the 6th house then the native suffers from consumption, weak lungs, chest and intestinal troubles. Too much talking and mental strain will cause health problems.

Mercury in the 7th house makes one intelligent, fond of good dress, has a pleasant appearance (feminine). He is famous. His wife is wealthy. (Mercury in this house makes one important, endows with a marriage partner with a very long tongue - whether the wife will talk wit or nonsense will depend upon the strength of Mercury).

Mercury in the 8th house makes one well known long-lived and head of a clan. He looks after his family very well.

Mercury in the 9th house makes the native, wealthy, religious and good in behaviour. He is scholar. He is expert in talk and loves to talk. (Fond of travelling: curious; scientific bent of mind).

Mercury in the 10th house makes one learned, strong, intelligent, and happy. He does good deeds and sticks to the truth. He will be successful in life. Whatever he takes up meets with early success.

(The native will possess some original talent, In this position success comes in teaching, preaching, banking and financial management. In Gemini, Libra and Aquarius endows with power of speech).

Mercury in the 11th house endows one with long life. The native with stick to his words. He will have much wealth, happiness and servants. (Help will come to him from friends who will be from the literary or scientific spheres. However if Mercury is weak then losses through them).

Mercury in the 12th house, makes one lazy, cruel, devoid of learning and poor. He is insulted and pitied by other. (Secret enemies bring about his downfall particularly in Taurus, Scorpio and Virgo. The enemies and Crafty. In other signs success in life and fluency in speech).

शोभावान् सुकृती चिरायुरभयो लग्ने गुरौ सात्मजो
वाग्मी भोजनसारवांश्च सुमुखो वित्ते धनी कोविदः ।

सावज्ञः कृपणः प्रतीतसहजः शौर्येऽघकृद्दुष्टधी-
बन्धौ मातृसुहृत्परिच्छदसुतस्त्रीसौख्यधान्यान्वितः ॥१४॥

पुत्रैः क्लेशयुतो महीशसचिवो धीमान् सुतस्थे गुरौ
षष्टे स्यादलसोऽरिहा परिभवी मन्त्राभिचारें पटुः ।
सत्पत्नीसुतवान्मदेऽतिसुभगस्तातादुदारोऽधिको
दीनो जीवति सेवया कलुषभाग्दीर्घायुरिज्येऽष्टमे ॥१५॥

ख्यातः सन् सचिवः शुभेऽर्थसुतवान् स्याद्धर्मकार्योत्सुकः
स्वाचारः सुयशा नभस्यतिधनी जीवे महीशप्रियः ।
आयस्थे धनिकोऽभयोऽल्पतनयो जैवातृको यानगो
द्वेष्यो धिक्कृतपवाग्व्यये वितनयः साघोऽलसः सेवकः ॥१६॥

Jupiter in different houses:

Jupiter in the first house endows one with good appearance, engaged in good deeds, long-lived and fearless. He has sons and happiness from them. (In Aries\, Leo and Sagittarius makes one generous, successful, a good friend, proud and haughty, firm and faithful; in Taurus, Virgo and Capricorn, Selfish, conceited, ostentatious and void of thought; in Gemini, Libra and Aquarius just, generous, even in temper, faithful, ready to help others with money and support; in cancer, Scorpio and Pisces; careless but generally fortunate in money matters unless Jupiter is retrograde. In Scorpio – ambitious and selfish. In general he desires public recognition of his good deeds. He thinks and works only on grand scale.

Jupiter in the 2nd house makes one intelligent, expert in speech (wins in discussions and debates) ; he has a good face and he gets good food (He controls others by controlling the finances. Generally looks after the financial side of a big organization).

Jupiter in the 3rd house makes one sinful, miser and he does not get respecting life. The native is crafty. However his brother occupies a position of trust and responsibility. He trusts his brothers. (He travels much inside the country. He has good relations with relatives and neighbours).

Jupiter in the 4th house endows the native with a good mother, friends, servants, sons and wife. He has plenty of grains etc. He lives happily (His old age is the best part of life. The father occupies a high position of honour).

Jupiter in the 5th house shows mixed results. The native is intelligent and he is a Minister to a king. He has sorrow on account of his sons (ie he has no sons or his sons die prematurely, or the area source of suffering or differences exists between the native and his son). In Sagittarius, Jupiter gives only daughters at times two. The result is based on the general principle that the significator of a thing, should not occupy the house which stands for it. Jupiter is significator of sons (male child) and 5th house also signifies children (similarly Venus is not good in the 7th house, Mars in the 3rd house etc.

Jupiter in the 6th house gives success over enemies; makes the native lazy; he gets insulted due to his own behaviour; however he is well versed in religious rites and clever.

Jupiter in the 7th house gives a good wife. He has good sons. He has good looks and he is generous than his father (the native raises to better position than that of his father. This position of Jupiter is very good to make one a lawyer – a Judge. He gets favour from people in better position. Jupiter in Capricorn in a male horoscope gives five wives).

Jupiter in the 8th house is not good. The native is without pride and serves others he is engaged in low type of jobs but is long lived. (We have found that Jupiter here makes one do such good deeds that he is long remembered. Jupiter in Cancer makes one religious but indicates danger of poison - food poisoning as soon as the periodic influence of Jupiter commences. The lower portion of the body becomes heavy).

Jupiter in the 9th house endows one with wealth, sons, and fame. He is always inclined to be engaged in religious deeds. He is a minister to a king.

Jupiter in the 10th house makes one extremely rich and loved by the king. The native behaves well and he is well known. (The native benefits through his father and he is a favourite to him).

Jupiter in the11th house endows one with wealth, long life and fearlessness. He has many Vehicles but limited family (less children).

Jupiter in the 12th house makes one hated by others. The native uses bad words, he is lazy, engaged in sinful activities, devoid of children and serves others (Jupiter if strong endows one with the ability to make even enemies turn into friends. He succeeds in life).

तनौ सुतनुदृक्प्रियं सुखिनमेव दीर्घायुषं
करोति कविरर्थगः कविमनेकवित्तान्वितम्।
विदारसुखसम्पदं कृपणमप्रियं विक्रमे
सुवाहनसुमन्दिराभरणवस्त्रगन्धं सूखे ॥१७॥

अखण्डितधनं नृपं सुमतिमात्मजे सात्मजं
विशत्रुमधनं क्षते युवतिदूषितं विक्लवम्।
सुभार्यमसतीरतं मृतकलत्रमाढ्यं मदे
चिरायुषमिलाधिपं धनिनमष्टमे संस्थितः ॥१८॥

सदारसुहृदात्मजं क्षितिपलब्धभाग्यं शुभे
नभस्यतियशःसुहृत्सुखितवृत्तियुक्तं प्रभुम्।
धनाढ्यमितराङ्गनारतमनेकसौख्यं भवे
भृगुर्जनयति व्यये सरतिसौख्यवित्तद्युतिम् ॥१९॥

Venus in different houses :

Venus in the Ascendent makes the native attractive to the eyes, good looking physical appearance, happy and long-lived. (The native is evergreen physically and mentally. The native is much beloved by women from he gains, fondness for pleasure, generous, well versed in fine arts.

Venus comparatively shows better effects in Gemini, Libra, Aquarius and Pisces. It does not show good results in Aries, Virgo, Scorpio and Capricorn. In Scorpio it makes one in fine arts – like music, paintings, etc. But reduces longevity.

Venus in second house gives success in life (If weak and ill aspected then the money is wasted on worthless things). The wealth comes from various sources and the native loves poetry. (It gives success in banking and financial management, softness in speech – a sort of purring sound).

Venus in the third house shows bad results. The native is miser, not good to look at, devoid of happiness, respect and property. At times he is without a wife. (Venus here inclines to illicit connections. The neighbour's daughter should be protected from these people. Fondness for singing and travelling.

Venus in the 4th house endows one with vehicles, good house, ornaments, clothes and luxury. (Good looking face, gain by inheritance and a happy old age).

Venus in the 5th house makes the native wealthy like a King. He has happiness from sons and he is intelligent. (Fondness for drinks and gambling. Good looking daughters who will be dutiful and loving. The native's children are endowed with artistic talents.

Venus in the 6th house makes the native poor. He will have no enemies. He will have illicit relationship with many women and he will be unhappy. (Many times Venus here gives intimate relationship with servants. Benefit from maternal aunts. He is fond of good dresses).

Venus in the 7th house reduces happiness from wife. The wife is good but does not live long. The native has connections with married women. He is wealthy.

Venus in the 8th house makes one long lived and wealthy. He owns much landed property. (The native inherits wealth and property but suffers from diabetic ailments).

Venus in the 9th house endows one with wife, sons and good friends. His fortunes rise due to the kindness of the king (people in better position). (He is religious and drawn more and more to Divine Love due to a woman pleasant journeys).

Venus in the 10th house, then the native is engaged in good work. He has happiness from friends. He gets respect, fame and occupies a seat of honour. (Such a person gets success in music and fine arts.

He meets women in connection with his work and falls in love with them. The native is pleasant even and agreeable, dislikes quarrels and others of every sort. He marries above his status (family status).

Venus in the 11th house endows the native with wealth, engaged in women and happiness from various sources. (Many good and sincere friends; friendship with musicians).

Venus in the 12th house gives pleasures of bed, wealth, prosperity and relationship with many women. (It is for extreme success in business. If Saturn associates then deceit and treachery and even one's own wife goes against him).

स्वोच्चे स्वकीयभवने क्षितिपालतुल्यो
लग्नेऽर्कजे भवति देशपुराधिनाथः
शेषेषु दुःखपरिपीडित्त एव बाल्ये
दारिद्र्यदुखवशगो मलिनोऽलसश्च ॥२० ॥

विमुखधनमर्थेऽन्यायवन्तं च पश्चा
दितरजनपदस्थं यानभोगार्थयुक्तम्।
विपुलमतिमुदारं दारसौख्यं च शौर्ये
जनयति रविपुत्रश्चालसं विक्लवं च ॥२१ ॥

दुःखी स्याद्गृहयानमातृवियुतो बाल्ये सरुबन्धुभे
भ्रान्तो ज्ञानसुतार्थहर्षरहितो धीस्थे शठो दुर्मतिः।
बह्वाशी द्रविणान्वितो रिपुहतो धृष्टष्च मानी रिपौ
कामस्थे रविजे कुदारनिरतो निःस्बोऽध्वगो विह्वलः ॥२२ ॥

शनैश्चरे मृतिस्थिते मलीमसोऽशंसोऽवसुः।
करालधीर्बुभुक्षितः सुहृज्जनवमानितः ॥२३ ॥

भाग्यार्थात्मजतातधर्मरहितो मन्द्र शुभे दुर्जनो

मन्त्री वा नृपतिर्धनी कृषिपरः शूरः प्रसिद्धोऽम्बरे।
बह्वायुः स्थिरसंपदायसहितः शूरो विरोगो धनी
निर्लज्जार्थसुतो व्ययेऽङ्गविकलो मूर्खो रिपूत्सारितः॥२४॥

Saturn in different houses:

Saturn* in Libra, Capricorn or Aquarius, in the Ascendent makes the native a king (head of a city or country). In other signs Saturn in the Ascendent causes sorrow in childhood, he is troubled by others and even afterwards he is poor, unhappy, lazy and has a shabby appearance.

In Gemini, Libra, Aquarius – thoughtful, tight fisted, sincere, devout in religion.

The native will interfere in others affairs especially when Saturn is in Libra . He is a nuisance to everybody due to his selfish and proud ways. In Cancer and Pisces – dull and dejected – suffers from cough, not good in character – revengeful. At times enthusiastic in religion. In Scorpio Crafty, cold and not to be trusted. In fact Saturn's position in the first house makes one shy, averse to society, stubborn, subtle for his own ends. Curious religious beliefs. Austere and averse to changes.

Saturn in the 2nd house makes one devoid of wealth and he follows the path of injustice. The native is not good to look at. However during the second part of life, the native will leave his birth place and settle down in a foreign country. He will get wealth, vehicles and luxurious things (away from birth place).

Saturn in the 3rd house makes the native intelligent and broad hearted. He has happiness from wife. He is lazy and sorrowful.

---

*(According to 'Man Sagri ' – Saturn in Meena or Dhanu shows very good results). (It makes the native timid, suspicious and fearful. At times contemplative and dutiful. Malicious. Envious. In Aries, Leo and Sagittarius – the native is free, straight, honest hand have tremendous hardworking abilities. Persistence, at time argumentative. In Taurus, Virgo and Capricorn – particularly Taurus dull and heavy with a cumbersome gait, malicious; in Virgo inquisitive, fretful but fond of jokes, in Capricorn – crafty, selfish, hard working, ambitious and ruthless. Cold blooded.

Saturn in the 4th house makes one devoid of house, vehicles and restricts happiness from mother. The native will be sickly in childhood. Saturn by placement in the house of happiness destroys it. (If Saturn is in Libra, Capricorn and Aquarius then judge the reverse. In other signs the old age is the most unhappy part of life. If Saturn owns the ascendant then the native earns wealth through agriculture, mining, agricultural equipments. He inherits wealth but his old age is troublesome).

Saturn in the 5th house makes the native a confidence trikster. He is always engaged in irreligious activities and always planning to bring about the ruins of others. He is devoid of learning, sons, wealth and happiness. He moves about freely and thinks in an abnormal manner.

(Saturn in Gemini, Virgo, Libra or Capricorn denies children or causes delays. In other signs destroys them or they are the cause of continual trouble and unhappiness to the native. Losses through speculation. However it is very good success in teaching. Strong desire to acquire knowledge in order to get recognition and respect in life).

Saturn in the 6th house makes the native fond of food (i.e. he eats much); he is wealthy; he is successful over his enemies; he is proud and behaves badly with elders.

(This is not good because Saturn cause sad and lingering sickness. In Taurus, Leo, Scorpio and Aquarius – danger of heart disease, gravel or stone, diptheria and throat troubles (particularly in Taurus) or bronchitis. In Gemini Virgo, Sagittarius and Pisces – indicate consumption, asthma, Cancer, bad legs, bowel and kidney complaint, breathing trouble or skin disease. In Aries, Cancer, Libra and Capricorn weak stomach, rheumatism, pains in the nerves, bad servants and looses through them. In Libra it causes defrangement of liver, hernia and trouble in the lower portion of stomach.

Saturn in the 7th house makes one engaged to a bad women. He is poor, walks on foot and unhappy. In early time walking on foot was taken as a measure of hardship. (If Saturn is strong then the wife is faithful). (Saturn makes the husband and wife possess money – he could be a widower or disparity in the age of husband and wife.

Very rarely the marriage turns out to be happy. It is bad for legal disputes, partnerships dealing with other. The native should work alone. In Gemini, Virgo, Sagittarius and Pisces - a second or even a third marriage. The wife is cold, reserved, melancholy and morose. Saturn at times causes delays in marriage or bad experience in early age.

Saturn in the 8th house makes one shabby in appearance. He suffers from piles etc. (Urinary troubles), dies due to hunger, devoid of wealth, and is neglected by his friends. He is cruel in thought. (The marriage partners is poor. He is constantly troubles and loses money or legacy due to the treachery of others).

Saturn in the 9th house makes one devoid of fortunes, children, father and religion. He is a bad person. (Head strong, thoughtful, reserved and contemplative. Fondness for Astrology and occult sciences. Loss through relatives by marriage. Danger in travelling by water. Saturn is always not bad in the 9th house. It draws one to Ascetic life. The native passes through crises after crises and becomes stronger. It is like gold when melted in fire losses its impurities and shines better. Saturn does the same here to the native. Saturn in Libra brings revolution religion. Strong Saturn in the house of religion – aspected or associated with Jupiter makes one religious and saintly indisposition.

His Holiness Swami Karpatriji Maharaj

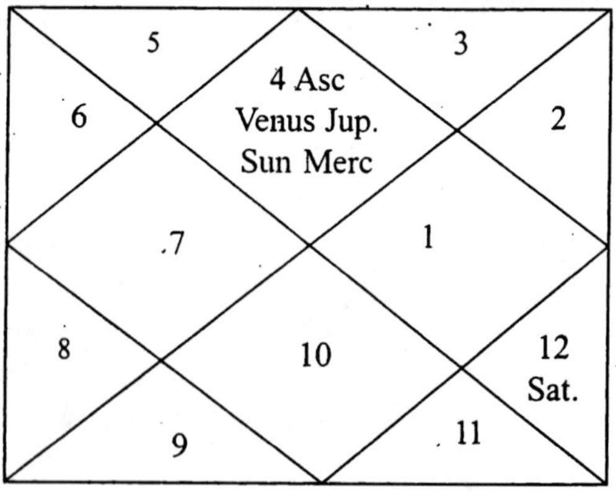

His Holiness Anandmayi Ma

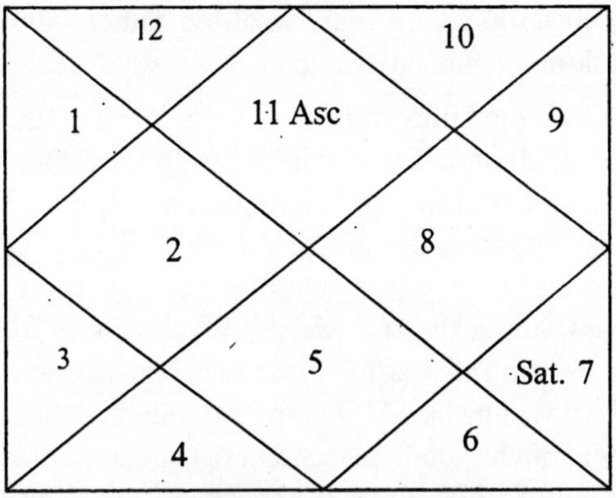

Srila Prabhupada Goswami

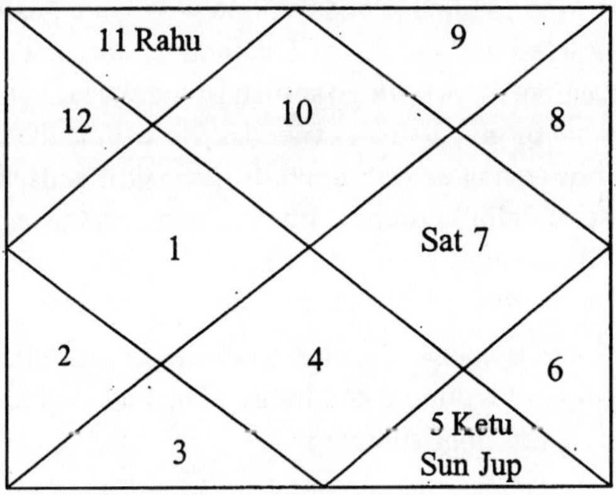

(1) His Holiness Swami Karpatriji Maharaj had Saturn in Pisces and Sun,. Jupiter, Venus, Mercury in Cancer in the first house. He even refused the seat of Shankracharya.

(2) His Holiness Anandmayi Ma had exalted Saturn in the 9th house. She is well known.

Four planets in the Ascendent has caused Sanyas Yoga in Swami Karpatriji's horoscope. Strong Saturn draws one to philosophical and religious life. He renounces the material things. Strong Saturn makes one like beautiful textured clothes (not rough and uneven).

Saturn in the 10th house shows very good results. The native is a king or Minister to a king, very wealthy, famous and brave. He is engaged in farming and agriculture.

(If Saturn is debilitated then success in early life followed by fall. Old age is full of misery and troubles. In Libra Saturn makes one religious. His Holiness Swami Prabhupad had Saturn in his 10th house in Libra. He started the International society for Krishna consciousness. He did concrete work in the religious path by spreading Krishna consciousness during the last twelve years of life. The natural age over which Saturn rules is 68th year and onwards and if Saturn is strong this part will go best. If Saturn is debilitated then 68th year and onwards it will not be good. In Mrs. Indira Gandhi's horoscope Saturn rules the 7th and 8th house and it is posited in the first house which means that it is good for incumbent's health and position.

Saturn in the 11th house endows one with good health, courage, wealthy, long lived and property. His income continues throughout his life. (The native loses through selfish friends). He should not stand surety for others or give loans to friends. He will be the loser Saturn in the 12th house makes one devoid of wealth, sons, honour and foolish. He has a deformed body (many times it is the legs which are defective). His enemies bring about his fall. (Saturn causes troubles through secret enemies. Troubles in the eyes and teeth.

The old age is spent in seclusion either in institutions or away from society – in old, dilapidated house. The native is liable to false accusations or even imprisonment.

लग्नेऽहावचिरायुरर्थबलावानूर्ध्वाङ्गरोगान्वित-
श्छन्नोक्तिुर्मुखरुग्घृणी नृपधनी वित्ते सरोष: सुखी।
मानी भ्रातविरोधकी दृढमति: शौर्ये चिरायुर्धनी
मूर्खो वेश्मनि दु:खकृत्ससुहृदल्पायु: कदाचित्सुखी॥२५॥

नासोद्यद्वचनोऽसुत: कठिनहृद्राहौ सुते कुक्षिरु-
ग्द्विट्क्रूरग्रहपीड़ित: सगुदरुक्छ्रीमांश्चिरायु: क्षते।

स्त्रीसंगादधनो मदेऽथ विधुरोऽवीर्य: स्वतन्त्रोऽल्पधी-
रन्ध्रे ऽल्पायुरशुद्धिकृच्च विकलो वातामयोऽल्पात्मज: ॥२६॥

धर्मस्थे प्रतिकूलवाग्गणपुरग्रामाधिपोऽपुण्यवान्
ख्यात: खेऽल्पसुतोऽन्यकार्यनिरत: सत्कर्महीनोऽभय: ।
श्रीमान्नातिसुतश्चिरायुरसुरे लाभे सकर्णमय:
प्रच्छन्नाघरतो बहुव्ययकरो रि:फेऽम्बुरुक्पीडित: ॥२७॥

Rahu in different houses :

Rahu in the Ascendant gives short life, wealth and strength. However the native has some disease in the uppper part of the body. (At times it is in the mind and the native is controlled by spirits living in the 4th dimensions. He should worship snakes to overcome troubles created by Rahu).

Rahu in the second house endows the native with an ability to talk in ambiguous language. He will speak in a secretive manner. In Astrology Rahu (the North Node of moon) is considered a thief and the second house is the house of speech. Rahu's position here makes the natives suffer from disease in the mouth, he speaks lies. He is angry by temperament and becomes wealthy with the king's wealth.

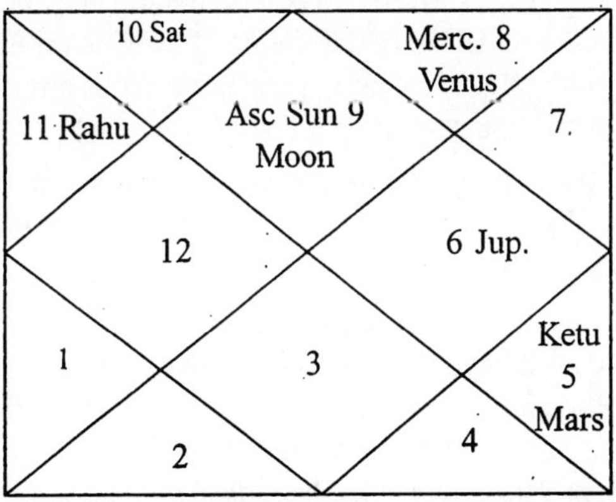

If Rahu is in the 3rd house then he is successful in diplomatic service. Rahu signifies foreigners, foreign countries, and wealth comes from there. Secondly wealth comes from people of different religion, community or where social disparity exists between the native. However he opposes and is also opposed by his brothers. (With this placement of Rahu the native, even if born in an ordinary family will become rich by virtue of his good fortunes and ability. This is the best position of Rahu).

Rahu in the 4th house makes one a fool, short lived, causes pains and sufferings to others. The native will rarely be happy. However Rahu gives many good friends.

Rahu in the 5th house makes one cruel in disposition, devoid of sons, and the native suffers from disease in the flanks (the lower portion of the stomach on the sides). The native speaks with a nasal tone.

Rahu in the 6th house makes the native wealthy and long lived. The native however suffers from urinary troubles. Such a person is troubled by enemies and other malefic planets.

Rahu in the 7th house destroys the wife. The native loses wealth due to illicit relationship with women from lower status of life (or belonging to other religion). The native is independent he is not very strong where potency is considered.

Rahu in the 8th house makes one suffer from wind troubles (gastric ailments etc.), short live, restless in mind and body, engaged in improper and mental work and he has few sons (children) (The native meets with trouble in foreign countries and at airports like loss of passports and important papers.

Rahu in the 9th house makes the native engaged in bad deeds. He always speaks the opposite words. However the native is the head of a clan, village or a city.

Rahu in the 10th house makes one engaged in bad deeds. He works for others; is fearless; he has few sons. However the native is famous. (Rahu in this position gives success through people in political power. If the native does not go in politics, he has friendship with politicians. His contacts are beneficial).

Rahu in the 11th house makes one suffer from disease in the ears. The native is wealthy and long lived. He has few sons and is engaged in sinful activities. (Rahu here causes frequent hospitalization or imprisonment. The native suffers from false accusations. Troubles from secret enemies).

Rahu in the 12th house shows bad results. The native suffers from disease caused by water (deficiency of water in the body, pleurisy or excess off water in stomach etc.). He spends money freely and is engaged in sinful activities. (Rahu here causes frequent hospitalization or imprisonment the native suffers from false accusation. Troubles from secret enemies.

लग्ने कृतघ्नमसुखंपिशुनं विवर्ण
स्थानच्युतं विकलदेहमसत्समाजम्।
विद्यार्थहीनमधमोक्तियुतं कुदृष्टिं
पातः परान्ननिरतं कुरुते धनस्थः ॥२८॥

आयुर्बलं धनयशःप्रमदान्नसौख्यं
केतौ तृतीयभवने सहजप्रणाशम्।
भूक्षेत्रयानजननीसुखजन्मभूमि-
नाशं सुखे परगृहस्थितिमेव दत्ते ॥२९॥

पुत्रक्षयं जठररोगपिशाचपीडां
दुर्बुद्धिमात्मनि खलप्रकृतिं च पातः।
औदार्यमुत्तमगुणं दृढतां प्रसिद्धिं
षष्ठे प्रभुत्वमरिर्दनमिष्टसिद्धिम् ॥३०॥

द्यूनेऽवमानमसतीरतिमान्त्ररोगं
पातः स्वदारवियुतिं मदधातुहानिम्।
स्वल्पायुरिष्टविरहं कलहं च रन्ध्रे
शस्त्रक्षतं सकलकार्यविरोधमेव ॥३१॥

पापप्रवृत्तिमशुभं पितृभाग्यहीनं
दारिद्र्यमार्यजनदूषणमाह धर्मे।
सत्कर्मविघ्नमशुचित्वमवद्यकृत्यं
तेजस्विनं नभसि शौर्यमतिप्रसिद्धम् ॥३२॥

लाभेऽर्थसंचयमनेकगुणं सुभोगं
सद्द्रव्यसोपकरणं सकलार्थसिद्धिम्।
प्रच्छन्नपापमधव्ययमर्थनाशं
रि:फे विरूद्धगतिमक्षिरुजं च पात: ॥३३॥

Ketu in different houses:

Ketu (the South Node of Moon) when posited in the first house makes the native suffer from deformity in body (and mind), devoid of happiness, a backbiter, fond of bad people (under the influence of gangsters, easily influenced by low type of people), ungrateful, not good to look at and belonging to mixed race. He has to face disadvantageous removals from his position. (The native is likely to suffer from burns on face).

Ketu in the second house makes one devoid of education and wealth. The native has bad eyesight (or disease in the eyes). He will speak bad words and will be fond of eating at others houses. (To depend on others for food is taken as a sign of children in the family).

Ketu in the 3rd house makes one long lived, strong, wealthy and famous. The native will be prosperous and will have happiness from wife. The native downs not get happiness from his brothers.

Ketu in the 4th house makes the native devoid of property, farm, mother and happiness. The native lives in the house of others (as a dependent). He is compelled to leave his place of birth.

Ketu in the 5th house destroys children. (Premature birth of children).

The native suffers from stomach ailments. He will be troubled by ghosts. Such type of people are bad by nature. They always think about bad things.

Ketu in the 6th house makes one generous, endowed with good qualities, firm, famous, occupy a seat of honour, successful over enemies. Such a person attains spiritual powers by propitiating Gods. (Ketu's position in 6th house creates 'Shukra –Hanta- Yoga' i.e. one who annihilates his enemies).

Ketu in the 7th house makes the native get insulted by others. The native indulges in clandestine relationship with prostitutes and low type of women. He does not get happiness from his own wife or he is separated from his own wife. He suffers from intestinal problems and weakness of semen. (Generally the native's wife is sickly. Difficulties through the second child or he suffers in life).

Ketu in the 8th house causes loss of loved ones. The native is short lived and quarrels with others. The native get hurts through arms and he is opposed in everything he wants to do.

Ketu in the 9th house makes one sinful, engaged in bad deeds, devoid of happiness from father, unfortunate, poor and he talks ill of good people. (Ketu here makes one religious. The wealth comes to him but he spends it all in the end).

Ketu in the 10th house prevents one from doing good deeds. He creates obstacles for others as well. He is however courageous, fiery and famous for his fighting qualities. He is engaged in bad deeds and dirt by the nature.

Ketu in the 11th house makes one wealthy and endowed with good qualities. He accumulates wealth and things of luxury. He gets success in every work he undertakes.

Ketu in the 12th house shows bad results. The native is engaged in sinful activities secretly. He spends money in his bad schemes. He loses his wealth.

He suffers from defects in the eyes and always follow in the footsteps of bad people. (The native is many times hospitalized or imprisoned. He has to face false accusation. Fortunately Ketu here gives liberation – more so if Jupiter also placed with it.

उदयर्क्षांशस्फुटतुल्यांशे निवसन् पूर्ण फलमाधत्ते।
शनिवद्राहुः कुजवत्केतुः फलदाता स्यादिह संप्रोक्तः ॥३४॥

We have already discussed the effects of planets in different house. We would add that if a planet is at the cusp of a house then it shows the maximum effect of that house. When we say the cusp then we are referring to the equal house division. If a planet is in the same degree as the degree of the Ascendant then it will show maximum results.

For example in Horoscope No.1 the Ascendent is one degree of Aries. Saturn is also one degree in the 5th house then Saturn will show very little results of the 5th house placement.

Mantreshwar emphasizes that a planet's full effect will depend upon its closeness to the cusp of the house. It will vary according to its distance from the cusp of the house. For example a planet which is at the middle of two cusps (in horoscope No.1 the Ascendant is one degree, in Aries is the mid point) then it will show very little results. From personal experience we found that the effect is over delayed so much so that the passes.

(There are many systems of house divisions. We have shown only equal house divisions).

Horoscope No.1

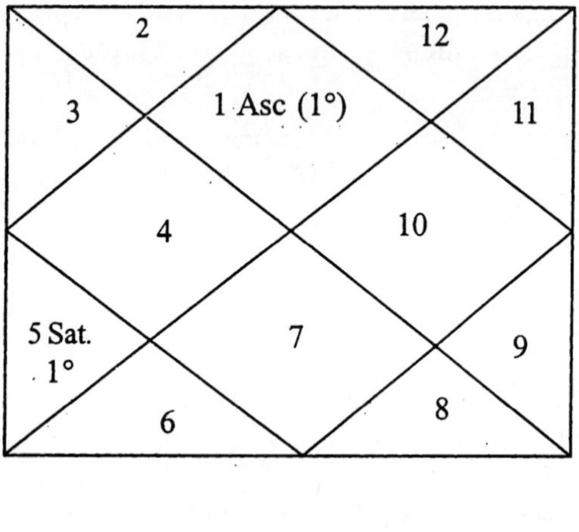

Horoscope No. 2

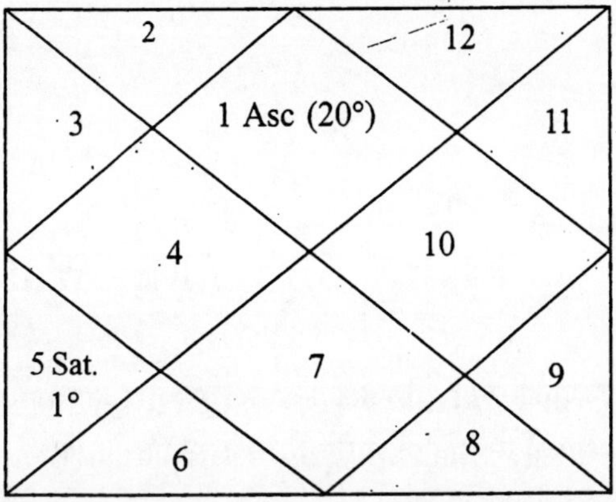

Astrologers are of the opinion that Rahu's effects are similar to Saturn's and Ketu's effects are like that of Mars.

भावसमांशकसंस्था भावफलं पूर्णमेव कलयन्ति।
न्यूनाधिकांशवशतः फलवृद्धिर्ह्रासता वाच्या ॥३५॥

The same matter that we have spoken of has been explained here. It should be observed as to how far away the planet to be considered is from the cusp of a house. The nearer it is to the cusp the more effect it will show. The farther it is from the cusp the lesser effect will be the result.

9

Rising Sign / Moon at Birth

वृत्तेक्षणो दुर्बलजानुरुग्रो भीरुर्जले स्याललघुभुक् सुकामी।
संचारशीलश्चपलोऽनृतोक्तिर्व्रणाङ्गिः क्रियभे प्रजातः ॥१॥

पृथूरुवक्त्रः कृषिकर्मकृत्स्यान-
    मध्यान्सौख्यः प्रमदाप्रियश्च।
त्यागी क्षमी क्लेशसहश्च गोमान्
    पृष्ठास्यपार्श्वेऽङ्कयुतो वृषोत्थः ॥२॥

श्यामेक्षणः कुञ्चितमूर्द्धजः स्त्रीक्रीडानुरक्तश्च परेङ्गितज्ञः।
उत्तुङ्गनासः प्रियगीतनृत्तो वसन् सदान्तः सदने च युग्मे ॥३॥

स्त्रीनिर्जितः पीनगलः समित्रो बह्वालयस्तुङ्गकटिर्धनाढ्यः।
ह्रस्वश्च वक्रो द्रुतगः कुलीरे मेधान्वितस्तोयरतोऽल्पपुत्रः ॥४॥

पिङ्गेक्षणः स्थूलहनुवशालवक्त्रोऽभिमानी सपराक्रमः स्यात्।
कुप्यत्यकार्ये वनशैलगामी मातुवधेयः स्थिरधीर्मृगेन्द्रे ॥५॥

स्रस्तांसबाहुः परिवत्तगेहै-
    संपूज्यते सत्यरतः प्रियोक्तिः।
व्रीडालसाक्षः सुरतप्रियः स्या-
    च्छास्त्रार्थविच्चाल्पसुतोऽङ्गनायाम् ॥६॥

चलत्कृशाङ्गोऽल्पसुतोऽतिभक्तो
देवद्विजानामटनो द्विनामा।
प्रांशुश्च दक्षः क्रयविक्रयेषु
धीरोऽदयस्तौलिनि मध्यवादी ॥७॥

वृत्तोरुजङ्घः पृथुनेत्रवक्षा
रोगी शिशुत्वे गुरुतातहीनः।
क्रूरक्रियो राकुलाभिमुख्यः
कीटेऽब्जरेखाङ्कितपाणिपादः ॥८॥

दीर्घास्यकण्ठः पृथुकर्णनासः
कर्मोद्यतः कुब्जतनुनृपेष्टः।
प्रागल्भ्यवाक्त्यागयुतोऽरिहन्ता
साम्नैकसाध्योऽश्विभवो बालढ्यः ॥९॥

अधः कृशः सत्त्वयुतो गृहीत-
वाक्योऽलसोऽगम्यजराङ्गनेष्टः।
धर्मध्वजो भाग्ययुतोऽटनश्च
वातार्दितो नक्रभवो विलज्जः ॥१०॥

प्रचछन्नपापो घटतुल्यदेहो
विघातदेक्षोऽध्वसहोऽल्पवित्तः।
लुब्धः परार्थी क्षयवृद्धियुक्तो
घटोद्भवः स्यात्प्रियगन्धपुष्पः ॥११॥

अत्यम्बुपानः समचारुदेहः
स्वदारगस्तोयजवित्तभोक्ता।
विद्वानन्कृतज्ञोऽभिभवत्यमित्रान्
शुभेक्षणो भाग्ययुतोऽन्त्यराशौ ॥१२॥

If Moon is in Aries or Aries rises at the time of birth, then the person will have round eyes, weak knees, is angry by temperament, but is afraid of water. He is fond of walking, active, and has scars of wounds in the body. Such a person is lustful by nature and eats very little. He likes to speak lies.

If at birth, Taurus rises, or is occupied by Moon, then the native will have a big face and huge thighs. He will be engaged in agriculture. If we divide his span of life in three parts, then the 2nd and 3rd parts will be happier. Such a person is fond of women. He forgives easily. He is endowed with property, vehicles, cows and other animals. The native has some type of mark on his back, face, or flanks. This sign is either a birthmark or a wound or a mole.

If Gemini rises or Moon occupies Gemini at birth, then the native will have black eyes and wavy hairs. He is interested in spending his time with the opposite sex. However he is intelligent, and understands the psychology of others. He has a high nose, and is fond of music and dancing. He likes to live in his own house (room) and would prefer to avoid walking on foot unlike the Aries rising people.

If Cancer rises or is occupied by Moon at birth, the native is under the thumb of women or is controlled by women. He has a heavy throat and is endowed with good friends. The native has a number of houses and is rich and he has a big waist. He is not tall. He is intelligent, fond of swimming and playing in water. He walks fast. He has few children (few sons). At times he is cunning (In the original sloka, the word 'vakra' is used, literary it means distorted or twisted body but here cunning is more appropriate).

If Leo rises or is occupied by Moon at birth then the native will have yellow eyes, fat chin and a big face. He will be proud, very hard-working endowed with great perseverance and fixed views. His mother loves him. He likes to roam about in the forest and hills. He is fiery by temperament and losses temper even on minor matters in which he should not be angry.

If Virgo rises or is occupied by Moon at birth, the native has purity of mind. He never leaves the path of truth, softly and uses endearing words. He has shyness in eyes and is good looking. He is learned and knows the scriptures well. He benefits from the wealth of others and as well as from the houses of others. His shoulders are bent and arms are loose. He has few sons.

When Libra rises, or is occupied by Moon at birth, then the native is a worshipper of Gods and Brahmins but he is restless and has a lean body. He is tall and expert in buying and selling loves justice and has tolerance. He works as a judge (or in a court). The native has generally two names. He has few children and is fond of travels. He rises in life in the later years.

If Scorpio rises or Moon occupies Scorpio, then the native has a big chest and very big eyes. The thighs and shin are round. He has signs of lotus in his palm and feet. In childhood he will not keep good health, and he does not get full happiness from father and Guru. He is engaged in cruel deeds and occupies a high positioning in the government i.e. a position of responsibility.

If at the time of birth Sagittarius rises, or Moon is in Sagittarius, then the person so born, will have big nose, ears, face, and throat. He is never idle and constantly busy in something or the other. He is an expert in speaking and can sacrifice anything. He is not very tall and while walking he bents forward. He is courageous and overcomes his enemies. They are physically strong and favourite of the ruler. He can be controlled only by logic. If we want him to do some work for us, we have to logically explain the merits and demerits of the work and only then he will take up the matter.

If Capricorn rises, or Moon occupies Capricorn at the time of birth then the native's lower portion of the body down below the knees is weak (not so well developed as the upper portion), but he has sufficient physical energy, mental power, and inner strength - a powerful soul. He will accept the opinion of others, but by temperament is easy going or lazy at times. There is disparity of age between him and his woman friend who is generally he marries older. Outwardly he appears to be very religious. He is fond of walking and is fortunate but has no shame. He is likely to suffer from diseases caused by disorder of wind in the body (or inhibitions due to bad experiences in early childhood).

If at birth Moon occupies Aquarius or Aquarius is the rising sign then the native will commit sins and it will remain secret. He has some wealth. He is fond of others' wealth is greedy and would like to possess it. He will tolerate pains and sufferings during travels but would cause mental anguish and pains to others. In subsequent years of life he will be heavy, like an earthen pot. He is fond of flowers and scented things; there are fluctuations in his finances. At times they have nothing and at other time they are flush with money.

If Moon occupies Pisces or Pisces rises at the time of birth then the native has a symmetrical proportionate body. He is good looking. He has a charming manner of looking at others. He is learned, and reciprocates good deeds. He is satisfied and interested only in his wife, (not interested in other women). He is fortunate. He benefits from the things, which come out of the water. These days we can also indicate that he can do well through export-import business shipping etc. The native overcomes his enemies and is victorious over them.*

राशेः स्वभावाश्रयरूपवर्णन्
ज्ञात्वानुरूपाणि फलानि तस्य।
युक्त्या वदेदत्र फलं विलग्ने
यच्चन्द्रलग्नेऽपि तदेव वाच्यम् ॥१३॥

ग्रहे सति निजोच्चगे भवति रत्नगर्भाधिपो
महीपतिकृतस्तुतिर्महितसंपदामालयः।
उदारगुणसंयुतो जयति विक्रमार्को यथा
नये यशसि विक्रमे वितरणे धृतौ कौशले ॥१४॥

स्वमन्दिरगते ग्रहे प्रभुपरिग्रहादायतिं
प्रभुत्वमपि वा गृहस्थितिमचञ्चलां प्राप्नुयात्।

---

*We have noticed from our experience some contradictory things. Pisces rising or Moon in Pisces can make one romantic, fond of drinking at times and he has fancied. *Grievances with others. They indulge in complaining all the time that others do not reciprocate their good gestures.

नवं भुवनमुर्वराक्षितिमुपैति काले स्वंके
जने बहुमतिं पुनः सकलनष्टवस्तुन्यपि ॥१५॥

ग्रहः सहृत्क्षेत्रगतः सुहृद्भिः
कार्यस्य सिद्धिं नवसौहृदं च।
सत्पुत्रजायधनधान्यभाग्यं
ददात्ययं सर्वजनानुकूल्यम् ॥१६॥

गते ग्रहे शत्रुगृहं निकृष्टतां
परान्नवृत्तिं परमन्दिरस्थितिम्।
अकिंचनत्वं रिपुपीडनं सदा
स्निग्धोऽपि तस्यातिरिपुत्वमाप्नुयात् ॥१७॥

नीचे ग्रहेऽधः पतनं स्ववृत्तेर्दैन्यं दुराचारमृणाप्तिमाहुः।
नीचाश्रयं कीकटदेशवासं भृत्यत्वमध्वानमनर्थकार्यम् ॥१८॥

ग्रहो मौढ्यं प्राप्तो मरणचिरात् स्त्रीसुतधनैः
प्रहीणत्वं व्यर्थे कलहमपवादं परिभवम्।
समर्क्षस्थः खेटो न कलयति वैशेषिकफलं
सुखं वा दुःखं या जनयति यथापूर्वमचलम् ॥१९॥

वक्रं गतः स्वोच्चफलं विदध्या
त्सपत्ननीचर्क्षगतोऽपि खेटः।
वर्गोत्तमांशस्थितखेचरोऽपि
स्वक्षेत्रगस्योक्तफलानि तद्वत् ॥२०॥

Whatever sign has to be considered we should fully take into account its characteristics, the appearances, caste etc. We should also consider whether the lord of the sign is strong or not i.e. which house it occupies, with which planet it conjoins with the which other planets are aspecting the sign. Side by side, if other planets occupy or aspect the sign then they should be all taken into account. Only after considering all the factors, we should draw our conclusion. The conclusions should also depend upon the country, the times prevailing, and the person concerned. Generally, fifty per cent effect is from the rising sign, and the other fifty per cent is from the Moon sign. For example, the same type of results has been given for Aries Rising, and the same if the Moon occupies aries. We have therefore given the interpretation of the twelve rising signs, as well as if Moon occupies those signs in one place only.

Now we give the effects of Planets if they are exalted, in the house of a friend etc.

If a planet occupies its of exaltation, then the person is the owner of or the lord of much property. Kings and rulers praise him and he owns precious items. The native is endowed with various good traits and earns name and fame, has perseverance and intelligence. He is well versed in diplomacy, generous and famous, like King Vikramaditya*. King Vikramaditya was a great scholar and is famous in Indian history for his love of poetry, patience, courage, as well as for his unparalleled judgements and religious aptitude.

When a planet occupies its own sign then during its periodic influence, the native enjoys high position, good home, and power on account of the patronage of famous and well known persons. The native stays in his home under comfortable circumstances. In ancient times it was considered a good indication if one lived happily in his own house and did not have to go out for earning his livelihood. The native with the configuration will get new house and will be the owner of new lands in which all varieties of crops grow. During the periodic influence of a planet in own sign the native commands respect and if he has already suffered losses during the earlier bad influences of malefic planet then he regains the lost things.

When a planet occupies a sign owned by his friend, then the person succeeds on his work with the help of his friends. He keeps

All these good effects will be realized only when the exalted planet is the owner of good house in a nativity, like the 5th or 9th and is well placed in a sign as well as in different vargas viz. navansha etc.

on making new friends. He is blessed with good sons, wife, happiness, wealth and all types of prosperity. He is fortunate and everyone is favourable inclined towards him. Now we give the effects of a planet, which is placed in the sign of an enemy.

If a planet occupies the house of an enemy, then the native is dependent upon others. He will be living in the house of others and will be poor. His enemies will constantly trouble him. Even his faithful friends will become his enemies *i.e.*, he does not benefit from friends, but on account of their behaviour he passes through pains and mental anguish. His enemies will cause him troubles.

When the native passes through the periodic influence of a debilitated planet then his social and financial status will fall. The effect of this is that he* keeps the company of bad people. He has a wavering mind. Due to bad influences and debts, he has to work as menial servant for low graded persons. He lives in bad surrounding and countries. He undertakes tiring journeys. He works and still is constantly insulted by his employers.

We are giving the effects of a planet, which is combust, or one which is posited in a neutral sign which is neither the house of a friends nor the house of an enemy.

A planet, which is very close to Sun within fifteen degree, is combust. A combust planet will show mostly malefic effects. (According to sages Mercury is an exception because it is never more than 28 degrees away from Sun).

(a) When the native passes through the periodic influences of a combust planet, he will pass through a difficult period of life a living Hell. He will lose his life or he will lose his wife, children, and wealth or they are out of his reach. He faces mental anguish on account of them. He will have to bear insults and accusations. He is defeated and suffers all types of miseries.

(b) When a planet occupies a neutral sign (which is owned neither by a friend nor by an enemy), then during the periodic influence of that Planet, the life is ordinary. Neither good things happen

*He will indulge in bad deeds, will be a low-grade person and live on the borrowings.

nor bad things take place. He may enjoy life a little bit and has minor sufferings only. He maintains a steady positions which is similar to what it was at the commencement of the periodic influence of the planet.

We give below the effects or retrograde and vargottam planet:

(a) Even if a planet occupies the house of an enemy, is debilitated or both, if it is retrograde then it will show good results as if it is exalted.

(b) If a planet is vargottam i.e. when a planet occupies the same sign and the same navansha, it is said to be vargottama then it will show extremely effects similar to a planet who is in its own sign.

We have dealt with the effects of planets when they occupy a sign of exaltation, own sign, the house of a friend, the house of an enemy, in a neutral sign, debilitated, combust, or vargottam.

Chart of Vargottam

A planet is Vargottam in between the following degree:

Sign	From		To	
	Degree	Mnts	Degree	Mnts.
Aries	0	0	3	20
Taurus	13	20	16	40
Gemini	26	40	30	00
Cancer	0	0	3	20
Leo	13	20	16	40
Virgo	26	40	30	00
Libra	0	0	3	20
Scorpio	13	20	26	40
Sagittarius	26	40	30	00
Capricorn	0	0	3	20
Aquarius	13	20	16	40
Pisces	26	40	30	00

Notes:

1. Where the word 'friend' is used, it refers to the natural friend. It is also a temporal friend then so much the better.
2. If a Planet is in the house of friend which is also its debilitated sign like Venus in Virgo as Mercury (the ruler of Virgo) is the friend of Venus, then the result of Venus will be like that of a planet which is debilitated.

   Those who are well versed in practicing Astrology, they remember by heart as to the degree where a planet is Vargottam however we have given the table of Vargottam, to enable the new Astrology lowers to decipher at a glance.

   It is easy to remember that in the immovable signs the first Navansha, in fixed signs the fifth Navansha (middle one) and in the dual signs, the last navansha is vargottam.
3. If a sign of 30 degrees is divided in a equal parts then each part will be of 3 degrees 20 minutes. This one section is called Navansha. 'Nav' is ninth and 'Ansha' is portion (part).
4. If a planet is debilitated or in the sign of an enemy out is 'vargottam' then it shows good results.
5. In the sign of exaltation, a vargottam planet shows the best effects. The good effect is reduced in descending order, if a planet is in own sign, in the sign of a great friend (a planet which is a natural as well as a temporary friend), in the sign of friend, in a neutral sign, in the sign of an enemy, or in the sign of debilitation. What will be the result should be decided after due consideration to all the points have been given?

10

The 7th House (The House of Marriage - Spouse)

शुभधिपयुतेक्षिते सुतकलत्रभे लग्नतो
विधोरपि तयोः शुभं त्वितरथा न सिद्धिस्तयोः।
सितान्व्ययसुखाष्टगैः खरखगैरसन्मध्यगे
सितेऽप्यथ शुभेतरेक्षितयुते च जायावधः ॥१॥

दारेशे सुतगे प्रणष्टवनितोऽपुत्रोऽथवा धीश्वरो
द्यूने वा निधनेश्वरोऽपि कुरुते पत्नीविनाशं ध्रुवम्।
क्षीणेन्दौ सुतगे व्ययास्ततनुगैः पापैरदारात्मजः
स्त्रीसंगाद्धननाशनं मदगयाः स्वर्भानुभान्वोर्वदेत्॥२॥

शुक्रे वृश्चिगे मदे मृतवधूः कामे वृषस्थे बुधे
स्त्रीनाशस्त्वथ नीचगे सुरगुरौ द्यूनाधिरूढे तथा।
जामित्रे झषगे शनौ सति तथा भौमेऽथवा स्त्रीमृति-
श्चन्द्रक्षेत्रगयोर्मदेऽर्किकुजयोः पत्नी सती शोभना॥३॥

अस्ते वास्तपतावसद्ग्रहयुते दृष्टेऽप्यसन्मध्यगे
नीचारातिग्रहेऽर्ककान्त्यभिहते ब्रूयात्कलत्रच्युतिम्।
कामे वा सुतभाग्ययोर्किलदारोऽसौ सपापे भृगौ
शुक्रे वा कुजमन्दवर्गसहिते दृष्टे परस्त्रीरतः॥४॥

भौमार्क्यस्ते भृगुजशशिनोर्दारहीनोऽसुतो वा
    क्लीबेऽस्ते वा भवति भवगौ द्वौ ग्रहौ स्त्रीद्वयं स्यात्।
द्वन्द्वर्क्षांशे मदपतिसितौ तस्य जायाद्वयं स्यात्
    ताभ्यां युक्तैर्गगननिलयैर्दारसंख्यां बदन्तु ॥५॥

स्त्रीसंख्यां मदगैर्ग्रहैर्मृतिमसत्खेटैश्च सद्भिः स्थितिं
    द्यूनेशे सबले शुभे सति वधूः साध्वी सुपुत्रान्विता।
पापोऽपि स्वगृहं गतः शुभकरः पत्न्याश्च कामस्थिता
    हित्वा षड्व्ययरन्ध्रपान्मदनगाः सौम्यास्तु सौख्यावहाः ॥६॥

भार्यानाशस्त्वशुभसहितौ वीक्षितौ वार्थकामौ
    तत्र प्राहुस्त्वशुभफलदां क्रूरदृष्टिं विशेषात्।
एवं पत्न्या अपि सति मदे चाष्टमे वास्ति दोषः
    सौम्यैर्दृष्टि सति शुभयुते दंपती भाग्यवन्तौ ॥७॥

चन्द्रे समन्दे मदगे पुनर्भूः
    पतिर्भवेद्वाप्यसुतो विदारः।
नीचारिभस्थैरशुभैर्मदे स्त्री-
    पुंसोर्मृत्तिः स्यान्निधने धने वा ॥८॥

लग्नात्कलत्रभवने समराशिसंज्ञे
    भावाधिपेऽपि च तथैव गतेऽसुरेड्ये।
सूर्याभितप्तरहिते सुतदारनाथे
    वीर्यान्विते तु जननं ससुतं कलत्रम् ॥९॥

कुटुम्बदारव्ययराशिनाथा
    जीवेक्षिताः कोणचतुष्टयस्थाः।
दारेश्वराद्वित्तकलत्रलाभे
    सौम्याः कलत्रं ससुतं सुखाढ्यम् ॥१०॥

लग्नास्तनाथस्थितभांशकोणे
नीचोच्चभे स्त्रीजननं च पत्युः ।
चन्द्राष्टवर्गेधिकबिन्दुराशौ
कलत्रजन्मेति तथा धवस्य ॥११॥

कामस्थाकामधिपभार्गवाना
मृक्षं दिशं शंसति तस्य पत्न्याः ।
शुक्रोऽस्तपो वा तनुनाथभांश-
त्रिकोणमायाति तदा विवाहः ॥१२॥

कलत्रसंस्थस्य कलत्रदृष्टे
र्दशागमेवाथ कलत्रपस्य ।
यदा विलग्नाधिपतिः प्रयाति
कलत्रभं तत्र कलत्रलाभः ॥१३॥

कलत्रनाथस्थितभांशकेशयोः
सितक्षपानायकयोर्बलीयसः ।
दशागमे द्यूनपयुक्तभांशक-
त्रिकोणगे देवगुरौ करग्रहः ॥१४॥

कलत्रनाथे रिपुनीचसंस्थे
मूढेऽथवा पापनिरीक्षिते वा
कलत्रभे पापयुतेऽथ दृष्टे
कलत्रहानिं प्रवदन्ति सन्तः ॥१५॥

If the 5th and 7th houses from the Ascendant* are occupied or receive aspect of benefic, or if the lords of the above houses aspect or are

*Ascendant and Moon are of equal important. Ideal placement of aspect is difficult to find and so mixed result ensue.

posited in their own houses, the lords of the 5th and 7th from Moon aspect or are posited in their own houses or if these houses are occupied or receive aspect of benefic then the native will get good results of these houses viz., he will have happiness from wife and children. If this is not so or if malefic occupy the 5th and 7th houses from Moon and Ascendant, then the native will be devoid of wife and children.

(a) If Venus is hemmed in between malefic. or

(b) If the 4th, 8th and 12th houses from Venus are occupied by malefic. or

(c) If Venus conjoins with or gets an aspect of malefic.

The results of these three combinations in the chart of a man is that the longevity of wife is reduced i.e. his wife will die. It will of course depend upon the intensity of the negative combinations as to how much he will suffer. The more the malefic combinations, the more he will suffer.

If the Lord of the 7th house is posited in the 5th house, then the native's wife will die, or he will have no sons. If the lord of the 5th or the 8th is posited in the 7th house, then also happiness does not come from wife and she has short life. If waning Moon occupies the 5th house and malefic occupy the 1st, 7th and 12th houses, then the native will be devoid of wife and children. If Sun and Rahu (North Node of Moon) are posited in the 7th house, then the native loses wealth on account of relationship with women. (He will spend his wealth on worthless women, and will be unfortunate after marriage).

(a) If Venus is posited in Scorpio in the 7th house; or

(b) If Mercury is posited in Taurus in the 7th house; or

(c) if Jupiter is posited in Capricorn in the 7th house; or

(d) If Saturn is in Pisces in the 7th house; or

(e) If Mars is in Pisces in the 7th house;

If anyone of the above yogas is in a chart, then the wife dies. If Cancer falls in the 7th house and Mars and Saturn are posited in it then the native will have a beautiful wife who will be of good character.

If the lord of the 7th house, or the 7th house is occupied, receive an aspect of a malefic, or is hemmed in between malefic, or if the lord of the 7th is debilitated, or is in the house of an enemy, or is combust, then the native will lose his wife. All the yogas, which have been given above, show the loss of wife. If Venus is placed together with a malefic in the 5th, 7th, or 9th house, then the wife will be sickly. She will have some deformity or the other in the body, and the native himself will be disturbed, emotionally upset, on account of above placements.

If Venus is in the Vargas of Mars or Saturn, or receive an aspect from either of these planets, then the native is involved with some other woman (not his wife).

If Mars and Saturn occupy the 7th house from Moon and Venus then the native will not have a wife. If neutral planets viz., Mercury or Saturn, are posited in the 7th house and two planets occupy the 11th house, then the native will have two wives. If the lord of the 7th house and Venus both of them occupy dual signs, and dual navansha, then the native will have two wives.

The number of planets which conjoin with the lord of the 7th and Venus will indicate the number of wives. It does not mean that the person will be legally married to many women. It is likely that he will have a wife, but other relationships will also prevail which are strong enough to be treated as marriage.

The number of wives also depends upon the number of planets who occupy the 7th house. The malefic planets indicate the number of wife who will die during the native's lifetime. Benefits planets will indicate the wives who will live. We have to consider the country, the time prevailing, and the person concerned before we interpret the marriage and relationship with many women. In Western countries people do have many other relationship, whereas in the eastern countries it is controlled on account of their culture. Mental attachments, and relationship which is strong enough to emotionally disturb a person, either physically or mentally, should be treated as marriage.

If the lord of the 7th house is benefic, strong, then the native will have a good and faithful wife who will be blessed with many sons. Even a malefic when it occupies the 7th house, which is its own house will indicate good results. Benefic who are the lords of

6th, 8th or 12th house, if posited in the 7th house, then they increase the efficacy of the have and the native will be blessed with a good wife.

If the 2nd or 7th house in a nativity receives an aspect by or occupied by malefic, then the wife dies. Out of these the malefic aspects are comparatively worse, particularly the aspect of Mars and Saturn. When we talk of aspects, the means the full aspect, i.e. the 4th and 8th and 7th aspect of Mars, the 3rd, the 7th, and 10th aspect of Saturn. Similarly, in the horoscope of a woman if a 7th or 8th or both the houses are conjoined with or afflicted by malefic, then it shows bad result to the husband.

However, if both* the 7th and 8th houses are occupied or receive aspect of benefic, or if benefic are connected with these houses, then the husband/wife will be fortunate.

If the horoscope of a Woman, Moon and Saturn occupy the 7th house, then she marries a second time. Rather, we should say more than one marriage. If the same yoga is in the horoscope of a man, then he will be devoid of wife and sons.

If a malefic occupy the 2nd, 7th and 8th houses and are in a debilitated sign or sign or an enemy then the life partner will not survive.

If an even sign falls in the 7th house and the lord of the 7th house and Venus are also in even signs and the lord of the 5th and 7th are strong and are not combust, then happiness from wife and children will come.

If the lords of the 2nd, 7th, and 12th houses are posited in a Trikona, i.e., the 5th or 9th house or occupy and angular position, and are aspected by Jupiter", If benefic are happy and he will be blessed with wife and children.

In the horoscope of a man, observe the signs and navanshas occupied by the lords of the 1st and 7th houses. This sign or the 5th and 9th signs from these navansha will be the Moon sign of wife, or

---

*Both the houses mean the 7th and 8th houses in a woman's horoscope and the 2nd and 7th houses in a man's horoscope.

the exaltation or debilitation sign of the lords of the 1st or 7th houses will be the sign occupied by Moon in the horoscope of the wife. Sometimes in the horoscope of man the maximum benefic points in the Moon's Ashtakvarga will indicate the Janmarashi (Moon sign) of wife.

In the horoscope of a man observe as to

(1) What sign falls in the 7th house;

(2) Which sign is occupied by the lord of the 7th;

(3) The sign occupied by Venus. It is likely that the native will marry a girl living in the direction indicated by one of the above. The 5th or 9th sign from the sign and Navansha occupied by the lord of the first, when transited by Venus, or by the lord of the 7th, then the marriage takes place.

When a person passes through the periodic influences of a planet which occupies or aspects 7th house or the lord of the 7th have, and the lord of the Ascendant transists the 7th house, then the native will be married.

Out of the lords of the sign and navansha occupied by the lord of the 7th house, Venus and Moon whichever is stronger when the native passes through the periodic influence (major or minor) of the strongest out of these four, and Jupiter transists the 5th or 9th house from the sign or navansha occupied by the lord of the 7th house, then the native will be married.

If the lord of the 7th house is in its sign of debilitation, combust, or in the house of an enemy, or aspected by malefic or if malefic occupy or aspect the 7th house, the 7th house is destroyed and happiness does not come from wife. This is the opinion of the learned.

11

The Nativity of Women

यद्यत्पुंप्रसवे क्षमं तदखिलं स्त्रीणं प्रिये वा वदे-
न्माङ्गल्यं निधनात् सुतांश्च नवमाल्लग्नात्तनोश्वरुताम्।
भार्तरं सुभगत्वमस्तभवनात्संगं सतीत्वं सुखात्
सन्तस्तेषु शुभप्रदास्त्वशुभदाः क्रूरास्तदीशं विना॥१॥

उदयहिमकरौ दौ युग्मगौ सौम्यदृष्टौ
सुतनयपतिभूषासंपदुत्कृष्टशीला।
अशुभसहितदृष्टौ चोजगौ पुंस्वभावा
कुटिलमतिरवश्या भर्तुरुग्रा दरिद्रा॥२॥
सद्राश्यंशयुते मदे द्युतियशोविद्यार्थवांस्तत्पति-
र्व्यत्यस्ते कुतनुर्जडश्च विधवा कितवो निःस्वो वियोगस्तयोः।
आग्नेयैर्मदनस्थितैश्च विधवा मिश्रैः पुनर्भूर्भवेत्
क्रूरेष्वायुषि भर्तृहन्त्यापि धने सन्तः स्वयं स्त्रीमृतिः॥३॥

सुतस्थेऽलिस्त्रीगोहरिषु हिमगौ चाल्पतनया।
यमारार्कांशर्क्षे मदनसदने सामयभगा।
सुखे पापैर्युक्ते भवति कुलटा मन्दकुजयो-
र्गृहेंऽशे लग्नेन्दू भृगुरपि च पुंश्चल्यभिहिता॥४॥

शुभक्षेत्रांशेऽस्ते सुभगजघना मङ्गलवती
विधाः सत्संबन्धेऽप्युदयसुखयोः साध्व्यतिगुणा।
त्रिकोणे सौम्याश्चेत्सुखसुतसंपद्गुणवती

बलोनाः क्रूराश्चेद्यपि भवति वन्ध्या मृतसुता ॥५ ॥
चन्द्रे भौमगृहे कुजादिकथितत्रिंशांशकेषु क्रमात्
दुष्टा दास्यसती सुशीलविभवा मायाविनी दूषणी।
शुक्रर्क्षे बहुदूषणान्यपतिगा पूज्या सुधीर्विश्रूता
ज्ञर्क्षे च्छाझवती नपुंसकसमा साध्वी गुणाढ्योत्सुका ॥६ ॥

स्वछन्दा भर्तृघातिन्यतिमहितगुणा शिल्पिनी साधुवृत्ता
चान्द्रे जेवे गुणाढ्य विरतिरतिगुणा ज्ञातशिल्पातिसाध्वी।
मान्दे दास्यन्यसक्ताश्रितपतिरसती निष्प्रजार्थार्किभे स्याद्
दुर्भार्या हीनवृत्ता धरणिपतिवधूः पुंविचेष्टान्यसक्ता ॥७ ॥

शशिलग्नसमायुक्तैः फलं त्रिंशांशकैरिदम्।
बलाबलविकल्पेन तयोरेवं विचिन्तयेत् ॥८ ॥

ज्येष्ठभ्रातरम्बिकां च पितरं भर्तुः कनिष्ठं क्रमात्
ज्येष्ठा ह्यासुरशूर्पजाश्व वनिता घ्नन्तीति तज्ज्ञा विदुः।
चित्रार्द्राभुजगस्वराट्च्छतभिषङ् मूलाग्नितिष्योद्भवा
वन्ध्या वा विध्वाथवा मृतसुता त्यक्ता प्रियेणाधना ॥९ ॥

चन्द्रास्तोदयभाग्यपाः सह शुभैः सुस्थानगा भास्वराः
पूज्या बन्धुषु पुण्यकर्मकुशला सौन्दर्यैभाग्यान्विता।
भर्तुः प्रीतिकरी सुपुत्रसहिता कल्याणशीला सती
तावद्भाति सुमङ्गली च सुतनुर्यावच्छुभाढ्येऽष्टमे ॥१० ॥

शीतज्योतिषि योषितोऽनुपचयस्थाने कुजेनेक्षिते
जातं गर्भफलप्रदं खलु रजः स्यादन्यथा निष्फलम्।
दृष्टेस्मिन् गुरुणा निजोपचयगे कुर्यान्निषेकं पुमान्
अत्याज्ये समये शुभाधिकयुते पर्वादिकालोज्भिते ॥११ ॥

Whatever yogas have been given for men should also be applied to the nativity's of women. Where the possibility that the Raja-yoga will not come to be fruitful, or it will not operate in the nativity of women, (for example women who are not themselves engaged in active work and career cannot expect to rise and occupy high position on their own), then the good results will be enjoyed by their husbands and the position of husband will improve. Similarly a man may have a yoga which indicates that he is likely to have many wives, but a similar planetary configuration in the horoscope of a woman will not be applicable, unless the background of a woman is such, (or she belongs to some Western countries) where more than one marriage can take place or secret affairs may take place. In some very conservative societies in India a woman marries only once in a lifetime. And even if she becomes a widow she will not marry again.

In the horoscope of a woman the 8th house is the house of conjugal happiness and longevity of the husband. The 9th house indicates son (and children) and the 1st house will give indication about her beauty and outward appearance. The husband should be considered from the 7th house (and whether she is fortunate for the husband or if she will have happiness from him). Desires for relationship with others and purity of character towards husband should be judged from the 4th house. If benefic occupy these houses, then the results will be good. If malefic occupy, then they will indicate negative results. However if a malefic occupies its own house, it will do good and not any bad results.

If in a woman's horoscope, Ascendant and Moon both occupy even signs and they receive aspect of benefic, then she will be blessed with good sons and husband. She will be gentle in behaviour and will possess wealth and ornaments. But on the other side if the rising sign and Moon are both in odd signs and receive aspect of or are conjoined with malefic, then she will be cunning she will behave rudely with her husband, she will be masculine in behaviour, difficult to be controlled and will be poor.

If the cusp of the 7th house* falls in a benefic sign and navansha and the cusp is also tenanted and aspected by benefic then the woman will have a good looking husband who is learned, well known, wealthy and famous but if the reverse holds good i.e. the cusp of the 7th house, has a malefic sign and navansha and the owner of the sign is a malefic, then she will have a deformed husband who will be a fool or extremely cunning and poor. She will lose her husband - due to separation or death.

If Mars occupies the 7th house, then she is likely to be a widow. If both benefic and malefic occupy the 7th house, then she is likely to marry again.

If malefic occupy the 8th house in a woman's nativity, then her husband is short-lived. But if malefic occupy the 2nd house from the Ascendant then she will die first i.e. she is outlived by the husband.

Our experience is that if in the horoscopes of a man and his wife both of them have Mars, Saturn, Rahu, Ketu and Sun of equal malefic influences then the negative effects in both the charts are neutralized i.e. they cancel each other.

If Taurus, Leo, Virgo or Scorpio falls in the 5th, then she will have few children.

If the cusp of the 7th house falls in the signs or navansha of Mars or Saturn, then she will have disease in private parts.

If malefic occupy the 4th house, then she will be bad of character.

If the Ascendant, Moon and Venus are in the signs and navansha of Mars or Saturn, then she will be fond of other men than her husband.

If the cusp of the 7th house falls in a benefic sign and benefic navansha, then the woman will have an extremely attractive upper portion of thighs. She will be blessed with conjugal happiness.

If the Rising sign, the 4th house and Moon are all benefic then she will be of good traits. If benefic occupy the 5th and 9th houses, then she will be happy and blessed with sons. She will be wealthy and endowed with good qualities. If weak malefic occupy the houses mentioned above then she will have no issues or her children will have short life.

Observe as to which is stronger, the Ascendant or the Moon and whichever is stronger then

(1) If it is an Aries or Scorpio, and is in the Trinshansha - (30th

portion of a sign) of Mars then she will be a bad woman: it is in the Trinshansha of Saturn. Then she will be a slave. If it is in the trinshansha of Jupiter, she will be gentle and wealthy in the trinshansha or Mercury; she will be attractive and will attract others to her. If it is in the trinshansha of Venus then she will have a fickle character and will not be faithful to husband. We would like to point out again that this faithfulness, character etc, should be considered only after taking the background of the person and the country.

(2) If it is in Taurus or Libra and is in the Trinshansha of Mars, then she will be a very bad character. If it is in the trinshansha of Saturn then she will have relationship with other's husband or she will marry a second time. In the trinshansha of Mercury then she will be learned. In the trinshansha of Venus then she will famous and widely known.

(3) If it is in Gemini or Virgo and it falls in the trinshansha of Mars then she will be a cheater. In the trinshansha of Saturn, she will be sexually cold, may be like a eunuch. In the trinshansha of Jupiter she will be pure and faithful, in the trinshansha of Mercury, she will have many good qualities. In the trinshansha of Venus, she will be enthusiastic for pleasure and luxuries.

(4) If it is in Cancer and it falls in the trinshansha or Mars, then the woman will be independent* and fond of roaming about according to her own desires. If in the trinshansha of Saturn then she is likely to destroy her husband. In the trinshansha of Jupiter she will be endowed with special attributes. In the trinshansha of Mercury, she will be expert in sculpture and painting, and anything, which requires dexterity of hand. In the trinshansha or Venus, she will always act in a 'gracious manner and good in behaviour.

(5) If it is in Sagittarius or Pisces and it falls in the trinshansha of Mars then she will be blessed with many good characteristics. If it is in the trinshansha of Saturn, then she will desire very little physical company of her husband. If it is in the trinshansha of

---

*Independence in women is a sign of laxity in character, not appreciated in the East.

Jupiter, she will be blessed with good qualities. If it is in the trinshansha of Jupiter, she will be blessed with good qualities. If it is in the Trinashansha of Mercury, then she will be an expert in fine arts. If it is in the trinshansha of Venus, then she is faithful and of good character.

(6) If it is in Capricorn or Aquarius and it also falls in the trinshansha of Mars then she is a slave. If it is in the trinshansha of Saturn, then she will be interested in other men. If it is in the trinshansha of Jupiter, then she will have control on her husband. In the trinshansha of mercury then she is fickle. If it is in the trinshansha of Venus, then she will be devoid of children and will be poor.

(7) If it is in Leo and it is also in the trinshansha of Mars, then she will be a bad wife. In the trinshansha of Saturn then she will have bad manners and will indulge in sinful activities. In the trinshansha of Jupiter, she will be married to a king or a big landlord. If it is in the trinshansha of Mercury, then she will be masculine (not like a woman) in behaviour. In the trinshansha of Venus, she is attracted to others.

If girl is born in certain constellations given below then she is supposed to bring difficulties to her family members:

(1) If a girl is born in Jyestha nakshtra, then immediately after marriage her husband's brother is likely to die.

(2) If a girl born in Aslesha nakshatra, then her mother-in-law dies.

(3) If in Mool nakashatra then she is bad for her father-in-law.

(4) If it is in the Vishakha nakshatra, then she is not good for the younger brother of her husband.

The girls whose birth star is Chitra, Ardra, Ashlesha, Shatbhisha, Jyestha, Mool, Kritika or Pusya are either devoid of children or become a widow or will have still-born children. They are destered by their husbands and are poor.*

---

*The results we have indicated above should not be considered alone, but in relationship with the strength of the full horoscope, For example, one factor may be a bit negative, but there may be other factors, which are positive. After considering all of them, we should draw a conclusion about her character.

If the lords of the Ascendant, seventh house, ninth house and the sign occupied by the Moon are well placed in the signs of benefic planets, and are not combust, then the girls so born will be fortunate, good-looking and she will be worshipped by her relatives. She will be engaged in doing charitable deeds. She will do things dear to her husband. She is good in character and soft-spoken. She will beget good sons. The more the number of benefic planets which aspect the 8th house, the longer her conjugal bliss will be. (The period of conjugal bliss depends upon the benefic who occupy the 8th house or aspect the 8th house).

When the menstrual period of a woman starts (not only for the first time, but any time in life) and Moon transits the 1st, 2nd, 4th, 5th, 7th, 8th, 9th, and 12th houses (from the rising sign), and receive and aspect from Mars, then she can conceive a child during that month. If Moon is not in such a position, then she will not conceive a child during that month.

If Moon is transiting the 3rd, 6th, 10th or 11th houses in the nativity of a man and receive an aspect from Jupiter, then one should have intercourse in order to get a child. He should avoid such periods, which are banned according to the Dharamshastras (Scriptures) and conventions.

In Dharamshastras it has been mentioned the dates which should be avoided for intercourse. For example, Ekadasi, Amavasya – When the longitude of Moon is 12 degree behind the longitude of Sun, the Amavasya commences and as soon as they are in the same longitude. then Amavasya is over, Full Moon (Purnima) is when Sun and Moon are 180 degree apart; or if it is the death anniversary of father or mother, or the fifteen days of the dark half assigned to the departed forefathers (Pitra-Paksha). The best time for intercourse is when the Ascendant receives the aspect of many benefic and when Moon is also aspected by benefic.

12

Children

सुस्था विलग्नशशिनोः सुतभेशजीवाः
सुस्थाननाथशुभदृष्टियुते सुतर्क्षे।
लग्नात्मपौ यदि युतौ च मिथः सुदृष्टौ
क्षेत्रे परस्परगतौ यदि पुत्रसिद्धि॥११॥

If the lord of the 5th house, the lord of the 5th from moon and Jupiter are well placed in a horoscope, and the 5th house receives the benefic rays of its lord and of benefic planets, viz., Jupiter and Venus, Secondly, the lord of the 4th, 9th, etc. who are benefic aspect the 5th house and the 5th house is devoid of the aspects of the lords of the 6th, 8th and 12th and the Lords of the Ascendant and the 5th are together, or have exchanged houses, or mutually aspect each other with friendly aspects (sextile, trine), then the native will be blessed with a son (will have a large family and happiness from children) i.e. All these combinations indicate children.

लग्नामरेड्यशशिनां सुतभेषु पापै
र्युक्तेक्षितेष्वथ शुभैरयुतेक्षितेषु।
पापोभयेषु सुतभेषु सुतेश्वरेषु
दुस्थानगेषु न भवन्ति सुताः कथंचित्॥२॥

Now we give below the combinations which denies children, or even if the children are born then they either live away from the native or are a source of misery to him or they have short life. Happiness does not come from children.

(1) If malefic planets occupy or aspect the 5th house from the rising sign, Moon and Jupiter and no benefic planets either aspect or occupy them.

(2) If the lords of the 5th house from Ascendant, Moon, and Jupiter are placed in the 6th, 8th or 12th from Ascendant (the 6, 8, 12th houses are called Dusthana).

(3) If the 5th house from the Ascendant Moon, and Jupiter are hemmed in between malefic planets. If a malefic owns the 5th house and is posited therein, then the native will have a son, but if a benefic owns the 5th house and is posited therein together with a malefic, then the native willl have a child, but the child will not live long. The purpose of mentioning is that if a malefic planet is in its own sign, it does not diminish its good effect. However, if it is in any other sign then it spoils the good effects of that house. If Taurus, Leo, Virgo or Scorpio falls in the 5th house, then the native will have few children, and that, too, in later years.

पापे स्वर्क्षगते सुते तनयभाक् तस्मिन् सपापे पुनः
पुत्राः स्युर्बहुलाः शुभस्वभवने सोग्रे सुते पुत्रहा।
संज्ञां चाल्पसुतर्क्षमित्यलिवृषस्त्रीसिंहभानां विदुः
तद्राशौ सुतभावगेऽल्पसुतवान् कालान्तरेऽसाविति ॥३ ॥

सूर्ये चाल्पसुतर्क्षगे निधनगे मन्दे कुजे लग्नगे
लग्नाष्टव्ययगैः शनीड्यरुधिरैश्चाल्पात्मजर्क्षे सुते।
चन्द्रे लाभगते गुरुस्थितसुतस्थाने सपापे भवे-
ल्लग्नेऽनेकखगान्विते तनयभाक्कालान्तरे यत्नतः ॥४ ॥

In this sloka different combinations have been given. If one of the 3 combinations given below is present in a nativity, then the native will have children after many efforts and that too in the later years of life.

(a) If Taurus, Leo, Virgo, or Scorpio falls in the 5th house and Sun is posited in it; Saturn occupies the 8th house, and Mars is in the rising sign.

---

*If there are planets in the 2nd and the 12th from a sign, then that sign is said to be hemmed in between planets.

(b) If Saturn is in the rising sign, Jupiter is in the 8th, and Mars is in the 12th house and Taurus, Leo, Virgo and Scorpio falls in the 5th house.

(c) Moon is in the 11th house, a malefic planet in the 5th house from Jupiter, and the Rising sign is occupied by many planets.

सूर्ये नान्युते सुतर्क्षसहिते चन्द्रस्य गेहे स्थिते
भौमे वा भृगुजेऽपि वा सति सुतप्राप्ति द्वितीयस्त्रियाम्।
मन्दे वा बहुपुत्रवाञ्च्छशिनि वा सौम्येऽपि वाल्पात्मजो
देवेड्ये बहुदारिका शशिगृहे तद्वत्सुताधिष्ठिते ॥५

(1) If Sun is posited all alone in the 5th house in Cancer.

(2) If only Mars is posited in the 5th house in Cancer.

(3) If only Venus is posited in the 5th house in Cancer, then the person gets a son from the second marriage. If Cancer falls in the 5th house and only Saturn occupies it then the native will be blessed with many sons. If Mercury is in Cancer in the 5th house, the person will have few sons. If Moon occupies the 5th house in Cancer and there is no other planet with the Moon, then the native will have few sons. If exalted Jupiter is posited in the 5th house, then the native will have many daughters.

सुखास्तदशमस्थितैरशुभकाव्यशीतांशुभि-
र्व्ययाष्टतनयोदयेष्वशुभगेषु वंशक्षयः।
मदे कविविदौ मतौ गुरुरद्धिरंबुस्थितैः
सुते शशिनि नैधनव्ययतनुस्थपापैरपि ॥६ ॥

If one of the four combinations given below are taken present then there are no descendents in the family.

(1) If the 4th house is occupied by malefic, Venus is in the 7th house, and Moon is in the 10th house.

(2) If the 1st, 5th, 8th and 12th houses are occupied by malefic.

(3) If Mercury and Venus are in the 7th house, Jupiter is in the 5th house and a malefic occupies the 4th house.

(4) If Moon is in the 5th house and malefic occupy the 1st, 8th, and 12th houses from the Ascendant.

पापे लग्ने लग्नपे पुत्रसंस्थे
धीशे वीर्ये वेश्मनीन्दावपुत्रः ।
ओजर्क्षेशे पुत्रगे सूर्यदृष्टे
चन्द्रे पुत्रक्लेशभाक् स्यादसूनुः ॥७॥

We give below 2 combinations, and if any one of them takes place, then the native will have no son, or even if he has a son, then the progeny is a source of sorrow.

(1) If a malefic is the Ascendant, the lord of the rising is in the 5th the lord of the 5th is in the 3rd, and the Moon occupies the 4th house, then the native does not have a son.

(2) If Moon is in odd* sign and odd navansha and receives an aspect from sun then there is no son or sorrows on account of him.

मान्दं सुतर्क्षं यदि वाऽथबोधं
मान्द्यर्कपुत्रान्वितवीक्षितं चेत् ।
दत्तात्मजः स्यादुदयास्तनाथ-
संबन्धहीनो विबलः सुतेश ॥८॥

We give below 2 other combinations. If any one of these takes place, then the native does not beget his own son, but will adopt a son.

(1) If Gemini, Virgo, Capricorn, or Aquarius falls in the 5th house, and Mandi** or saturn aspect or as posited in the 5th house.

(2) If the lord of the 5th house is devoid of strength, that is debilitated or placed in the 6th, 8th, or 12th, or is hemmed in between malefic; Side by side the lord of the 5th is not connected with the lord of the 1st or the 7th house.

---

*Aries, Gemini, Leo, Libra, Sagittarius and Aquarius are odd signs.

**"Mandi" is also known as "Gulik".

नीचारिमूढोपगते सुतेशे
रि:फरिरन्ध्राधिपसंयुते वा।
सुतस्य नाश: कथितोऽत्र तज्ज्ञै:
शुभैरदृष्टे सुतभे सुतेशे ॥९॥

If the lord of the 5th house is debilitated, occupies the house of any enemy, is set or is posited with the lord of the 6th, 8th and 12th, then the children are destroyed. However if the lord of the 5th and the 5th house have the aspect of benefic, then the children will survive.

सुतनाथजीवकुजभास्करेषु वै
पुरुषांशकेषु च गतेषु कुत्रचित्।
मुनयो वदन्ति बहुपुत्रतां तदा
सुतनाथवीर्यवशत: सुपुत्रताम् ॥१०॥

If the lord of the 5th house, Jupiter, Mars, and Sun, (wherever they may be) occupy male navanshas then according to the sages the native will be blessed with many sons.

If the lord of the 5th is strong, then the children will be good and religious, but if the lord of the 5th is weak, then they will be a constant source of misery.

पुंराशयंशेऽ धीश्वरे पुंग्रहेन्द्रै-
र्युक्ते दृष्टे पुंग्रहे पुंप्रसूति:।
स्त्रीराश्यंशे स्त्रीग्रहैर्युक्तदृष्टे
स्त्रीणां जन्म स्यात्सुतर्क्षे सुतेशे ॥११॥

In order to judge whether a person will have daughter or sons, we give below the following:

If the 5th house falls in a male sign* and male navansha, and male planets aspect or occupy the 5th house, and the lord of the 5th house also occupies a male sign and navansha, receives an aspect of

---

*Odd signs are male and even signs are female signs.

other male planets or is posited with other male planet then the native will have many sons.

However if the 5th house falls in a female sign and female navansha, and female planets (like Venus, Moon and Mercury) and occupy or aspect the 5th house, and the lord of the 5th house is also posited in the sign and navansha of a female is aspected by female planets, then the native will have more daughters.

Generally these principles may not be found in toto in a horoscope and so only mixed effect will be visible.

बलयुक्तौ स्वगृहांशेष्वर्कसितावुपचयर्क्षगौ पुंसाम् ।
स्त्रीणां वा कुजचन्द्रौ यदा तदा संभवति संभवति गर्भः ॥१२ ॥

If in the horoscope of a man, Sun and Venus are strong in their own sign and own Navansha, and are transiting the 3rd, 6th, 10th or 11th houses from the rising sign, and in the horoscope of a woman, Mars and Moon are also situated in their own house and navanshas, and are strong as well as transiting through the 3rd, 6th, 10th or 11th, then the woman is likely to conceive a child.

अशत्रु नीचरिनवांशकैः सुतै
सुतेशयुक्तैरपि तैस्तथाविधैः ।
सुतर्क्षगैर्वा गुरुभादिनांशकात्सुते
फलैः पुत्रमितिर्विचिन्त्यते ॥१३ ॥

In this slokas, it has been indicated as to how many sons will be born. We have to observe which planet or planets occupy the 5th house, or are posited with the lord of the 5th house and out of all those, how many of them are debilitated or in a friend's or in an enemy navansha. Similarly, we have to assess the planet or planets in the 5th house from Jupiter and the lord thereof whether Jupiter and the lord of the 5th from it are in the navansha of a friend or not. Simultaneously we should also see the navansha occupied by Sun, and the planets which are in the 5th house from that navansha, the planet which owns the 5th house from that navansha - whether all of them are in the navansha of friends or not.

In this sloka it is indicated how to observe from a horoscope if a man/woman is capable of having a child or not. We will consider the horoscope of a man for this purpose. In the horoscope of a man add the longitudes* of sun, Jupiter and Venus. By adding all these we get an odd sign and navansha, then it is to be understood that the person has the full capacity for having a son (male child). If we find that only one of them (sign or navansha) is odd, and the other one is even, then the indication is that it will give mixed results. If both the sign and the navansha are even, then conclude that the man doesn't have the capacity to produce a male child and some type of deficiency is present in the semen.

Similarly, when we have to consider the horoscope of a woman, then we should add the longitudes of Moon, Mars and Jupiter. If the sun total gives an even sign and even Navansha then the girl is capable of given births. If odd, then there is only limited capacity to have children, but if both of them are odd, then she will be incapable of conceiving a child.

जीवेन्दुक्षितिजस्फटैक्यभवने युग्मे च युग्मांशके
स्त्रीणां क्षेत्रबलं वदन्ति सुतदं मिश्रे प्रयासात्फलम्।
भास्वच्छुक्रगुरुस्फटैक्यभवनेप्योजांशकेऽप्योजभे
पुंसां बीजबलं सुतप्रदमिमं मिश्रे तु मिश्रं वदेत्॥१४॥

पञ्चाघ्नाच्छशिनः स्फुटादिषुहतं भानुस्फुटं शोधये-
न्नीत्वा तत्र तिथिं सिते शुभतिथौ पुत्रोऽस्त्ययत्नादपि।
कृष्णे नास्ति सुतस्तिथेर्बलवशद्ब्रू याद्द्वयोः पक्षयोः
दर्शे च्छिद्रतिथौ च विष्टिकरणे न स्यात् स्थिराख्ये सुतः॥१५॥

We give below a second method. Multiply the longitude of Sun by 5; we should also multiple the longitude of Moon by 5. Now deduct the product so obtained for Sun from that of the Moon. The result will be called the resultant tithi• for children. Tithi is the difference

---

*Sign, degree, minute and seconds.

•For further knowledge about tithi please refer to pages 38, 39 of the "Sugam Jyotish Praveshika".

between the longitude of sun and the longitude of Moon. Half of a tithi is called a Karan. When we know the difference between Sun and Moon then we can also know the Karan.

We have explained above the method of to find tithi and karan (Tithi is also called a lunar day). If this resultant tithi is a benefic tithi, during the waxing Moon (Bright half) then it should be considered that the native will have a son without much efforts. But if the tithi falls in the dark half of Moon (waning Moon) then the possibility of having a child is reduced. We should decide whether a tithi is benefic or not only after considering the strength of that tithi. If the tithi is an amavasya, or if this gives us some tithi which is not good (chidra) then happiness from children is reduced. We should also take into account the karan. If the karan is vishti, chtuspada, kinstugna, nagav or sakuni even then happiness from children is curtailed. The name of the karanas in order are bava, balava, kaulava, taitila, gara, vanij, visti, sakuni, chatusada, naga and kinstugna.

Santan dosha Parihar

How to remove obstacles and get children?

विष्टिः स्थिरं वा करणं यदि स्यात्
कृष्णं यजेत् पौरुषसूक्तमन्त्रैः ।
पष्ठ्यां गुहाराधनमनमत्र कार्यं
यजेच्चतुर्थ्यां किल नागराजम् ॥१६ ॥

रामायणस्य श्रवणं नवम्यां
यद्यष्टमी चेच्छ्रवणव्रतं च ।
चतुदर्शी चेद्यपि रुद्रपूजा
स्याद्द्वादशी चेत्स्मृतमन्नदानम् ॥१७ ॥

तृप्तिं पितृणमिह पञ्चदश्यां
कृष्णे दशम्याः परतोऽतियत्नात् ।
पक्षत्रिभागेष्वपि नागराजं
स्कन्दं च सेवेत हरिं क्रमेण ॥१८ ॥

We have mentioned above that if the tithi is either an amavasya or an chidra tithi then the results will not be good. What is a 'chidra Tithi'. The 4th, the 6th, the 8th, the 9th, the 12th and the 14th day after amavasya, or after the full Moon are called chidra tithi. These are considered inauspicious in the above context.

We have already pointed out that if from the calculations we get a malefic tithi and karan then it denies happiness from children. We now indicate as to what should be done to overcome these malefic influences.

If by the above method the 'Karan' is Visti, (it is also called Bhadra), chatushpada, nagav, kinstughna or sakuni then we should worship Lord Krishna by reciting all the mantras of Purushsukta. If we get the 6th day from amavasya or from full Moon, then we should worship Kartik Swami. If we get the 4th tithi then we should worship the Nagaraja, the head of the snakes. If we get the 9th day, then we should hear Ramayana and recite it.

If it is the 8th day then one should fast during the month of Shravana, (during the rainly season). If the tithi is chaturdashi, the 14th day, then one should worship Rudra (Lord Sankara), and if it is the 12th day, then in order to overcome the bad effects one should donate corn and feed the poor. If the tithi comes to be amavasya, (the dark day), or the full Moon (Purnima), one must perform Shradha and do such things which satisfy the departed forefathers. If the tithi is 10th day, the 11th day, the 12th, the 13th, the 14th day of the dark half or amavasya then one should undertake intensely all the above measures in fact the sages have considered the full dark half of Moon as inauspicious and it is said that from the first day of the new Moon to the 5th day of the new Moon if we get tithi then we should worship Nagaraja, the god of snakes. If we get any tithi from the 6th day of the dark half to the 10th day of the dark half, then one should worship Kartikswami, son of Lord Siva. If we get any day during the dark half from Ekadasi (the 11th day) to the complete dark half, then one should worship and sing praises of Hari (Lord Vishnu).

पुत्रेशो रिपुनीचगोऽस्तमयगो रिःफाष्टमारिस्थित
स्तद्वत्पुत्रगृहस्थितोऽपि यदि वा दुःस्थानपस्तद्वशात्।

पुत्राभावनिदानमेव कथयेत् तत्खेचराक्रान्तभ-
प्रोक्तैर्दैवतभूरुहैरपि मृगैः सन्तानहेतुं वदेत् ॥१९॥

If the lord of the 5th house is in the sign of an enemy, debilitated, combust of posited in the 6th, 8th or 12th house from the rising sign, then there will be obstacles in begetting children. Similarly, if any planet is debilitated, in the sign of an enemy, combust, or is the lord of the 6th, 8th, or 12th house and is posited in the 5th house, then the native will have difficulties through his children or will not have any children at all. The intensity of obstacles will depend upon the number of negative combinations mentioned above.

The planet, which is obstructing from having children, will give a clue as to what have we done in the previous births. When we know that the planet obstructing, is in a particular sign then we should take appropriate measures to pacify the gods tree or spirits indicated by that sign.

द्रोहाच्छंसुपर्णयोर्नहि सुतः शापात्पितृणांरवे
रिन्दोर्मातृसुवासिनीभगवतीकोपान्मनोदोषतः।
स्वग्रामस्थितदेवतागुहरिपुज्ञात्युत्थदोषात्कुजे
शापाद्बालकृताद्बिलालवधतः श्रीविष्णु कोपाद्बुधे ॥२०॥

पारंपर्यसुरप्रियद्विजगुरुद्रोहात्फलाढ्यद्रुम-
च्छेदाद्देवगुरौ तथा सति भृगौ पुष्पद्रु मच्छेदनात्।
साध्वीगोकुलजातदोषवशतो यक्ष्यादिकामेन सा
मन्देऽश्वत्थवधाद्रुषा पितृपतेः प्रेतैः पिशाचदिभिः ॥२१॥

स्वर्भानौ सुतगे सुतेशसहिते सर्पस्य शापात्तथा
केतौ ग्राह्मणशापतश्च गुलिके प्रेतोत्थशापं वदेत्।
शुक्रेन्दू गुलिकान्वितौ यदि वधूगोहत्तिमाहुः सुते
जीवो वाथ शिखी समान्दिरिह चेंद्भू देवहत्याऽसुतः ॥२२॥

We give the reason why different planets cause obstacles in child birth:

(1) If we find that Sun is posited in the 5th house or is delaying child birth, then it should be understood that we have offended Shiva and Garuda and due to the ill feelings of the forefathers, we are not getting children.

(2) If Moon is the cause of obstacles then it should be understood that we have caused mental anguish or suffering to mother or to married woman or due to the anger of the Goddess Parvati.

(3) If Mars is causing obstacles in child birth, it means that we have caused some disobedience to Lord Kartikswami, or to the god of the village, or on account of the curses of enemies or relatives (brothers/sisters) to whom we have caused sufferings.

(4) If Mercury is causing obstacles, then it should be understood that we have killed a cat, or awe have killed many fish, or broken the eggs of birds of the curses of young children, or due to the anger of Lord Vishnu.

(5) If Jupiter is obstructing child birth, either in this life or in the previous birth, we have cut down fruit trees in full bloom, or insulted the family priest or Guru (Brahmins).

(6) If we find that Venus is the cause of obstacles in child birth, then it should be understood that the native has cut down green trees full of flowers of has caused some suffering to a cow, or incurred the curses, of a pure married woman. In this case Yakshini's ill - will is preventing children. Yakshanis are the entities that live in the 4th dimension. They live with Kuvera, the God of (treasures) wealth, who has infinite wealth in his treasures and lives below Mount Kailash.

(7) If Saturn is afflicted in the horoscope, then the native has the sin of cutting the Pipal trees (a particular type of tree on which Ghosts are supposed to reside) and the child birth is delayed on account of the curses of Ghosts, Spirits and Yamaraja.

(8) If Rahu (the North Node of Moon) is in the 5th house, or by association spoils the lord of the 5th house, then the reason is that due to the curses of a snake child birth is blocked.

(9) If it is on account of Ketu, the South Node of Moon, then the cause is that we have stolen the money and gold of a Brahman.

If Mandi is in the 5th house or with the lord of the 5th house then due to the curses of a ghost, children are denied.

(10) If both Moon and Venus are placed with Mandi in the horoscope, then it should be considered that the native has killed a cow or a young woman in his previous birth.

(11) If we find that South Node of Moon (Ketu) and Jupiter are posited in the 5th house with Mandi then the native has killed a Brahman in his previous life and so children are not born to him.

एवं हि जन्मसमये बहुपूर्वजन्म-
कर्मार्जितं दुरितमस्य वदन्ति तज्ज्ञाः ।
तत्तद्ग्रहोक्तजपदानशुभक्रिया-
भिस्तद्दोषशान्तिमिह शंसतु पुत्रसिध्द्यै ॥२३ ॥

This way planets in a horoscope indicates as to the sins one has committed in his previous birth which are obstructing child birth. It is necessary for the birth of a son, that whichever planets are causing obstacles, should be pacified by Japa, worshiping of Gods, donating the materials and various other things mentioned for that planet, as well as wearing of appropriate gem stones. [The horoscopes of birth husband and wife should be considered]. After the negative effects are eliminated then child birth can take place.

सेतुस्नानं कीर्तनं सत्कथायाः
पूजां शंभोः श्रीपतेः सद्व्रतानि ।
दानं श्राद्धं कर्जनागप्रतिष्ठां
कुर्यादेतैः प्राप्नुयात्सन्ततिं सः ॥२४ ॥

In the above Slokas it has been mentioned that different types of benefic activities a person should perform in order to overcome the malefic influences. In the present Sloka we give details of what one should resort to in order in eliminate the effect of Karmas.

One must bathe in the sea, do sankirtana, listen to the sacred stories (recite the stories in Srimad - Bhagavatam, the Gita and other religious texts). One must worship Lord Shiva and Lord Vishnu and do fastings on Ekadashis. One should donate different materials and pacify the forefathers by doing shraddha, should feed snakes with milk and install the statue of Nagaraja the serpent god. This will enable him to overcome the obstacles.

लग्नास्तपुत्रपतिजीवदशापहारे
पुत्रेक्षकस्य सुतगस्य च पुत्रसिद्धिः।
पुत्रेशराशिमथवा यमकण्टकर्क्षं
जीवेगते तनयसिद्धिरथांशभे वा॥२५॥

During the major or the minor periodic influences of one of the following, one is likely to be blessed with a son.

(1) The Lord of the Ascendant.

(2) The Lord of the 7th house.

(3) The Lord of the 5th house.

(4) Jupiter

(5) The planet which aspects the 5th house.

When Jupiter in transit through the 9th or the 5th house from the sign or navansha occupied by the lord of the 5th house or YamaKantak then also the native is likely to be blessed with a son.

लग्नाधीशः पुत्रनाथेन योगं
स्वोच्चे स्वर्क्षे चारगत्या समेति।
पुत्रप्राप्तिः स्यात्तदा लग्ननाथः
पुत्रर्क्षं वा याति धीशप्तभं वा॥२६॥

When the lord of the Ascendant (in transit). (i) Conjoins with the lord of the 5th house, (ii) is transiting its exaltation sign or (iii) is transiting its own sign, then the person can be blessed with a son.

If the lord of the rising sign passes through the 5th house, or the sign occupied by the lord of the 5th, then the period is favourable for the conception of a child.

विलग्नकामात्मजनायकानां योगात्समानीय दशां महाख्याम्।
सुतस्थतद्वीक्षकतत्पतीनां दशापहारेषु सुतोद्भवः स्यात्॥२७॥

We give below another method to find the appropriate time for the birth of a child.

Add together the sign, degrees, minutes and seconds of the lords of the 1st house, 7th house, and 5th house. We should next find which particular constellation is indicated by the sum total of the above. When the native passes through the major periodic influence of the lord which rules the above constellation and the minor period of one of the planet which (i) occupy the 5th house, (ii) or aspects the 5th house, (iii) or the lord of the 5th house, then he will be blessed with a child.

सुतपतिगुर्वोरथवा तद्युक्तराश्यंशकाधिपानां वा।
बलसहितस्य दशायामपहारे वा सुतप्राप्तिः ॥२८॥

Another method which indicate child-birth is given over here. Find the strongest planet out of the following:

(i) Lord of the 5th, (ii) the Lord of the sign occupied by the lord of the 5th, (iii) the navansha lord of the sign occupied by the lord of the 5th, (iv) Jupiter; (v) the lord of the sign occupied by Jupiter; and (vi) the lord of the navansha occupied by Jupiter. The strongest planet out of the above will give a son during its major or minor periodic influence.

जीवे तु जीवात्मजनाथभांशक-
त्रिकोणगे पुत्रजनिर्भवेन्नृणाम्।
अथान्यशास्त्रेण च जन्मकालतो
निरूपयेत्सन्ततिलक्षणं बुधः ॥२९

Another method of knowing the time of child birth is given below:

Look at the 5th house from Jupiter. Consider now the sign and navansha occupied by the lord of the 5th from Jupiter. When Jupiter transits the 5th and 9th house from that sign and navansha, then one is blessed with a son. This is on the basis of transit. Some texts however states that the time of child birth should be arrived at only from the radical position of planets at the time of birth.

जन्मनक्षत्रनाथस्य प्रत्यर्याक्षाधिपस्य च।
स्फुटयोगं गते जीवे त्रिकोणे वा सुतोद्भवः ॥३०॥

Look to the nakshatra occupied by the Moon. Add the longitudes (sign, degree, minutes and seconds) of the lord of that nakshatra and the lord of the 5th nakshatra from the Moon's nakshatra, when Jupiter transits that sign (and degree, minutes and seconds) or the 5th or 9th from the sign the child birth take place.

निषेकलग्नाद्दिनपस्तृतीये
राशौ यदा चारवशादुपैति।
आधानलग्नादथवा त्रिकोणे
रवौ यदा जन्म वदेन्नराणाम्॥३१॥

Time for Child Birth

When will the child be born?

(1) When sun transits the 3rd sign from the sign occupied by Moon in which the child conceived.

(2) When Sun transits the 5th or the 9th sign from the sign rising at the time of conception.

आधानलग्नात्सुतभेशजन्म
भाग्येऽपि वा पुण्यवशाच्च वाच्यम्।
आधानलग्ने शुभदृष्टियोगे
दीर्घायुरैश्वर्ययुतो नरः स्यात्॥३२

If the birth is in the 9th or 5th from the sign rising at the time of conception, then it should be concluded that this birth is on account of the good deeds committed by the native.

If the rising sign at the time of conceiving is strong and benefic occupy it or aspect it, then the child born, will be long-lived and prosperous. The Ascendant at the time of conceiving is called 'the Adhan Lagna'.

तत्कालेन्दुद्वादांशे मेषात्तावति भेऽपि वा।
तस्मात्तावति भे वापि जन्मचन्द्रं वदेद्बुधः ॥३३॥

Calculate the longitude of the Moon and its 12th division when the child was conceived. Next count the same number of 12th division from Aries onwards and whichever sign comes, will be the sign occupied by Moon at birth.

प्रश्नात्मजस्वीकरणोपनीतिकन्याप्रदानाभिनवार्तवेषु।
आधानकालेऽपि च जन्मतुल्यं फलं वदेज्जन्मविलग्नतश्च ॥३४॥

Whatever principles related to children have been mentioned from the nativity should also be used from the following:

(i) The Horary chart i.e. the chart calculated for the time of asking a question,

(ii) The time of adopting a child.

(iii) The time of the Upanayan, the sacred thread ceremony.

(iv) The time of marriage of a girl.

(v) The horoscope calculated for the time when a girl commences her first menstrual period.

(vi) The horoscope erected for the time of conceiving.

In all the above types of horoscopes, equal importance should be given both to the Ascendant and the Moon chart (sign occupied by Moon should be used as the first house).

13

Ayur Bhav(Longevity)

जाते कुमारे सति पूर्वमार्यै
रायुर्विचिन्त्यं हि ततः फलानि।
विचारणीय गुणिनि स्थितेतद्
गुणाः समस्ताः खलु लक्षणज्ञैः ॥१॥

केचिद्यथाधानविलग्नमन्ये शीर्षोदयं भूपतनं हि केचित्।
होराविदश्चेतनकाययोन्योर्वियोगकालं कथयन्ति लग्नम् ॥२॥

आद्वादशाब्दान्नरयोनिजन्मना–
मायुष्कला निश्चययितुं न शक्यते।
मात्रा च पित्रा कृतपापकर्मणा
बालग्रहैर्नाशमुपैति बालकः ॥३॥

आद्ये चतुष्के जननीकृताघै
र्मध्ये च पित्रार्जितपापसङ्घैः।
बालस्तदन्त्यासु चतुःशरत्सु
स्वकीयदोषैः समुपैति नाशम् ॥४॥

When a child is born then first of all his age should be determined and after that other factors should be attended to. When we mention the word age, it does not mean how old is he at present because we already know the child is just born. But it is related to the longevity, the life span of the child, whether he has long life, medium life or what? If there are other Rajayogas in the horoscopes, then with the help of astrologers they should be discussed after his longevity has been determined.

What time is to be taken as the time of birth? Some people take the time as the time when the child comes into the womb. Other people take the time when (i) the head comes out from the body of the mother and that is considered the main time. But still some people are of the opinion that (ii) when the full body comes out that should be taken as the time of birth because the child has come into being. (iii) The other opinion of Astrologers is that when the emblical cord is cut, that should be taken as the time of birth. Because then the child is suppose to have an independent identity and is separate from the mother.

Until the age of 12, the longevity can not be established with firmness and determination. The reason is that even though mathematical process indicates that the child will have long life but until the age of 12, he has to bear the karmas of his father and mother. Due to the bad deeds, sinful activities of the parents not only in this life time but in the past life, can cause danger and death to a child in early part of life. The indication of these will be available in the horoscope of mother and father. Due to certain planets in the chart of a child called 'Balarishta', life span is affected in early part of life i.e. in childhood.

Until four years of age, it is mother sins which may cause untimely demise of a baby. From the age of five years to the age of eight years it is due to sinful deeds of father that the child may not live and then the next four years between 9 to 12 years the child is affected by his own deeds of the previous life and does not survive. So until the age of twelve years first to four years are due to the destiny of the mother, the next four from that of the father, and the last four by the deeds in the past life of the child himself will affect him.

तद्दोषशान्त्यै प्रतिजन्मतार-
माद्वादशाब्दं जपहोमपूर्वम्।
आयुष्करं कर्म विधाय ताता
बाल चिकित्सादिभिरेव रक्षेत् ॥५॥

अष्टौ बालारिष्टमादौ नाराणां
योगारिष्टं प्राहुरतिंशति स्यात्।
अल्पं चाद्वात्रिंशतं मध्यमायु-
श्चायप्तत्याः पूर्णमायुः शतान्तम् ॥६॥

नृणां वषशतं ह्यायुस्तस्मिंस्त्रेधा विभज्यते।
अल्पं मध्यं दीर्घमायुरित्येतत्सर्वसम्मतम् ॥७॥

Every year during the lunar date of birth of the child (according to the cycle of the Moon), religious rites including Japa, fire sacrifice etc. for pacifying the ill effects of the deeds of the previous life should be performed. This should be done until the age of twelve years is attained. It is also highly recommended for the father that in order to preserve the life of the child, he should consult doctors and use other methods of increasing the longevity and the health of the child.

From birth to eight years is called the Balaristhta*. From the age of eight years to twenty years is called the yogarishta. From twenty years to thirty-two years of age is called short life (Alpayu). From thirty-two years to seventy years medium life- Madhyayu. From seventy year to 100 years and more is called Dheergayu or Poornayu.* long life.

मृत्युः स्यादि्दनमृत्युरुग्विषघटीकालेऽथ तिष्येऽबुभे
तातम्बासुतमातुलान्पद्रवशात्त्वाष्ट्रे च हन्यात्तथा
मूलर्क्षे पितृमातृवंशविलयं तस्यान्त्यपादे श्रियं
सार्पे व्यस्तमिदं फलं न शुभसम्बन्धं विलग्नं यदि ॥८॥

If the birth of a child is in Dinmrityu - Death of the day, "or Dinrog" (disease) or in the "Vish Ghatikaal", then the child will die very early.

---

*The planetary configurations in a horoscope which can cause sickness and death to children is called Balarishta.

For example– Waning Moon which is weak is in the 6th or 8th house. Then the lunar date, day of the week, constellation, planet etc. which cause negative things, are called 'Yogarishta'.

1. Din Mirtyu

What is 'Dinmrityu' - like this is a name called Dinmrityu. Mrityu means- Death, Din means- Day. This is a combination of particular quarter of a constellation and the birth time. If the birth is in the constellation of Dhanistha and Hasta, the first quarter; The second quarter of the constellation Vishakha and Ardra; The 3rd quarter of Uttra Bhadrapada and Aslesha; and the 4th quarter of Bharani and Mool, and the birth is in the day time then it is called Dinmrityu. If the birth is at night then this negative matter does not apply.

2. Din Rog

This also is a combination of the time of the birth and particular quarter of a constellations Aslesha. The first quarter of Aslesha and Uttra Bhadrapadh; the second quarter of Bharani and Mool; The third quarter of Uttara Phalguni and Sravana and the fourth quarter of Swati and Mrigsiras and if the birth is in the day time then it is called Din Roga. If the birth is at night then this does not apply.

3. Vish Gahtis

In every constellation four Ghatikas. (1 Ghaties = 24 minutes) is called the 'Vish Ghati Kaal'. Vish means- 'poison' and Ghati is a method of measurement of time and Kaal means 'duration'. These are given below:

Constellation		Ghaties
Ashwini	-	50-54 Ghaties.
Bharani	-	24-28 Ghaties.
Krittika	-	30-34 Ghaties.
Rohini	-	40-44 Ghaties.
Mrigsiras	-	14-18 Ghaties.
Ardra	-	21-25 Ghaties.
Punarvasu	-	30-34 Ghaties.
Pushya	-	20-24 Ghaties.
Aslesha	-	32-36 Ghaties.
Magha	-	30-34 Ghaties.
Purva Phalguni	-	20-24 Ghaties.

Uttara Phalguni	-	18-22 Ghaties.
Hasta	-	21-25 Ghaties.
Chitra	-	20-24 Ghaties.
Swati	-	14-18 Ghaties.
Vishakha	-	14-18 Ghaties.
Anuradha	-	10-14 Ghaties.
Jestha	-	14-18 Ghaties.
Mool	-	56-60 Ghaties.
Purvashad	-	24-28 Ghaties.
Uttarashad	-	20-24 Ghaties.
Sarwan	-	10-14 Ghaties.
Dhanishta	-	10-14 Ghaties.
Satabisaj	-	18-22 Ghaties.
Purva Bhadrapada	-	16-20 Ghaties.
Uttra Bhadrapada	-	24-28 Ghaties.
Revati Bhadrapadth	-	30-34 Ghaties.

These are for the 27 constellations. The Vish Ghati Kaal is supposed to prevail when in the constellation of Ashwini 50 Ghaties are over and the next 4 Ghaties are prevailing i.e. until the 54 Ghaties. Similarly it should be understood at all places.

If the birth is in the first quarter of Pusya - Purvashad or Chitra then it may cause death of the child's father; If the birth is in the second quarter of the constellations mentioned above then the death of mother can happen. If the birth is in the third quarter then the child may not survive; and if it is in the fourth quarter then the native's Maternal Uncle may die. If the ascendant is not connected with benefic planets and birth is in the Mool or Aslesha Constellation then the following is the result.

Mool (1st Quarter)	Aslesha (4th Quarter)	Death of father
Mool (2nd Quarter)	Aslesha (3rd Quarter)	Death of Mother.
Mool (3rd Quarter)	Aslesha (2nd Quarter)	The entire family is destroyed.

Mool (4th Quarter)	Aslesha (1st Quarter)	Increase of wealth and prosperity.

पापाप्तेक्षितराशिसन्धिजनने सद्यो विनाशं ध्रुवं
गण्डान्ते पितृमातृहा शिशुमृतिर्जीवेद्यदि क्ष्मापतिः ।
जातः सन्धिचतुष्टयेऽप्यशु भसंयुक्तेक्षिते स्यान्मृति-
मृत्योर्भागगते च सा सति विधौ केन्द्रेऽष्टमे वा मृतिः ॥९॥

If the birth is at the juncture of two signs and the sign is also occupied by malefic or receives aspect of malefic then early death of the child should be concluded. If the birth is in Gandanta then the death of father, mother or the child himself takes place, and if the child survies then his propsperity and life is like that of a king.

In between Aries and Pisces i.e. end of Pisces and beginning of Aries of in the middle of Cancer and Leo, in the middle of Scorpio and Sagittarius. All these are called Gandanta.** What is a juncture or Middle? It means where one sign is ending and the second sign is commencing could be exactly the 30 degrees or the beginning of the Zero (0). These children who are born in the joint of two signs when the malefics also conjoin with or aspect the joints of two sign, they do not live long.

If Moon is in an angle or in the 8th house and is in the part of death then also the child dies early. In which sign and in which Navansha, Moon and the ascendant are said to be in the part of death. This has been explained in the next two slokas.

चान्द्रं रूपं लोकशूरो वरज्ञः
कुड्ये चित्रं भाग्यलोके मुखानाम् ।

---

1. Please see our Book 'Sugam Jyotish Praveshika'.

2. Sign- In the original Sloka it is not mentioned if it is the sign rising or it is the sign occupied by Moon. Our opinion is that it is related to sign rising i.e. the ascendant.

**One opinion is that the Ascendant, Sun and Moon all of them should be at juncture.

मेने राज्यं मुत्युभागाः प्रदिष्टा
मेषादीनां वर्णसंख्यैर्हिमांशोः ॥१०॥

दानं धेनो रुद्र रौद्री मुखेन
भाग्या भानुर्गोत्र जाया नखेन।
पुत्री नित्यं मुत्युभागाः क्रमेण
मेषादीनां तेषु जाता गतायुः ॥११॥

In which part or in what degrees the ascendant or the Moon should be posited to be called in the 'part of death' has been given in Table below.

Moon Part (Degree)	Ascendant Parts (Degree)	Signs
26	8	Aries
12	9	Taurus
13	22	Gemini
25	22	Cancer
24	25	Leo
11	14	Virgo
26	4	Libra
14	23	Scorpio
13	18	Sagittarius
25	20	Capricorn
5	21	Aquarius
12	10	Pisces

If at birth Moon or the ascendant are in these degree then the child is short lived.

रन्ध्रे केन्द्रेषु पापैरुदयनिधनगैर्वाथ लग्नास्तयोर्वा
लग्नेऽब्जेवोग्रमध्ये व्ययमृतिरिपुगे दुर्बले शीतभानौ।
क्षीणेन्दौ साशुभे वा तनुमदगुरुधीभाजि रन्ध्रास्तागोग्रै-
मृत्युः स्यादाशु केन्द्र न यदि शुभखगाः सद्युतिर्वीक्षणं वा ॥१२॥

In the following combinations also death takes place early.

1. Malefic in angles or in the 8th house.
2. Malefic in the ascendant and in the 8th house.
3. Malefic in the ascendant and in the 7th house.
4. The ascendant and Moon is hemmed in between Malefic.
5. Weak Moon in the 6th, 8th or 12th houses.
6. Waning Moon with Malefic in the 1st, 5th, 7th or 9th house and
7. Ugra or Malefic in the 7th and 8th houses.

In the seven conditions given above the child dies early. But if benefic conjoin with or aspect it (ascendant, moon or malefic) then or if benefic planet are in angles then the Yogas which are supposed to cause early death are neutralised.

जन्मेशोऽथ विलग्नपो यदि भवेद्दुस्थोऽबलो वत्सरै-
स्तद्राशिप्रमितैश्च मारयति तन्मासैर्दृगाणधिपः ।
अंशेशो दिवसैस्तथा यदि मृतिर्द्वित्र्यादियोगान्बहू-
नाचोच्य प्रवदेत्सुताष्टमगतैः पापैरिष्टं शिशोः ॥१३ ॥

1. If lord of the 1st and lord of the Moon sign are weak and are place in dusthan which is the 6th, 8th or 12th house, then the numerical number of the sign in which such ascendant lord or the lord of the Moon sign is placed gives the age of the child i.e.-

For	Aries	-	1year,
For	Taurus	-	2 years,
For	Gemini	-	3 years and

   this way the counting should be done.

2. If the decanet lord of the ascendant or the Moon sign are weak and placed in 6th, 8th or 12th house, then in whatever sign they are the child lives upto the number of months indicated by the number of the sign.

   For example-

In Aries	-	1 month,
Taurus	-	2 months,
Gemini	-	3 months and so on.

3. If the Navansha lord of the ascendant or the Navansha lord of the Moon sign is weak and placed in 6th, 8th or 12th house, then the child lives only upto the days indicated by the number of sign in which these are placed.

In the above as to three combinations which is the strongest should be considered and also observe, which are the malefic planets in the 5th and 8th from the ascendant, and then the consideration of the longivity of the child should be done.

लग्नेद्वोस्तदधीशयोरपि मिथो लग्नेशरन्ध्रेशयो-
द्रेक्काणत्स्वनवांशकादपि मिथस्तद्द्वादशांशात्क्रमात्।
आयुर्दीर्घसमाल्पतां चरनगव्द्यंगैश्चरेऽ स्थिरे
ब्रूयाद्द्वन्द्वचरस्थिररुभयभैः स्थास्नुद्विदेहाटनैः ॥१४॥

See if the following are movable, fixed or dual?

(a) The decanet sign of ascendant and the decanet sign of Moon. If both of them are in movable sign or one is in a fixed sign and the other one in a dual sign then the native will have long life. If both of them are in fixed signs or one is in a movable and other one in dual sign then short life. If both are in dual signs or one is in a movable sign and the other one in a fixed sign then medium life should be inferred.

(b) Here the Navansha sign of the lord of the ascendant and the Navansha sign of Moon sign are considered. If both are in movable signs or one is in fixed and the other one is dual then long life. If both are in fixed or one is in movable and the other one is in dual sign then short life. If both of them are in dual signs or one is in movable and other one is in fixed sign then medium life.

(c) Here the dwadashansha signs occupied by the lords of the ascendant and 8th house are considered. If both the signs are movable or one is fixed and the other is a dual sign then long life. If both are in fixed sign or one is in movable and other one is in dual sign then short life. If both are in dual signs or one is in a movable and the other one is in fixed sign then medium life.

After taking into consideration all the three mentioned above the majority decision should be decided.*

लग्नाधीशशुभाः क्रमाद्बहुसमाल्पायूंषि केन्द्रादिगाः
रन्ध्रेशोग्रखगास्तथा यदि गता व्यस्तं विदध्युः फलम्।
जन्मोशाष्टमनाथयोरुदयपच्छिद्रेशयोमैंत्रतो
भास्वल्लग्नपयाश्चियरायुरहितेऽल्पायुः समे मध्यमः ॥१५॥

If the lord of the ascendant and all the benefic plancts are in angles then the native has long life; If they are into succeedent houses then medium life, and if they are in cadent houses then short life. If lord of the 8th house and all the malefics are in angles then short life in succeedent houses then medium life, and in cadent houses then long life.

See if the following are mutual friends, neutrals or enemies;

(a) The lord of the Moon sign and the lord of the 8th sign occupied by Moon with each other.

(b) Lord of the 1st and the lord of the 8th with each other.

(c) Lord of the 1st and Sun with each other.

If they are mutual friends then long life; if they are neutrals then medium life, and if they are enemies then short life.

लग्नाधिपो लग्ननवांशनायको
जन्मेश्वरो जन्मनवांशनायकः।
स्वस्वादिष्टमेशाद्यपि चेद्बलान्विता
दीर्घायुषः स्युर्विपरीतमन्यथा॥१६॥

If the lord of the ascendant is stronger then its 8th house lord, if the lord of the Navansha falling in the ascendant is stronger then its 8th lord, the lord of the the Moon sign is stronger then its 8th lord; and the Navansha occupied by Moon if its lord is stronger then its

*Comments- If the three indications which have been considered in Sloka No. 14 are all different then according to Gemini Padhati the longevity should be considered. For the method propagated by Gemini, please see-page-126 of Sugam Jyotish Praveshika.

lord of the 8th then long life to the native. But if lord of the ascendant etc. are comparatively weaker then the lord of their 8th house then short life.

The principle that has been given above for that we will also need the Navansha Chart besides the birth chart. The following four should be stronger then their own lord of the 8th house.

1. Lord of the first (Ascendant).
2. Lord of the Navansha falling in the ascendant.
3. The lord of the sign occupied by Moon at birth.
4. Lord of the Navansha occupied by Moon

Only then long life should be concluded.

लग्नेश्वरादतिबली निधनेश्वरोऽसौ
केन्द्रस्थितो निधनरिः फगतैश्च पापैः।
तस्यायुरल्पमथवा यदि मध्यमायु-
रुत्साहसंकटवशात्परमायुरेति ॥१७॥

If compared to the lord of the Ascendant, the lord of the 8th is very strong and is placed in an angle i.e. in the 1st, 4th, 7th or 10th and the malefic are in the 8th or 12th houses, then the native has short life or will have only medium life; even if he attains long life, his life will be in danger like he may be sick and will have constant problems.

नरोऽल्पायुर्योगे प्रथमभगणे नश्यति शने-
र्द्वितीये मध्यायुर्यदि भवति दीर्घायुषि सति।
तृतीये निर्याणं स्फुटजशनिगुर्वर्कहिमगून्
दशां भुक्तिं कष्टापि वदति निश्चित्य सुमतिः ॥१८॥

Add together the sign, degree, minute and seconds of the following planets. Sun, Moon, Jupiter and Saturn.

Illustration:

In the example horoscope we have the four planets-

Sun-	7 signs,	26 degrees.
Moon-	11 signs	20 degrees.

Jupiter	6 signs	14 degrees.	
Saturn -	0 sign	7 degrees.	
Total	26	7	or 2 signs, 7 degrees.

So we get 26 signs, 7 degress or 2 signs and 7 degrees i.e. the 7 degrees of Gemini. If the native has short life then when Saturn comes in transit to Gemini in the first cycle in the horoscope and when it comes to exactly the 7 degrees of Gemini, then death will come to the native. If it is medium life then when Saturn comes during the second time to the 7 degrees of Gemini then death will come, and if the native has long life then when Saturn in transit comes, third time to the 7 degrees of Gemini then death will take place. When consideration of this transit is taken at that time the major and minor periods of the planet under which the native is passing through should also be considered.

सपापो लग्नेशो रविहतरुचिर्नीचरिपुगो
यदा दुःस्थानेषु स्थितिमुपगतो गोचरवशात्।
तनौ वा तद्योगो यदि निधनमाहुस्तनुभृतां
नवांशाद्द्रेक्काणाच्छिशिरकरलग्नादपि वदेत् ॥१९॥

If the lord of the 1st house is placed with a malefic and debilitated or in the sign of an enemy and is simultaneously combust then when in transit it goes to the 6th, 8th or 12th or comes to the 1st house or has a relationship with the 1st then, death comes to the native. This principle about the lord of the 1st which has been mentioned above, should also be applied to the lord of the Navansha of the ascendant, the lord of the Decanet in the ascendant as well to the lord of Moon sign*.

शशी तदारूढगृहाधिपश्च
लग्नाधिनाथश्च यदा त्रयोऽमी
गुणाधिकाः सद्ग्रहदृष्टियुक्ता
गुणाधिकं तं कथयन्ति कालम् ॥२०॥

When Moon, the lord of the Moon sign and the lord of the ascendant, all three of them, are strong in transit and are aspected by benefic then that period will be an excellent period for the native. Here it should also be considered that the lord of the ascendant, Moon and the lord of the Moon sign i.e. the dispositer of the Moon, wherever they are posited in the birth chart are also receiving benefic aspect from the transiting planets.

For example– If some one has Leo rising and Sun is in Scorpio then not only when Sun in transit is strong but the radical Sun should also receive a beneficial aspect from Jupiter and other benefic planets.

लग्नाधिपोऽतिबलवानशुभैरदृष्टः
केन्द्रस्थितः शुभखगैरवलोक्यमानः ।
मृत्युं विहाय विदधाति स दीर्घमायुः
सार्द्धं गुणैर्बहुभिरूर्जितराजलक्ष्म्या ॥२१ ॥

If the lord of the 1st house is very strong, does not receive any aspect from malefic, is posited an angle and is receiving aspect from benefic, then such a strong lord of the 1st house obstructs Marak Planets, (Fatal Planets) and besides long life it also confers various attributes like wealth, prosperity and luxuries.

सर्वातिशाय्यतिबलः स्फुरदंशुजालो
लग्ने स्थितः प्रशमयेत् सुरराजमन्त्री ।
एको बहूनि दुरितानि सुदुस्तराणि
भक्त्या प्रयुक्त इव चक्रधरे प्रणामः ॥२२ ॥

If strong Jupiter is posited in the ascendant (it should not be combust) then it nullifies many negative effects like, if only one time a person with respect bows to lord Vishnu pays his humble obesiance then many calamaties and danger are wipedout.

*In Sloka No. 19 many things have been mentioned. When in transit planets come to the 6th, 8th, 12th or 1st house but generally planets always keep on transiting these houses. Therefore in our view if some one is sick or we have to consider in a pin point manner his longevity then only this sloka should be used.

मूर्तेस्त्रिकोणगमकण्टकेषु रवीन्दुजीवर्क्षनवांशसंस्थ: ।
सुकर्मकृन्नित्यमशेषदोषान्मुष्णाति वर्द्धिष्णरनुष्णरश्मि: ॥२३ ॥

If the birth is during the bright half i.e. the waxing Moon and Moon is placed in the 1st, 4th, 5th, 7th, 9th, 10th or 11th house and is also in Navansha in Cancer, Leo, Sagittarius or Pisces, then it nullifies many negative things in the chart and is beneficial.

केन्द्रत्रिकोणनिधनेषु न यस्य पापा
लग्नाधिप: सुरगुरुश्च चतुष्टयस्थौ ।
भुक्त्वा सुखानि विविधानि सुपुण्यकर्मा
जीवेच्च वत्सरशतं स विमुक्तरोग: ॥२४ ॥

If in the horoscope of a person there are no malefic in an angle or trine or in the 8th house and the lord of the 1st house and Jupiter are in angular position then such a person is engaged in doing Punya Karma. He enjoys many types of happiness and lives to 100 years of age in good health.

श्रीपत्युदीरितदशाभिरथाष्टवर्गात्-
यत्कालचक्रदशायोडुदशाप्रकारात् ।
सम्यक्स्फुटाभिहतया क्रिययाप्तवाक्या-
दायुर्बुधो वदतु भूरिपरीक्ष्या च ॥२५ ॥

If a horoscope according to the learned Gurus, calculation of planets, periodic influences of planets and all types of mathematical calculation given by Sripathi, as well as Ashtakvargas, Kalchakra Dashas etc. should be considered thoroughly and then longevity should be decided.

14

Decision about Disease

रोगस्य चिन्तामपि रोगभावस्थितैर्ग्रहैर्वा व्ययमृत्युसंस्थैः ।
रोगेश्वरेणापि तदन्वितैर्वा द्वित्र्यादिसम्वादवशाद्वदन्तु ॥१ ॥

In this chapter, disease, death, previous birth and next life have been considered.

1. The type of disease should be decided from the planets given below:

   (a) The planet posited in the 6th house.

   (b) The planet in the 8th house.

   (c) The planet in the 12th house.

   (d) The lord of the 6th house.

   (e) The planet conjoined with the lord of the 6th house.

   When a common type of disease is indicated after examining and taking into account all the factors and the various planets only then a correct and logical conclusion should be drawn as to the type of disease which might affect the native.

पितोष्णज्वरतापदेहतपनापस्मारहृत्क्रोडज-
व्याधीन्वक्ति रविर्दृगार्त्यरिभयं त्वग्दोषमस्थिस्रुतिम् ।
काष्ठाग्न्यस्त्रविषार्तिदारतनयव्यापच्चतुष्पाद्भयं
चोरक्ष्मापतिधर्मदेवफणभृद्भूतेशभूतं भयम् ॥२ ॥

निद्रालस्यकफातिसारपिटकाः शीतज्वरं चन्द्रमाः

श‍ृङ्ग्यब्जाहतिमग्निमान्द्यमरूचिं योषिव्द्यथाकामिला: ।
चेत:शान्तिमसृग्विकारमुदकाद्भीतिं च बालग्रहाद्
दुर्गाकिन्नरधर्मदेवफणभृद्यक्ष्याश्च भीतिं वदेत् ॥३ ॥

तृष्णासृक्कापपित्तज्वरमनलविषास्त्रार्तिकुष्ठाक्षिरोगान्
गुल्मापस्मारमज्जाविहतिपरुषतापमिकादेहभङ्गान् ।
भपारिस्तेनपीडां सहलसुतसुहृद्वैरियुद्धं विधत्ते
रक्षोगन्धर्वघोरग्रहभयवमनीसूनुरूर्ध्वाङ्गरोगम् ॥४ ॥

भ्रान्तिं दुर्वचनं दृगामयगलघ्राणोत्थरोगं ज्वरं
पित्तश्लेष्मसमीरजं विषमपि त्वग्दोषपाण्ड्वामयान् ।
दु:स्वप्नं च विचर्चिकाग्निपतने पारुष्यबन्धश्रमान्
गन्धर्वक्षितिहर्म्यवाहिभिरपि ज्ञो वक्ति पीडां ग्रहै: ॥५ ॥

गुल्मान्त्रज्वरशोकमोहकफजान् श्रोत्रार्तिमोहामयान्
देवस्थाननिधिप्रपीडनमहीदेवेशशापोद्भवम् ।
रोगं किन्नरयक्षदेवफणभृद्विद्याधराद्युद्भवमं
जीव: सूचयति स्वयं बुधगुरूत्कृष्टापचारोद्भवम् ॥६ ॥

पाण्डुश्लेष्ममरुत्प्रकोपनयनव्यापत्प्रमेहामयान्
गुह्यस्यामयमूत्रकृच्छ्रमदनव्यापत्तिशुक्लस्रुतिम् ।
वारस्त्रीकृतदेहकान्तिविहतिं शोषामयं योगिनी–
यक्षीमातृगणाद्भयं प्रियसुहृद्भङ्गं सित: सूचयेत् ॥७ ॥

वातश्लेष्मविकारपादविहतिं चापत्तितन्द्राश्रमान्
भ्रान्तिं कुक्षिरुगन्तरुष्णभृतकध्वंसं च पार्श्वाहतिम् ।
भार्यापुत्रविपतितमङ्गविहतिं हृत्तापमर्कात्मजो
वृक्षाश्मक्षतिमाह कश्मलगणै: पीडां पिशाचादिभि: ॥८ ॥

स्वर्भानुर्हृदि तापकुष्ठविमतिव्याधिं विषं कृत्रिमं
पादार्तिं च पिशाचपन्नगभयं भार्यातनूजापदम्।
ब्रह्मक्षत्रविरोधशत्रुजभयं केतुस्तु संसूचयेत्
प्रेतोत्थं च भयं विषं च गुलिका देहार्तिमाशौचजम्॥९॥

When sun signifies any sickness, then the following types of disease can occur, or in other words sun signifies the following disease and sufferings.

Troubles due to bile, High fever. Burning Sensation (and heat) in the body. Epilepsy. Heart problems. Eye problems. Sickness involving portion below naval and/or wombs (in females). Skin problems. Disease related to the bones. Fears from enemies. Danger from woods. Pains and danger from fire, arms, or poison. Sufferings and insults from wife and sons. Danger from thieves and cattle. Fear of snakes. Fear from Kings, Yama and Rudra.

Moon causes the following diseases and sufferings:

Sleeping sickness (too much sleep, no sleep viz. Insomnia, or walking during sleep. Laziness. Phlegm. Dysentery. Wounds, carbuncle. Fever due to cold or malaria. Fear from animals with horns or animals resulting in Water (crocodiles etc.) Digestive Problems due to liver. No appetite or (fear of food like anorexia). Mental anguish due to women. Jaundice. Blood disorders (impurities of blood). Fear from water. Mental fatigue. Fear (or curse) of Durga - Kinnar - Yama - Snakes and Yakshini.

Mars causes the following diseases and problems:

Thirst (desire to drink water all the time). Problems due to Pitta or Vat disorders. Fever due to excessive bile, fear from fire, poison or arms. Leprosy. Eye disease. Appendicitis or wounds inside the stomach. Loss of blood. Lack of substances inside bones - disease related to bones. Itching. Skin problems (uneven skin and patches or black heads). Deformity or loss of a portion of body. Fear from kings, fire and robbers. Quarrels with brother, friends and sons. Fighting with Enemies. Fear of Rakshas (Demons), Gandharvas and malefic planets and disease on the upper portion of body.

Mercury gives the following disease and sufferings:

Mental derangement, illogical thinking, no rationality, mental apprehensions, unnecessary fear, loss of memory, forgetting the right things and remembering wrong facts and figures – all these are signs of a weak mind. To utter bad and insulting remarks. Eye problem. Throat problems. Disease related to nose. Disease arising out of the disorder of Vata, Pitta, Kapha, Kapha. Sickness due to poisoning. Skin disease. Jaundice (Liver problems). Bad dreams and itching. Fear of getting burnt; the native behaves harshly with others or others threat him this way. Hard work, nervous breakdown. Disease due to Gandharva.

All these take place due to Mercury

Now we speak of disease and problems arising due to Jupiter:

Ulcer, Appendicitis, Typhoid Fainting - these diseases are caused due to phelgm disorders, Phlegm is ruled by Jupiter. Ear disease, problems related to temples - court cases involving temple trust, property etc. Troubles due to the curse of Brahmins. Legal cases or disputes related to a treasure, trust or banks and financial institutions. Troubles created by Vidyadhars, Yaksha - Kinnars, Gods or Bad behaviour towards Gurus, Respected persons and elders, or result of not doing ones duties towards these persons – will bring negative results during the major and minor periods of Jupiter or due to transit of Jupiter.

Now we speak of the type of disease and problems due to Venus:

Yellow appearance due to anemia. Disease caused by disorder of vat and kapha (Wind and phlegm) - Eye problem, urinary problems. Venereal and gynecological disease. Prostrate problems, Syphilis etc. Semen disorder. Impotency. Lack of luster on the face and weakness in body due to excessive indulgence in Sex. Weight loss. Fear from yogini, yakshini and Matrikas. If Venus is causing troubles than break in friendship also occurs.

Now we deal with the disease and troubles, which occur on account of Saturn:

Disease due to disorder of vat and kapha (Wind and Phlegm). Lameness or pains in legs. Tiredness due to excessive work (mal nutrition - problems). Mental apprehension and fears which has no basis (The same as is indicated by Mercury). Disease in wombs (Hanks). Dryness inside the body. Trouble on account of servants - servants leave the job or are treacherous. Problems related to wife and sons. Injury in some part of body. Mental anguish, injury due to a tree or stone. Troubles cause by bad spirits and calamities.

Now we talk of the suffering and disease worries on account of Rahu:

Heart problem. Heat in the heart (or Jealousy). Leprosy. Bad mental thinking - bad ideals. Mental derangement - fears. Disease due to poison - reaction of medicine, allergy etc. Pains in legs of injury. Problems to wife and sons or troubles on account of them. Fears from serpents and bad spirits.

Now the physical and mental problems and sufferings due to Ketu is as followers:

Trouble on account of fight with Brahmins and Shatriyas, fear from enemies.

Now we speak of troubles on account of 'Gulik'. If Gulik is in the 6th house or placed with the lord of the 6th house then sickness in the body, death of a relative or fear from Ghosts.

मन्दारान्वितवीक्षिते व्ययधने चन्द्राणौ चाक्षिरुक्
शौर्यायाङ्गिरसो यमारसहिता दृष्टा यदि श्रोत्ररुक्।
सोग्रे पञ्चमभे भवेदुदररुग्रन्ध्रारिनाथन्विते
तद्वत्सप्तमनैधने सदगुरुच्छुक्रे च गुह्यामयः ॥१०॥

षष्ठेऽर्केऽप्यथवाष्टमे ज्वरभयं भौमे च केतौ व्रणं
शुक्र गुह्यरुजं क्षयं सुरगुरौ मन्दे च वातामयम्।
राहौ भौमनिरीक्षिते च पिलकां सेन्दौ शनौ गुल्मजं
क्षीणेन्दौ जलभेषु पापसहिते तत्स्थेऽम्गुरोगं क्षयम्॥११॥

Now we give some more combinations of various types of disease.

(1) It Sun and Moon are placed in the 2nd or 12th house and they receive an aspect of Mars and Saturn then eye disease occurs. Here one should be kept in mind that is Sun and Moon are together and they receive full aspect from Mars and Saturn then possibility of total loss of that eye exists (vision or otherwise). The 2nd house indicates right eye and if the yoga is in the 12th house then it will be the left eye which will be affected.

Similarly if out of Sun or Moon anyone is in the second or 12th house and either Mars or Saturn aspect them then the disease will affect the right or left eye depending upon if Sun or Moon is in 2nd or 12th house. The 2nd and 12th house are called the house indicating eyes. If only one out of Mars and Saturn aspect them (when Sun or Moon is posited therein) then the evil will be much less compared to the simultaneous* aspect of Mars and Saturn both.

This is our experience. We have also noticed that if instead of Sun or Moon, malefic are in the 2nd or 12th house and other malefic aspect them then also loss of vision takes place.

(2) If the 3rd and the 11th houses and Jupiter receive aspect of or are conjoined with Mars then disease related to Ears (hearing) takes place. The third house indicates the right ear and the 11th house controls the left ear. Hearing (word), touch, sight rasa (taste) and smell. These five are related to the five elements i.e. Earth, Water, Fire, Wind and Ether. Fire is the element of Sun and Mars, water is the element of Moon and Venus, earth is the element of Mercury, the Wind or Vayu is the element of Saturn and Ether (Akash tatwa) that of Jupiter. The significator of 'Shabdha' is Akash and as the element 'Akash' is related to Jupiter so if Jupiter is aspected (with full aspect) or is conjoins with Mars and Saturn either by anyone or both then disease of the Ears or deafness follows. Here it should be logically decided as

---

*The concentrated simultaneous aspect of Mars and Saturn on any house or for that matter on any planet diminish the good effects and the evils increase and unless there is a strong counter benefic aspect.

to the intensity of the problem. The weaker the 3rd and 11th houses or the more the aspect or association of malefic with them or with more the malefic getting associated with these houses and Jupiter (Jupiter being the ruler of 'Shabdha') the result will be that much more intense and ear problems will be so much the worse. Mars rules 'Pitta' (bile) so its association or aspect will indicate wound, pimples, bursting of blood vessels in and around ears.

Saturn rules Vayu so it will bring in problems in the ear due to Vat disorders. Vat, pitta and Kapha are the three doshas according to 'Ayurved' the imbalance of which creates various types of disease in the body.

(3) Mars in the 5th house gives stomach problems. Any malefic viz., Sun, Mars, Saturn, Rahu, Ketu) if placed in the 5th house causes pains and problems in stomach. The fifth house indicates stomach.

(4) Venus if placed in the 7th or 8th house then it causes semen related problems or urinary diseases.

(5) If the lord of 6th or 8th is in the 7th house or the lord of the 6th is in the 8th house then there will be disease related to private parts. The 7th house then rules the lower portion of stomach including private parts, and the 8th rules the canal track. If a malefic or the lords of the 6th – 8th are placed in a house, then they create disease in that part of the body which is indicated by the house.

   (1) If Sun is in the 6th or 8th house then it can cause fever (high temperature).

   (2) If Mars or ketu is in the 6th or 8th house then it gives wounds (injury, boils, scar etc.)

   (3) Venus in the 6th or 8th house gives private organ related disease (like urinary problems, diabetes, syphlice, and V.D.).

   (4) Jupiter in the 6th or 8th house gives T.B. etc.

   (5) Saturn in the 6h or 8th house gives disease due to the disorder of Vat, mal nutrition, and breathlessness.

(6) Mars and Rahu in the 6th or 8th house or if Mars aspect the 8th house then Carbuncle, injury urinary problems and impurity of blood.

(7) Moon and Saturn together in the 6th or 8th house causes, tumours on the left side of stomach), spleen enlargement. Disease related to it.

(8) If waning Moon, with a malefic is in the 6th or 8th house in a watery Sign* then it cause water in stomach or other parts of body or TB. etc.

जातो गच्छति येन केन मरणं वक्ष्येऽथ तत्कारणं
रन्ध्रस्थैस्तदवेक्षकैर्बलवता तस्योक्तरोगैर्मृतिः ।
रन्ध्रर्क्षोक्तरुजाथवा मृतपतिप्राप्तर्क्षदोषेण वा
रन्ध्रेशेन खरत्रिभागपतिना मृत्युं वदेन्निश्चितम् ॥१२ ॥

ग्रहेण युक्ते निधने तदुक्तरोगैर्मृतिर्वाऽथ तदीक्षकस्य ।
ग्रहैर्विमुक्ते निधनेऽथ तस्य राशेः स्वभावोदितदोषजाता ॥१३ ॥

अग्न्युष्णज्वरपित्तशस्त्रजमिनाश्चन्दो विषूच्यम्बुरु-
ग्यक्ष्मादि क्षितिजोऽसृजा च दहनक्षुद्राभिचारायुधैः ।
पाण्ड्वादि भ्रमजं बुधो गुरुरनायासेन मृत्युं कफात्
स्त्रीसङ्गोत्कथरुजं कविस्तु मरुता वा संनिपातैः शनि ॥१४ ॥

कुष्ठेन वा कृत्रिमभक्षणाद्वा
राहुर्विषाद्वाथ मसूरिकाद्यैः ।
कुर्याच्छिखी दुर्मरणं नराणां
रिपोर्विरोधादपि कीटकाद्यैः ॥१५ ॥

---

*According to 'Horasar' CH I, Sl # 8 Cancer, Scorpio, Capricorn and Pisces are Watery signs.

लग्नादष्टराशेः स्वभावदोषोद्भवं वदेन्मृत्युम्।
निधनेशस्य नवांशस्थितराशिनिमित्तदोषजनितं वा ॥१६॥

पैत्त्यज्वरोष्णैर्जठराग्निनाजे
वृषे त्रिदोषैर्दहनाच्च शस्त्रात्।
युग्मे तु कालश्वसनोष्णशूलै-
रुन्मादवातारुचिभिः कुलीरे ॥१७॥

मृगज्वरस्फोटजशत्रु जं हरौ
स्त्रियां स्त्रियागुह्यरुजा प्रपातनात्।
तुलाधरे धीज्वरसंनिपातजं
प्लीहालिपाण्डुग्रहणीरुजालिनि ॥१८॥

वृक्षाम्बुकाष्टयुधजं हयाङ्ग
मृगे तु शूलारुचिधीभ्रमाद्यैः।
कुम्भे तु कासज्वरयक्ष्मरोगै
र्जले विपद्वा जलरोगतोऽन्त्ये ॥१९॥

पापर्क्षयुक्ते निधने सपापे
शस्त्रानलव्याघ्रभुजङ्गपीडा
अन्योन्यदृष्टौ व्ययशुभौ सकेन्द्रो
कोपात्प्रभोः शस्त्रविषाग्निजैर्वा ॥२०॥

सौम्यांशके सौम्यगृहेऽथ सौम्य-
सम्बन्धगे वा क्षयभे क्षयेशे।
अक्लेशजातं मरणं नराणां
व्यस्ते तदा क्रूरमृतिं वदन्ति ॥२१॥

Cause of Death

Now we speak of the reason of death and how it will come to pass

(a) (1) The planet in the 8th house or the planet posited in the 8th house out of these the strongest planet will be the planet responsible for death. The native will get the disease indicated by that strongest planet. The 8th house is the house of longevity. We have already mentioned above, the various diseases that fall under a particular planet.

(2) In case no planet is posited in the 8th house is the house of longevity. We have already mentioned above, the various diseases that fall under a particular planet.

In the above case either the matters (disease) which fall under the 8th house or the sign or the house occupied by the lord of the 8th house, will indicate the disease and cause of death. For example if the lord of the 8th house, will indicate the disease and cause of death. For example if the lord of the 8th house is in the 5th house then from stomach problems, in the 4th house it will indicate heart (or breast problems): if the lord of the 8th house is Sun or Mars then from bile, Saturn indicates wind (Vayu) disorders etc. The lord of the 22nd decanet from the decanet of the Ascendant – is also the indicator of death. The combinations related to the 8th house if they are not applicable then the disease indicated by the lord of the 22nd Decanet from the decanet of the Ascendant - any one of those disease will be the cause of death.

(b) The 13 sloka in a manner is the elaboration of the 12th sloka because it also clearly states that the strongest planet which aspect or are posited in the 8th house will indicate the disease (Dosha) which may cause death. If there is no such planet then the sign in the 8th house (and its lord) will indicate the disease which will be the cause of death.

(1) Sun - Fire, high temperature, biles or arms (weapons).

(2) Moon - Cholera, Edema (in this disease water accumulates in hands, feet and other places), TB. Etc. – are the causes of terminating life.

(3) Mars - From burns (Electric shocks, lighting, fire, etc. all under this, blood impurities or due to loss of blood, black magic (Jadoo, Tantra, etc.), and liver problems. - these will be caused by Mars.

(4) Mercury - Jaundice, anemia; confusion or muddled thinking, disease related to the nervous system (nervous breakdown). Liver does not function properly resulting in Low hemoglobin, lack of substance in the blood system.

(5) Jupiter - Rules phlegm. Causes death due to excess or disorder of it. Does not give any pains.

(6) Venus - When it is the cause of death then the reason is that too much indulgence in sex reduces the amount of semen and as such the body becomes weak and lustreless due to lack of resistance to disease. Urinary disorders and diseases connected with private parts fall under Venus.

(7) Saturn - paralytic stroke, vat disorders etc. are the cause of death.

(8) Rahu - Leprosy and food poisoning, eating rotten or infected food, due to snake bite or poisonous insect bite resulting in infection in the body, pimples, tumours etc. - All these are the cause of death.

(9) Ketu - When it causes death then it is a horrible death or sudden death like accident (disaster) in train, car, falling down from a house, due to being crushed or murdered – any one of these. Due to the opposition of enemies, due to insect bite resulting in septic or an insect or poisonous matter entering the system through food. These are some of the causes of death.

(c) (i) The disease or doshas which are indicated by the 8th house from the Ascendant, the lord of the 8th house or the planets which are placed in it or aspect it - all of them fall in this).

(ii) The disease or dosha indicated by the lord of the navansha in which the Lord of the 8th house is placed.

(d) Mention has been made above as to the disease dosha indicated by various signs. What dosha/disease is indicated by planets has been given. Now we will speak of the disease indicated by different signs on their own (natural disease).

(1) Aries - Disease due to excess of bile resulting in fever; heat (due to warm weather) like heat stroke, sunburns etc; low digestive power (due to low metabolism or otherwise).

(2) Taurus - Disorders due to Tridoshes (Vat - Pitta - Kapha), due to weapons, burns from fire.

(3) Gemini - Disease related breathing (lungs are affected) Asthama, sudden piercing pains due to bile.

(4) Cancer - Lunacy, Mental aberrations, Vat disorders, lack of appetite (anorexia).

(5) Leo - Death due to wild animals, Fever, wounds, danger due to enemies.

(6) Virgo - Due to women, disease in private parts (urinary troubles) danger due to falling down from height.

(7) Libra - Brain fever, lack of control on mind due to high temperature, meningitis.

(8) Scorpio - Spleen, Dysentery, Jaundice.

(9) Sagittarius - Due to a tree – while cutting it or due to falling down from it Water, Due to wood (Due to getting hurt or struck by wood or while cutting wood) danger from weapons.

(10) Capricorn - Appendictis, colic pain, tumour or wound in stomach, no appetite mental apprehensions or derangement due to nervous system or due to a disease when control on mind is lost.

(11) Aquarius - Cough, fever, TB.

(12) Pisces - Due to drowning, danger from water; water borne disease.

(e) If the lord of the 8th house is a malefic and malefic are also placed in the 8th house (or even if one malefic is in the 8th house), then sufferings occur on account of weapons, fire, Tigers, Snakes etc. If two malefic in angles aspect each other then death takes place due to the anger (unhappiness) of the

Government, weapons (fire arms), poison, fire etc.

(f) (1) If the lord of the 12th house is posited in a benefic sign or in the navansha owned by a benefic or is placed together with a benefic.

(2) The lord of the 12th house is benefic and a benefic is posited in the 12th house then there are no pains or sufferings at the time of death. If the conditions are reversed i.e. (i) The lord of the 12th house is placed in the sign or navansha owned by a malefic or is placed with a malefic. (ii) A malefic is posited in the 12th house and is aspected or owned by a malefic then the death comes with pains and sufferings.

Now the condition in between when one life ends and the next life will commence (birth).

स्वोच्चे स्वमित्रे सति सौम्यवर्गे
व्ययाधिपे चोर्ध्वगतिं ससौम्ये
विपर्ययेऽद्योगतिमेव केचित्-
ऊर्ध्वास्यशीर्षोदयराशिभेदात् ॥२२ ॥

केलासं रविशीतगू भृगुसुतः स्वर्गं महीजो महीं
वैकुण्ठं शशिजो यमो यमपुरं वद्ब्रह्मलोकं गुरुः ।
द्वीपान् भोगिवरः शिखी तु निरयं सम्प्रापयेत्प्राणिनः
सम्बन्धव्द्ययनायकस्य कथयेत्तत्रान्त्यराश्यंशतः ॥२३ ॥

धर्मेश्वरेणैव हि पूर्वजन्म
वृत्तं भविष्यज्जननं सुतेशात् ।
तदीशजातिं तदधिष्ठितर्क्ष
दिशं हि तत्रैव तदीशदेशम् ॥२४ ॥

स्वोच्चे तदीशे सति देवभूमिं
द्वीपान्तरं नीचरिपुस्थलस्थे ।

स्वर्क्षे सुहृद्भे समभे स्थिते वा
सम्प्राप्नुयाद्भारतवर्षमेव ॥२५॥

आर्यावर्तं गीष्पतेः पुण्यनद्यः
काव्येन्द्वोश्च ज्ञस्य पुण्यस्थलानि।
पङ्गोर्न्द्यिा म्लेच्छभूस्तीक्ष्णभानोः
शैलारण्यं कीकटं भूमिजस्य॥२६॥

स्थिरे स्थिरांशधिगतः सपापः
पृष्ठोदयेऽधोमुखभे च संस्थः।
तदीश्वरो वृक्षलतादिजन्म
स्यादन्यथा जीवयुतः शरीरी॥२७॥

लग्नेशितुः स्वोच्चसुहृत्स्वगेहान्
तदीश्वरो याति मनुष्यजन्म।
समे मृगाःस्युर्विहगाः परस्मिन्
द्रेक्काणरूपैरपि चिन्तनीयम्॥२८॥

तावेकराशौ जननं स्वदेशे
तौ तुल्यवीर्यौं यदि तुल्यजातौ।
वर्णो गुणस्तस्य खगस्य तुल्यः
संज्ञोदितैरेव वदेत्समस्तम्॥२९॥

(A) 1. If the lord of the 12th house is in its sign of exaltation, in the sign of a friend, is in benefic Vargas in Hora, Dreshkana i.e Decanet, Saptamansh, Navansh, Dwadashansa and Trinshansh etc. or is placed with a benefic then the native in over upwards after death i.e. towards heaven.* But if the

*The belief is that Heaven is situated above Earth and Hell is below - deep down under.

lord of the 12th is in a sign of an enemy, or debilitated sign, or is in the Vargas of the malefic or conjoins with malefic, then the native after death goes to the bottom i.e. towards the hell.

2. Some learned persons are of the opinion that if in the 12th house the sign is- Urdhawasya or the lord of the 12th house is in the Urdhawasya sign then after death the person goes up (upper portion) i.e. to heaven otherwise he goes downwards towards hell.

3. Some others are of the opinion that the signs rising from the head first, are the significator of Urdhagati i.e. to the upper regions and the signs rising with the tail first, are significator of the downwards movements. The signs– Gemini, Leo, Virgo, Libra, Scorpio and Aquarius are the signs which rise head first and the signs– Aries, Taurus, Cancer, Sagittarius and Capricorn rise with the feet first. Pisces rises both ways and is called Ubhayodaya.

(B) 1. What happens after death? What is the condition after the soul departs from the body? Where does the Soul go to?

(i) From the planets or planet in the 12th house.

(ii) The Navansha in the 12th house and

(iii) The planet situated in the Navansha which falls in the 12th house or other planets in the 12th house.

(iv) The planet or planets with which the lord of the 12th sign is associated with, these should be considered about the conditions after death.

2. If Sun or Moon fulfil the conditions mentioned above then the native goes to Kailash. The abode of Lord Shiva, after death.

If Mars is the planet indicating or describing the condition after death then the native will be reborn on earth very soon.

If Mercury, then the native goes to abode of lord Vishnu, 'Vaikuntha';

Jupiter indicates that the Atma will go to 'Brahmalok'.

Venus takes one to Heaven and Saturn to the abode of lord Yama (Yama Loka).

Rahu makes a person born in other islands like–away from the island where the person dies (foreign countries) and Ketu draws one to Hell after death. The next birth or where a person will go after death have been considered from the 12th house.

3. Now we speak of how to judge what a person was in his previous birth before he was born on this earth?

   The ninth house is the house which indicates about the previous birth. What will be the condition after death has been described above. To which lokas, the Soul– the Atma goes to after death and then in that loka after the Punya Karmas are finished i.e. he has enjoyed the result of his good deeds in the life time then according to the Bhagwat Gita-

   "क्षीणे पुण्ये मर्त्य लोक विशान्ति"** In which part of earth he will be born, what will be his condition, in what manner or what kind of body he will be in, should be considered from the fifth house.

4. About the caste or the country etc., in what direction a person existed in his previous life or where he will be born in the next life. All these should be considered from the 9th house, from the lord of the 9th house, the planet or planets posited in the 9th house. (all these for previous birth); From the 5th house, from the lord of the 5th house, from the planet or planets posited in the 5th house, the birth in the next life, should be judged.

   If the planet indicating the next birth is exalted in sign then in the Dev Bhoomi the abode of the Gods i.e. Heaven,

   If it is in the sign of an enemy or is debilitated then in another island.(foreign country).

   If the planet indicating is in own sign or in the sign owned by a friend then after death the birth will be in Bhartvarsh

i.e the present India. (or in the same country where a person was born before).

(C) Now we speak, of which planet has special relationship with which part of India.

(i) Sun– Mountains, hills and forest.

(ii) Moon– Holy Rivers, where taking a dip in those rivers gives Punya, good things of life and the sins are wiped out viz. Ganga, Yamuna, Narmada, Godawari etc. (These are the name of the rivers).

(iii) Mars– Keekat Desh, Daridra and Kuntsith Desh. One part of (present) Bihar is also known as Keekat Desh.

(iv) Mercury– Indicates birth in a Holy place. Those which are called Teerth like- Shri Rameshwaram, Shri Rangam, Dwarka, Ayodhya, Varanasi etc.

(v) Jupiter– Indicates Aryavarth- Himalayas and Vindhya which extends from the North to the South and then from the East to the West the Sea is the boundary.

(vi) Venus– Indicates the same places which are indicated for Moon.

(vii) Saturn– Not good places or places where people of different religions like– Muslim or Christians or low class of people live.

(D) In the Sloka No. 24 above we have talked about the previous birth.

Now in the same sequence we point out that the planets which have been mentioned in the previous Slokas–24 above and if those planets are posited in a fixed sign or fixed Navansha, and side by side they are also placed in a sign which rises with the feet first and is also an Adhomukh Rashi then the previous birth was in the form of a tree or a climber. These are considered from the 9th house; or if we have to consider the 5th house and these configuration are present (which have been mentioned) then the next birth will be in the form of a tree or climber.

If the Navansha is not fixed, and the sign is also not the sign rising feet first, then the birth would be in the form of a human being i.e. Urdhawasya Rashi sign and sign rising with head first, movable sign, movable navansha etc. (all these if related to the 9th house then the previous birth was in the form of a human being).

If all these thing are related to the 5th house, then the next life will be in the form of a human being.

Here we would like put up a note. This is a book which is now in English but the Hindu Philosophy, the Vedic Traditions talks of the Births– previous birth, present birth and re-births. It does not agree with the thinking that if you are born in this life– That's all. That's finished. No. There are birth and there will be births again and again till a person attains liberation or is detached from 'Maya'- the matters and charms of life so that he need not come back for the settlement of his Karmas.

2. When we talk about the human being i.e the form of a human, it means both man and woman and will be applicable to both. The opinion of the traditional Hindu Philosophy and this is our opinion too that if a person is born as a male in one life time, then he will always be born as a male in other lives and a woman will always be born as woman in all, her lives. Man- Prana and Woman- Prana i.e. Yosha Prana - this is the speciality of the 'Prana'.

(E) 1. If the lord of the 9th house is placed in a sign which is the exaltation sign of the ascendant lord or is the own sign of the ascendant lord, then the native was in his previous birth a human being.

2. If the lord of the 5th is in the exaltation or own sign of the lord of the ascendant then the rebirth will be as a human being.

3. If the lord of the 9th house is in a sign which is the neutral sign of the lord of the ascendant i.e. neither a friend nor an enemy, then the native in his previous birth was in the form of an animal.

4. If the lord of the 5th house is in a sign which is the neutral sign of the lord of the ascendant then in his next life he will be an animal.

5. If the lord of the 9th house is in a sign which is the debilitated sign or the sign of an enemy of the lord of the ascendant then the native in his previous birth was a bird.
6. If the lord of the 5th is in a sign which is owned by an enemy or the sign of debilitation of the lord of the ascendant then the native's rebirth will be in the form of a bird.

(F) In the Sloka -28 above the consideration of the lord of the 9th or of the lord of the 5th has been given. It should also be considered in which decanet the lord of the 9th or the lord of the 5th are placed. What is the form of this decanet?

1. If the lord of the 9th and the lord of the 5th are placed together in one sign then the previous birth as well as the next birth will be in the same place or country.
2. If the lord of the 9th and the lord of the 5th both are of equal strength then the native was of the same caste in his previous life and will be born in the same caste in the next life.
3. In the 1st Chapter - we have described in details the caste, the attributes etc. of various planets. When describing the previous birth these should be used in relation to the lord of the 9th house and when speaking of the next birth, (next life after death) then the details should be described according to the caste, the qualities etc. of the lord of the 5th house. Planetary formation, caste, temperament, nature etc. has already been described in the 1st Chapter.

The principles to know about the past and future births has been given according to the theory. These may not be so useful from the practical point of view. This is an interesting subject from the angle of philosophy. In the book 'Karma Vipak' description of previous birth have been given in details. But it can not be taken for granted as to the authenticity of the correctness of those because there is no way logically or mathematically verify them. There is no way or no method which can guarantee if the description are correct.

15

Bhava Chinta (Houses Analysis)

CONSIDERATION OF HOUSES

भावाः सर्वे शुभपतियुता वीक्षिता वा शुभेशै-
स्तत्तद्भावाः सकलफलदाः पापदृग्योगहीनाः।
पापाः सर्वे भवनपतयश्चेदिहाहुस्तथैव
खेटैः सर्वैः शुभफलमिदं नीचमूढारिहीनैः ॥१॥

तत्तद्भावात् त्रिकोने स्वसुखमदनभे चास्पदे सौम्ययुक्ते।
पापानां दृष्टिहीने भवनपसहिते पापखेटैरयुक्ते।
भावानां पुष्टिमाहुः सकलशुभकरीमन्यथा चेत्प्रणाशं
मिश्रं मिश्रैर्ग्रहेन्द्रैः सकलमपि तथा मूर्तिभावदिकानाम् ॥२॥

नाशस्थानगतो[१] दिवाकरकरैर्लुप्तस्तु यद्भावपो[२]
नीचारातिगृहं[३] गतो[४] यदि भवेत्सौम्यैरयुक्तेक्षितः[४]।
तद्भावस्य विनाशनं वितनुते तादृग्विधोऽन्योऽस्ति चेत्
तद्भावोऽपि फलप्रदो न हि शुभश्चेन्नाशमुग्रग्रहः ॥३॥

लग्नादिभावाद्रिपुरन्ध्ररिःफे
पापग्रहास्तद्भवनादिनाशम्।
सौम्यास्तु नात्यन्तफलप्रदाः
स्युर्भावादिकानां फलमेवमाहुः ॥४॥

यद्भवनाथो रिपुरन्ध्ररि:फे
दु:स्थानपो यद्भवनस्थितो वा।
तद्भावनाशं कथयन्ति तज्ज्ञा:
शुभेक्षितस्तद्भवनस्य सौख्यम् ॥५॥

भावाधीशे च भावे सति बलरहिते च ग्रहे कारकाख्ये
पापान्त:स्थे च पापैररिभिरपि समेतेक्षिते नान्यखेटै:।
पापैस्तद्बन्धुमृत्युव्ययभवनगतैस्तत्त्रिकोणस्थितैर्वा
वाच्या तद्भावहानि: स्फुटमिह भविह द्वित्रिसंवादभावात् ॥६॥

तत्तद्भावपराभवेश्वरखरद्रेष्काणपा दुर्बला
भावार्यष्टकामगा निजदशायां भावनाशप्रदा:।
पापा भावगृहात् त्रिशत्रुभवगा: केन्द्रत्रिकोणे शुभा:
वीर्याढ्या: खलु भावनाथसुहृदो भावस्य सिद्धिप्रदा: ॥७॥

1. In this 15th chapter the good and ill effect of houses has been analyzed. When consideration of any house has to be done then the following principles should be applied.

The houses where benefic planets are posited, the houses which receive the aspect of benefic planets they give good results. The house where the lord of a sign is posited itself then good results are realized. If a house receives the aspect of its own lord then it gives good result. Where the aspect is full then full results, if the aspect of a planet is only ¾ then the result will also be 75%, if the aspect is only half the effect is also 50 % and if it is ¼, the result will also be ¼.

One commentator has commented that the lords of good houses if they aspect any other house, then they will bring prosperity related to that house. But our opinion is that the word benefic is in the context of a natural benefic planet – and not on account of the lordship of good houses.

For example, for Aries rising, the lord of the 9th and lord of the 10th Saturn is and will act as a benefic but on its own, it is a malefic. For Libra rising people Jupiter is a natural benefic but as the owner of 3rd and 6th house, it will not be called a benefic. Our opinion is that the writer of Phaldeepika wanted to clarify the benefic and malefic planets according to their basic nature.

If a malefic is the ruler of a particular house and is also posited over there then it will increase the efficacy of that house and will not destroy it. Similarly if a malefic aspects its sign which it owns with full aspect then it improves the house. But some sentences that has been mentioned as to the planet behaving in a totally benefic manner will only be applicable when the planet is neither debilitated, combust, nor posited in the house of an enemy. Out of these three 'doshas' (negative points), if any one or more are present, then the planet's power to generate benefic effect is destroyed or is reduced to a great extent.

2. The house, which is to be considered, look at that house as the ascendant and then examine from that house. If the lord of the house is posited in 1st, 4th, 2nd, 5th, 7th, 9th and 10th houses from the house under consideration then benefic effect will be felt.

If in the above mentioned houses from the house under consideration benefic planets are posited then the prosperity of the house will be the result. It should be noted the 1st, 2nd, 4th, 5th, 7th, 9th, 10th receive the aspect of only benefic and malefic are not posited in them. If only benefic are posited in respect to these houses then full benefic effect will be the result. If all the planets posited in or throwing aspect are malefic then the total result will be a malefic. If some are positive and others are malefic then the effect will also be mixed i.e. something good something bad. For consideration of any house examine different places from it. See if benefic or malefic are posited in them and only then final conclusion should be drawn.

For example let us consider the 2nd house in a horoscope. The sign over there is Virgo. Now use Virgo as the 1st house, and then the 2nd house from this is Libra, the 4th house from this is Sagittarius the 5th house is Capricorn, the 7th house is Pisces and in same manner the 9th and 10th house from it. We find that Venus is in Libra, which is the second house. In the 7th house from Virgo, Jupiter is there, in the 9th house from Virgo Moon is posited. As these are natural benefic and so their placement in the houses mentioned above will increase the good effects. The native will be rich. In similar manner, other planets and houses should be examined.

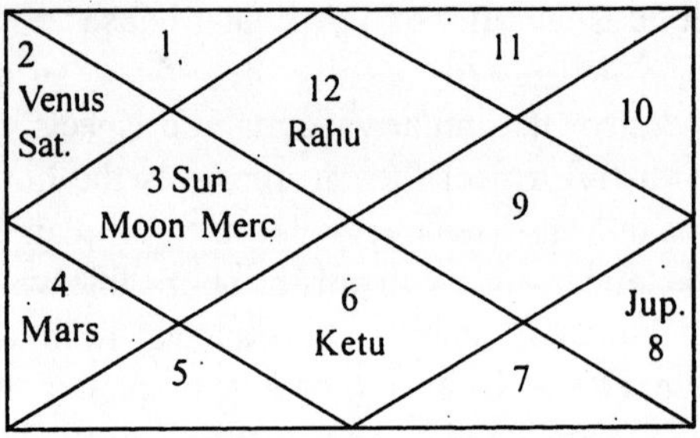

3. If the lord of a particular house (1) is in the 8th house or (2) if the lord of the particular house is combust due to closeness of sun (3) is posited in its sign of debilitation (4) is in the sign of an enemy or is not conjoined with or receives aspect from benefic, then the house is destroyed i.e. there will be no happiness in relationship to the matters indicated by that house. On the other hand extreme sufferings and sorrow related to it. Some people are of the opinion that if the lord of a house under consideration, is in the 8th house from it and if it simultaneously in the 6th, 8th and 12th from the Ascendant then the house of which that particular planet is the lord will be spoiled. If any benefic planet is debilitated or in the house of an enemy or combust and is posited in a house then the house in which this planet is placed or the house which this planet aspect then it will spoil the house. It will also destroy the good effects of the planet it is associating with. If it is a malefic planet, debilitated or combust or in the house of an enemy, or is posited in a house and is not conjoined with or aspected by benefic, then it will totally and with great intensity destroy the house. For example* in the horoscope given above Mars is debilitated in the 5th house. It however receives an aspect from Jupiter which is in the 9th house otherwise Mars would have spoiled the 5th house much more. Due to the aspect from Jupiter, the malefic effect of Mars is reduced. However as Mars is debilitated so the native's two older sons did not survive

and the native himself suffered from water in the stomach. He did not have much happiness from the side of children.

4. If malefic are posited in the 6th, 8th and 12th houses from a house, which is to be considered then they destroy the house. For example if you have to consider the 7th house, then the 6th house from the 7th is 12th, 8th house from it is the 2nd house from the 7th; the 12th house from the 7th is the 6th house and if malefic are in all these three places then it will destroy the 7th house which the house of spouse or partnership.

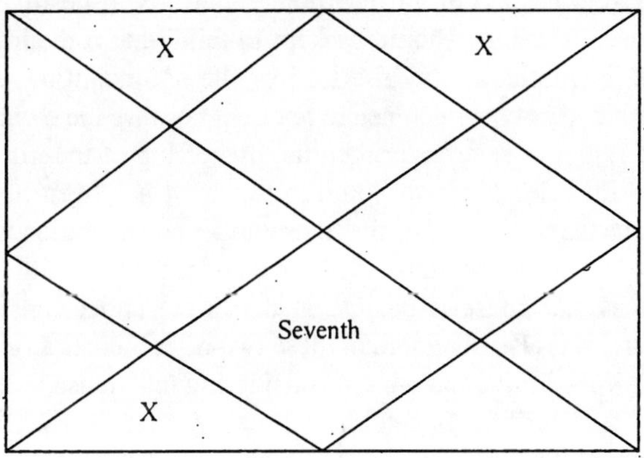

We repeat that if 12th house, 2nd house and 6th house are afflicted due to the placement of malefic and then the house of marriage is destroyed. Whatever house has to be considered, the 6th, 8th and 12th house from it should be examined and if benefic are there then even they are not able to impart strength to that house what to talk of the malefic. For example consider the 7th house and look to the 6th, 8th and 12th houses from it. Jupiter is posited over there but Jupiter in such a position will not be able to impart much strength to the 7th house. The question is why so? It is so because from these houses it will not be able to aspect the house with full aspect. If Jupiter or any benefic is in the 12th house from the ascendant then it will aspect the 7th house with ¾ aspect only but in the 6th from the 7th , being the house of the enemy it will not be in good position.

5. Whichever house has to be considered if the lord of that house

is posited in the 6th, 8th or 12th house from the ascendant then this house is spoiled. This is a general rule. For example if the lord of the 1st house is posited in the 8th then the physical structure will be weak or the native will be generally sick. If lord of the 7th house is in the 8th house then it reduces the conjugal bliss. But there are some exceptions to these rules (for this see chapter 6, Sloka-57). Whichever house is under consideration and in that house if the lord of a trik* is posited, or then, it will reduce the good effect of the house. For example, if the lord of the 8th house is posited in the 10th house then it will destroy the 10th house. One thing should be kept in mind that if the lord of the trik is simultaneously the lord of the ascendant as well then there will not be much negative effect because the ownership of the 1st house is stronger then the ownership of the trik this is a general rule. The two conditions which has been mentioned above that is the lord of the house under consideration is posited in a bad house then this is not good and if the lord of the dusthan that is bad house is posited in the house under consideration then this is also not good. In these two rules there is an exception that if the house that we are considering that house receives the aspect of benefic planets then some good results related to that house will be realized.

6. How does happiness related to a house or the negativity related to it is experienced? This we give below:-

   (1) If the house, the lord of the house and the significator of that house is weak.

   (2) If the house, the lord of the house and the significator of that house is hemmed in between malefic, or is posited or aspected by malefic, or with enemy planets then it is not good and simultaneously it should also not aspected or conjoined with benefic.

   (3) The house which is under consideration count from that house the 4th, 5th, 8th, 9th and 12th and if these are occupied by malefic.

---

*Trik is 6th, 8th and 12th house from the ascendant.

We have mentioned above that the house, the lord of the house and the significator* of the house - these three should be considered before arriving at a conclusion. If out of these three, two or more negative combinations exist, then the house is destroyed. For example, if wife is to be considered and the 7th house, the lord of 7th and the significator of the 7th of which is Venus are without strength and side by side the 4th and 8th from Venus have malefic, then undoubtedly the native's first wife will die or his marriage breaks up. The purpose of mentioning is that if many negative signs are present then the full yoga will take place*.

Planet	House
Sun	I
Jupiter	II
Mars	III
Moon and Mercury	IV
Jupiter	V
Saturn and Mars	VI
Venus	VII
Saturn	VIII
Sun and Jupiter	IX
Sun, Mercury, Saturn and Jupiter	X
Jupiter	XI
Saturn	XII

Sun is the significator of I house, Jupiter is the significator of the II house etc.

7. Which planet destroys a house and which bring positive effects to a house – this is mentioned below:-

The following are the factors by which a house is destroyed.

(i) The lord of the 8th house from the house under consideration.

---

*We give below the significator of the 12 houses.

(ii) The lord of the 22nd decanet from the house under consideration.

(iii) If the lords of 6th, 7th and 8th houses from the house under consideration, are weak.

These planets in their major and minor periods destroy the house under consideration. Now we indicate the factors, which bring strength to a house.

(i) If malefic occupy the 3rd , 6th, and 11th from the house under consideration then during their periods they bring happiness related to that house.

(ii) If benefic planets are posited in the 1st, 4th, 5th, 7th, 9th and 10th houses from the house under consideration then the house will prosper.

(iii) The enemies of the lord of the house, which is to be considered they will in their major and minor periods will destroy and give ill effects related to that house. The planets which are the friends of the lord of that particular house under consideration and if these friends are strong then they will give strength and the house will prosper during their major and minor periods.

An example of the last principles enunciated is given below:

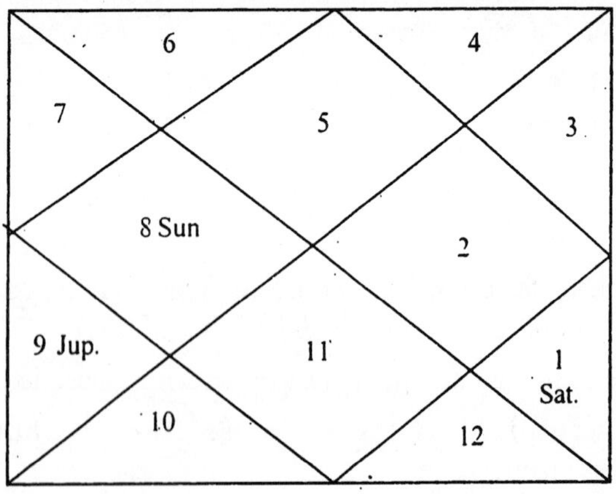

The horoscope given above has Leo rising, Sun in Scorpio in the 4th house, Jupiter in Sagittarius in the 5th house, Saturn in

Aries in the 9th house. For example look to the above horoscope and suppose we have to examine the 1st house then Saturn is the enemy of Sun then in the major and minor period of Saturn there will be ailments related to the body. Jupiter is the friend of Sun so during the major and minor periods of Jupiter, there will be contentment of body.

राश्तोर्जन्मविलग्नयोर्धृतिपतिर्मृत्युस्थतद्वीक्षकौ
मन्दः क्रूरदृगाणपो गुलिकपस्तैर्युक्तराश्यंशपा।
राहुश्चैष सुदुर्बलः स जनने भावानभीष्टस्थितः
पापालोकितसंयुतो निजदशायां भावनाशावहाः ॥८॥

8. The following planet in their major and minor period destroy the house.

(i) The lord of the third house from the ascendant

(ii) The lord of the 3rd house from Moon

(iii) The planet posited in the 8th house

(iv) The planet which aspect the 8th house

(v) Saturn

(vi) The lord of the 22nd dreshkan (decanet).

(vii) The lord of house where mandi is posited

(viii) The 7 planets (which have been mentioned above) in whichever sign and Navansha they are in, the lord of those signs and Navansha.

(ix) If Rahu is weak and is posited in the 8th and 12th house or if it conjoins with a malefic or receives an aspect from a malefic.

This has not been mentioned as to which house or the efficacy of which house is destroyed. But looking back to the slokas enunciated earlier the malefic wherever they are posited or whichever house they aspect or if they are posited with some planets then they destroy those houses or planets. Their placement or aspect should apply the same principles that malefic, destroy the house and the planets they associate with.

भावस्योदयपाश्रितस्य कुशलं यद्भवपेनोदय-
स्वामी तिष्ठति संयुतोऽपि कलयेत्तद्भावजातं फलम्।
दुःस्थाने विपरीतमेतदुदितं भावेश्वरे दुर्बले
दोषोऽतीव भवेद्बलेन सहिंते दोषाल्पता जल्पिता ॥९ ॥

9. The house where the lord of the first i.e. the lord of the ascendant is posited the efficacy of that house improves for the better. If the lord of the ascendant is posited with the lord of a Bhava (house) then also the efficacy of that lord of the Bhava increases i.e. the benefic effect increases. We have mentioned above that in whichever house the lord of the first is posited it increases the benefic effects. If the lord of any house is posited in a Dusthan then the result is negative and if the planet in the dusthan, is also weak then much worse should be expected. However if it is strong then the negative effect will dimnish.

यद्भावेष्वशुभोऽपि वोदयपतिस्तद्भाववृद्धिं दिशे-
द्दुःस्थानाधिपतिः स चेद्यदि तनोः प्राबल्यमन्यस्य न।
अत्रोदाहरणं कुजे सुतगते सिंहे झसे वा स्थिते
पुत्राप्ति शुभवीक्षिते झटिति तत्प्राप्तिं वदन्युत्तमाः ॥१० ॥

10. In this sloka it has been mentioned that the lord of the first house whether it is a benefic or a malefic, wherever it is posited it increases the positive effect of the house. It is an authentic principle of astrology that the 6, 8, and 12 are dusthan and these are not good houses. Now the question arises that if the lord of the first and is benefic and simultaneously if it is also the lord of the 6th or 8th then what type of effect it will show.

The answer to this question is that if a planet is the lord of the first house and simultaneously, is also the owner of the 6th or 8th then the main effect will be that of the first house and it will show benefic effect. Take for example Scorpio ascendant, Mars is the lord of the 1st and 6th house or for Aries ascendant, Mars is the lord of the 1st and 8th houses. If this Mars is posited in the 5th house then will it as being the lord of 6th or 8th cause sufferings to the children or as it is the lord of the 1st posited in the 5th it will show good effect related to children? The answer to this is that Mars as lord of the 1st or 6th or Mars as lord of the 1st and 8th if posited in the 5th house and receives aspect of benefic planet then it brings happiness from sons and the children are born at an early age.

द्विस्थानाधिपतित्वमस्ति यदि चेन्मुख्यं त्रिकोणर्क्षजं
तस्यार्द्ध स्वगृहेऽथ पूर्वमुभयोर्यत्तद्दशादौ वदेत्।
पश्चाद्भावमिहापरार्द्धसमये युग्मे गृहे युग्मजं
त्वोजस्थे सति चौजभावजफलं शंसन्ति केचिज्जना: ॥११॥

11. If any planet owns two houses then it will show more effect of the house of which is its mooltrikone. Which sign is the mooltrikone of a planet has been mentioned earlier (see page no. 5). For example for Leo rising horoscope Jupiter rules the 5th and 8th houses. The fifth house is a trine and it is a benefic house. The 8th house is not good. In this case the mooltrikone sign of Jupiter being the 5th house, the main effect in the horoscope will be of the lordship of the 5th house. The lordship of the 8th house will have only 50% effect i.e. the lordship of the fifth house if it has 16 units of effect then the lordship of the 8th house will show only eight units of malefic effects. In this manner the periodic influence of Jupiter as the owner of these two houses, one a benefic the other a malefic, will be both. The good effect will be one and the negative effect will be half of it.

In the example horoscope that we have given Jupiter will show the effect of the lordship of the 5th as well as the lordship of the 8th. Here we also should decide as to which result lordship would come first? The answer is that as counted from the ascendant, the sign which comes first the effect of that sign will be first, and the sign which comes afterwards the effect of that sign will follow it. But Mantreshwar Maharaj himself writes that some other learned persons are of the opinion that if a planet is posited in an odd sign, then out of its both signs, the one which is odd the effect of that odd sign will be felt first, and the effect of the second sign will follow. However if a planet is posited in an even sign then out of its both signs, the sign which is even that will show its effect first, and the effect of the odd sign rulership will come afterwards.

यद्भावेशस्याधिशत्रु ग्रहो वा
योवा खेटो बिन्दुशून्यर्क्षयुक्तः ।
तत्तपाके मूर्तिभावादिकानां
नाशं ब्रूयाद्दैववित्प्राश्निकाय ॥१२॥

12. In this sloka it has been mentioned as to which houses will be destroyed in the major or minor periodic influences of a particular planets. In this connection two things exists.

(a) During the major and minor periodic influences of a planet, which is a great enemy of the lord of a house, the house will be destroyed.

(b) If a planet in its own Ashtakvarga has no benefic points in a house i.e. devoid of any benefic points than during the major and minor period of the planet, ill effects related to that house will be felt.

The meaning of this is that suppose the periodic influence of Saturn is there and in the Saturn's ashtakvarga the 5th house is devoid of any shubh bindus then in the major and minor periodic influences of Saturn there wil! be suffering related to the 5th house.

(c) One another commentator has mentioned that suppose Leo is the ascendant and in the Sun's ashtakvarga Pisces is devoid of any benefic points, then the planets which are posited in Pisces, will cause physical sufferings during their periods. According to this view the house which is to be considered, look to the ashtakvarga of the lord of the house. If it is devoid of any benefic points then a planet posited in that sign during its major and minor periods will give the ill effect related to that house.

स्वोच्चे सुहृत्क्षेत्रगतो ग्रहेन्द्रः
षड्भिर्बलैर्मुख्यबलान्वितोऽपि ।

सन्धौ स्थितः सन्नफलप्रदः स्यात्
एवं विचिन्त्यात्र वदेद्विपाके ॥१३॥

भावेषु भावस्फुटतुल्भाग-
स्तद्भावजं पूर्णफलं विधत्ते।
सन्धौ फलं नास्ति तदन्तराले
चिन्त्योऽनुपातः खलु खेचराणाम् ॥१४॥

Even if a planet is exalted or posited in the sign of a friend and even if it is endowed with shadbalas (six types of strengths) but if that planet is in the mid point i.e. in the middle of two cusps then that planet becomes incapable of giving results. While predicting this view should be kept in mind.

The planets which are on the cusp of a house they show full results and those planets which are on the mid point they show zero result i.e. that not show any results. If planets are somewhere in between the cusp of a house and the midpoint then the nearer they are to the cusp, the more effect they will show related to that house. If a planet is closer to the midpoint then the result of that planet is substantially reduced.

If we have to be more thorough then mathematical calculation by the rule of three should be done. For example, suppose there is a spread out of 15 degrees between the cusp of a house and the midpoint then a planet which is 5 degrees away from the cusp of a house will show 2/3rd effect; exactly on the cusp it will show full effect, and a planet which is 5 degrees away from the midpoint will be able to give only 1/3rd effect. This is so because 15 when divided from 5 gives 1/3rd.

सुर्यादात्मपितृप्रीाावनिरुजां शक्तिं श्रियं चिन्तयेत्
चेतोबुद्धिनृपप्रसादजननीसंपत्करश्चन्द्रमा।
सत्वं रोगगुणानुजावनिरिपुज्ञातीन्धरासूनुना
विद्याबन्धुविवेकमातुलसुहृद्वाक्कर्मकृद्बधनः ॥१५।

प्रज्ञावित्तशरीरपुष्टितनयज्ञानानि वागीश्वरात्
पत्नीवाहनभूषणानि मदनव्यापारसौख्यं भृगोः।
आयुर्जीवनमृत्युकारणविपद्भृत्यांश्च मन्दाद्वदेत्
सर्पेणैव पितामहं तु शिखिना मातामहं चिन्तयेत्॥१६॥

In these slokas which matters should be decided from which planets has been given. From Sun consideration of *Atma* – the soul, father, authority, health, strength and Lakshmi i.e. wealth from Moon *Mana* i.e. emotional nature, intellectual abilities, patronage of king, mother and property. From Mars *Satva* i.e. courage, valour, disease good attributes, brother, earth, enemies, kinsmen like cousins etc. should be considered. Education, relatives, discrimination, maternal uncle, friends, speech, ability to work and accomplish things should be considered from Mercury.

In Sanskrit sloka the word *Karma* has come that these should be considered from Mercury. Is Mercury the planet which rules *Karma*? What is the meaning of this? Mercury is the planet which controls the nervous system and when the nervous system is strong the person is engaged and busy in work. His tendency to work is strong he is busy in work. If the nervous system is weak then the person is not hard working and his desire to work does not arise and when the strength to work is weak then the interest to work is also not there. The 10th house is the house of career, the type of work one is supposed to do. *Karma* and work being related to 10th house and Mercury is also one of the significator of the 10 house.

Knowledge, wealth, physical strength and development and sons are considered from Jupiter. The significator of wife, vehicles, ornaments, relationship between men and women and happiness is Venus. Longevity, livelihood, the cause of death, the cause of sufferings and calamities and service should be considered from Saturn. From Rahu consideration for grand father (from father's side), and from Ketu maternal grandfather as well as father's mother should be considered.

द्युमणिरमरमन्त्री भूसुतः सोम सौम्यौ
गुरुरिनतनयारौ भार्गवो भानुपुत्रः।

दिनकरदिविजेज्यौ जीवनभानुज्ञमन्दाः
सुरगुरुरिनसूनुः कारकाः स्युर्विलग्नात् ॥१७॥

When anything has to be considered the astrologers generally look to the lord of the house and the house involved but whatever the importance of the house and the house involved, the same importance should be assigned to the significator. For example if we have to see about marriage and we find that the 7th house, the lord of the 7th are not good. However if Venus is very strong then happiness and contentment will come from wife. *Vice versa* if the lord of the 7th and the 7th house are good but Venus is weak then due to the lack of strength of Venus that much happiness will not come from wife. Which planet signifies what persons have been mentioned in the previous slokas. Now the same is repeated in relation to the house the planets signifies which planet or planets which signify any particular house. In a nativity there are 12 houses and the following are the significators of the 12 houses respectively.

Sun	I house
Jupiter	II house
Mars	III house
Moon and Mercury	IV house
Jupiter	V house
Mars and Saturn	VI house
Venus	VII house
Saturn	VIII house
Jupiter and Sun	IX house
Sun, Mercury, Jupiter and Saturn	X house
Jupiter	XI house
Saturn	XII house

सुहृदरिपरकीयस्वर्क्षतुङ्गस्थितानां
फलमनुपरिचिन्त्यं लग्नदेहादिभावैः ।
समुपचयविपत्ती सौम्यपापेषु सत्यः
कथयति विपरीतं रिःफषष्ठाष्टमेषु ॥१८॥

If we want to consider the effect of a planet then we should observe in which house (from the ascendant) it is posited, whether it is in the sign of a friend or in own sign or in its exalted sign or in the sign of an enemy. According to Satyacharya, if benefic are posited in a house then they increase the efficacy of the house and the house in which the malefic are that house loses its good effect. However the results are just the opposite when the 6th, 8th and 12th houses are considered.

पापग्रहाः षष्ठमृतिव्ययस्था-
स्तद्भाववृद्धिं कलयन्ति दोषैः।
शुभास्तु तदभावलयं हि
तस्माच्छत्र्वादि भावोत्फलप्रणाशः ॥१९॥

If malefic are posited in the 6th ,8th ,or 12th houses from the ascendant then they increase the negative effect of those houses. If on the other hands benefic are there in the 6th ,8th , or the 12th then they reduce the negativity of the house. Therefore if benefic are placed over there in the 6th , 8th , and 12th it is much better. Although Mantreshwar Maharaj has said that benefic in trik (6th 8th and 12th) destroy the evil effect of the house but they themselves get afflicted and are not able to show their full radiant and benefic effect during their major and minor periodic influences.

भावस्य यस्यैव फलं विचिन्तयं
भावं च तं लग्नमिति प्रकल्प्य।
तस्माद्व्ददेद्द्वादशभावजानि
फलानि तद्रूपधनादिकानि ॥२०॥

In this sloka we speak of something new.

Whichever Bhava is to be considered then make a new horoscope keeping that Bhava as the I house (ascendant) and then consider it in the manner a general horoscope or a nativity is considered. For example if we have to decide about the daughter-in-law in a horoscope then the 5th house from the ascendant is the house that gives indication about the son. The 7th house from the 5th i.e. the 11th house will tell us about the daughter-in-law. Or take another example if we want to know about the finances of wife then as we look consider wife from the 7th house then the 2nd from it rules the wealth of wife. We will make the 8th house as the ascendant and then consider the situation as far as wealth of wife. To consider the younger brother of wife look to the 9th house which is the 3rd from the 7th . This should be made the ascendant and then consideration for one's brother-in-law is done. Similarly any Bhava should be made into an ascendant to consider the other Bhavas from that Bhava. This is clear from the example given above.

> एवं हि तत्कारकतो विचिन्त्यं
> पितुश्च मातुश्च सहोदरस्य।
> तन्मातुलस्यापि सुतस्य पत्यु-
> र्भृत्यस्य सूर्यादिखगस्थितर्क्षात्॥२१॥

Now we speak of another matter. If we have to consider the matters related to father then as sun is the significator of the father then, make that house where Sun is posited as the ascendant. The 2nd from the sun will tell about his wealth, the 3rd will tell about the father's younger brother and this way the 12 houses will speak of the father and all matters about him. For consideration of the mother the sign where Moon is posited at birth should be taken as the ascendant. The brother should be considered from the house where Mars is placed. Make that house as the ascendant and other houses should be examined from it.

If consideration for the maternal uncle has to be done then Mercury being a significator of the maternal brothers and sisters then that should be taken as the ascendant and when the houses should be examined. For Son, Jupiter should be taken as the ascendant and then the other houses should be examined for, about the wife make the sign where Venus is posited as the ascendant and then consider it. Similarly about the servant, the sign where the Saturn is posited should be made into an ascendant and then the 12 houses should be considered as to their good or bad effects.

सूर्यस्थितर्क्षाज्जनकस्वरूपं
वृद्धिं द्वितीयेन तु तत्प्रकाशम्।
तद्भ्रातरं तस्य गुणं तृतीयात्-
तन्मातरं चापि सुखं चतुर्थात्॥२२॥

बुद्धि प्रसादं सुतभाच्च षष्ठा-
त्पीडा पितुर्दोषमरिं च रोगम्
कामं मदं तस्य तु सप्तमेन
दुःखं मृतिं मृत्युगृहात्तदायुः॥२३॥

पुण्यं शुभं तत्पितरं शुभेन
व्यापारमस्यैव हि कर्मभावात्।
लाभं ह्युपान्त्यात् क्षयमन्त्य-
भावाच्चद्रादिकानां फलमेवमाहुः॥२४॥

The sign in which Sun is posited, consider the appearance of father, the 2nd house from it consider the wealth of father and his fame. From the 3rd house from Sun, the father's brother and his attributes, i.e. his qualities can be considered. The happiness of father and father's mother from the 4th house, from Sun, the 5th house from the Sun sign will tell about the intellectual abilities and happiness of father. The 6th house from the Sun sign will speak of the negative effect, enemies and disease of the father. The 7th from the Sun sign will tell about love life (wife), the 8th from the Sun will speak of the unhappiness, longevity and death.

The 9th house from the Sun sign will tell about the father's spirituality his benefic and good points and father's father i.e. the grand father and the 10th house from the Sun sign will give indication of his business and work. The 11th house from the Sun sign will indicate gains of father and the 12th from it will speak of the losses, which may occur to him. We have taken the position of the Sun in a sign and then counted from it the different houses to know about the different departments of the father. In the same manner the radical

Moon should be considered as the ascendant and then different matters of the mother should be judged from the various houses from it. From the different houses from the sign occupied by Mars all about the brothers can be decided. Similarly Mercury and other planets should be respectively taken into account to know about other relatives and people in one's life.

तत्तद्भावात्कारकादेवमूह्यं
तत्तन्मातृभ्रातृपित्रात्मजाद्यम् ।
तस्मिन् भावे कारके भावनाथे
वार्योपेते तस्य भावस्य सौख्यम् ॥२५ ॥

Therefore, if consideration for father, mother, brother, maternal uncle, son, wife, servants, etc. has to be done then take into account the house, the lord of the house and the significator the house all the three of them. If all the three i.e. the house, the lord of the house and the significator of them are strong then happiness related to that Bhava (house) will take place.

धर्मे सूर्यः शीतगुर्बन्धुभावे
शौर्ये भौमः पञ्चमे देवमन्त्री ।
कामे शुक्रश्चाष्टमे भानुपुत्रः
कुर्यात्तस्य क्लेशमित्याहुरन्ये ॥२६ ॥

Some people are of the opinion that Sun in the 9th house, Moon in the 4th house, Mars in the 5th house, Jupiter in the 5th house, Venus in the 7th house and Saturn in the 8th house destroy the happiness of that house. We think that to some extent this is correct that the *Karak* is placed in the house it signifies destroys it and in many horoscopes we have found it to be true particularly with the position Venus in the 7th house and that of Jupiter in the 5th house.

लग्नेश्वरो यद्भवनेशयुक्तो
यद्भावगस्तस्य फलं ददाति ।
भावे तदीशे बलभाजि तेन
भावेन सौख्यं व्यसनं बलोने ॥२७ ॥

The lord of the ascendant gives the effect of the house it is posited in, or of the lord of a house with which it conjoins. If the house and its lord are strong then happiness in relation to that house is experienced. If they are weak then there is sufferings in the matters related to that house.

यद्भावप्रभुणा युतो बलवता मुख्याङ्गगो लग्नप-
स्तद्भावनुभवं वितनुते यद्भावगस्तस्य च।
संयुक्तो बलहीनभावपतिना निन्द्याङ्गभाजां फलं
कुर्यात्तद्विपरीतमेवमुदितं सर्वेषु भावेष्वपि॥२८॥

In the ashtakvarga of the lord of the 1st house, those houses which have more benefic points and the lord of those houses are also strong and they are posited with the lord ascendant then good results can be expected regarding that house. But if in the ashtakvarga of the lord of the ascendant a house has few benefic points and the lord thereof is also weak and even if the lord of the house is with the lord of the ascendant even then there will be no good effect related to that house will come. Similarly, all the houses should be considered.

Some persons suggest that we should look only to the lord of a house, if it is strong or weak. For this sloka, the consideration of ashtakvarga is not needed but we have used it, as it is a mathematical analysis of a house.

दु:स्थानपस्तदितरस्वगृहस्थिश्चेत्
स्वक्षेत्रभावफलमेव करोति नान्यत्।
मन्दो मृगे सुतगृहे यदि पुत्रसिद्धिः
षष्ठाधिपत्यकृतदोषफलं च नात्र॥२९॥

If a planet is the owner of two signs and one sign is in a benefic place in the nativity and the second sign is a dusthan, but if the owner of that house is in the sign which is a benefic position then the planet will give the good effect of ownership of that house it is posited in. It does not give the negative effects of being the owner of the dusthan. For example, for Virgo ascendant, look to Saturn which is posited in the 5th house in Capricorn and although it is the lord of the 5th and 6th so it should be half good and half bad yet according to Mantreshwar Maharaj, according to this sloka it will only give the result of the ownership of the 5th house and will always give good results. It will bless the native with sons and will not show any negative effects as the owner of the 6th house.

राशौ स्थितिर्मिथो योगो दृष्टि: केन्द्रेषु संस्थिति: ।
त्रिकोणे वा स्थिति: पञ्चप्रकारो बन्ध ईरित: ॥३० ॥

In this sloka relationship* or connection between planets are indicated. The relationship between planets is of five types.

(1) Exchange of houses between two planets. Suppose 'A' is in the sign of 'B' and 'B' is in the sign of 'A' then it is an exchange of signs (house).

(2) When two planets are together in one sign

(3) When two planets mutually aspect each other with full aspect.

(4) When two planets are in angular position.

(5) When two planets are in a trine.

Then the two planets are related.

Then this is relationship between the planets.

---

*This relationship is needed to make correct judgement of the minor periods of planets in the major period of a planet. This is also needed to decide if a planet or planets are creating rajayogas.

16

Dwadash Bhavphal

The Interpretation of the 12 Houses

लग्ननवांशपतुल्यतनुः स्याद्वीर्ययुतग्रहतुल्यतनुर्वा
चन्द्रसमेतनवांशपवर्णः कादिविलग्नविभक्तभगात्रः ॥१॥

लग्नेशे केन्द्रकोणे स्फुटकरनिकरे स्वोच्चभे वा स्वभे वा
केन्द्रादन्यत्रसंस्थे निधनभवनपे सौम्ययुक्ते विलग्ने।
दीर्घायुष्मानधनाढ्यो महितगुणयुतो भूमिपालप्रशस्तो
लक्ष्मीवान् सुन्दराङ्गो दृढतनुरभयो धार्मिकः सत्कुटुम्बी॥२॥

सत्संबन्धयुते कलेवरपतौ सद्ग्रामवासोऽथवा
सत्सङ्गः प्रबलग्रहेण सहिते विख्यातभूपाश्रयः।
स्वोच्चस्थे नृपतिः स्वयं स्वगृहगे तज्जन्मभूमौ स्थितिः
सञ्चारश्चरभे स्थितिः स्थिरगृहे द्वन्दं द्विरूपं फलम्॥३॥

विख्यातः किरणोज्वले तनुपतौ सुस्थे सुखी वर्धनो
दुःस्थे दुःख्यसदृक्षनीचभवने वासो निकृष्टस्थले।
स्वस्थो जीवति शक्तिमत्युदयभे वर्द्धिष्ण रूर्जस्वलो
निःशक्तौ निहतो विपद्भिरसकृत्खिन्नो भवेदातुरः॥४॥

अर्थस्वामिनि मुख्याभावजुषि सत्स्वर्थे कुटुम्बश्रिया
सर्वोत्कृष्टगुणो धनी च सुमुखी स्याद्दूरदर्शी नरः।

सम्बन्धे सवितुर्द्वितीयपतिना लोकोपकारक्षमां
विद्यामर्थमवाप्नुयादथ शनेः क्षुद्राल्पविद्यारतः ॥५ ॥

जैवे वैदिकधर्मशास्त्रनिपुणो बौधेऽर्थशांस्त्रे पटुः
शृङ्गारोक्तिोपटुर्भृगोर्हिमरुचेः किञ्चित्कलाविद्भवेत्।
कौजे क्रूरकलापटुश्च पिशुनो राहौ स्थिते लोहलः
केतौ भ्रश्यदलीकवाग्धनगतैः पापैश्च मूढोऽधनः ॥६ ॥

बन्धो यदि स्यात्तनुशौर्यनाथयो-
रन्योन्यराशिस्थितयोर्बलढ्ययोः।
धैर्य च शौर्यं सहजानुकूलतां
प्राप्नोत्ययं साहसकार्यकर्तृताम् ॥७ ॥

शौर्यपे बलिनि सद्ग्रहयुक्ते कारकेऽपि शुभभावमुपेते।
भ्रातृवृद्धिरथ वीर्यविहीने दुःस्थिते भवति सोदरनाशः ॥८ ॥

आयुग्मराशौ यदि कारकेशौ
गुर्वर्कभूसूनुनिरीक्षितौ चेत्।
आजो गृहः स्याद्यपि विक्रमाख्यः
पुंभ्रांतरस्त्वंशवशद्भवेयुः ॥९ ॥

दुःस्थाने सुखपे शशिन्यपि सतां योगेक्षणैर्वजिते
पापान्तःस्थितिमत्यसद्ग्रहयुते दृष्टे जनन्या मृतिः।
एतौ द्वावपि वीर्यगौ शुभयुतौ दृष्टौ शुभैर्बन्धुगै-
र्मातुः सौख्यकरौ विधोश्च सुखगैः सौम्यैर्वदेत्तत्सुखम् ॥१० ॥

लग्नेशे सुखगेऽथवा सुखपतौ लग्ने तयोरीक्ष्णे
योगे वा शशिनस्तथा यदि करोत्यन्त्यां स्वमातुः क्रियाम्।

अन्योन्यं यदि शत्रुनीचभवने षष्ठाष्टमे वा तयो-
मातुर्नोपकरोति नाशसमये बन्धस्तयोर्वा न चेत् ॥११॥

मातृभावोक्तवद्वाच्यं पितृभ्रातृसुतादिषु।
भावकारकभावेशलग्नेश्वरैर्वदेत् ॥१२॥

सुस्थौ सुखेशभृगुजौ तनुबन्धुयुक्ता-
वान्दोलिकां जनपतेश्वरतां विधत्तः।
स्वर्णाद्यनर्घ्यमणिभूषणपट्टशय्या-
कामोपभोगकरणानि च गोगजाश्वान् ॥१३॥

दुस्थे: सुखेशे कुजसूर्ययुक्ते
सुखेऽपि वा जन्मगृहं प्रदग्धम्।
जीर्णं तमोमन्दयुतेऽरियुक्ते
परैर्हृतं गोक्षितिवाहनाद्यम् ॥१४॥

सौम्यर्क्षांशे सौम्ययुक्ते पञ्चमे वा तदीश्वरे।
वैशेषिकांशे सद्भावे धीमान्निष्कपटी भवेत् ॥१५॥

स्थितिः पापाना वा, द्विषति बलयुक्तारिपतिना
युतो वा दृष्टो वा, यदि रिपुगृहे वा तनुपतिः।
अरीशः केन्द्रे वाऽयशुभखगसंवीक्षितयुतो
रिपूणां पीडां द्राग्भृशमपरिहार्यां वितनुते ॥१६॥

षष्ठेश्वरादतिबलिन्युदयाधिनादे
सौम्यग्रहांशसहिते शुभदृष्टियुक्ते।
सौख्येश्वरेऽपि सबले यदि केन्द्रकोणे-
ष्वारोग्यभाग्यसहितो दृढगात्रयुक्तः ॥१७॥

शत्रुनाथे तु दुःस्थाने नीचमूढारिसंयुते
तस्माद्बलाढ्ये लग्नेशे शत्रुनाशं रबौ शुभे ॥१८॥

यद्भावेशयुतो वैरिनाथो यद्भवसंश्रितः।
षष्ठस्थितो यद्भावेशस्ते भावाः शत्रुतां ययुः ॥१९॥

सत्संबन्धयुते सप्तर्क्षे तदीशे बलान्विते।
पतिपुत्रवती साध्वी भार्या सर्वगुणर्वृता ॥२०॥

केन्द्रादन्यत्र रन्ध्रेशे लग्नेशाद्दुर्बले सति।
नाधिर्न विघ्नो न क्लेशो नृणामायुश्चिरं भवेत् ॥२१॥

धर्मे कुजे वा सूर्ये वा दुःस्थे तन्नायके सति।
पापमध्यगते वाऽपि पितुर्मरणमादिशेत् ॥२२॥

दिवा सूर्ये निशा मन्दे सुस्थे शुभनिरीक्षिते।
धर्मेशे बलसंयुक्ते चिरं जीवति तत्पिता ॥२३॥

मन्दारयोः शीतरुचौ च सूर्ये
त्रिकोणगे तज्जननीपितृभ्याम्।
त्यक्तो भवेच्छक्रपुरोहितेन दृष्टे
तनूजोऽस्ति सुखी चिरायुः ॥२४॥

शनिर्भाग्यधिपः स्याच्चेच्चरस्थो न शुभेक्षितः।
सूर्ये दुःस्थानगेऽप्यन्यपितरं ह्युपजीवति ॥२५॥

धर्मे तदीशे वा मन्दयुक्ते दृष्टेऽपि वा चरे।
जातो दत्तो भवेन्नूनं व्येशे बलशालिनि ॥२६॥

नभसि सुभखगे वा तत्पतौ केन्द्रकाणे
बलिनि निजगृहोच्चे कर्मगे लग्नपे वा।
महितपृथुयशाः स्याद्धर्मकर्मप्रवृत्तिः
नृपतिसदृशभाग्यं दीर्घमायुश्च तस्य ॥२७॥

ऊर्जस्वी जनवल्लभो दशमगे सूर्ये कुजे वा महत्
कार्यं साधयति प्रतापबहुलं खेशश्च सुस्थो यदि।
सव्यापारवतीं क्रियां वितनुते सौम्येषु सच्छलाघितां
कर्मस्थेष्वहिमन्दकेतुषु भवेद्दुष्कर्मकारी नरः ॥२८॥

लाभेशे यद्भावनाथयुक्ते यद्भावगेऽपि वा।
भावं तदनुरूपस्य वस्तुनो लाभगैरपि ॥२९॥

व्ययस्थितो यद्भावेशो व्ययेशो यत्र विष्ठति।
तस्य भावस्यानुरूपवस्तुनो नाशमादिशेत् ॥३०॥

1. (A) The physical appearance of a native is according to the lord of the Navansha of the ascendant or it will be like that of the strongest planet in the chart. The varna that means the colour and complexion of the native will be according to the lord of the navansha occupied by Moon.

The 12 signs starting from Aries onwards indicate the different parts of body of the Kalpurush, the Supreme Lord. There are the twelve parts of the Supreme Lords, and so from ascendant to the twelve house, are the twelve portions of the Kalpurush.

Here Mantreshwar Maharaj points out that if the ascendant is a big sign then a benefic in the ascendant will give big and beautiful appearance to the head.

Similarly the body and the part of the body which is indicated by the portions of the Kalpurush will be according to the sign and planets posited in them.

(B) If the lord of the ascendant is in an angle or trine, is not combust and is either exalted, or in own sign and benefic are placed in the ascendant; in this manner if the ascendant and the lord of the ascendant both are strong and the lord of the 8th house is in any other house except in an angle then the native so born will be long lived, wealthy, praised by others, endowed with good qualities, favourite of the kings, possess laxmi, endowed with good and beautiful body, strength and not afraid of others, religious and spiritual, and comes from a good family.

(C) If the lord of the ascendant is related to benefic then he resides in a well established place, village (city etc.). He has the association of gentle and good people. If the lord of ascendant is with or associated with a powerful planet then a native gets the patronage of a famous king. This reasoning suggests that if the lord of the ascendant is in a Dusthan, 6th, 8th or 12th then the native will reside in a cheap place and if it is associated with debilitated and weak planets then the native will have the companionship of low class of people. If the lord of the ascendant is exalted then the native is a king. If the lord of the ascendant is in its own sign then the native keeps on residing in an around his birth place. If the ascendant lord is in a movable sign then the native does not live in one place for a long time i.e. changes keep on taking place in his place of residence. If the lord of the ascendant is in a fixed sign then the native will live in a place for a long time and if it is in a dual sign then the native will live in two or more places. Sometime he lives in two places and travels in between them frequently.

(D) If the lord of the ascendant is endowed with light and powerful i.e. far away from Sun and is endowed with illumination i.e. not combust then the native becomes famous. If ascendant lord is in good houses then the native is happy and attains high position. But if it is in a debilitated sign, in the sign of a malefic or in dusthana then the person resides in cheap houses and places.

If the lord of the ascendant is strong and placed in a Susthan (in a good house) then the native will be happy, endowed with ability to take initiatives, attains high status, has good life but if the ascendant lord is weak then such a person is surrounded by calamities and dangers. He is mentally disturbed due to different diseases i.e. all the time he is attacked by sickness or dangers and spends an unhappy life. In these Slokas the importance of the lord of the ascendant, if it is strong or weak and it is placed in good houses or in dusthana, has been described.

2. (A) If the lord of the 2nd house is in the 1st and benefic are in the 2nd then the native is endowed with extraordinary qualities, wealthy, has a good looking face, has foresight and has an excellent family.

If the lord of the 2nd is associated with Sun then the native is engaged in doing charity to others, is learned and wealthy. If the lord of the 2nd house has relationship with Saturn then the native is not educated or learns insignificant things and he will acquire very little education.

(B) If the lord of the 2nd house is associated with Jupiter then such a person is a Scholar of Veda and Scriptures. He is learned. If it is associated with Mercury then he is an expert in economics.

If with Venus then he is an expert in decorations, fine arts, literature and kamashastra etc.

If Moon is associated with the lord of the 2nd house then the native is expert in some arts.

If with Mars then he is a person of cruel arts, a butcher, killer etc. and is also engaged in backbiting.

If Rahu is in the 2nd house or is with the lord of the 2nd then there is problem in speech like– stammering or unclear speech and if Ketu is there in the 2nd house then also the

---

In the Sloka No. 5 and Sloka No. 6 above, we have given the results of the combination of the lord of the 2nd house with different planets. There results will also operate in the periodic influences of planets which are associated with the 2nd house. This is our opinion.

native either speak lies or stammers. If malefic are in the second house then the native is a fool and poor.

3. (A) If the lord of the 1st house and the lord of the 3rd house are related or they exchange signs i.e. strong lord of the 1st house is in the 3rd house and a strong 3rd lord is in the first, then the native is engaged in work which requires courage and is endowed with patience, is brave and loves his brothers and sisters.

(B) If the lord of the 3rd house is strong, is placed with benefic and the lord of the significator of the 3rd house is also strong and is placed in a good house then there is increase and prosperity for the brothers. But if the significator and the lord of the 3rd are weak and placed in dusthana then the brothers are destroyed.

(C) If the Lord of the 3rd and the significator of the 3rd house i.e. Mars both of them, are in odd signs and are aspected by Jupiter; Sun and Mars* and there is an odd signs in the 3rd from the ascendant then the Navansha already traversed in the 3rd house will give the number of brothers that the native will have.

If the 3rd house in this case is in the 4th Navansha then there will be four brothers.

4. (A) If in a horoscope lord of the 4th house and Moon are placed in dusthana and they do not get any association of benefic nor an aspect of a benefic but are placed in between malefic, or are with malefic or aspected by malefic, then the native's mother will have an early death.

But if all the other things are different from the ones mentioned above i.e. the lord of 4th and Moon are strong, are associated or aspected by benefic, or benefic are placed in the 4th house then there is happiness from mother. If there are benefic from the 4th house from Moon then happiness comes from mother.

---

*Only the lord of the 3rd house can receive an aspect from Mars. Mars can not aspect itself.

(B) If lord of the 1st house is in the 4th and the lord of the 4th is in the 1st and Moon joins them or aspect them then the native is able to perform the last rites of his mother. If both of them the lord of the 1st and the lord of 4th are placed in the 6th or 8th from each other are in the sign of each other's enemy, or in the debilitated sign of each other, or there is no relationship between them, then the native is not able to perform the last rites of his mother.

(C) In the manner the 4th house and the significator of mother Moon are considered in the same manner father, brother, sons etc. are also considered from the house and the planet which signifies them. It should be analysed how they are related with the ascendant, the lord of the ascendant, house, lord of the houses and significator. All these things should be considered to arrive at a judgement.

For example - If the ascendant and the lord of the ascendant are strong and the 5th house, the lord of the 5th and the significator of son which is Jupiter, are friends then the native have happiness and love from children. If the lord of the 1st and the lord of the 5th are enemies or are placed in the 6th, 8th from each other or are placed in the sign of enemy of each other, or debilitated sign of each other, then there will be no love lost between the father and his sons.

(D) The native gets a planquin from the king, if the lord of the 4th house and Venus are in the ascendant or in the 4th house or if both of them are in good houses and are not debilitated, or combust, or any other defects, then he will have a number of vehicles and will enjoy them. He will have gold, costly ornaments, comfortable beds, silken clothes, cow and luxurious items of many type, elephants, horses and happiness from all these.

If the lord of the 4th house is placed in a dusthan and Sun and Mars are with the lord of the 4th house then the native's place of living is destroyed in fire.

If Rahu and Saturn are in the 4th house then his residence will be old and depalidated. If there are planets which are enemy to the lord of the 4th house, in the 4th house, then the native's property, vehicles and lands, will be stolen and taken away by other people.

5. (A) If the 5th house is in the sign and Navansha of benefic planet and the 5th house is associated with benefic or benefic are placed in it then the native will be intelligent, simple and of good character.

If the lord of the 5th house is placed in a good house and is in the vaisheshikansha then similar effect should be drawn. In Sanskrit the word- 'Saumya' is used, it has two meanings- a benefic and the other one is Mercury. One Commentator has interpreted it as Mercury but in our opinion the word Saumya should be a benefic.

6. (A) There are certain combinations which are given below, if they are present then the native has serious troubles on account of enemies and he is unable to get rid of them.

(1) If malefic are in the 6th house.

(2) The lord of ascendant is associated with or aspected by a strong lord of the 6th house.

(3) Lord of the 6th house is associated with or aspected by a malefic and is placed in an angle.

In the original Sanskrit text there is another meaning of it as well that if the lord of the 1st is in the 6th house then also the native is troubled by his enemies. If the lord of the 1st house is also associated with a strong lord of the 6th or is aspected by it then the troubles are much more intense.

(B) If the lord of the 1st house is of excess strength then the lord of the 6th and the lord of the 1st is in the sign and Navansha of a benefic, has the association or aspect from benefic and the lord of the 4th, with strength, is place in an angle or trine then the native will have a strong built, healthy and fortunate.

(C) If the lord of the 6th is placed in dusthan (6th, 8th or 12th), in the sign of its debilitation, or in the sign of an enemy, or is combust and compared to the lord of the 6th house, the lord of the ascendant is stronger and Sun is placed in the 9th house then the native is victorious over his enemies and his enemies are destroyed. There is a slight difference in interpretation also in Sanskrit which means instead of Sun being in the 9th house, the meaning will be if benefic are in the 6th, then the native is victorious over his enemies.

(D) 1. The lord of the 6th house associated with the lord of any sign.

2. The lord of the 6th house in whichever house it is posited.

3. The lord of the any house which is placed in the 6th house.

All three of these will create enmity.

For example- If the lord of the 6th house is in the 5th house or if the lord of the 5th is posited in the 6th house or if the lord of the 5th and 6th are together, then the native's children will be his enemies.

7. If the lord of the 7th house is associated with benefic and the lord of the 7th house is strong then the wife will be endowed with all good qualities, good in character and will have sons.

8. If the lord of the 8th house is placed any other house except in angles and the lord of the 8th comparatively is weaker then the lord of the ascendant, then there is no mental problems, obstacles no sorrows and sufferings, and the native lives long.

9. (A) If Sun and Mars are in the 9th house and the lord of the 9th is placed in dusthan or is hemmed in between malefic, then the native's father dies early i.e. his father will have short life.

(B) If the birth is during the day time and Sun is placed well in a good house and is associated with benefic and the lord of the 9th house is strong then the native's father has long life. If the birth is at night and Saturn is placed in a good house and is associated with benefic and the lord of the 9th is also strong then the native's father has long life.

(C) If Sun and Moon are in the trine from Saturn and Mars then the child's parents will desert him, but if on them (Sun and Moon), the aspect of the Jupiter is there then the child will be happy and long lived.

(D) If Saturn as lord of the 9th house is posited in a movable sign and is not aspected by benefic and Sun is in a dusthan then the native is brought up by someone else other than his father.

(E) If there is a movable sign in the 9th house and it is occupied by Saturn or if Saturn aspect it or the lord of the 9th house is posited in a movable sign and is associated with Saturn being together or getting the aspect of Saturn, if out of these two combination anyone takes place and simultaneously the lord of the 12th is strong then the child so born will be adopted by someone else.

10. (A) If benefic are placed in the 10th house and the lord of the 10th is strong and is posited in own sign as well as in trine or angle, or the lord of the Ascendant is in the 10th and strong, then the native's fortunes are like that of a king and he is long lived. His fame spreads throughout and by nature he is engaged in religious and good activities.

(B) If Sun or Mars is posited in the 10th house then the native will be full of valour and popular and if the lord of the 10th house is placed in a good house then by great influence achieves his goals. If benefic are placed in the 10th house then the native uses such methods of business that he is praised by others. However if Saturn, Rahu or Ketu are in the 10th house, then the native so born is engaged in bad and sinful activities.

11. (A) 1. With whichever lord the lord of the 11th house is posited.

2. In whichever house the lord of the 11th is placed.

3. Whichever planet or the lord of whichever house is

posited in the 11th house, then the conclusion should be drawn that the gains will be from the metal and things which falls under those three lords or planets.

For example - If the lord of the 11th house is posited in the 5th house or the lord of 5th is posited in the 11th or lord of 11th and lord of the 5th are placed together then education (like- teaching) also sons, intellectual abilities, speculation will be sources of benefit. This is so because these things are considered from the 5th house. Similarly if the lord of the 11th house and the lord of the 7th are together, or if the lord of the 7th is posited in the 11th house or if the lord of 11th house is in the 7th then gains come from wife, working in partnership or from business activities.

12. The lord of whichever house is posited in the 12th house or the lord of the 12th house wherever it is placed, then that house will indicate the type of losses.

    For example- If the lord of the 4th house is in the 12th house then the expenses and losses through vehicles or loss of property and lands.

    If the lord of the 12th house is in the 5th then through sons or speculation loss of money should be judged.

BHAVA SIDDHIKAAL

(The timings of the fruitfulness of a house)

When will be the fruitfulness or realisation of a house?

भावेशस्थितभांशकोणमपि वा भावं तु वा लग्नपो
लग्नेशस्थितभांशकोणमुदयं वाऽयाति भावाधिपः ।
संयोगेऽपि विलोकनेऽ च तयोस्तद्भावसिद्धिं तदा
ब्रूयात्कारकयोगतस्तनुपतेर्लग्नाच्च चन्द्रादपि ॥३१ ॥

The realisation of the effect of a house will be during any of the times given below-

(i) When the lord of the 1st house transits a trine from the sign and navansha of any house then the matters of that house will be realised.

(ii) When the lord of a house in transit comes to the house or the Navansha, occupied by the lord of the ascendant or transit in trine to the house or Navansha where the lord of the ascendant is.

(iii) When the lord of the ascendant and the lord of a house aspect each other or are together. (in transit)

(iv) When the significator of a matter comes in transit to the house where the lord of the ascendant or the lord of the Moon sign is placed.

(v) When the lord of the ascendant transit the house which is to be considered.

In the same manner these things should also be considered from Moon.

यद्भावेशास्थतर्क्षांशत्रिकोणस्थे गुरुर्यदा।
गोचरे तस्य भावस्य फलप्राप्तिं विनिर्दिशेत्॥३२॥

Observe which is the sign and the Navansha occupied by the lord of a house about which consideration has to be done. When Jupiter transits a house which is in trine to that sign or the Navansha then good effects of that house takes place or is realised.

लग्नारिनाथयोगे तु लग्नेशद्दुर्बले रिपौ।
तदा तद्वशगः शत्रु र्विपरीतमतोऽन्यथा॥३३॥

When lord of the 1st and the lord of the 6th combine in transit then what is the effect? If lord of the 6th is weak compared to the lord of the 1st then the native overcomes his enemies and if the lord of the 6th is stronger compared to the lord of the 1st, then the native is controlled and defeated by his enemies.

यद्भावपस्य तनुपस्प भवत्यरित्वा-
तत्कालशत्रु वशतोऽरिमृतिस्थितो वा।
स्पर्धा तदा तदतु तेन च गोचरस्थ-
स्तद्वत्सुहृत्वमपि संयुतिमैत्रतश्च॥३४॥

The lord of any particular house and the lord of the ascendant if they are temporary or natural enemies or if they are in 6th and 8th from each other, then whenever in transit they conjoin then enmity or quarrels or jealousy related to that house should be understood. The other side is, if the lord of the 1st or the lord of any house are temporary or natural friends and in transit, when the lord of the ascendant and the lord of that house are conjoined, then happiness, new friendship, good things and fruitfulness related to that house should be judged.

In the coming 23rd Chapter—A horoscope is presented where the lord of 1st is Sun and the lord of the 6th is Saturn. These two are natural enemies and here they are temporary enemies also. They are in the 6th, 8th from each other as well. Therefore whenever there will be a combination of Sun and Saturn in transit, then there will be troubles and sufferings created by enemies. In the same horoscope Sun is the lord of the ascendant and Jupiter is the lord of the 5th house both are natural friends and they are temporary friends also, so whenever Sun and Jupiter will conjoin in transit then good happenings related to the 5th house will take place.

लग्नेशयद्भावपयोस्तु योगो
यदा तदा तत्फलसिद्धिकालः ।
भावेशवीर्ये शुभमन्यथान्य-
ल्लगनाच्च चन्द्रादपि चिन्तनीयम् ॥३५ ॥

Whenever the lord of the 1st house in transits conjoins with the lord of any particular house then realisation and good effect of that house will be there i.e. that house will prosper. Suppose one person wants to buy land or property and asks a question as to when he will gain a house or land. Then see if in the horary chart or in a horoscope, there is going to be a conjunction of the lord of the 1st and the lord of the 4th then the event will materialise. Whenever combination of the lord of the 1st and lord of the 4th takes place then that person will have gain of a house or land. But it is possible only if the lord of the 4th is strong. Whenever the lord of a house is strong then good events related to that house takes place. On the other hand if the lord of a house is weak then even if there is a conjunction of the lord of the 1st with that lord of the house which is weak, there will be no realisation. Side-by-side we should also consider the major and minor periodic influence through which one is passing.

We have mentioned above how to consider the fruitfulness of a house from the birth chart and lord of the ascendant, in the same manner consideration should be done from the sign occupied by Moon *viz.* that Moon sign should be treated as ascendant.

17

Niryana Prakarana (The Timing of Destruction)

तत्तद्भावादष्टमेशस्थितांशे तत्त्रिकोणगे।
व्ययेशस्थितभांशे वा मन्दे मद्भावनाशनम् ॥१॥

If consideration has to be done about the timing when a house will stop operating then look to the Lords of the 8th and 12th houses from that particular house. If we have to consider the destruction of the first house i.e. death, then look to the position of the Lords of the 8th and 12th house. When Saturn in transit comes to the sign and Navansha where the Lords of the 8th house or 12th house (from the house in consideration) are posited then there will be the destruction of the house. When Saturn in transit also comes to the 9th and 5th house from the places mentioned above then also it destroys the house in question.

For example look to the horoscope provided subsequently in the chapter related to 'Ashtakrage. Suppose we have to find as to when the 10th house (service or father) will be destroyed? The 10th house has Taurus. The 8th house from it is Sagittarius and its Lord is placed in Libra and in Aquarius Navansha- so when Saturn transits Aquarius Navansha in Libra or in the Aquarius Navansha of Aquarius (trine from Libra) or in the Aquarius Navansha of Gemini then destruction of the 10th house will take place i.e. loss of job, work or sickness (or death) to father.

Placement of Saturn when death comes.

In this Sloka we mention where Saturn will be at the time of death.

रन्ध्रेशो गुलिको मन्दः खरद्रेक्काणपोऽपि वा।
यत्र तिष्ठति तद्भांशत्रिकोणे रविजे मृतिः ॥२॥

See in which signs and Navansha the following planets are:

1. Lord of the 8th house
2. Gulik
3. Saturn
4. The Lord of the 22nd decante from the Ascendant.

When Saturn in transit goes to the sign and Navansha, mentioned above or in the 9th and 5th from it then the native's death takes place.

उद्यद्दृगाणनाथस्य तथा रन्ध्राधिपस्य च।
रन्ध्रद्रेक्काणपस्यापि भांशकोणे गुरौ मृतिः ॥३॥

See where the following are placed—

1. The Lord of the Decante in which the Ascendant is,
2. Lord of the 8th house.
3. The Lord of the 22nd decante from the Ascendant. The above three in whichever signs and Navansha are or the signs in the 9th and 5th from them, whenever Jupiter transits these, then death occurs.

स्वस्फटद्वादशांशे वा रन्ध्रेशस्थनवांशके।
लग्नेशस्थनवांशे वा तत्त्रिकोणेऽपि वा मृतिः ॥४॥

See where the following are posited in the birth chart—

1. The Sun's Dwadashansha sign
2. The Navansha (sign) of the Lord of the 8th house
3. The Navansha (sign) of the Lord of the Ascendant. When Jupiter and Sun comes in transit to these signs or to the signs in trine (9th and 5th) to the above signs then the native's death occurs.

In these Slokas the timings that are indicated due to the transit of Saturn, Jupiter, and Sun does not mean that the native will definite die then, as Saturn comes to the same place after 30 years, Jupiter after 12 years and Sun every year. The purpose of mentioning these transit is that if the native's is also passing through the major or minor periodic influence of a planet (and is also of the age) which is a "Markesh" (endowed with power to destroy) then only it should be decided as to the year, month etc. according to the above method (transits).

रन्ध्रप्रभोर्वा भानोर्वा भांशकोणं गते विधौ।
मृतिं वदेत्सर्वमेतल्लग्नाच्चन्द्राच्च चिन्तयेत् ॥५ ॥

When the Moon in transit comes to the signs or Navansha where the Lord of the 8th is posited or where Sun is placed or to the signs in trine (5th, 9th) from the above mentioned signs, then the native can die. The principles that have indicated from the Ascendant, the same should also be applied from the sign occupied by Moon (Radical Moon as Ascendant).

लग्नेशहीनयमकण्टकभांशकोणं
प्राप्तेऽथवा शनिविहीनहिमांशुभांशम्।
याते गुरौ स्वमरणन्त्वथ राहुहीन-
भूसूनभांशकगुरौ सहजप्रणाशः ॥६ ॥

1. Subtract the sign, degree, minute of 'Yama Kantaka' from the sign, degree, minutes of the Lord of the Ascendant whatever is the balance call it 'A'.
2. Subtract the sign, degree, minute of the Moon from that of Saturn call the balance 'B'.

The above mentioned 'A' and 'B' in whichever signs or Navansha are and the signs and Navansha in trine from them, when Jupiter comes in transit to these then the native's death occurs.

Subtract the Longitudes (signs, degree, minutes) of Mars from that of Rahu call it - 'C'. When Jupiter comes in transit to the signs, Navansha where 'C' is or to the signs and Navansha in the 9th to these, then the native's brother can die.

भानोः कण्टकवर्जितस्य भवनांशे वा त्रिकोणे गुरौ
तातो नश्यति कण्टकोनगुलिकर्क्षांशत्रिकोणे शनौ।

अर्कोनेन्दुगृहांशकोणगगुरौ चन्द्रोनमन्दात्मज-
क्षेत्रेंऽशेऽप्यथवा त्रिकोणेगृहगे मन्दे जनन्या मृति ॥७ ॥

Subtract the longitude (sign, degree, minute) of Yama Kantak from the Longitude of Sun. The balance be called 'A'. The sign and Navansha where 'A' is, will be badly affected and lead to the death of father by the transit of Jupiter through them. The same will be the result when Jupiter comes in transit to the 9th and 5th from them.

Subtract the longitudes of Mandi from the longitude of Yama Kantak- call the remainder as 'B'. When Saturn comes in transit to the sign and Navansha of 'B' or in trine (9th, 5th) from it, then the death of father can take place.

Subtract the longitude of Mars from that of Sun– call the balance as 'C'. When Jupiter in transit comes to the sign and Navansha where 'C' is or in trine to them then the death will come to the native's mother.

Deduct the longitude of Mandi from that of the Moon call the balance 'D'. When Saturn comes in transit to the sign and Navansha of 'D' or in trine to it then the death of mother occurs.

वदेत्प्रत्यरिनक्षत्रनाथाच्च यमकण्टकम् ।
त्यक्त्वा तद्भवने कोणे गुरौ पुत्रविनाशनम् ॥८ ॥

Deduct the longitude of Yama Kantak from the Lord of the 5th constellation from the birth star (constellation of Moon at birth). Whatever is the balance– when Jupiter in transit comes to that sign or in trine to it then the death of son take place.

लग्नार्कमान्दिस्फुटयोगराशेरधीश्वरो यद्भवनोपगस्तु ।
तद्राशिसंस्थे पुरुहूतवन्द्ये तक्कोणगे वा मृतिमेति जातः ॥९ ॥

Add together the (i) Longitude of Ascendant (ii) Longitudes of Sun (iii) Longitude of Mandi whatever is the total then see as to where the Lord of that sign is. When Jupiter comes to the place occupied by the Lord of the above mentioned sign or in trine to them then the native's own death can take place.

मान्दिस्फुटे भानुसुतं विशोध्यं
राश्यंशकोणे रविजे मृतिः स्यात्।
धूमादिपञ्चग्रहयोगराशि-
द्रेक्काणयातेऽर्कमुते च मृत्युः ॥१०॥

(i) Subtract the longitude of Saturn from that of Mandi then when Saturn in transit comes to that sign or in trine to it then the native's death will take place.

(ii) Add together 'Dhoom' etc. all the five upagrahas. Look to the sign and Decante which comes after adding them. When Saturn transit them then the native's death takes place.

विलग्नमान्दिस्फुटयोगभांशं
निर्याणमासं प्रवदन्ति तज्ज्ञाः।
निर्याणचन्द्रो गुलिकेन्दुयोगो
लग्नं विलग्नार्किसुतेन्दुयोगः ॥११॥

1. Add together the longitude of the Ascendant and longitude of Mandi. The total will indicate the month of death i.e. when Sun in transit comes to that sign then the native's death will take place.

2. The sign which comes by adding together the longitudes of Moon and Mandi, will indicate that Moon will be in that sign at the time of death.

3. The sign which comes by adding together the longitudes of Ascendant, Mandi and Moon will be the Ascendant at death.

मान्दिस्फुटोदितनवांशगतेऽमरङ्घे
तद्द्वादशांशसहिते दिननाथसूनौ।
द्रेक्काणकोणभवने दिनपे च मृत्यु
र्लग्नेन्दुमान्दियुतभेशगतोदये स्यात् ॥१२॥

In this Sloka conclusion about death is based on Mandi.

1. Look to the Navansha of Mandi and when Jupiter comes in transit to this sign.

2. Look to the Dwadashansa of Mandi and when Saturn in transit comes to the same sign;

3. Look to the Decante of Mandi and when Sun in transit passes through that sign or in trine (9-5) to that sign then the native's death will take place. What will be the Ascendant at the time of death? Add together the longitudes (sign, degree, minutes) of Ascendant, Moon and Mandi. See where the Lord of the sign, which comes from the total, is placed. The sign occupied by the above mentioned lord will be the Ascendant rising at death.

गुलिकं रविसूनुं च गुणित्वा नवसंख्यया।
उभयोरैक्यराश्यंशगृहगे रविजे मृतिः ॥१३॥

Add together the longitudes of Mandi multiplied by 9 and the longitudes of Saturn also multiplied by 9. Whatever the sign and Navansha that comes from this total then when Saturn in transit comes to this, will indicate the time of death.

स्फटे विलग्ननाथस्य विशोध्य यमकण्टकम्।
तद्राशिनवभागस्थे जीवे मृत्युर्न संशयः ॥१४॥

Subtract the longitudes of Yama Kantak from that of the Ascendant. See what sign and Navansha comes. When Jupiter in transit comes to the sign and Navansha then the native will without doubt meet his death.

षष्ठावसानरन्ध्रेशस्फुटैक्यभवनं गते।
तत्त्रिकोणेपगे वाऽपि मन्दे मृत्युभयं नृणाम् ॥१५॥

Add together the longitudes of the Lords of the 6th, 8th and 12th houses. Whatever the sign comes then death will take place when Saturn comes in transit to that sign or in transit to the signs in trine (5th, 9th) from it.

उद्यद्दृगाणपतिराशिगते सुरेड्ये
तस्य त्रिकोणेमपि गच्छति वा विनाशम्।
रन्ध्रत्रिभागपतिमन्दिरगेऽथ मन्दे
प्राप्ते त्रिकोणमथवास्य वदन्ति मृत्युम् ॥१६॥

Look as to where the Lord of the decante in which the Ascendant is. When Jupiter transits over the lord of that decante or in the 5th-9th (trine) to it then fear of death exists. This is in relation to the transit of Jupiter. Now in the same Sloka we mention the fear of death due to the transit of Saturn. See the dreshkana on the cusp of the 8th house- and the position of its lord. When Saturn in transit passes through the signs owned by the lord of the dreshkana or in trine to these signs then fear of death exists.*

विलग्नजन्माष्टमराशिनाथयोः
खरत्रिभागेश्वरयोस्तयोरपि।
शाङ्कमान्द्योरपि दुर्बलांशक-
त्रिकोणगे सूर्यसुते मृतिर्भवेत्॥१७॥

Observe as to which is the weakest out of the following pairs–

1. The Lord of the 8th house from the Ascendant or the lord of the 8th house from Moon.
2. The lord of 22nd decante from the Ascendant and the lord of the 22nd decante from Moon.
3. Moon and
4. Mandi.

Out of all these four, look to the Navansha of the weakest. When Saturn in transit passes through this Navansha or in the 5th and 9th from it, then the fear of death exists.

लग्नाधिपस्थितनवांशकराशितुल्यं
रन्ध्राधिपस्य गृहमापतिते घटेशे।
तस्मिन्वदेन्मरणयोगमनेकशास्त्र-
संक्षुण्णखिन्नमतिभिः परिकीर्तितं तत्॥१८॥

---

*In the original Sloka the word 'रन्ध्र त्रिभाग पति मन्दिरगेऽथ' has come. It can have two meanings. The lord of dreshkana (decante) in the 8th house– in whichever sign it is in, then when Saturn passes through this sign or in trine to it then the fear of death exists.

Look to the Navansha occupied by the lord of the Ascendant. Call this 'a'. The sign occupied by the lord of the 8th house - call this 'b'. Measure the distance between Aries and 'a' call this 'c'. When Saturn in transit goes from 'b'' to that much distance indicated by 'c' then the possibility of death exists. For example suppose 'a' is Leo and 'b' is 'Scorpio then 'a' is, if counted from Aries is the 5th sign. Then Pisces will be the 5th sign from Scorpio which is 'b'. Therefore when Saturn passes through Pisces then death can take place.

This is the opinion of those learned scholars who have studies various Shastras (Scriptures).

शशङ्कसंयुक्तदृगाणपूर्वतः
खरत्रिभागेशगृहं गतेऽपि वा।
त्रिकोणगे वा मरणं शरीरिणां
शशिन्यथ स्यात्तनुरन्ध्ररिःफगे ॥१९ ॥

Now we take up as to where Moon will be at the time of death. In this Sloka it has been stated that Moon can be posited in any one of the following places at death:–

1. When Moon comes in transit to the decante occupied by it at birth.
2. In the sign of the lord of the 22nd decante as counted from the decante occupied by Moon at birth.
3. In thc 5th and 9th signs from the signs mentioned above in (1) and (2).
4. In the Ascendant.
5. In the 8th house from the Ascendant.
6. In the 12th house from the Ascendant.

निधनेश्वरगतराशौ भानाविन्दौ तु भानुगतराशौ।
निधनाधिपसंयुक्ते नक्षत्रे निर्दिशेन्मरणम् ॥२० ॥

If Sun in transit is passing through the sign where the lord of the 8th house is posited and Moon (a) in transit is passing through the sign where the radical Sun (Sun at birth) is posited (b) or Moon in transit is in the same constellation where the lord of the 8th house in birth chart, is posited, then the native can die.*

यो राशिर्गुलिकोपेतः तत्त्रिकोणेगते शनौ।
मरणं निशिजातानां दिविजानां तदस्तके ॥२१॥

Observe in which sign Gulik is posited in case the native is born at night. (between Sun set to Sun rise). When Saturn passes through signs in trine to the sign occupied by Gulik then the native's death can take place. If the birth is during the day time then when Saturn comes to the 7th sign from the sign occupied by Gulik then the death of the native will take place.

गुरुराहुस्फुटक्यस्य राशिं यातो गुरुर्यदा।
तदा तु निधनं विद्यात्तत्त्रिकोणगतोऽथवा ॥२२॥

When Jupiter passes through the sign which comes after adding together the longitudes of Jupiter and Rahu or in trine to it (sign) then death can occur.

अष्टमस्य त्रिभागांशपतिस्थितगृहं शनौ।
तदीशनवभागर्क्षं गते वा मरणं भवेत् ॥२३॥

1. When Saturn in transit comes to the sign occupied by the lord of the decante which is on the cusp of the 8th house, then death comes.
2. When Saturn transits the Navansha which is the Navansha occupied by the lord of the 8th house, then death occurs.

जन्मकाले शनौ यस्य जन्माष्टमपतेरपि।
राशेरंशकरराशेर्वा त्रिकोणस्थे शनौ मृतिः ॥२४॥

---

*When a person is passing through the major and minor periods of 'Markesh' (the lord that kills) and also taking into account the transit of Saturn and Jupiter- when they indicate death- only then consideration of the transit of Sun and Moon be done. It is so because Moon in one month and Sun in one year traverses through all the signs.

1. The sign and Navansha occupied by Saturn in the nativity- then when Saturn comes in transit to these signs or in trine to these signs then death takes place.
2. The lord of the sign in which the radical Moon is– see in which sign and Navansha it is in, then when Saturn comes in transit to these signs or in trine to them then death occurs.
3. When Saturn comes in transit to the sign or Navansha occupied by the lord of the 8th house or in trine from them then death occurs.

निशीन्दुराशौ जेज्जन्म मान्दिभेंऽशें शनौ मृतिः ।
दिवार्कभे चेत्तद्द्यूनत्रिकोणे वा शनौ मृतिः ॥२५॥

1. If the birth is at night then when Saturn transits the sign and Navansha in which the radical Moon or Mandi is placed.
2. If the birth is during the day time (from Sun rise to Sun set) then when Saturn goes through the sign and Navansha occupied at birth by Sun or transits the signs in the 5th, 7th or 9th from it.

रन्ध्रेश्वराद्यावति भे मान्दिस्तावति भे ततः ।
शनिश्चेन्मरणं ब्रूयादिति सद्गुरुभाषितम् ॥२६॥

Count the distance (signs and degrees) between the Lord of the 8th house and Mandi. When Saturn comes in transit to the same distance (signs and degree) from Mandi then the death comes to the native. This is the saying of the Saintly Gurus. (सदगुरू)

जन्मकालीनभृगुजात्कामशत्रु व्यये रवौ ।
मरणं निश्चितं ब्रूयादिति सद्गुरुभाषितम् ॥२७॥

See in which sign Venus is placed. When Sun in transit passes through the 6th, 7th or 12th from it then death comes. This happens thrice in a year therefore as we have said earlier that only when the full 'Marak Yoga' is operating only then this Sloka should be considered.

तिष्ठन्त्यष्टमरिःफषष्ठपतयो रन्ध्रत्रिभागेश्वरो

मान्दिर्यद्भवनेषु तेष्वपि गृहेष्वार्कीड्यसूर्येन्दवः ।
सर्वे चारवशात्प्रयान्ति हि यदा मृत्युस्तदा स्यान्नृणां
तेषामंशवशाद्वदन्तु निधनं तत्तत्त्रिकोणेऽपि वा ॥२८ ॥

See as to where in the horoscope the following are:–

1. Lord of the 8th house
2. Lord of the 12th house
3. Lord of the 6th house
4. The lord of the Decante on the cusp of the 8th house.
5. Mandi.

When in transit Saturn, Jupiter, Sun and Moon are passing through them then the native can die, or the above mentioned lords and Mandi in whichever Navanshas (or in the 5th and 9th from them) then when Saturn, Jupiter, Sun and Moon are passing through them then the possibility of death exists.

18

Two Planets Together

The Effect of Two Planets Together

What is the effect and results if two planets are placed together in a horoscope has been discussed in this Chapter.

तिग्मांशुर्जनयत्युषेशसहितो यन्त्राश्मकारं नरं
भौमेनाघरतं बुधेन निपुणं धीकीर्तिसौख्यान्वितम्।
क्रूरं वाक्पतिनान्यकार्यनिरतं शुक्रेण रङ्गयुधै-
र्लब्धस्वं रविजेन धातुकुशलं भाण्डप्रकारेषु वा ॥१॥

कूटस्त्र्यासवकुं भपण्यमशिवं मातुः सवक्रः शशी
सज्ञः प्रश्रितवाक्यमर्थनिपुणं सौभाग्यकीर्त्यान्वितम्।
विक्रान्तं कुलमुख्यमस्थिरमतिं वित्तेश्वरं साङ्गिरा
सस्त्राणां ससितः क्रियादिकुशलं सार्किः पुनर्भूसुतम् ॥२॥

मूलादिस्नेहकूटैर्व्यवहरति वणिग्बाहुयोद्धा ससौम्ये
पुर्यध्यक्षः सजीवे भवति नरपतिः प्राप्तवित्तो द्विजो वा।
गोपो मल्लोऽथ दक्षः परयुवतिरतो द्यूतकृत्सासुरेज्ये
दुःखार्तोऽसत्यसन्धः ससवितृतनये भूमिजे निन्दितश्च ॥३॥

सौम्ये रङ्गचरो बृहस्पतियुते गीतप्रियो नृत्याविद्
वाग्मी भूगणपः सितेन मृदुना मायापटुर्लम्पटः।

सद्विद्यो धनदारवान् बहुगुणः शुक्रेण युक्ते गुरौ
ज्ञेयः श्मश्रुकरोऽसितेन घटकृज्जातोऽन्नकारोऽपि वा ॥४॥

असितसितसमागमेऽल्पचक्षु-
र्युवतिसमाश्रयसम्प्रवृद्धवित्तः।
भवति च लिखिपुस्तकचित्रवेत्ता
कथितफलैः परतो विकल्पनीयाः ॥५॥

1. If Sun and Moon are together at birth then the native is an expert in working with machines and Sculpture and in work connected with stones like a Mason. Sun and Mars together then he indulges in sinful acts. Sun and Mercury in one sign then he is an expert, intelligent, famous and happy. Sun and Jupiter in one sign then he is cruel and works for other people. Sun and Venus together then he is expert in dance, music, cinema like film line, dramatics and also he earns wealth from teaching scriptures. Sun and Saturn together then the person is good in working with iron, steel and also with work connected with pots and vessels.

2. If Moon and Mars are in one sign then the native makes money from wine, by being a shopkeeper, by making pots and pans which are made by mixing two or more metals. This is not a good combination for happiness from mother. If one's mother lives then he is not obedient to her.

3. When Moon and Mercury are together then the native speaks sweet and endearing speech. He is expert in making money *i.e.* he is an expert in Financial Management, and mathematics. He has good comprehension. He is well known, famous and fortunate. When Moon and Jupiter are together then a person is strong, achieves success, becomes the head of his family, very wealthy and has good mental ability but he has a fluctuating and changeable disposition. Moon and Venus together indicates success in work connected with garments, clothes. When Moon and Saturn are together then a person is the son of a women who has married a second time. We are of the opinion that this combination will not apply to those Hindu cultural families where second marriage is not permitted.

4. When Mars and Mercury are together then a person benefits from work connected with roots, herbs, plants, trees, skin of trees etc., as well as from oil, ghee, smooth materials, medicine etc. The person is a wrestler or a boxer. When Mars and Jupiter are together then the native is the head of a city, king or a rich Brahmin. When Mars and Venus are together then he is the owner of a herd of cows, wrestler, interested in other's women, gambler and clever. When Mars and Saturn are together then the native is unhappy, does not keep his promises *i.e.* he is liar and gets a bad name.

5. When in any horoscope Mercury and Jupiter are together then the native is good and expert in work, in dramas, works on the stage like singing, acting and is an expert in dance or the art of dancing. When Mercury and Venus are together then a person is an orator, owner of lands, head of a Sect or Counsellor, When Mercury and Saturn are together then the native is extremely clever, confidence trickster, and a womanizer.

6. If Jupiter and Venus are in one house, then the person is endowed with good education, wealth, many women and good qualities. When Jupiter and Saturn are together then a person works as a Barbar, maker of pots and a good cook. This is the opinion of Mantreshwar Maharaj. Our opinion is that Jupiter is the planet of knowledge and Saturn is the planet of Sanyas. When Jupiter and Saturn are together then the native is introvert.

7. When Venus and Saturn* are together then the native has some problems in vision (eye sight). The prosperity and property of such a person increases when he takes the patronage of a (older or old) woman. At times they are attracted to women which are older. The person is a good writer and an expert in drawing or writing books etc. We have given above the planetary combination of two planets together. When more then two planets are together then the effect given above should be logically blended.

---

*This combination gives wealth from antiques, old properties, renovation and success in calligraphy.

भूपो विद्वान् भूपतिर्भूपतुल्य-
श्चन्द्रे मेषे मोषको निर्धनश्च।
निस्स्वः स्तेनो लोकमान्यो महीशः
स्वाढ्यः प्रेष्यश्चापि दृष्टे कुजाद्यैः ॥६॥

युग्मस्थेऽयोजीविभूपज्ञधृष्टा-
श्चन्द्रे दृष्टे तन्तुवायोऽधनी ॥
स्वर्क्षे योधप्राज्ञसूरिक्षितीशा
लोहाजीवो नेत्ररोगी क्रमेण ॥७॥

राजा ज्योतिर्विद्धनाढ्यो नरेन्द्रः
सिंहे चन्द्रे नापितः पार्थिवेन्द्रः।
दक्षो भूपः सैन्यपः कन्यकायां
निष्णात स्याद्भूमिनाथश्च भूपः ॥८॥

शठो नृपस्तौलिनि रुक्मकार
श्चन्द्रे वणिक् स्यात्पिशुनः खलश्च।
कीटे नृपो युग्मपिता महीशः
स्याद्वस्त्रजीवी विकृताङ्गवित्तः ॥९॥

धूर्तो हयाङ्गे स्वजनं जनेशं
नरौघमाश्रित्य शठः सदम्भः।
भूपो नरेशः क्षितिपो विपश्चि-
द्धनी दरिद्रो मकरे हिमांशै ॥१०॥

कुभेऽन्यदारनिरतः क्षितिपो नरेन्द्रो
वेश्यापातिर्नृपवरो हिमगौ नृमान्यः।
अन्त्येऽघकृत्पटुमतिर्नृपतिश्च विद्वान्
दोर्षकदृग्दुरितकृच्च कुजादिदृष्टे ॥११॥

1. If Moon is posited in Aries then the effect of the aspect of Sun, Mars, Mercury, Jupiter, Venus and Saturn on it will be respectively as follows:-

    1. Poor
    2. King
    3. Learned Person
    4. King
    5. Like a King
    6. Thief.

    If Moon is posited in Taurus, the effect of the aspect of Sun, Mars, Mercury, Jupiter, Venus or Saturn on it will be respectively as follows:-

    1. Servant
    2. Poor *i.e.* without wealth
    3. Thief
    4. Respected among the public
    5. King and
    6. Wealthy

    If Moon is in Gemini and it receives the aspect of Sun, Mars, Mercury, Jupiter, Venus and Saturn then the effect respectively will be as follows:-

    1. Poor
    2. One engaged in work connected with iron and steel
    3. King
    4. Learned person
    5. Courageous
    6. Weaver or engaged in the work of clothes

4. When Moon is in Cancer and Sun, Mars, Mercury, Jupiter, Venus and Saturn has aspect on it, then the following will be the result respectively.

    1. Disease of the eyes

2. Soldier
3. Scholar
4. Intelligent Person
5. King and
6. One who earns livelihood with work connected with Iron.

5. When Moon is in Leo, the aspect of different planets on it will be as follows:-

1. Aspect of Sun makes one a king.
2. Mars makes one king.
3. Makes one a person knowing astrology.
4. Jupiter's aspect makes one very rich.
5. Venus makes one king and
6. Saturn makes one a Barbar.

Those people who are not Barbars they do work which is similar to that of a Barbar. We can say in the present times - those working in Beauty Saloon, Beautician, massage etc.

6. When Moon is placed in Virgo and Sun, Mars, Mercury, Jupiter, Venus and Saturn has aspect on it, then the following will be the result respectively-

1. King
2. Clever person
3. King
4. Commander-in-Chief
5. Very intelligent and Clever and
6. Owner of lands and properties.

7. When Moon is in Libra the aspect of Sun etc. will be as follows-

1. From Sun it makes one a villian.
2. Mars makes a person a bad person (like a devil)
3. From Mercury a king.
4. From Jupiter a goldsmith.
5. From Venus a person engaged in trading.

6. From Saturn a backbiter.

8. When Moon is in Scorpio and different planets aspect it then from Sun it makes one poor; from Mars a king; from Mercury then he is the father/mother of twins; from Jupiter a king, from Venus then he earns his livelihood from garments. Saturn's aspect makes one deformed in the body.

9. When Moon is in Sagittárius and it receives aspect of a planet, then the result of the aspect of Sun, Mars, Mercury, Jupiter, Venus and Saturn is respectively as follows:-

   1. Proud (Arrogant)
   2. Cunning
   3. Landlord of many people, (has many slaves).
   4. From Jupiter a king or one under whom many people live.
   5. Venus makes one the patron of others and
   6. Saturn's aspect makes one a bad person.

10. When Moon is in Capricorn and is aspected by any planet then from the Sun a person is poor, 'from Mars a king; When Mercury aspect's then a big king; With Jupiter owner of lands like a king; Venus makes one intelligent and learned and Saturn makes one wealthy.

11. When Moon is in Aquarius and is aspected by different planets then the result will be as follows:-

   1. Sun makes a person worshipped, proud and famous.
   2. Mars makes one indulge with other women.
   3. Mercury owner of lands.
   4. Jupiter a big king
   5. From Venus favourite of prostitutes.
   6. King of kings.

12. Moon when posited in Pisces and is aspected by any planet then the following is the result:-

   1. From Sun it makes one who is engaged in doing dirty and bad acts.

2. With Mars a shameful person.
3. Mercury intelligent.
4. Jupiter makes one a king.
5. Venus a Scholar.
6. Saturn a person who always finds faults with others.

When Moon is in different Navanshas then what are the results of the aspect of different planets on it.

Moon in different Navansha and the aspect of planet on it

आरक्षको वधरुचिः कुशलश्च युद्धे
भूपोऽर्थवान्कलहकृत्क्षितिजांशसंस्थे।
मूर्खोऽन्यदारनिरतः सुकविः सितांशे
सत्काव्यकृत्सुखपरोऽन्यकलत्रगश्च ॥१२॥

बौधे हि रङ्गचरेकवीन्द्रमिन्त्र-
गेयज्ञशिल्पनिपुणः शशिनि स्थितेंऽशे।
स्वांशेऽल्पगात्रधनलुब्धतपस्विमुख्यः
सत्रीप्रेष्यकृत्यनिरतश्च निरीक्ष्यमाणे ॥१३॥

सक्रोधो नरपतिसंमतो निधीशः
सिंहांशे प्रभुरसुतोऽतिहिंस्त्रकर्मा।
जीवांशे प्रथितबलो रणोपदेष्टा
हास्यज्ञः सचिवविकामवृद्धशीलः ॥१४॥

अल्पायो दुःखितः सत्यपि स्वे
मानासक्तः कर्मणि स्वेऽनुरक्तः।
दुष्टस्त्रीष्टः कोपनश्चर्किभागे
चन्द्रे भानौ तद्वदिन्द्वादिदृष्टे ॥१५॥

1. If at birth Moon is in the Navansha of Mars *i.e.* in Aries or Scorpio and is aspected by Sun, Mars, Mercury etc. then the result respectively will be as follows:-
    1. Defender.
    2. Interested in killing and butchering
    3. Expert in warfare
    4. King
    5. Wealthy
    6. Quarrel some.
2. When Moon is in the Navansha of Venus *i.e.* in Taurus or Libra, then the aspect of the planets on it in order are:-
    1. Fool
    2. Interested in other's Women.
    3. Mercury makes one an excellent poet.
    4. From Jupiter an excellent poetry writer and great writer.
    5. From Venus always engaged in getting luxuries of life.
    6. From Saturn illicit connections with other's women.
3. When Moon is in the Gemini or Virgo and other planets aspect then the result in order are—
    1. From Sun one who is engaged in the work of drama, cinema etc.
    2. With Mars - thief.
    3. Mercury makes a person - poet.
    4. Jupiter aspect a minister to a king.
    5. From Venus expert in music and singing.
    6. From Saturn an expert in sculpture and a mechanic.
4. When Moon is in Cancer and is aspected by planets the results in order are as follows:-
    1. A pygmy or person with a very small structure.
    2. Mars makes one greedy.

3. Mercury makes one a Tapaswi *i.e.* a hard working person (highest) position.
4. Jupiter makes one occupy the main (highest) position.
5. Venus makes one work under a woman.
6. Saturn makes one engaged in own business and work.

5. Moon in Leo Navansha and if aspected by different planets then the results in order is:-

1. Sun- makes one angry. Always getting irritated very quick and fast.
2. Mars- enables one to get patronage of a king.
3. Mercury - a treasurer or wealthy.
4. Jupiter - a high position (Officer).
5. Venus- without issues (without sons).
6. Saturn - engaged in cruel acts and a killer.

6. When Moon is in Sagittarius or Pisces Navansha and other planets aspect it then-

1. Sun - makes a person famous because of his power.
2. Mars- makes one a commander or one whose orders are obeyed by an army.
3. Mercury- an expert in making others laugh, endowed with sense of humour.
4. Jupiter- a minister to a king.
5. Venus - without emotional desires.
6. Saturn - behaves like an old person.

7. When Moon is in Capricorn or Aquarius Navansha and different planets aspect it then the result is as follows-

1. From Sun - very few children.
2. With Mars- unhappy.
3. Mercury - arrogant and proud.
4. Jupiter- busy is own work.
5. Venus- lover of a low class bad woman.

6. Saturn makes one angry.

Note: The result which has been indicated due to the position of Moon in different Navanshas and receiving the aspects of other planets, the same type of result should be drawn when Sun is in those Navanshas and is aspected by different planets. For example– If Sun is in Sagittarius Navansha and is aspected by Moon then the result will be the same which applies when Moon is in Sagittarius Navansha and is receiving the aspect of the Sun which is 'Fame due to one's power' or take another example– When Moon is in Libra Navansha and is aspected by Saturn then the result is shown as that the person will keep relationship with other's women. The same will apply when Sun is in Libra Navansha and receives the aspect of Saturn *i.e.* the person will have illicit connections with other's women.

सूर्यादितोऽत्रांशफलं प्रदिष्टं
ज्ञेयं नवांशस्य फलं तदेव।
राशीक्षणे यत्फलमुक्तमिन्दो-
स्तद्द्वादशांशस्य फलं हि वाच्यम्॥१६॥

The result which has been stated in Sloka No. 12 to Sloka No. 15 are due to the placement of Moon in different Navansha and the aspect of different planets on that Moon. From Sloka No. 6 to Sloka No. 11 the results indicated has been due to the placement of Moon in different signs and when receiving the aspect of other planets. Now we speak of something new. Suppose Moon is in Aries and is aspected by Jupiter. The results which will be there due to this position, will also take place when Moon in Dwadashansha is in Aries. (Dwadashansha is the 12th part) and is aspected by the Jupiter *i.e.* if it is placed in the sign or it is placed in the Dwadashansha then the aspect of different planet will be the same. So the same results (which has been given for different signs from Sloka No. 6 to Sloka No. 11) should be interpreted if Moon is placed in different Dwadashansha and receives aspect of different planets.

वर्गोत्तमस्वपरगेषु शुभं यदुक्तं
तत्पुष्टमध्यलघुताऽशुभमुत्क्रमेण।

वीर्यान्वितोंऽकशपतिर्निरुणाद्धि पूर्व
राशीक्षणस्य फलमंशफलं ददाति ॥१७॥

When Moon is Vargottam *i.e.* in the same sign and same Navansha then the result which has been indicated above will be intensive. If Moon is in own Navansha then compared to Vargottam, the results, the benefic results will be a little less and if is in another Navansha then the benefic result will be much less. If some negative result has been indicated and Moon is Vargottam then due to Vargottam its effects the malefic result will be very little and at times may totally subside. In own Navansha the negative result will be ordinary and in enemy Navansha the result will be extremely bad. The purpose of pointing all this is that Vargottam increases the positive effects, the beneficial effects and reduces and mitigates the evil effects. If Moon is in a Navansha of an enemy then it reduces the benefic effects and intensifies the malefic effects.

Now we say a second thing. Two results of Moon has been stated:-

1. When it is placed in a sign and is being aspected by a planet.
2. When it is in a Navansha and aspected by a planet.

Now we point out that if the lord of the Navansha occupied by Moon is strong, then the results of the Navansha will dominate over the result of the sign. The result of the sign will not be that much *i.e.* the lord of the Navansha is strong, then we should attached more importance to the Navansha.

19

Dashaphal (The Effect of the Periodic Influence of Planets)

भक्त्या येन नवग्रहा बहुविधैराराधितास्ते चिरं
सन्तुष्टाः फलबोधहेतुमदिशन्सानुग्रहं निर्णयम्।
ख्यातां तेन पराशरेण कथितां संगृह्य होरागमात्
सारं भूरिपरीक्ष्यातिफलितां वक्ष्ये महाख्यां दशाम् ॥१॥

Parashar Muni worshipped the Nava Grahas the nine planets in various manners and by getting satisfied the Nava Graha's, the nine planets blessed him with the 'Divyagyan' the enlightened knowledge as to what type of effect the Dasha of any planet will show. After examining time and again the truthfulness of the predictive principles of the dashas of Maharishi Parashar and verifying the authenticity of those principles I, Mantreshwar, am - presenting the substance of those periodic influences of planets that have been stated by Maharishi Parashar.

Now we will speak of the effects Dashas as well as how to calculate the dashas and the balance of any dasha at birth.

अग्न्यादितारपतयो रविचन्द्रभौम-
सर्पामरेड्यशनिचन्द्रजकेतुशुक्राः।
तेने नटः सनिजया चटुधान्यसौम्य-
स्थाने नखा निगदिताः शरदस्तु तेषाम् ॥२॥

The constellation occupied by Moon at birth will indicate the years of the Dasha of a planet and which other dashas will follow This will be clear from the table given further:-

Nakshatras	Nakshatras	Nakshatras	Planets	Years of Dasha
(9 Rows)				(these are fixed yrs.)
1. Krittika	Uttra Phalguni	Uttrashada	- Sun	6
2. Rohini	Hasta	Shravana	- Moon	10
3. Mrigsiras	Chitra	Dhanishta	- Mars	7
4. Ardra	Swati	Shatbhisa	- Rahu	18
5. Punarvasu	Vishakha	Porva-bhadrapada	- Jupiter	16
6. Pusya	Anuradha	Uttara-bhadrapada	- Saturn	19
7. Aslesa	Jyestha	Revati	- Mercury	17
8. Magha	Moola	Ashwini	- Ketu	7
9. Poorva-phalguni	Porvashada	Bharani	- Venus	20

ऋक्षस्य गम्या घटिका दशाब्द-
निघ्ना नताप्ता स्वदशाब्दसंख्या।
रूपैर्नगैः संगुणयेन्नतेन
हतास्तु मासा दिवसाः क्रमेण ॥३॥

How do we calculate the balance of the periodic influence of any planet at birth? Look to the constellation of the Moon at birth and for how much longer it will remain in that constellation. The measurement of time is in Ghatis and Palas.

1 Ghati = 24 Minutes and 60 Palas make 1 Ghati.

How much longer (in Ghatis) Moon will remain in that constellation? Multiply that number (of Ghatis) by the year of the Mahadasha of the planet and then divide it by 60. Then the balance will come out. We will explain this by giving an example.

Suppose at birth the balance of constellation Punarvasu was 20

Ghatis. We have stated in Sloka No. 2 above that when birth is in Punarvasu constellation then the periodic influence commences with that of Jupiter. So the birth is in the mahadasha of Jupiter. What was the balance of the Jupiter's period? This we will work out as shown as under:-

20 - (twenty) (which is the Ghatis remaining to be traversed) x 16 (which is the total years of Jupiter's period) and divide this by 60. So we get $20 \times 16/60 = 16/3 = 5$ years and 4 months as the balance. In the statement of Mantreshwar Maharaj and in the treatise of other Astrological Books, the difference is that according to Mantreshwar the division should always be with sixty but in other Books of Astrology the division is done from the total duration of the constellation. See - Sugam Jyotish Praveshika, 10th Chapter by Pt. Gopesh Kumar Ojha. We will explain this below. According to the method stated by Mantreshwar and other Indian Astrological method, there is a little difference in finding the balance of the period of a planet at birth. The following difference exist between the methods.

1. The system invogue add together the Ghatis and Palas in a Nakshatras traversed by Moon and the balance of Ghatis and Palas remaining in the same Nakshatra that will give the duration of the total Ghatis say 'A'. In the constellation the remaining Ghatis and Palas call this - 'B'.

Now suppose that the birth is in the period of Jupiter, then what is the balance dasha? Suppose in 'A' it is 16 years, then in it is 16/A in B, $16/A \times B/1$. After processing this the year, month and days will come.

in 'A' it = 16 yrs.

in 1 is = 16/A

in 'B' is = $16/A \times B/1$

According to Mantreshwar we have $16/60 \times B/1$. The difference is that in this the total duration of the constellation is not taken into account. 'A' is always 60 ghatis. Only 'B' changes and the mathematical calculation are done based on 'B' that gives the balance of the period.

रविस्फुटं तज्जनने यदासीत्
तथा विधश्चेत्प्रतिवर्षमर्कः।
आवृत्तस्यः सन्ति दशाब्दकानां
भागक्रमात्तद्दिवसाः प्रकल्प्याः ॥४॥

In this Sloka we have indicated what type of year should be taken in a mahadasha. Whether the lunar year of 360 days or the year of the constellation or the Solar year. In some part in South of India, particularly in Kerala the year taken in account is the Lunar year of 360 days but according to the above Slokas the position of Sun *i.e.* the sign, degree, minute and seconds of the Sun is considered *i.e.* when . Sun after completing a full cycle, comes back to the same sign, degree, minutes and seconds that should taken as one year. This is called a Solar Year or Saur Varsha and this year should be used in the calculation of the Mahadashas. The 12th part of this solar year is the month and the 30th part of the month is the day. This should be understood. In most places the Solar year is used in calculating the major and minor periods of planets.

भानुः करोति कलहं क्षितिपालकोप-
माकस्मिकं स्वजनरोगपरिभ्रमं च।
अन्योन्यवैरमतिदुःसहचित्तकोपं
गुप्त्यर्थधान्यसुतदारकृशानुपीडाम् ॥५॥

क्रौर्याध्वभूपैः कलहैर्धनाप्तिं
वनाद्रिसंचारमतिप्रसिद्धिम्।
करोति सुस्थो विजयं दिनेश-
स्तैक्ष्ण्यं सदोद्योगरतिं सुखं च ॥६॥

मनःप्रसादं प्रकरोति चन्द्रः
सर्वार्थसिद्धिं सुखभोजनं च।
स्त्रीपुत्रभूषाम्बररत्नसिद्धिं
गोक्षेत्रलाभं द्विजपूजनं च ॥७॥

बलेन सर्वं शशिनस्तु वाच्यं
पूर्वे दशाहे फलमत्र मध्यम्।
मध्ये दशाहे परिपूर्णवीर्यं
तृतीयभागेऽल्पफलं क्रमेण॥८॥

भौमस्य स्वदशाफलानि हुतभुग्भूपाहवाद्यैर्धनं
भैषज्यानृतञ्चनैश्च विविधैः क्रौर्यैर्धनस्यागमः।
पित्तसृग्ज्वरबाधितश्च सततं नीचाङ्गनासेवनं
विद्वेषः सुतदारबन्धुगुरुभिः कष्टोऽन्यभाग्ये रतः॥९॥

सौम्यः करोति सुहृदागममात्मसौख्यं
विद्वत्प्रशंसितयशश्च गुरुप्रसादम्।
प्रागल्भ्यमुक्तिविषयेऽपि परोपकारं
जायात्मजादिसुहृदां कुशलं महत्त्वम्॥१०॥

धर्मक्रियाप्तिममरेन्द्रगुरुर्विधत्ते
संतानसिद्धिमवनीपतिपूजनं च।
श्लाघ्यत्वमुन्नतजनेषु गजाश्वयान-
प्राप्तिं वधूसुतसुहृद्युतिमिष्टसिद्धिम्॥११॥

क्रीडासुखोपकरणानि सुवाहनाप्ति
गोरत्नभूषणनिधिप्रमदाप्रमोदम्।
ज्ञानक्रियां सलिलयानमुपैति शैक्र्यां
कल्याणकर्मबहुमानमिलाधिनाथात्॥१२॥

पाकेऽर्कजस्य निजदारसुतातिरोगान्-
वातोत्तरान्कृषिविनाशमसत्प्रलापम्।
कुस्त्रीरतिं परिजनैर्वियुतिं प्रवास-
माकस्मिकं स्वजनभूमिसुखार्थनाशम्॥१३॥

कुर्यादहि: क्षितिपचोरविषाग्निशास्त्र-
भीतिं सुतार्तिमतिविभ्रमबन्धुनाशम्।
नीचावमाननमतिक्रमतोऽपवादं
स्थानच्युतिं पदहतिं कृतकार्यहानिम् ॥१४॥

विधुंतुदे शुभन्विते प्रशस्तभावसंयुते
दशा शुभप्रदा तदा महीपतुल्यभूतिदा।
अभीष्टकार्यसिद्धयो गृहे सुखस्थितिर्भवे-
दचञ्चलार्थसंचया: क्षितौ प्रसिद्धकीर्तय: ॥१५॥

पाथोनमीनालिगतस्य राहो-
र्दशाविपाके महितं च सौख्यम्।
देशाधिपत्यं परवाहनाप्ति-
र्दशावसाने सकलस्य नाश: ॥१६॥

केतोर्दशायामरिचोरभूपै:
पीडा च शस्त्रक्षतमुष्णरोग:।
मिथ्यापवाद: कुलदूषितत्वं
वाह्वेर्भयं प्रोषणमात्मदेशात् ॥१७॥

1. (A) In this Sloka the result of the Sun's period is mentioned. Here the effect of Sun is not good. It looks that this will be so if Sun is the lord of a bad house or is placed in a wrong place like in track. Then the bad effect will manifest itself. Sun in its period creates quarrels; sudden anger of the king, disease in the family and makes a person wander about. In the past sudden travel to distance places was supposed to be troublesome. Creates mutual jealousy and quarrels with close people. In the mind anger and intolerance, loss of secret wealth and grains from fire; fears from the law and suffering to wife and sons.

   (B) If Sun is in a good place, good position in the nativity then the gain of wealth comes from cruelty, travelling, from the pleasure of kings and fighting or quarrels (it means from legal cases and disputes). The native wanders around in forests and hills and gains fame and becomes well known. The native is constantly engaged in new methods of earnings. There is penetration in his temperament and work and he receives victory and happiness.

2. (A) In the Moon's period the mind is happy. All types of realisation of work and gain of wealth. Food and in take of food is happily done. Gains of wife, sons, ornaments, garments, clothes, jewels, gems, cow and agricultural lands. The native honours Brahmins and worship them.

(B) The above mentioned effect will be fully realised only when Moon is strong. From the first day till the 10th day of the waxing Moon *i.e.* when Moon is increasing in light, during these ten days Moon is of medium strength so the effect of the Moon will be only medium. For the next 10 days *i.e.* from the 11th day of the waxing Moon till the 5th day of the waxing Moon, Moon is of full strength so during these days it will show the full benefic results and in the last 10 days *i.e.* from the 6th day of the waning Moon till amavasya. Moon gradually becomes weaker and weaker so during these days it will show very little benefic effect. According to another opinion upto the 5 days it is very weak then from 6th to 10th days it is medium strength and from 10th to 15th days it is of full strength. This is during the Mahadasha of the Moon.

3. (A) If the native is passing through the periodic influence of Mars then gain of wealth comes from fire, kings, war etc. The native also gains through speaking lies from treachery, from medicine and various types of cruel acts.

During the period of Mars the native suffers from access of piles, Blood disorders, fever, feverishness etc. He developes relationship with low types of women. He will have differences with his own son, wife, relatives and religious Gurus. He will be engaged in bringing good fortunes to others act like a king maker *i.e.* from his efforts other people will benefit.

4. When the period is of Mercury then meeting with friends takes place. A person has happiness himself. Scholars praise him. Fame and publicity comes. He gains name and blessings of the Guru's. In his speech there is persuation and power *i.e.* automatic expressions come to him and he expresses his opinion in a very authoritative and correct manner. In the Mahadasha of Mercury the native is engaged in good deeds of life and he receives happiness from wife, sons, friends and relatives and gains importance.
5. **Jupiter:** In the period of Jupiter a person is engaged in doing religious deeds. He has gain of children or happiness from children; Kings and people in authority pay homage and honour to him. Other famous people and well known people will also praise him. He gains elephants, horses and vehicles. His desires of the heart are fulfilled. He gets kindness from his wife, sons, friends and is constantly in touch with them.
6. During the Mahadasha of Venus the person gains luxurious items of enjoyment, high class of vehicles, cow, gems, ornaments, wealth, enjoyment from women, knowledge *i.e.* from things which increases knowledge, travelling by water. Honours from the kings or the government. In the period of Venus good deeds take place in the house like marriages, celebrations etc.
7. In the Mahadasha of Saturn the native's wife or sons suffer from disease. He himself suffers from 'vata' disorder loss of agriculture and he speaks filthy languages.* He is engaged and falls in love with a bad woman. He is separated from his family members and sudden losses of relatives, lands, happiness and wealth. Our opinion is that these negative effect will happen in the period of Saturn when it is very weak and badly placed in a chart."

---

*"A person when he is passing through the periodic influences of a planet gets the shadow of that planet on to his body and mind. If one is passing through the periodic influence of a benefic planet then he utters good words. In the influence of a planet which is a malefic, a person utters sarcastic remarks, illogical words and filthy speech which does not have any sense."

8. A. In the Mahadasha of Rahu there is a fear from rulers, thieves, poison, fire and weapons; suffering from children, mental anguish of a high order and uneasiness in the mind; loss of kinsmen, insults from low people defame. Some type of bad deed takes place which causes misfortunes and bad name. Loss of place, residence or service. Whatever work one takes up results in losses failure and setbacks in position.**

   B. In the 14th Sloka above, the negative effect of the periods of Rahu has been mentioned. In the present Sloka it is stated that if Rahu is with a benefic and well placed in a good house, then the Mahadasha of Rahu gives exceptionally good results. The native's prosperity is equal to a king. All the works he undertakes are successful. He lives happily in his own residence. He accumulates wealth with strength and he is famous on the earth.

   C. If Rahu is in Virgo, Scorpio or Pisces then we mention special points to be considered during the Mahadasha of Rahu. If out of these three signs, Rahu is in any one of them, then the native becomes the ruler of place he lives in i.e. he rises to the top position and gets much happiness. He will have a palanquin. All these good things happen as long as the dasha continues but in the last phase of the dasha particularly in the end, all and every thing that is attained in the Rahu's period is wiped out.

9. In the Mahadasha of Ketu there is trouble from enemies, thieves and the kings. Some type of disease related to heat and bites in the body, danger of getting hurt from weapons. Such type of disease where heat is felt viz., pimples, worms, dropsy, heat-storkes etc. In the Mahadasha of Ketu the native's family gets the blame and loses prestige. There is danger of fire, unnecessary blame on self of certain things in which the native is not involved. He may have to be an outcast and leave his country of birth.

**In the original Sanskrit Sloka the word 'Padhati' is used, which can have two meanings. (i) setback in one's position (ii) or injuries to feet. Here we think the first one is more authentic.

This way after speaking about the Mahadasha's of the nine planets— Sun etc. in order, we go to the interpretation of the nine planets in the sequence they come in the Vimshotari Mahadasha.

अथ तरणिदशायां क्रौर्यभूपालयुद्धै-
धर्नमनलचतुष्पात्पीडनं नेत्रताप: ।
उदरदशनरोग: पुत्रदारार्तिरुच्चै-
र्गुरुजनविरह: स्याद्भृत्यानाशेऽर्थहानि: ॥१८॥

शिशिरकरदशायां मन्त्रदेवद्विजोर्वी-
पतिजनितविभूति: स्त्रीधनक्षेत्रसिद्धि: ।
कुसुमवसनभूषागन्धनानारसाप्ति-
र्भवति खलविरोध: स्वक्षयो वातरोग: ॥१९॥

क्षितितनदशायां क्षेत्रवैरक्षितीश-
प्रतिजनितविभूति: स्यात्पशुक्षेत्रलाभ: ।
सहजतनयवैरं दुर्जनस्त्रीषुक्ति-
र्दहनरुधिरपित्तव्याधिरर्थोपहानि: ॥२०॥

असुरवरदशायां दु:स्वभावोऽथवा स्या-
दतिगहनगदार्ति: सूनुनार्योर्विनाश: ।
विषभयमरिपीडावीक्षणोद्ध्वर्वाङ्गरोग:
सुहृदि कृषिविरोधो भूपतेर्द्वेषलाभ: ॥२१॥

अमरगुरुदशायाम्बराद्यर्थसिद्धि:
परिजनपरिवारप्रौढरत्यर्थमान: ।
सुतधनसुहृदाप्ति: साधुवादप्तपूजा
भवति गुरुवियोग: कर्णरोग: कफार्ति: ॥२२॥

रवितनयदशायां राष्ट्रपीडाप्रहार-
प्रतिजनितविभूतिं प्रष्यवृद्धाङ्गनाप्तिः।
पशुमहिषवृषाप्तिः पुत्रदारप्रपीडा
पवनकफगुदार्तिः पादहस्ताङ्गतापः ॥२३॥

शशितनयदशायां शश्वदाचार्यसिद्धि-
र्द्विजजनितधनाप्तिः क्षेत्रगोवाजिलाभः।
मनुवरसुरपूजा वित्तसंधातसिद्धिः
प्रभवति मरुदुष्णश्लेष्मरोगप्रपीडा ॥२४॥

शिखिजनितदशायां शोकमोहोऽङ्गनाभिः
प्रभुजनपरिपीडा वित्तनाशोऽपराधः।
प्रभवति तनुभाजां प्रोषणं स्वीयदेशा-
द्दशनचरणरोगः श्लेष्मसन्तापनं च ॥२५॥

भृगुतनयदशायामङ्गनारत्नवस्त्र-
द्युतिमिधिधनभूषावाजिशय्यासनाप्तिः।
क्रयकृषिजलयानप्राप्तवित्तागमो वा।
भवति गुरुवियोगो बान्धवार्तिर्मनोरुक् ॥२६॥

In the Sloka No. 5 to Sloka No. 17. The general order of planet like— Sun, Moon, Mars, Mercury, Jupiter, Venus, Saturn, Rahu and Ketu has been mentioned and in the same manner the tendency of each planet to show their effect was outlined.

Now in Sloka's 18th to 26th, according to the Vimshotri Mahadasha the order of the dasha is Sun, Moon, Mars, Rahu, Jupiter, Saturn, Mercury, Ketu and Venus and in this order the tendencies of the planets as to what type of effect they show has been mentioned. In the 19th Chapter the influence of planets as to how they manifest themselves during their periods has been discussed twice and we are of the opinion that the following mystery lies behind it.

1. From Sloka No. 5 to 17 the interpretation of the planets that has been given are the general tendencies of the planets. As is the case in the Yogini Dashas that the Yogini Dashas of benefic planets the effect is benefic, and in the Yogini Dasha of malefic planets, ill-effects manifest themselves. According to another opinion, in the other types of dashas viz. Ashtottari etc. the effect and result should be interpreted according to that mentioned in Sloka No. 5 to Sloka No. 17.
2. In the Sloka 18th to Sloka 26th the order of the planet has been kept as it is in the Vimshotri Mahadasha. There are certain specific points in the Vimshotari Mahadasha.

For example: The lord of the 11th which is a house gains has been called a malefic. Not only this it has been called the worst malefic out of the three houses like the 3rd, 6th and 11th houses. The lord of the 6th is mentioned as more malefic than the lord of the 3rd and the lord of the 11th is even more malefic then the lord of the 6th house. The second speciality is that if a benefic planet is the lord of an angle which is the 1st, 4th, 7th and 10th, then it does not show benefic results. But if a malefic owns an angle then it does not give malefic or ill-effects.

The question is that whether the lord of the 1st should also be taken into account for all this. It is a very debateable point but the full good effect comes when the lord of the 1st is a malefic? So, in these the general rules should not be applied that a benefic planet will show benefic effect and a malefic will show malefic effect. Due to this reason from Sloka No. 5 to 17 the result should be applicable to different type of periodic influences like— the Astottari, Yogini, Kalachakara dashas etc. Here the rule is that in the periodic influence of a malefic planet the effect will be malefic and the periodic influence of a benefic planet only benefic results will manifest. But when we have to consider the Vimshotari Mahadasha and what type of effect it will show, then Sloka No. 18 to Sloka No. 26 should be taken into account and the interpretation should be according to the principles indicated in these Slokas.

Now we give the effect of the various Mahadashas. It would be useful for Vimshotari Mahadashas.

1. When a native is passing through the periodic influence of Sun then gain of wealth comes through cruelty and courage, through kings or from war. Danger from fire and cattles. Burning sensations in the eyes, disease connected with stomach and teeth, the son and wife suffers from sickness or some other types of sufferings, loss of wealth, servants and employees cause problems, separation or death to elderly people like— father, uncle etc. In the present Slokas the negative effect of Sun has been mentioned. This will only take shape when Sun is badly placed and does not have strength in chart. There are always certain types of specialities related to different planets. When a planet is weak then ill-effects connected to those things over which it rules will be felt. When it is strong and well placed then the matters which fall under the planet will show gains.

2. In the periodic influence of Moon, there are gains of luxuries and nice things through various types of Mantras, Gods, Brahmins and Kings. How can one attain Ashwarya and Luxuries through Mantras? It means that either the person should perform and do the Japas himself to attain prosperity or he gains wealth as 'Dakshina' from the people he will do the Mantras for. In the Mahadasha of Moon, gain of wife, women, wealth and agricultural lands. Gain of flowers, garments, ornaments, scented materials and different types of Rasa— Juice. Opposition from bad characters, loss of wealth, body and disease connected with access of vata. In the present slokas both the good and bad effect of the Moon has been mentioned. If Moon is strong and well placed in a good house, is the owner of a good house, then benefic results will ensue. If Moon is weak, placed in a 'dusthan' 6th, 8th, 12th then the negative and ill effect will be more.

3. During the period of Mars the gains are from lands, from enmity and happiness is received through Kings, gain of cattles and agricultural lands but enmity with own brothers and sons, interest in women of fickle characters, blood disorder *i.e.* impurities of blood and disease related to heat in the body, danger from fire, disorder of biles and loss of wealth, takes place.

4. During the Mahadasha of Rahu the native's temperament becomes bad and cruel *i.e.* the native's loses his tolerance and danger

from some types of serious, sickness, loss of wife and sons, danger from poison, troubles and suffering created by enemies, disease in the eyes and head; psychological problems, opposition from friends and in work connected with agriculture, enmity with kings *i.e.* unpleasantness of kings resulting in losses or danger from the law.

5. Now we speak of the result of the periodic influence of Jupiter. When the Jupiter's period is running then gain of new clothes. Increase in the number of servant and family members, The prestige increases, gain of sons like—birth of a child, wealth increases and increases in the number of friends, people praise him and he receives honour and recognition from well place and high class people. But it causes loss of elderly people like father etc. sickness in ears and disease arising out of disorder of phlegm. Any type of disease can take place with the excess of phlegm.

6. In this Sloka the effect of Saturn's period has been discussed. When one is passing through the Saturn Mahadasha then there is likely to be some type of calamity in the country one lives in or the country is engaged in war or fighting is going on due to which wealth is gained.

   For Example: During the war time, people make money in the black market or during the time of famine people earn more money by engaging in illegal activities. In the period of the Mahadasha of Saturn one gains servants, gain of an older women (A women who has crossed her young age) Relationship developes with her. Millions of people pass through Saturn's period but relationship with an old women does not happen for everyone. Here the meaning of old should be taken as a women who is of more age than the native and if in the birth chart Saturn indicates this type of relationship or indicates illicit relationship then this will be effective. At times we have seen that if a person is older and he is in the Saturn's period then he gets attracted to very young women where the age disparity is 18th to 20th years and more. During the Mahadasha of Saturn gain of cattles, buffalo, ox, etc. but the wife and sons pass through bad times and they suffer. The native himself suffers from vata disorder, arthritis, rheumatic, cough and cold. There are disease like piles, fistula etc. and there is burning sensation constantly in the hands and feet.

7. During the Mahadasha of Mercury the native constantly gains Acharya Siddhi. Acharya Siddhi has two meanings *i.e.* (1) The native gains success and learning from his Gurus or (2) the native himself becomes a Guru and that way he attains fame. In the period of Mercury gain of agricultural lands, horses and money from Brahmins. The natives comes in contact with high class and well placed people. He is engaged in worship of Gods and gains substantial wealth. Mercury is the ruler of the three gunas vata, pitta and cough and during this period of Mercury there is suffering and disease related to the excess of any of these, or any two or all the three gunas.

8. In the periodic influence of Ketu very bad results ensue. Due to women there is much involvement and sufferings and emotional distress. A person feels tense in the heart and it is called big sorrow and mental anguish. Mental derangement when a person loses his logic - this may happen during the Mahadasha of Ketu.

   The native's suffers from women and rich people or his officers or employer cause him harm and problems. The native gets involved with wrong people and as such is involved in shameful activities. His wealth is lost. He may have to leave his country and wander around. He suffers from disease caused by phlegm and disease in the legs and teeth.

9. In the Mahadasha of Venus the native get gems, garment, clothes, luster on the face, underground treasures, wife, women, wealth, luxurious items, horses, beds and sofas. Buying and selling goods, agriculture or shipping and import and export through water, wealth is gained. In the Mahadasha of Venus the benefic results are indicated, but it can cause separation or death to elderly people *viz.*, father, mother etc. There are worries and problems to relatives.

In this 19th Chapter the good and ill-effects, that has been discussed, from them conclusion should be drawn as to when the benefic result will take place and the negative effects will be of what type? Only for knowledge and direction these slokas should be taken into account. These should be blended with logic and experience and then conclusion be drawn. If in the birth chart the benefic are more and the planet is a benefic then mostly it will give benefic results and if it is supposed to give ill-effects then the ill-effects will be of a very light magnitude. When a planet is not well placed *i.e.* is in a trick 6th, 8th, 12th or is the lord of the negative house then the malefic effects will increase and the positive results will subside. Beneficial and ill effects are due to the following reasons:

1. Whether a planet is a natural benefic or a natural malefic.
2. The lordship *i.e.* which houses it owns.
3. In which house it is placed.
4. With what planets it conjoin with.
5. What planets are aspecting it.
6. The planet under consideration is it strong in Dashvargas and Astakvargas.
7. Whether it is combust.

After all these things are considered then conclusion should be drawn, if a planet will show good effects or ill-effects or mixed results.

Now we state some principles of how to judge a nativity as is given in the Book - 'Bhavarth Ratnakar'.

'Bhavarth Ratnakar' is written by Sh. Ramanujacharya. The initial sloka of 'Mangla Charan' which has been given in the beginning of the Book indicates that the author of this Jyotish Granth— 'Bhavarth Ratnakar' and the famous 'Mahapravartak' of Vaishnav Sampradai Sh. Ramanujacharya was one and the same. If they are two different Ramanujacharya even then it does not make any difference in the waitage of this book because there are certain principles which have been written in these books, and these are not available in other books of Astrology. The learned readers will themselves analyze this. The name of the Book 'Bhavarth Ratnakar'. Now Ratnakar has two meanings (1) Ratno Ka Akar— That means the 'collection of Jewels' and (2) Sea.

In this predictive Astrology there are many precious Gems *i.e* why the name of Ratnakar which depicts the sense of the Book.

Ratnakar means 'Samudra' - The Waves. So this book has been divided into different Tarang in different waves instead of chapters and names viz., first tarang, first waves, dutiya tarang, second wave etc. In all there are 14 waves. If we give the original Sanskrit text and its meaning (in the Hindi language) then the present book will become too big and time consuming, so here only the substance of the book is given.

ARIES RISING

1. If a person has the rising sign as Aries and there is a relationship between the lords of the 4th and the 5th then it is a Rajyoga. The lord of the 4th house is Moon and Sun is the lord of the 5th house and this relationship between Sun and Moon is a Rajyog. If both of them are in the 7th from each other then the birth will be near the full Moon as such Moon will be quite powerful and this will be a beautiful combination, a strong Rajyog. During Amawasya Sun and Moon are in one sign but the waning Moon so close to Sun is not very strong. One another Astrological Book is of the opinion that any ascendant may be rising if Sun and Moon both of them are in Leo, or in Cancer or, Sun in Cancer and Moon in Leo then the native's body is weak and thin looking. If these two are simultaneously aspected by malefic planets or any other bad yoga is there, then a person can have tuberculosis (T.B.).

2. Venus, being the ruler of the 2nd and 7th house, is a 'Markesh' if Aries is rising. But it should not be taken for granted that Venus will definitely kill. First of all the longevity of the native should be calculated to ascertain if he has short or medium or long life. At whatever age the 'Marak' planets take effect, then in that period the major period of Venus and minor period of Saturn, or in the minor period of any other malefic, it can be a marak (fatal). Wherever we have used the word Marak *i.e* fatal, then it should always be considered, if the native has short life, medium life or long life.

3. For Aries rising people Jupiter is the ruler of the 9th and 12th house and such a Jupiter if placed in the 10th house *i.e* in his sign of debilitation then it can be a marak. A planet which can be fatal during its major or minor period.

4. In Aries ascendant, Saturn and Jupiter even if they have any connection then only from this combination the Rajyog does not take place. Here the saying is that Saturn is no doubt the ruler of the 10th and Jupiter is the ruler of the 9th. Still this yoga has not been considered as good. For other planets a connection between 9th and 10th lords is a very good Raj Yog. But the reason here is that Saturn together with the 10th ownership also rules the 11th house and 'Brashpati' simultaneously rules the 12th. So the combination of the lord of 9th and 10th here loses its beneficial effects.
5. The Aries rising native suffers from small pox, worms, pimples, scars and danger from weapons. The reason is that Mars being the owner of Aries is prone to create these things.
6. When Mars is with the lord of the 6th house or 8th house then it causes danger or getting hurt in the head during its Mahadasha and Antardasha or can cause blood pressure so that the disease connected with the brain occurs or death* due to some other problem related to head.
7. In the horoscope of Aries rising natives, if Venus the ruler of the 2nd house is placed in the 12th house then it is a benefic. The reason is that in the 12th house here Venus goes to Pisces and it is the exalted sign of Venus. Besides this the 12th house is also the house from which we judge luxuries beds, enjoyment and if Venus is placed here it is quite powerful and happy and gives extraordinary luxurious things of life. So for Aries rising people Venus in the 12th is suppose to be good but this is a bye-law of the general principle (in the case of the Venus). The general rule is that if the lord of the 2nd house which is the house of wealth is placed in the 12th house then it causes destruction of wealth. So it has been said 'Meshe Tatashya Dhanko Vaisthopy Kavisubha Itarakhtu Jatashya Vaistha Dhankosubha..

---

*Where the word death comes it should not be understood that the native will die. It can also mean intense sufferings equal to death. (For Aries rising, Mars being the ruler of the 8th itself can not be with the lord of the 8th, so if it is with the lord of the 6th then these things can happen).

मेषे जातस्य धनपो व्ययस्थोपि कविश्शुभ: ।
इतरर्क्षेतु जातस्य व्ययस्थ: धनपोऽशुभ: ॥७॥

8. For Aries rising people the combination of Mars and Venus is mixed. This combination is good and bad both. It is good because it is a relationship between the lord of 1st and the lord of the 2nd house. So it is an excellent combination for gain of wealth and it will show great significance in the chart. But side by side as they are the rulers of the 7th and 8th houses like— Venus rules the 7th and Mars rules the 8th, so this combination can have 'Marak' effect as well. Marak as we have said is 'fatal' i.e. one which kills.

9. For Aries rising people— Mars, Jupiter and Venus are together in the 2nd house then this combination of the three definitely gives a good Yoga*.

10. If Aries is rising and Mars the ruler of the 1st house is placed in the 3rd house with Jupiter and Venus, then this is not a yoga giving combination.

11. Aries rises and Mars and Jupiter are both in the 4th house, then definitely it is a combination which is a Raj Yog and good effect comes. Here one things should be kept in mind that in the 4th house for Aries rising people Cancer is the sign and although it will be the debilitated sign of Mars yet because Jupiter is exalted here which is posited with Mars so the bad effect of the debilitation of Mars goes away. It nullifies the debilitation effects. Another things is that the lord of the 1st and the lord of the 9th, both simultaneously will aspect the 10th house and they are in an angle so this is a good combination.

12. If Aries is the ascendant and Mars is in the 5th house then the Mahadasha of Mars definitely will give yoga (Rajyoga) rise in life etc.

---

*The planet which shows full benefic effects....either due to the rulership of good houses or on account of benefic association with other planets then it result in yoga for beneficial results.

मेषे जातस्यहि कुजः पञ्चमस्थो भवेद्यदि।
कुजदायेचसंप्राप्ते योगदश्चभवेद्ध्रवम् ॥२ ॥

13. When Aries is the rising sign and Jupiter is placed in the 11th house then in the periodic influence of Jupiter- *'Avayoga' occurs *i.e.* during the Mahadasha of Jupiter there is no rise in life but this placement of Jupiter causes, downfall and setbacks.

14. For Aries rising people if Mars and Mercury are together placed in the 6th house then in the Mahadasha of Mercury or Mars the native suffers from blood disorders, injuries, worms, pimples etc. Although Mercury here in Virgo which is the 6th house for Aries rising is exalted yet due to the combination of the lord of the 1st and 6th this is not a good yoga.

15. If Aries rises and Mars and Venus are together in Libra in the 7th house then the native from his own strength and valour improves his luck. The destiny improves and he also earns some wealth. The purpose of stating is that this is a good yoga but not that it gives a huge amount of wealth.*

16. When Aries rises and Mars is in the 8th house then it does not give a good effect. The 8th house is Scorpio and Mars is the ruler of this sign but being in dusthana 6th, 8th and 12th are called dusthan bad house, in dusthan it does not confer a yoga. But if Sun and Venus are also placed with Mars then the native is able to earn some wealth. Our opinion is that this type of person with Mars, Sun and Venus in the 8th house may get disease related to private parts like—fistula, piles and other types of sickness related to the eyes. Sudden death will happen. Although Bhavarth Ratnakar has stated that this is being the combination of the lord 1st, lord of 2nd, the lord of 5th and the lord of the 7th so some wealth will come but placement of the lord of the 7th in the 8th and then three planets in 8th (not a good house) is not good. Due to Venus in the 8th house the native will have disease related to disorder of the semen, urinary problems and destroys

---

*Avayoga is the opposite of Yoga. Yoga means a good combination. The good effect. Avayoga means the one which does not give good effects.

happiness from women. Not much happiness from even once own wife.

17. If Aries is the ascendant and Sun, Mars as well as Jupiter, Venus are placed in the 9th house, secondly Saturn is in Libra in the 7th house, then there is a special Yoga. Lord of the 1st, 5th, 7th, 9th and 2nd are together and that also in the 9th house which is the house of the fortune, and then the lord of the 10th (which indicates Raja, Kingdom, success in career) is also exalted so this is called a special Yoga.

18. If Aries is the ascendant and Sun, Venus are in the 1st house but Jupiter does not aspect them then Venus is not a Yoga giving planet.

19. (a) Aries rises and Jupiter aspects Venus, then Venus does not confer a Yoga.

    (b) Aries is the ascendant and Jupiter aspects Sun then definitely it is a Yoga giving aspect. We have talked above of two different interpretations of the aspect of Jupiter the result are different. The reason seems to be that Jupiter and Sun are friends. And the aspect of Jupiter on Sun is benefic but Venus and Jupiter on the other hand are enemies. So the aspect of Jupiter on Venus, does not give nice results. Although both are benefic so bad results can not be much but beneficial effect is reduced.

20. For Aries rising people if Sun, Mercury and Venus all three of them are posited in the 11th house, then their dasha's bring increase in fortunes.

21. For Aries rising people Sun in the first house in Aries and Moon is the 4th house in Cancer then defiantly it is a Raja Yoga.

22. If a person has Aries rising and Sun, Jupiter and Venus are in the 10th house then in their dashas he will take a holy dip in that Ganges. (Ganga).

Note: The special combinations which has been mentioned for the Aries rising people they are generally not available in the other books of Astrology.

For example– The mutual aspect between Venus and Jupiter

according to Maharishi Parasar is taken as a good factor, good and beneficial because one is the lord of an angel and the other is the lord of a trine. But in section 19 above this Yoga is indicated to be no good. In Bhavarth Ratnakar there are special Yogas. This is the speciality and use of it.

TAURUS ASCENDANT

1. If Taurus rises then Saturn inspite of it being the lord of the 9th and 10th is not a Yoga Karak. Neither without the connection of Sun and Mercury any Raja Yoga takes place. The original Sanskrit Sloka is as follows:

   वृषभजातस्यच शनिः भाग्यकर्मेश्वरोऽपिवा।
   सूर्यसोमसुताभ्याम् वा न युक्तो नैव योगदः ॥

   A. Commentator has translated it and commented on it as if Taurus is the ascendant and Saturn inspite of being the lord of the 9th and 10th house is not a Yoga Karak. Sun and Mercury even if posited in the 1st house does not give any Raja Yoga. Our opinion is that if Saturn does not join hands with Sun and Mercury then it does not give Yoga on its own.

2. If Taurus is the Lagna, Rahu is in the 10th house or Mars and Jupiter in Capricorn in the 9th house, then the native bathes in Ganges.

3. If Taurus rises and Moon is in the 4th house and that Moon receives the full aspect of Jupiter and Mercury then this Moon gives an excellent Yoga *i.e.* gives beneficial results. For Taurus rising people Moon is the ruler of the 3rd house. Generally the ruler of the 3rd house is taken as a Paapi- a Malefic. Jupiter is the ruler of 8th and 11th house so it is also a malefic by ownership. Generally speaking if a Paapi aspect another Paapi then there is a Paapa Yoga, bad Yoga. But if in the 'Shadbal' six types of strength it is strong then Mercury and Jupiter's aspect is always supposed to be a good aspect. On the basis of this Jupiter's aspect on Moon is benefic. Mercury being the ruler of the 2nd and 5th house for the Taurus rising people is also a Markesh but

due to its ownership of the 5th house it has become a benefic. So the aspect of Mercury on Moon which is in the 4th house is taken as a benefic aspect. The other reason is that in the 4th house Moon has one after one out of one directional strength and one Roop due to the angular position. Therefore Moon is taken as a benefic.

4. If Taurus is rising and Mars is in the 7th house in Scorpio then Mars confers good results.

5. If Sun and Saturn are in Pisces then the native is long lived and fortunate. Here Saturn is the lord of the 9th and 10th houses and Sun being the Lord of the 4th so this is a combination of the lord of the 4th, 9th and 4th and 10th so this is a good relation 'Labhesarwe Prasastha'. According to this principle Sun and Saturn are well placed in the 11th house which in this case is Pisces.

6. If Taurus is the ascendant and Mercury, Jupiter in any house are together or they aspect each other then it is a wealth giving Yoga. Mantreshwar Maharaj as said that if the lord of the 8th house which here is Jupiter if it get relationship with any other house then it is not good. In Jataka Deshmarg an excellent Book of Jyotish (Astrology) Chapter - 10 (Sloka - 34).

   It has been stated that 'Asthamesh' the lord of the 8th if it aspects any planet or any lord of any house if placed in the 8th, then the planet is spoiled. This is a natural question as to how Jupiter being the lord of the 8th and 12th, its aspect on Mercury or getting conjoined with Mercury can create a Yoga for wealth. The answer is that Jupiter is the 11th lord and Mercury is the lord of the 2nd so the combination of these two will be wealth conferring Yoga. There placement in different houses will give different types of results. If Mercury is in Virgo, as the lord of the 2nd and 5th, in exalted situation in the 5th and Jupiter as the lord of the 11th, in Pisces in own sign then the aspect of Mercury and Jupiter on each other will be best. The amount of wealth is also good if Mercury being the lord of the 2nd house is posited in the 2nd and Jupiter lord of the 8th house is in the 8th house. If both of them are together in the 12th house then how can they show the same type of results. So logic should be applied to their position, as to the sign and house they are in.

7. The combination for wealth which has been mentioned above in No. 6 if Mars has a relationship with Mercury and Jupiter then the Yoga is nullified *i.e.* Mercury or Jupiter or both if they have the aspect of Mars, 4th aspect, 7th or 8th aspect then or if Mercury, Jupiter are also posited simultaneously with Mars then the Yoga for wealth does not occur. The reason is that Mars rules the 12th house. The 12th house indicates expenses and loss of money or expenses so the lord of the 12th, when it is in contact with the lord of the 11th house or with the lord of the 2nd house then it destroys the Yoga for collection of wealth. Whether it aspects either one or both of them. 8 and 9 if Taurus is rising Mars, Jupiter and Mercury are together then during the period of Mercury the native will take loan or will become indebt to others.

   In the above case the Mahadasha of Mars is the one which gives wealth. If Mercury is in angle then also wealth comes in the period of Mercury. The period of Jupiter is mixed *i.e.* some times gain of wealth and at time loss of wealth. Why the period of Mars has been said to be good here? Mars is the ruler of the 7th and 12th houses in this condition- being the lord of the 7th Mars is called good because according to Parasar if the lord of an angle is a malefic then it does give benefic results. Here it should also be considered as to where Mars is posited?

   For example: If Mars is in its sign of exaltation in Capricorn then it will be in the 9th house and it will give good results. It will not show good results to that extent if it is debilitated. If it is in own sign of Aries in the 12th house then also it will not show that much good effect as when it will do when exalted and placed in the 9th house. If it is in the 8th house then the insurance money of husband *i.e.* the husband dies and a woman gets the insurance money. It is not good at all for the health of husband. As the lord of the 7th house and if posited in the 6th then there will be constant differences and quarrels with husband. All these things should be considered. If in the nativity of a man it is in the 6th house, then there will be quarrels with wife.

10. If Mercury and Venus are in the 1st house and Jupiter is in the 7th house then the Mahadasha of Mercury will be of a very high quality Yoga creating dasha. Here the reason is that the lord of the 1st house, the lord of the 2nd house and the lord of the 5th house they are together. Venus is the lord of the 6th as well, but if a planet is the lord of the 1st and lord of 6th or if a planet is lord of the 1st and simultaneously lord of the 8th it does not get negative effect due to the ownership of the 6th or 8th house. The aspect of Jupiter intensifies the effect of the combination of Mercury and Venus.
11. If Mars and Venus are in the Taurus ascendant and Jupiter is in the 9th house in Capricorn then in the periodic influence of Mercury and Jupiter the native will have a very fortunate period.
12. If Mars, Mercury and Saturn are in the 9th house and Rahu is in the 10th house in Aquarius then in the periodic influence of Mars and Rahu the native takes a holy dip in Ganges.
13. In Taurus ascendant the period of Venus is good. This is a general rule. The reason is that Venus is the lord of the 1st and the 6th house. Being the lord of the 1st it does not get the negative effect of the simultaneous ownership of the 6th. Parashar has also written that for Aries rising people Mars even though it is the lord of 8th house also will show good effect and Venus for Taurus rising people even though the owner of the 6th as well will show good effect. During the period of Venus money is gained and the fortunate time commence.
14. If Moon is in the Taurus ascendant then the native does not get any special money giving Yoga. But if it is in any other sign, then Moon in the 1st house brings in good fortunes.

GEMINI ASCENDANT

1. If Gemini is the rising sign and Sun, Mercury are in Leo in the 3rd house then Mercury gives the effect of a Yoga and the period of Mercury is good. According to Parashar, Chapter—23, Sloka-3, Sun and Mercury's combination is an excellent Yoga. In this context please see Chapter—16, Sloka-7 of the present Book where the combination of the lord of the 1st and the lord of the 3rd is mentioned as a good combination.

2. In the horoscope of a person with Gemini rising, Moon, Mars and Venus if posited in the 2nd house then the period of Venus confers wealth.

3. If Gemini is the ascendant and Mars is in the 2nd house in Cancer and Moon and Saturn are in the 8th house in Capricorn where Saturn is in its own sign of Capricorn then the results of Saturn's Mahadasha is mixed *i.e.* good results as well as bad results. In the Mahadasha of Mars wealth comes there is no doubt about it.

4. For Gemini ascendant, Mars and Saturn in the 2nd house, Moon in the 8th house then in the periodic influences of Saturn and Mars wealth is destroyed, property is destroyed and losses occur. But still some source of income remains.

5. For Gemini ascendant rising persons, Moon being the ruler of the 2nd house is a Markesh but does not act as one (is not fatal).

6. For Gemini ascendant persons if Moon and Mars are in the 11th house, *i.e.* the house of gains, then or of the lord of the 9th house, Saturn is posited in the 9th itself in Aquarius then this is a special combination which confers wealth.

7. For Gemini ascendant Jupiter and Saturn in the 9th house then in the major period and minor period of these planets the native takes a dip in the holy Ganges. Jupiter is a planet which confers spirituality and in its Dasha and Antardasha *i..e.* in the major and minor periods religious activities viz. bathing in the Ganges are natural but Saturn also does the same here. The reason of this principle is that in a horoscope with Gemini rising the 9th house is Aquarius and Saturn being the owner of this sign will be in its own sign in the 9th house. The principle of astrology is that if a malefic is posited in a house then it destroys and spoils a house but if a malefic is in own sign then it does not destroy the house and increases the good effect of that house. Secondly all planets give good results in the 9th house.

"पापोऽपि स्वगृहस्थश्तेद् भाववृद्धिं करोत्यलम्" – According to this principle the 9th house has Saturn in it but being the ruler of that house Aquarius himself it does not spoil it but increases the efficacy of the house. The 9th house is the house from which spiritual and religious activities are seen so the result of Saturn will be bathing in ganga and this type of religious activities, are indicated.

8. Mercury in Aries in the 11th house causes opposition and differences with elder brothers.

CANCER ASCENDANT

1. In Cancer rising Horoscopes Jupiter does not confer any special Yoga.
2. For Cancer rising people Mars is the Yogakarak. Mars if posited in Aries in the 10th house or in Scorpio in the 5th house then definitely it gives yoga *i.e.* gives a special rise in life.
3. If Venus is in the 2nd house or in the 12th house then it confers big Yoga. In other houses it does not give Yoga.
4. If Moon, Mars and Jupiter are in the 2nd house and Sun and Venus are in the 5th house then the native is wealthy and fortunate.
5. If Venus and Mercury are in the 5th house then periodic influence of Mercury confer Yoga. In the previous pages where we have given the Yogas of Bhavarth Ratnakar there the word Yoga stands for good Yoga *i.e.* during this period rise in status, rise in prestige, gain of wealth, success etc. are the good results.
6. For Cancer rising people Moon, Mercury, Venus in the 11th house, Jupiter in the 1st house, Sun in the 10th house are great Yoga giving planets. The native is courageous endowed with good qualities and a well known king.
7. When Sun and Mars are in the 10th house for Cancer rising people then the native is wealthy but the period of Jupiter is a fatal (marak) period.
8. If Mercury and Venus are in the 12th house then there is a special good effect (a raja yoga) during the mahadasha of Venus.
9. If Moon and Jupiter are in the 1st house then the native is famous and fortunate. This is a special Rajyoga .

Bathing in Ganges in the Hindu tradition is supposed to be one of the best manner of spiritual purity and attainment of 'moksha' (liberation after death).

10. If Moon in Cancer is in the 1st house and Mars in Capricorn is in the 7th house then this is a Raj Yog.
11. If Moon is in Cancer in the ascendant and exalted Saturn is in Libra in the 4th house it is a Raj Yoga.
12. For Cancer rising people Moon in the Ascendant and Sun in the 10th house in Aries is a Raj Yoga.
13. If Mercury and Jupiter are in the 11th house; Saturn, Rahu are in the 5th house, then during the Mahadasha of Rahu benefic results ensue and the native takes a dip in the holy Ganges.

LEO ASCENDANT

Now we give the Yogas which are effective when Leo is the rising sign.

1. When the ascendant is Leo and Sun, Mars and Mercury are in one place then the native is very wealthy.

   Here the combination of the lords of the 1st and 2nd; the lord of 1st and the lord of the 11th creates Yoga for wealth. For Leo rising people Mars is ruler of an angel and trine. So it is a Yogakarak. Therefore the combination of Sun, Mars and Mercury these three is an excellent Yoga for wealth. Sun, Mars combination is the Yoga of lord of the 1st, 4th and 9th houses, so this is a very strong Yoga.

2. If Sun, Mercury and Jupiter are together then also great wealth comes to the native. Sun and Mercury together are wealth giving factors. The reason of which has been mentioned above that they are the lord of the 1st, 2nd and 11th houses. Jupiter here being the lord of the 5th house also creates a Yoga with lord of the 1st, 2nd, 5th and 11th. So this should definitely be a combination which confers wealth.
3. If only Sun and Mercury are together then the fortunes are some what less.
4. If Jupiter and Venus are together then they do not create any yoga but rather they nullify any yoga if it exist. This is the opinion of Astrologers.

5. If the ascendant is Leo and Venus is in Libra in the 3rd house, then Venus is a benefic. But if Venus is placed in the 10th house then it will be a paapi and will not give good effect. Why the writer of Bhavarth Ratnakar has mentioned this we are not able to understand as to how a planet which is posited in its own sign is destroying the house. This is true that if a benefic is the lord of an angel then it does not give good results and if a malefic is the lord of an angel then it does good. But whatever even if a planet is a benefic or a malefic if it is posited in own sign, then it should increase the efficacy of that sign. Besides this Venus in this position creates one of the five Maha Pursha Yogas viz. Malavya Yoga which is a very excellent yoga. Therefore we do not agree with this view of the Bhavarth Ratnakar.

   In our opinion, the strength of Venus, its relationship with other planets, and the aspect of other planets on it should be considered. The only thing that we are able to understand that in the 10th house, Venus does not have any directional strength which is very little or Zero here.
6. If Leo is the ascendant then the combination of only the 9th lord and 10th lord *i.e.* Mars and Venus does not give any Yoga.
7. For Leo ascendant if Sun, Mars and Mercury are in the 1st house then during the period of Mercury increase of fortunes, prosperity and wealth takes place.
8. For Leo ascendant if Mars is in Cancer with Saturn then during the period of Saturn it gives Yoga.

VIRGO ASCENDANT

Now we speak of the Yoga which are there in the nativities of persons with Virgo rising.

1. If Virgo is the ascendant and Sun has a relationship with Venus or Moon then in the period of Sun wealth is gained.

In many yogas that has been given for Cancer ascendant people, in all the places it is not written if Cancer is the ascendant, but all these yogas should be understood for Cancer ascendant people.

2. If Sun is related to Venus then in the period of Venus the native loses all his money. Probably Venus as the lord of the 2nd house is combust or the lord of the 2nd is in relationship with the lord of the 12th which is the house of expenses and losses *i.e.* why this inference is drawn.

3. If Sun and Moon are related then the period of Moon gives mixed result *i.e.* some times good, some times bad, some things are good, other things are not so good in various departments of life.

4. If Moon and Venus are in the 7th house, Jupiter is in the 11th house, Sun is in Aries then in the period of Jupiter and Venus the person has four or five living wives *i.e.* a person has many wifes and four or five of them are live. Such a person lives like a king and his prosperity is that of a king and he will have all the luxuries of life. In olden when many wifes were supposed to be a sign of prosperity and happiness and luxury then this yoga has been written. But these days according to the different laws prevailing in many countries more then one marriage is not a legal thing. So either this Yoga may not take effect or a person may have many paramour and mistresses. However if Moon and Venus are together in Pisces in the 7th house then Venus is exalted and the lord of the 7th Jupiter is in the 11th house which is its sign of exaltation, aspect with full aspect the 7th house. Such a person will have a wife who will be beautiful, endowed with charm and good qualities and will also come from a respected and high family. This is so because the lord of the 7th house is exalted and such a person will have benefit from marriage or his fortunes smile after marriage. Sometimes the wife does not bring in wealth directly but her luck shines and brings prosperity and luxuries to the husband. The lord of the 7th house here is in the house of gain and the lord of the house of gain is in the 7th house. Because of the mutual exchange of houses, both the houses and both the planets become strong.

5. If Virgo is the ascendant and Jupiter and Venus are together in the 4th house then in the period of the Jupiter and Venus there is good Yoga.

6. For Virgo ascendant persons Saturn in the house of gains which

is the 11th house then the period of Saturn will give benefic results.

LIBRA ASCENDANT

Now we give below some Yoga which applies to people with Libra rising.

1. For Libra ascendant person Saturn is the Yoga Karak.
2. Jupiter although it rules the 3rd and 6th houses for Libra ascendant people yet it does give a good Yoga.
3. Mars being the ruler of the 2nd and 7th house, so Mars will be a Paapi, a malefic but it is not a marak, it does not kill. In our opinion if other combinations are present then only judgement should be drawn if the period of Mars will be fatal or not.
4. If ascendant is Libra and (i) if Jupiter and Venus are together—this is one, (ii) if Jupiter and Venus aspect each other, (iii) if they are receiving aspect from Mars and Saturn simultaneously or (iv) they are in the signs of Mars and Saturn, then in the major period of Jupiter and the minor period of Venus or in the major period of Venus and minor period of Jupiter, the native will suffer from wounds, small pox and skin problems etc.
5. For Libra rising if Sun, Mercury and Venus are in the first house in Libra then the native will be rich and fortunate. Generally speaking Sun in Libra is supposed to be ill-placed as this is the sign of debilitation of Sun. "Prithiyashas" has written in his book 'Horasar' that if Sun is in the 10th degree in Libra then it destroys hundreds of Raja Yogas. Here in Bhavarth Ratnakar it has been stated that the additional Yoga of Venus and Mercury with Sun in the 1st house is an excellent Raj Yoga.
6. If Libra is the ascendant and Sun and Mercury are in the 12th house and Saturn aspect them then the native's father will be fortunate and will have medium life.
7. When Libra is the ascendant Sun, Mercury and Saturn have a relationship with Mars then the native will be very fortunate.
8. If Libra is the ascendant, Sun, Mercury, Saturn has a relationship with Moon then the native is very fortunate.

9. For Libra ascendant, Mercury, Venus and Saturn are in the 1st house and Moon and Mars are in the 7th house, then in the period of Mercury the native becomes rich.

10. If in the horoscope of a person with Libra ascendant, Jupiter is in the 8th house, Saturn is in the 9th house, and Mars and Mercury together are in the 11th house then this is a special Rajyoga.

11. The Moon is in the 1st house in Libra, Jupiter is in the 6th or 12th house then in the period of Saturn a person becomes very fortunate.

12. For Libra Ascendant, Venus in the 1st house is a Markesh (is fatal).

13. Mars although it rules the 2nd and 7th house, still it is not a Markesh.

    In No. 3 and No. 5 above the Yoga which has been given we have explained our own opinion. Here Venus is the lord of the 1st house and as far as his Marak Dosh is concerned Parashar in his Book has written that at times even the lord of the 1st house can be a Marak. Venus as it is the lord of the 1st and 8th houses, so it should not have the bad effect of being the ruler of the 8th house. But at times all the principles of Astrology are not that logical.

14. If Saturn is in the 1st house and Moon is in the 10th house then it is a Raja Yoga.

15. If Mars, Mercury, Jupiter and Venus are in Libra and Rahu is in the 10th house, then in the Mahadasha of Rahu the person goes on pilgrimage and takes a holy dip. These beneficial results take place."

SCORPIO RISING

Now we give below some Yogas of people when Scorpio Ascendant is rising.

1. In the horoscope for Scorpio rising people the combination of Mercury and Jupiter has been mentioned as a wealth giving Yoga of high intensity.

2. If Scorpio is the ascendant then Jupiter's placement in the 3rd house, makes the person very generous by nature.
3. If Sun, Mercury and Venus are in the 7th house, then in the periodic influence of Mercury the Raj Yogas operates and the native becomes famous all around.
4. Jupiter and Mercury are in the 5th house in Pisces and Moon is in Virgo in the house of gains *i.e.* if 11th house then the native is very rich and fortunate.
5. If Moon is in Cancer with Jupiter and Ketu in the 9th house, then the Mahadasha of Ketu is ordinary but the period of Jupiter is very propitious.

SAGITTARIUS ASCENDANT

Now we give some Yogas for the natives who have Sagittarius rising.

1. If Sagittarius is the ascendant and Saturn is posited in the 5th house, then the Mahadasha of Saturn is Yoga giving Mahadasha *i.e.* gives benefic results.
2. If Sagittarius is the ascendant then Saturn in the 11th house in Libra confers Yoga. In any other ascendant Saturn in the 11th house is not Yogakarak, does not create Yoga. We do not agree with this opinion because in "Saravali", Chapter-6, Sloka-4, all planets in the 11th house are endowed with benefic effect and give gain of wealth. It has been said "Labhe Sarway Prasastha" *i.e.* in the house of gains that's the 11th house even if they are benefic planets or malefic, all the planets are welcome *i.e.* they are good. So in this manner only Saturn in Libra in the 11th according to Bhavarth Ratnakar is the Yoga giving planet and if it is in other signs in the 11th then it does not give a yoga this is against the established principle.

'In Sanskrit language the word "Ghat" is printed- the meaning of this is that in Aquarius, Mars, Mercury, Jupiter and Saturn are placed and Rahu is in the 10th house then benefit of having holy dips is the result. If we do not accept this as Ghat but the meaning of Ghat is used as Libra then the meaning that has been given above will be the correct one.

3. For Sagittarius ascendant Sun and Venus is in the 9th house in Leo, Saturn in Aquarius in the 3rd then in the Dasha of Saturn special wealth comes and the fortunes smile on the native.

4. For Sagittarius ascendant, Mars and Sun in the 3rd house in Aquarius, and Rahu in the 9th house, then during the period of Rahu the native goes to holy places to take a dip.

CAPRICORN RISING

Now we give below certain Yogas for people who have Capricorn as the ascendant.

1. If Capricorn is the ascendant then Mercury is the Yoga giving planet *i.e.* the Mahadasha and the Antardasha of Mercury shows good results.

2. For Capricorn ascendant, Jupiter in the 1st house and if that Jupiter is aspected by Venus, and Mercury is in the 8th house then the native is long lived but is poor.

3. For Capricorn ascendant Venus in the 5th house in Taurus is a Yoga giving planet. But in the 10th house it is not a Yoga giving planet.

4. If Moon is in the 5th house and Jupiter aspects that Moon, and if Mercury and Venus are simultaneously in the ascendant then it is a very strong Raj Yog.

5. If Jupiter is in the ascendant, and Mars and Venus are in the 11th house then during the Jupiter's period the native gains wealth through brothers or he takes away the wealth of his brothers.

6. For Capricorn ascendant if Sun, Moon and Mercury are in the 1st house, and Mars and Venus are in the 12th house then also the native's luck rises on account of his brothers as well as due to his own efforts and hard work he also earns wealth. The native's own as well his brother's fortunes smile due to this planetary combination.

7. Mercury and Saturn together in the 9th house makes the native very fortunate.

---

*Here Saturn is exalted.

8. Rahu and Jupiter in the 12th house gives a very excellent Yoga and the Mahadasha of Rahu is very fortunate and brings in fortune.
9. If Mars is in Capricorn in the 1st house, Moon in Cancer in the 7th house then this is an excellent Yoga. This is also a Raj Yog.

AQUARIUS ASCENDANT

Now we give the Yogas which operate for Aquarius Ascendant persons.

1. If Aquarius is the lagna the combination of the lord of the 9th and 10th house *i.e.* Mars and Venus together does not create a Raj Yoga *i.e.* if there is no other planet involved and only Mars and Venus have a relationship the Raj Yog does not take effect.
2. If Venus is in the 12th house then it does not give a Yoga.
3. If Sun and Venus are in the ascendant and Rahu is in the 10th house then the good effect and Yoga takes place during the periods of Rahu and Jupiter.
4. If Sun and Mars are in the 8th house then in their dasha the native has sorrows, sufferings and unhappiness. But the period of Mercury is a Yoga giving dasha.

5&6. If Jupiter is in the 1st house in the ascendant and Saturn is in the 2nd house, then the period of Jupiter will give mixed results *i.e.* sometimes good and sometimes bad. But the Mahadasha of Saturn gives very good results.

7. If Saturn and Venus are in Sagittarius in the 11th house then the Mahadasha of Venus gives good Yoga.
8. If Sun, Mercury and Jupiter are in the 3rd house then the Mahadasha of Sun will be a benefic Raj Yog Karak period.

PISCES LAGNA

Now we gives some results for the Pisces rising people.

1. If the ascendant is Pisces or Aquarius and Venus is in the 12th house then it does not confer any Yoga. But if it is any other rising sign except Pisces or Aquarius then Venus in the 12th house shows good effect.

2 (A) *Saturn in the 12th house is a Raj Yog Karak planet. But if Moon is in the 12th house, then the native is without wealth.

B. In 'A' above and in the same context we speak when there is the minor period of the Moon in the major period of Jupiter then the effect is very little.

3. If Jupiter is in the 5th house then the native's have many daughter and very few sons and at times no sons.

4. If Moon is in the 2nd house, Mars is in the 5th house then in the period of the Moon, wealth is gained.

5. If Jupiter is posited in 6th house, Venus in the 8th house Saturn in the 9th house, and Moon and Mars are placed in the 11th house then it is an excellent combination. The native is fortunate.

6. If Moon, Mars and Mercury are in Capricorn in the 11th house, then gain of wealth, property and Vehicles. It is an excellent combination for these things.

7. If Moon and Saturn are in the 1st house, Mars is in the 11th house, Venus is in the 6th house, then during the Mahadasha of Venus the fortunes smile on the native.

8. If Moon, Mars, Mercury and Jupiter are in the 4th house then during the major and minor periods of these planets the native attains fame and his fortunate time commences. But if the lord of the 3rd house and 8th house (which is Venus here) is also with these four planets then the Yoga is destroyed.

9. If Jupiter is in Sagittarius in the 10th house then definitely it is a Yoga creating placement.

10. When Moon is in Taurus, Sun in Leo, Mercury in Virgo, Venus in Libra, Jupiter in Sagittarius, Mars in Capricorn and Saturn in Aquarius then it is a very fortunate placement and the luck shines very much. If the placement of seven planets which has been

---

*Here the meaning should be taken as that for Pisces rising people Saturn in the 12th house confers Yoga. In many places these things have not been repeated that if the ascendant is this particular one. But it should be inferred under which consideration these Yogas have been given and accordingly judgement should be taken. It should not be universally applied for all the ascendants.

described above does not exist but only five planets are in such position then also the native is very fortunate.

We have added some Yogas from Bhavarth Ratnakar an ancient predictive astrological Book and from that we have given twenty two combination of Aries ascendant, fourteen for natives of the Taurus ascendant, eight for Gemini; rising, thirteen those who have Cancer lagna, eight for those who have Leo rising, six for natives who has Virgo as the ascendant, fifteen for the people with Libra ascendant, five for the Scorpio ascendant, four for the Sagittarius rising people, nine for the Capricorn ascendant, eight for Aquarius rising people and ten for those who have Pisces rising. This way we have given 122 combination keeping in view that the readers of the Phaldeepika, besides knowing the principles which has been enunciated in Phaldeepika should also have other authentic view point of an excellent treatise like Bhavarth Ratnakar so that they can get help in arriving at better judgement.

20

Antardasha Phal (Influence of Minor Periods of Planets)

Major and Minor Periods and their Special Effects

In this chapter, the benefic or ill effects which has been described if the Lord of a house is strong, should be applied both to the Mahadasha and Antardasha *i.e.* both to the major and minor periods of a planet.

भावेश्वरेण प्रबलेन येन यद्यत्फलं हीनबलेन येन।
यदानुभोक्तव्यमनन्यसम्यक्संसूचयिष्यत्यथ संग्रहेण ॥१॥

If the Lord of a house is strong then what is the effect and if it is weak *i.e.* without strength then what result should be expected and at what time these will be applicable has been described in a nutshell.

लग्ने बलिष्ठे जगति प्रभुत्वं सुखस्थितिं देहबलं सुवर्चः।
उपर्युपर्यभ्युदयाभिवृद्धिं प्राप्नोति बालेन्दुवदेष जातः ॥२॥

पाकेऽर्थनाथस्य कुटुम्बसिद्धिं
सत्पुत्रिकाप्ति सुखभोजनं च
प्राप्नोति वाग्जीविकया धनानि
वक्ता सदुक्तिं सदसि प्रशस्ताम् ॥३॥

शौर्ये सवीर्ये सहजानुकूल्यं
सन्तोषवार्ताश्रवणं च शौर्यम्।

सेनापतित्वं लभतेऽभिमानं
जनाश्रयं सद्गुणभाजनत्वम् ॥४॥

बन्धूपकारं कृषिकर्मसिद्धिं स्त्रीसङ्गमं वाहनलाभमेति।
क्षेत्रं गृहं नूतनमर्थसिद्धिं स्थानंप्रशस्तं च सुखेशदाये ॥५॥

पुत्रप्राप्तिं बन्धुविलासं नृपतीनां
साचिव्यं वा धीशदशायां बहुमानम्।
प्राज्यैर्भोज्यैर्मृष्टमिहाश्नाति ददाति
श्रेयस्कार्यं सज्जनशस्तं स विदध्यात् ॥६॥

रिपून्निहन्ति साहसैररीश्वरस्य वत्सरे।
अरोगतामुदारतामधृष्यतामतिश्रियम् ॥७॥

सम्पाद्य वस्त्राभरणानि शय्यां
प्रीतो रमण्या रमतेऽतिवीर्यः।
करोति कल्याणमहोत्सवादीन्
सन्तोषयात्रां च मदेशदाये ॥८॥

ऋणविमोचनमुच्छ्रितिमात्मनः
कलहकृत्यनिवृत्तिमुपैति सः।
महिषपश्वजभृत्यजनागमं
वयसि रन्ध्रपतेर्बलशालिनः ॥९॥

स्त्रीपुत्रपौत्रैः सहबन्धुवर्गै-
र्भाग्यंश्रिय चानुभवत्यजस्रम्।
श्रेयांसि कार्याण्यवनीशपूजां
भाग्येशदाये द्विजदेवभक्तिम् ॥१०॥

यत्कार्यमारब्धमुपैत्येनेन
तस्यैव सिद्धिं सुखजीवनं च।
कीर्तिं प्रतिष्ठां कुशलप्रवृत्तिं
मानोन्नतिं कर्मपतेर्दशायाम् ॥११॥

ऐश्वर्यमव्याहतमिष्टबन्धु-
समागमं भृत्यजनांश्च दासान्
संसारसौभाग्यमहोदयं च
लभेत लाभाधिपतेर्दशायाम् ॥१२॥

व्ययेशितुर्वयस्यतिव्ययं करोति सज्जने।
अघौघनाशिनीं शुभक्रियां महीशमान्यताम् ॥१३॥

1. If the Lord of the first house is strong then during the periodic influence of the Lord of the first house the native's influence and authority increases in the world, he lives happily. The health is good *i.e.* during the periodic influence of the Lord of the Ascendant the native has strength and does not get disease. There is luster on the face. The luster on the face indicates that the mind and body are both in good shape. As the second day of the waxing moon increases every day and attains luster in the same manner, the native constantly rises to prosperity and in status when he is in the Dasha of a strong Lord of the Ascendant.

2. If the Lord of the second house is strong then what is the result has been described below.

   During the Dasha of the Lord of the second house the native's family increases. He gets good daughters. He gets food easily. He earns wealth due to his voice and power of speech that is he gets livelihood and wealth where speech is more used. Either he speaks endearing sentences and words so all people praise him in meetings or he is a good lawyer where logic and power of speech is utilised or he is a professor and has convincing ability. In short the second house is the house of the speech, wealth and family and good results related to these matters are realized.

3. If the Lord of the third house is strong, then during its Dasha there is love and affection with brothers and sisters. Good news is received. Courage and Valour increases. The native is the leader of a community or a general. Other people help him and co-operate with him. Many good traits develop in him and the native's presitge, honour and status increases.

4. If the 4th house and its Lord are strong, then during the periodic influence of the Lord of the 4th house the native does good for his relatives, success comes in work connected with agriculture. He enjoyes the company of his wife and gain vehicles. He gets farms, houses, wealth, success and mansions to live in *i.e.* they come to him. The meaning is that he has promotion and/or he moves to a new residence or acquires property.

5. If the Lord of the 5th house is strong then during its 'Mahadasa', birth of Son or Grand children. He lives happily with his relatives. Becomes Minister to a King and gets a lot of honour. The natives does good deeds and gentleman praise him. He enjoys varieties of tasteful food himself and also feeds others.

   In Sloka No. -15 subsequently, where the Lord of the second house has been considered, the consideration of 'Patrika' *i.e.* letters has been mentioned and not putrika, (daughters).

6. If the Lord of the 6th house is strong then during its period the native defeats his enemies on account of his courage. He is healthy. He is generous and becomes very powerful and enjoys wealth *i.e.* no one can subdue him and he leads a luxurious life.*

7. When the Lord of the seventh house is strong then the native will get new clothes, ornaments and enjoys life, happily with his

---

*In the original Sloka ' the word 'Satputrikaptim' is used, but no where it is written that from the 2nd house, consideration of daughters be done. Definitely family is considered and it falls under the second house. Probability is that instead of 'Satputrikaptim' the original Sloka has 'Satpatrikaptim' that will mean that benefic correspondence is received.

*Those who read only 'Laghuparasharee" they think that the period of the Lord of the 6th house is always bad but this is a wrong interpretation. When a planet is strong then it shows good results related to houses it owns- all the times.

wilfe. His strength constantly increases. There are auspicious events in his house *i.e.* marriage and other goods events take place. He travels and he is satisfied with his travels *i.e.* the cause for which he is travelling will be fruitful. From the seventh house, happiness from wife and travels are considered. So in the Mahadasha of a strong Lord of the 7th house, the native gets full happiness from the matters which fall under the 7th house.

8. If the Lord of the 8th house is strong then the native will pay back his debts *i.e.* he will not owe money to others. He is promoted in his work. If he has some type of fight or legal dispute with others then it ends. Increase in the number of buffalow, animals, goats and servants for him.**

9. If the Lords of the 9th house is strong then the native in the company of his wife, sons, grandsons, brothers and relatives, constantly enjoys wealth *i.e.* with his family members he has a luxurious life. In the Mahadasa of the Lord of the 9th house he worships Gods and Brahmins. He is praised and honoured by Kings and he is engaged in good deeds. From the 9th house, wealth and fortunes are considered. So when the Lord of the 9th house is strong then during its periods increase in fortunes as well as increase of wealth.

10. If the 10th house and the Lord of 10th house are strong then during the Mahadasha of the Lord of the 10th house whatever work the natives undertakes, he achieves success in that and his life is full of happiness. His prestige increases and he gets fame. He is busy in good deeds and acquires a high status.

11. In the period of Lord of the 11th house which is strong constant increase of luxuries. The relatives with whom he has good terms they visit him and there is increase in the number of employees and servants. Much affluence and fortunes come to him.

12. In the period of the Lord of the 12th house which is strong the

---

**Generally the period of the Lord of the 8th house is always considered to bring sufferings and sorrows but 'Mantreshwar Maharaj' has said that if the Lord of the 8th house is strong then during its period the native gets out of problems and he acquires instruments of happiness.

native spends much money on good people. In the dasha of a strong lord of the 12th house definitely expenses increase, but these expenses are related to good work and not in bad deeds. The native is honoured from the King and people. Such people do good deeds so their sins are destroyed.

वक्रगस्य निजतुङ्गसुहृत्-
सुस्थानगस्य दशाफलमेवम्।
शत्रुनीचगृहमौढ्यषडन्त्य-
छिद्रगस्य तु फलान्यपि वक्ष्ये ॥१४॥

The results which has been given above for Sloka No. 2 to Sloka No. 13 will be effective only when the Lord of the house is placed in a good place and is exalted or in own sign or is retrograde. If the Lord of the house is in the sign of an enemy, or debilitated combust or posited in the 6th, 8th or 12th, in any of these dusthan, then the planet will show bad results. In short it should be remembered that the Lord of any sign gives good effect if it is well placed and strong itself and if the lord of a house is weak or ill placed and not in good shape then it will give bad result. What ill effects the lord of a house can give, have been given below—

दु:स्थे लग्नपतौ निरोधनमुपैत्यज्ञातवासं भयं
व्याध्याधीनपरक्रियाभिगमनं स्थानच्युतिं चापदम्।
जाड्यं संसदि वाक्कुटुम्बचलनं दृष्पत्रिकां दृग्रुजं
वाग्दोषं द्रविणव्ययं नृपभयं दु:स्थे द्वितीयाधिपे ॥१५॥

दुश्चिक्याधिपतौ सहोदरमृतिं कार्ये दुरालोचना-
मन्त:शत्रु निपीडनं परिभवं तद्गर्वभङ्गं वदेत्।
मातृक्लेशमरिष्टमिष्टसुहृदां क्षेत्रगृहोपप्लुतिं
पश्वश्वादिविनाशनं जलभयं पातालनाथेऽबले ॥१६॥

वीर्योने प्रतिभापतौ सुतमृतिर्बुद्धिभ्रमं वञ्चना-
मध्यवानं ह्युदरामयं नरपते: कोपं स्वशक्तिक्षयम्।

चोराद्भीतिमनर्थतां च दमनं रोगान् बहून्दुष्कृतिं
भृत्यत्वं लभतेऽवमानमयशः षष्ठेशदाये व्रणम् ॥१७॥

जामातुर्व्यसनं कलत्रविरहं स्त्रीहेत्वनर्थागमं
द्यूनेशे विबलिन्यसत्यभिरतिं गुह्यामयं चाटनम्।
रन्ध्रेशायुषि शोकमोहमदमात्सर्यादिमूर्च्छोच्छ्रितिं
दारिद्र्यं भ्रमणं वदेदपयशोव्याधीनवज्ञां मृतिम् ॥१८॥

पूर्वोपासिदेवकोपमशुभं जायातनूजापदं
दौष्कृत्यं स्वगुरोः पितुश्च निधनं दैन्यं शुभे दुर्बले।
यद्यत्कर्म करोति तत्तदफलं स्यान्मानभङ्गो नभो-
भावे दुर्गुणतां प्रवासमशुभं दुर्वृत्तिमापन्नाताम् ॥१९॥

श्रवणमशुभवाचां भ्रातृकष्टं सुतार्तिं
भवपवयसि दैन्यं वञ्चनं कर्णरोगम्।
बहुरुजमपमानं बन्धनं सर्वसम्मत्-
क्षयमपरशशीवाऽऽयाति रिःफेशदाये ॥२०॥

1. If the Lord of the 1st house is afflicted with one or more of the four faults given above* then during the periodic influence of the Lord of the 1st house the native may have to go to prison or underground *i.e.* he may be imprisoned or may fall into such bad situation that he have to hide himself from public eye; he will be constantly in fear and will suffer from mental anguish and physical ailments. Physical ailments are related to the body disease viz. physical deformities, diseases, trouble etc., and mental anguish are worries of some types or the other. If the Lord of the 1st house is placed in 'dusthan' or is weak then during the periodic influence of such Lord of the 1st house, the native will be engaged in some type of sad rites like- death of

*Footnote sign of an enemy; debilitated; combust; or in the 6th, 8th or 12th house.

some one, or something negative or the other. He will be displaced from his status and may lose his house and he is constantly surrounded with problems.

2. If the Lord of the 2nd house is spoilt then during the periodic influence of that Lord, if the native gets a chance to speak in public, then suddenly he might stammer or lose his speech due to nervousness. He will not be able to control his speech, his family is in bad situation and will break. He suffers from disease of the eyes. He had problem in speech (due to disease in mouth or ulcers or he resorts to sarcastic remarks) money is lost, fear from Kings and people in authority. He gets unpleasant letters. When considering the 2nd house all those things should be considered which fall in 2nd house.

3. If the Lord of the 3rd house is spoilt* then death of brother or sister takes place. The native himself is blamed for certain things for which he is not responsible. He is troubled by secret enemies. He is defeated. He is demoted from his position and loses respect. In the periodic influence of the Lord of the 3rd house which has no strength, is weak and spoiled, the above results will take place.

4. If the Lord of the 4th house is weak then during its periodic influence the mother suffers. His dear ones and friends are in trouble, loss of farm houses and residential properties. His cattle and horses are destroyed, danger from water. From the 4th house water is also considered. Therefore if the Lord of the 4th house is badly situated then fear from water is indicated.

5. If the Lord of the 5th is weak then during its periodic influences the native will lose his son like— death or suffering for the Son. He is confused, he is taken for a ride *i.e.* he is cheated, he wanders around for no reason, he has to walk on feet and he suffers from stomach problems. Anger from the Kings and the native spends his strength without any results.

6. If the Lord of the 6th house is spoilt then there is danger from thieves, poverty and such events which gives suffering. The

---

*Weak, combust, debilitated etc.

native is suppressed by others and suffers from disease. The native commits sinful acts or other people misbehave with him. The native will serve others and is constantly insulted and gets bad name. He gets wounds and boils in the body.

7. If the Lord of the 7th house is weak then during the Mahadasha of that Lord the Son-in-laws suffers. The native is separated from his wife and he suffers much on account of his wife. If the Lord of the 7th house is weak then during its periodic influence the native enjoys speaking lies, suffers from disease in the private parts and he travels around without any aim or accomplishment.

8. If the Lord of the 8th house is in bad shape then during its periodic influence poverty, sufferings, fears, tiring journeys, bad name, mental anguish, physical problems, insults etc. come to the native, even death can occur. In the period of the lord of the 8th house which is weak, sorrow, disappointment in love, pride, jealousy and due to dropsy the mind is under pressure. 'Moorcha' is a Sanskrit word which means dropsy. It causes much mental pressures.

9. If the Lord of the 9th house is weak then during its period the native's wife and son, they face dangers. He becomes lusterless, down and out, mentally and physically. The native's father separates from him or death comes to him. He resorts to bad deeds and death to some elderly person in the family. The 9th house is the house of religion so during the period of a weak Lord of the 9th house— dangers, calamities, sufferings and various types of negative things take place. This should be understood that all these are due to some type of sins, committed in the past towards the God who has been worshipped before.

10. If the Lord of 10th house is weak then what will be the results? The 10th house is the house of career and if the Lord hereof is weak, then during its period whatever work a man is engaged in all of them go in vain. The native is engaged in low type of activities. He has to be out of his house and so he suffers. Bad happenings in and around him take place. In short the native's life is full of sufferings, failures and insults. He does not get any recognition.

11. If the Lord of the 11th house is weak and has no strength, then the brother suffer, the son is sick, the native is cheated. He suffers diseases of ears. He becomes weak physically, mentally and financially. During this 'Mahadasha' or in the minor period of a weak Lord of the 11th house*, bad news is received. Here we would like to draw attention to one more side that from the 3rd house the younger brother is considered, and from the 11th the older brother. From the 3rd house the right ear and from the 11th house, the left ear.

12. If the Lord of 12th house is weak then the native suffers from various disease, is insulted, is imprisoned and like the waning Moon of the dark half his wealth is slowly destroyed.

    If the Lord of a house is strong then the periodic influence of that Lord gives benefic effect and if the Lord of a house is weak then during its period negative results occur. When undertaking prediction of any periodic influence of a planet, it should be seen as to which house or houses it own, also if it is weak or strong.

संज्ञायां यदगाच्च कारकविधिश्लोकेषु यज्जल्पितं
कर्माजीवनिरूपितं फलमिदं यद्रोगचिन्ताविधौ।
यद्यस्येक्षणयोगसंभवफलं भावेशयोगोद्भवं
भावेशैरपि भावगैरपि फलं वाच्यं दशायामिह ॥२१॥

When predicting the periodic influence of a planet the following things should be kept in view.

1. Whatever attributes of signs/planets etc. mentioned in the 1st Chapter.
2. What things a planet signifies, which have been given in 2nd Chapter..
3. What type of work comes under which planet and the manner of the livelihood in the 5th Chapter.
4. The type of disease and mental anxiety which falls under different planets and has been mentioned in Chapter 14th.

---

*At times death of mother.

The effects when two planets are placed together or aspect each other, or when the Lords of two houses are together, or the ownership of a house, or how a planet is posited in a house. All these should be thoroughly considered and only then the periodic influence of that planet should be interpreted.

All these subjects has been analysed from the Chapter -15 to Chapter -20.

वर्गोत्तमांशस्थदशा शुभप्रदा
मिश्रैव सा चास्तमिते च नीचगे।
मृत्युव्यारीशदशापहारयो-
स्तत्र स्थितस्याप्यशुभं फलं भवेत् ॥२२॥

If a planet is 'Vargotham' then it shows great benefic results. If a planet is 'Vargotham' but simultaneously that planet is in its sign of debilitation or combust, then the results will be mixed, good and bad both. Consider the Lord of the 6th, 8th or 12th houses. If the major period is of one of the Lords and the minor period is of any other Lord then this period will show very bad results. Similarly if any planet is posited in the 6th, 8th or 12th and its major period is running then the minor period of any other planet who is also posited in 'trik' is very bad.

क्रूरग्रहस्यैव दशापहारे
त्रिपञ्चसप्तर्क्षपतेर्विपाके।
तथैव जन्माष्टमनाथभुक्तौ
चोरारिपीडां लभतेऽतिदुःखम् ॥२३॥

During the major periodic influence of a malefic and in the minor period of a planet, which is the ruler of the 3rd, 5th or 7th constellation from the birth star, there is possibility of theft in the native's house. He suffers from enemies and he is miserable. Which planet is the ruler of which 'Nakshatra' has been mentioned before. Suppose a person is born in the constellation 'Revati'. Then 'Revati', 'Ashwini', 'Bharani' and so on, Bharani is the 3rd constellation, 'Rohini' is the 5th constellation and 'Ardra' is the 7th constellation from 'Rohini'. The

Lord of 'Bharani' is 'Venus', the Lord of 'Rohini' is 'Moon' and the Lord of 'Ardra' is 'Rahu'. In this way if there is the periodic influence of a malefic *i.e.* the major period of a malefic say 'Saturn' then the minor periods of 'Venus' 'Moon' and 'Rahu' will cause sufferings.

Similarly if the major period is that of a malefic then the minor periods of the Lord of the 'Moon' sign or the Lord of the 8th house from the 'Moon' sign, is troublesome. It causes sufferings and troubles created by thieves, enemies and sorrows.

शनेश्वतुर्थी च गुरोस्तु षष्ठी
दशा कुजाह्योर्यदि पञ्चमी सा।
कष्टा भवेद्राश्यवसानभाग-
स्थितस्य दुःस्थानपतेस्तथैव ॥२४॥

The following periods cause problems.

1. If the major period of the Saturn is the 4th period.
2. If the major period of Jupiter is the 6th dasha.
3. If the periods of Mars or Rahu is the 5th one.
4. If a planet is in the 30 degree of a sign *i.e.* in last degree of any sign, then the period of that planet.
5. The Lord of 'trik' *i.e.* 6th, 8th and 12th.

If a person is born in the periodic influence of the 'Mars' then the 'Saturn' period will be the 4th period for him *i.e.* Mars 1st dasha, Rahu 2nd dasha, Jupiter 3rd and Saturn will be the 4th. If a person is born in the periodic influence of 'Venus', then the Rahu dasha will be the 5th 'Mahadasha' and the 'Jupiter' will be the 6th periodic influence. Similarly if a person is born in the period of 'Ketu' then the period of the Mars being the 5th period for him, will not be a good period.

ऊर्ध्वास्यतुङ्गभवनस्थितभूमिजस्य
कर्मायगस्य हि दशा विदधाति राज्यम्।
जित्वा रिपून्विपुलवाहनसैन्ययुक्तां
राज्यश्रियं वितनुतेऽधिकमन्नदानम् ॥२५॥

If Mars is posited in a sign which is 'Urdmukh' and which coincides with 'Capricorn' and is simultaneously the 10th or 11th house from Ascendant, then the period of the Mars, bestows 'throne' to the native. Such a person annihiliates his enemies *i.e.* victorious over his enemies and is a General or Commandar of an army. He enjoys wealth of a kingdom and many people are under his patronage. This is a special 'Rajayog' which has been mentioned above. In this 'Rajyog' three things should be there.

1. Mars should be exalted.
2. Should be placed in the 10th or 11th house.
3. It should be in a 'Urdmukh Rashi'. What is a 'Urdmukh Rashi"? This has been explained in Sloka No. 8 in the first chapter.*

स्वोच्चस्थितो भृगसुतो व्ययकर्मगो वा
लाभेऽपि वाऽस्तरहितो न च पापयुक्तः ।
तस्याब्दपाकसमये बहुरत्नपूर्णो
धीमान्विशालविभवो जयति प्रशस्तः ॥२६ ॥

This is a special 'Rajyog' connected to 'Venus'. If Venus is posited in 'Pisces', 'Libra' or 'Vrishabha' in the 10th or 12th house or even in the 11th house but should neither be with a malefic nor combust, then in the periodic influence of such a 'Venus', the native becomes very rich, endowed with luxurious items, gold etc. He is praised in this world and he enjoys life. This is the effect during the major period of Venus.*

Now we speak of the periods of planets which are in their sign of debilitation, or are posited in the 6th or 8th house. Generally it is

*This is the results in the period of Mars.

*In the Mool Sloka 'Swochastith' this word has been used. Own sign or exalted sign, if we take this meaning then 'Venus' is in— 'Taurus', 'Libra' or 'Pisces'. In any one of them will show the results given above, but if we take it as the exalted sign only, then the above mentioned 'Yoga' will take place only if 'Venus' is posited in 'Pisces'. We are with the second opinion. Other planets are not considered so good in the 12th house, but 'Venus' in the 12th house gives enjoyment of life and is very auspicious. It also gives great success in work also.

understood that benefic planets wherever they are placed are good. Then the question is if benefic planets are posited in the 6th or 12th house will they show benefic results? There is a proverb related to 'Astrology;

"Papashaste Vitalabham Prakuryu".

So will Papagraha (malefic) show good result in the 6th house? The answer to these doubts have been clarified in the Sloka given below—

नीचारिषष्ठव्ययसंश्रिता हि
शुभाः प्रयच्छन्त्यशुभानि सर्वे।
शुभेतरास्त्वेषु गताः प्रयच्छ-
न्त्यमोघदुःखानि दशासु तेषाम्॥२७॥

If benefic planet are debilitated in the sign of enemy, posited in the 6th or 12th house then they will show ill effect and those planet which are not benefic *i.e.* those which are malefic if they are debilitated, sign of an enemy, or are posited in the 6th or 12th house then what type of result they will show? They will produce intensified sufferings during their periods. The word 'Amogh' has been used which literally means such sufferings from which there is no respite and it is difficult to get out of it.

Until now we have been talking of the results of the major and minor periodic influences. We now speak the result of minor periods in the following Sloka.

दशेशशत्रोररिगेहभाजो
लग्नेशशत्रोरपि वाऽथ भुक्तौ।
शत्रोर्भयं स्थानलयः तदास्य
स्निग्धोपि शत्रुत्वमुपैति नूनम्॥२८॥

If the minor period is of a planet which is

(i) The enemy of the planet who's major period is running.

(ii) Or is posited in the sign of an enemy.

(iii) Or posited in the 6th house.

(iv) Or is the enemy of the Lord of the 1st house, then during such a minor period there is fear of enemies, fear of loss of place *i.e.* one may lose his job and status or may lose his property (residence). This minor period is really bad, full of troubles and even one's friends become his enemies.

This should also be considered that the Lord of the minor period is not posited in the sign owned by the enemy of the Lord of the major period.

यद्भावगः पाकपतिर्दशेशात्-
तद्भावजातानि फलानि कुर्यात्।
विपक्षरिःफाष्टमभावगश्चेद्-
दुःखं विदध्यादितरत्र सौख्यम् ॥२९॥

Observe where the planets who's major and minor periods are in the offing are placed. If counted from the lord of the major period, the Lord of the minor period is in the 6th, 8th or 12th house from it, then this period will be full of sufferings and sorrows.

If the Lord of the minor period is placed in any other house from the lord of the major period but not in the 6th, 8th and 12th, then it is good. One new thing has been mentioned in this Sloka *i.e.* while taking into account the Lords of the major and minor periods of influence then they should not only be considered separately but their placement from each other should also be taken into account *i.e.* the Lord of the minor period should not be in the 6th, 8th and 12th from the Lord of the major period.

The house occupied by the Lord of the minor period from the Lord of the major period the effect of that house will be felt. If the Lord of the minor period from the major period is in the 9th house

---

*In the original Sloka the word "Arigehbhajo' has come which can be interpreted in two ways:-

1. Posited in house of an enemy.
2. The enemies are considered from the 6th house so if posited in the 6th from the ascendant. We have given both the meanings when commenting on the above Sloka.

then it will increase fortunes, if it is posited in the 10th house then it will bring upliftment in position and status. In the 11th house gains.- The principle is that not only the Lord of the minor period should be considered from the ascendant or from the 'Moon' but also from the Lord whose major period is in the offing.

स्वोच्चत्रिकोणस्वहितारिनीचे
पूर्णं त्रिपादार्द्धपदाल्पशून्यम्।
क्रमाच्छुभं चेदशुभं विलोमात्
मूढे ग्रहे नीचसमं फलं स्यात्॥३०॥

If a planet is exalted then it shows full benefic result. If a planet is in its 'Moolatrikon', then it shows three fourth good effect.

If a planet is in own sign then it shows half benefic results.

If a planet is in the sign of a friend then its effects is one fourth.

If a benefic planet is in the sign of an enemy then it will show very little good effect and if a benefic planet is posited in its sign of debilitation then the good results will be almost nil.

If a malefic is debilitated then it will show 100% negative effects. If a malefic is in the sign of an enemy then it will show 75% malefic effect.

If a malefic is in the sign of a friend then only 50% bad results.

If a malefic is in own sign then only 25% ill effects.

If a malefic is in the "Moolatrikon" sign then it will show only one eighth negative results and if a malefic is exalted then the bad effect will be almost nil.

If a planet is combust then it shows the effect as if it is posited in its sign of debilitation.

मन्दमान्द्यगुखशरन्ध्रपाः-
तन्नवांशपतयोऽपि ये ग्रहाः।
तेषु दुर्बलदशा पृतिप्रदा
कष्टभे चरति सूर्यनन्दने॥३१॥

Observe which is the weakest out of the following-

(a) Saturn, (b) Mandi, (c) Rahu, (d) The Lord of 22nd decanet from the ascendant, (e) Lord of the 8th house and (f) The Lord of 'Navansha' in which the planets which has been mentioned from a to e above.

Out of the above whichever is the weakest, the periodic influence of that planet is equal to death and at times actual death comes, if 'Saturn' in transit is also unfavourable.

मृतीशनाथस्थितभांशकेशयोः
खरत्रिभागेश्वरयोर्बलीयसः
दशागमे मृत्युपयुक्तभांशक-
त्रिकोणगे देवगुरौ तनुक्षयः ॥३२॥

Observe (A) the Lord of the sign in which the Lord of the 8th house is placed and (B) the Lord of the 'Navansha' in which the Lord of the 8th house is, out of these two which is stronger. Similarly see which one (C) the Lord of 22nd decanet from the ascendant or (E) The lord of the decanet falling in the ascendant. Out of these two which is stronger?

In the periodic influence of the stronger planet mentioned above, and if Jupiter is transiting one of the following places then death comes.

1. The sign occupied by the lord of the 8th house.
2. The Navansha sign occupied by the Lord of the 8th house.
3. In the 9th and 5th from (1) and (2) which has been mentioned above.

चतुष्टयस्थ गुरुजन्मलग्नपा
भवन्ति मध्ये वयसः सुखप्रदाः।
क्रमेण पृष्ठोभयमस्तकोदय-
स्थितोऽन्त्यमध्यप्रामिषु पाकदः ॥३३॥

Now we mention another thing. If any planet is in a sign which rises head first then it starts to show its good influence from the beginning of the period. If a planet is in a sign which rises from the feet first then it shows its special effect at the end of the dasha. If a planet is in a sign which rises both ways then it shows its effects during the middle portion of the dasha. For example- If a dasha is of 18 years. Then the middle portion will be eventful. Which 'Rasi' rises with the feet first or head first or both ways has been described in chapter— 1 Sloka No. 8. Here one thing is specially mentioned that according to the opinion in 'Phaldeepika', Gemini is a sign which rises both ways. Another things has been mentioned at other places about these signs and this is indicated here. If a malefic occupies a sign which rises feet first then it shows much ill effect but if it is a benefic planet then the bad effect is less. In signs which rise with the head first, the benefic planets posited in them show their full benefic results and malefic show reduced malefic effect. In signs which rises both ways the result are mixed.

यद्भावगो गोचरतो विलग्नात्-
दशेश्वरः स्वोच्चसुहृद्गृहस्थः ।
तद्भावपुष्टिं कुरुते तदानीं
बलान्वितश्चेज्जननेऽपि तस्य ॥३४॥

Look through which house from the Ascendant a planet, whose 'Mahadasha' is running, is passing through. This is a new thing which has been described in this Sloka. A planet whose 'Mahadasha' is running when it goes into different houses from the ascendant then its dasha will show different results.

If the Lord of the periodic influence is strong in the nativity then when it transits during its periodic influence, in its signs of exaltation, own sign or a sign of friend then in whichever house it is transiting from the ascendant then it increases the efficacy of that house. Suppose in a horoscope 'Rahu' is strong and when the Rahu's Mahadasha is in the offing then if by transit, it is in the 11th house from the ascendant then it will give financial gains, when it will be in the 10th house from the ascendant then it will give upliftment in the status. When it will be in the 9th house then it will bring good fortunes and betterment in luck. So the Lord of a 'Mahadasha' by its transit will give different results and this should be logically decided.

बलोनितो जन्मनि पाकनाथो
मौढ्यं स्वनीचं रिपुमन्दिरं वा।
प्राप्तश्च यद्भावमुपैति चारात्-
तद्भावनाशं कुरुते तदानीम् ॥३५॥

In the Sloka above it has been mentioned that if the Lord whose dasha is in progress is strong in a nativity and is also strong in transit then what types of benefic results it does.

Now we speak of a planet which is weak in a nativity and if during transit it is also weak then what is the ill effect it causes.

If a planet whose dasha is in the offing is devoid of strength in a horoscope and during the transit it passes through its sign of debilitation, or in the sign of its enemy, or is combust due closeness to Sun then in whichever house it is from the ascendant then it causes ill effects related to that house.

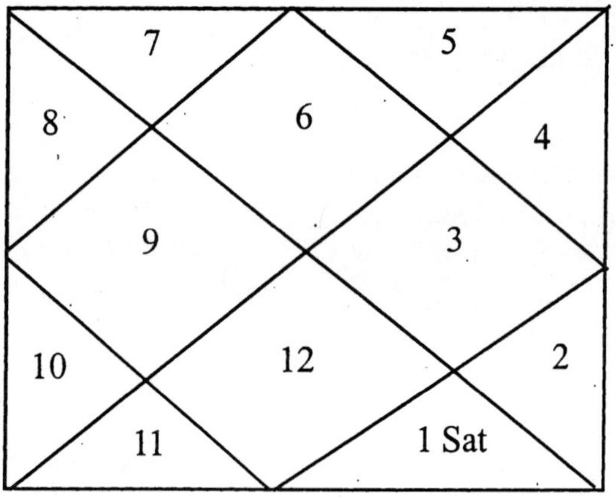

Chart with 'Virgo' rising and Saturn debilitated in the 8th house. Suppose the ascendant is Virgo, Saturn is in the 8th house. It is debilitated and as such weak and suppose it is the 'Mahadasha' of

*In the original Sloka at many places "Pakprabhu" or "Paknath", this word has been used. So the principles which will apply to the major periodic influence of a planet will also be applicable to the minor periodic influence of planets.

Saturn and Saturn is transiting through Leo, Sun is the enemy of Saturn and so when Saturn is transiting in Leo then being in the 12th house from the ascendant it will indicate ill effect related to the 12th house.

दशेशस्य तुङ्गे सुहृद्भे दशेशात्
त्रिषट्कर्मलाभत्रिकोणस्तभेषु।
यदा चारगत्या समायाति चन्द्रः
शुभं संविधत्तेऽन्यथा चेदरिष्टम् ॥३६॥

Now we give below the different houses from the 'Dashanath' where Moon in transit, shows good results.

(A) When Moon transits the sign of exaltation of the planet whose dasha is running.

(B) In the signs of friends of the planet whose dasha is running.

(C) In the 3rd, 5th, 6th, 7th, 9th, 10th and 11th from the planet whose dasha is running.

All the above is related to the radical position of the dashanath. Moon generally is in a sign for two and a quarter days. Suppose we have to find from the angle of the planet whose dasha is running if Moon will show some good results? Then see if Moon is in transit passing through the above mentioned houses. If Moon is transiting in other signs then during that period the benefic result of the 'Dashanath' will not be realised.

पाकप्रगोचरतः स्वनीचं
मौढ्यं यदायाति विपक्षभं वा।
कष्टं विदध्यात्स्वगृहं स्वतुङ्ग
वक्रं गतः सौख्यफलं तदानीम् ॥३७॥

If a planet whose dasha is invoke whether it is the major period or the minor period and if it is in transit passing through the sign of its debilitation or the sign of an enemy or due to proximity of the Sun, is combust then in such cases, it will show negative effects and will cause sufferings.

Generally these things has been mentioned in Sloka -35 above. The only difference is that in Sloka — 35 it has been added that the planet whose dasha is invoke is also devoid of strength at birth, but the same thing has not been repeated in Sloka No. 37. The conclusion is that the planet whose 'Mahadasha' is running if in transit it is combust or is passing through a sign which is not his friend or own sign or exaltation sign but on the other hand owned by its enemy or sign of debilitation. Then it creates sufferings.

Now take the second view - The planet whose major or minor period is running when it goes to its sign of exaltation, own sign, or is retrograde then it shows good results.

Why retrograde? Because when a benefic is retrograde then it shows much better effects.

पाकेशस्य शुभप्रदस्य भवनं तुङ्ग प्रपन्ने यदा
सूर्ये तत्फलसिद्धिमेति गुरुणाऽप्येवं फलं चिन्तयेत्।
नीचं कष्टफलप्रदस्य च दशानाथस्य वैरिस्थलं
प्राप्ते भास्वति गोचरेण लभते तस्यैव कष्टं फलम्॥३८॥

If a planet is capable of giving beneficial results then during its major or minor period when will it show its benefic results? The benefic results will be when Sun in transit goes to the sign of exaltation of the planet whose major or minor period is running or if Jupiter transit through the sign of exaltation of the planet whose major or minor period is running. Suppose in a horoscope 'Venus' is to give benefic results and its major or minor period is running. The exaltation sign of Venus is Pisces. In this case when Sun transits Pisces or Jupiter in transit passes through Pisces then benefic results will occur.

Now take another view:

In a horoscope the planet which is supposed to give ill results and its major or minor period is running then when will some special negative things happen? This will be when Sun in transit goes to the sign of debilitation or in the sign of an enemy of that planet, then there will be miseries.

येन ग्रहेण सहितो भुजगाधिनाथ-
स्तत्खेटजातगुणदोषफलानि कुर्यात्।
सर्पान्वितः स तु खगः शुभदोऽपि कष्टं
दुःखं दशान्त्यसमये कुरुते विशेषात् ॥३९ ॥

Rahu collects the good and bad qualities of the planet it conjoins with and shows similar effect. See the horoscope given here with Cancer rising and Rahu and Venus in the 4th house in Libra. Whatever effect, good or bad of Venus, the same type of effect Rahu will give.

In this Sloka two sections has been mentioned. Secondly it has been said that the planet with Rahu will get the negativity of Rahu. Even if it is a great benefic it causes suffering especially at the end of its Mahadasha. If in a horoscope, Rahu is with Venus and when the periodic influence of Venus will be over then great suffering will result in. Venus is benefic still it will show sufferings. The purpose of mentioning it is that Rahu is snake and it infects the planet with its poison.

द्वावर्थकामाविह मारकाख्यौ
तदीश्वरतत्र गतो बलाढ्यः ।
हन्ति स्वपाके निधनेश्वरो वा
व्ययेश्वरो वाऽप्यतिदुर्बलश्चेत् ॥४० ॥

The 2nd house and the 7th house are called Marak Places. *i.e.* the house which is 'fatal'. If the Lords of these houses are placed in these houses or other planets are placed in these houses and are strong then in their periodic influence they cause death. If the Lord of the 8th house or 12th house are also very weak then even their periodic influence that can give death.

केन्द्रेशस्य सतोऽसतोऽशुभशुभौ कुर्याद्दशा कोणपाः
सर्वे शोभनादास्त्रिवैरिभवपा यद्यप्यनर्थप्रदाः ।
रन्ध्रेशोऽपि विलग्नपो यदि शुभं कुर्याद्रविर्वा शशी
यद्येवं शुभदः पराशरमतं तत्तद्दशायां फलम् ॥४१ ॥

If the Lord of an angle is a benefic then it shows ill effects and on the other hand if the Lord of angle is a malefic it will give good results. The Lord of trine from the ascendant *i.e.* the Lord of the 9th or 5th house from the ascendant, always gives benefic results. The 1st house *i.e.* the ascendant is both an angle as well as a trine. So the Lord of 1st is always a benefic. The Lords of the 3rd, 6th and 11th houses even if they are benefic they give negative effects. If the Lord of the 1st house is simultaneously the Lord of the 8th also, this is possible when the ascendant is Aries or Libra, then it is a benefic. If the Lords of the 8th house are Sun or Moon then also it gives good results, this is possible when the rising signs are Sagittarius or Capricorn. The conclusion from all this is that except for Aries, Libra, Sagittarius and Capricorn rising people, for all other ascendants the Lord of the 8th causes bad results. This is the opinion of ' Parashar'. The planets show their effect in their periodic influences.

कोणाधीशः केन्द्रगः केन्द्रपो वा
कोणस्थश्चेद् द्वौ च योगप्रदौ स्तः ।
द्वावप्येतौ भुक्तिकाले दशाया-
मन्योन्यं तौ योगदौ सोपकारौ ॥४२ ॥

Similarly the Lords of 3rd, 6th and 11th houses whether they are Paapa or not has been explained in the book, in details.

1. If the Lord of a trine is in an angle or the Lord of an angle is in a trine then these two are Yoga giving planets. If the major period is of one of them and the minor period is of the other then they show benefic results. This way they exchange Yoga with each other and strengthen each other.

न दिशेयुर्ग्रहाः सर्वे स्वदशासु स्वभुक्तिषु ।
शभाशुभफलं नृणामात्मभावानुरूपतः ॥४३ ॥

In the Sloka No. 41 above the word 'Tattaddashayam Phalam'

*We have given the effect of the Lords of the angle and trine in details in "Sugam Jyotish Praveshika" an astrological book by Pt. Gopesh Kumar Ojha.

i.e. the planet gives their results in their major period. The question is do they give their full effect in their minor period as well? The answer is no. The same thing has been explained in this Sloka that Sun etc. all the planets in their own major period and in their minor period, do not give good or bad results to human beings. Then when do they give their full effect? This has been explained in the next Sloka.

आत्मसम्बन्धिनो ये च ये ये निजसधर्मिण: ।
तेषामन्तर्दशास्वेव दिशन्ति स्वदशाफलम् ॥४४ ॥

In one's own major period when the minor period is of a planet which is related or is of similar nature, then the planet show its good or bad effect. What is a related planet or what is a relationship between planet? See Chapter-15 Sloka No.30. What is a planet with similar nature?

(A) The planets which are 'Yoga Karak' like themselves are of similar nature.

(B) The benefic planets are of similar nature.

(C) The malefic are of similar nature.

केन्द्रत्रिकोणनेतारौ दोषयुक्तावपि स्वयम् ।
सम्बन्धमात्राद्बलिनौ भवेतां योगकारको ॥४५ ॥

The Lord of an angle and trine even if they are afflicted with negative qualities but if they are related with each other then they give Yoga.

What is the meaning of being afflicted or endowed with Dosha?

For example– For Aries rising people, Saturn is the Lord of the 10th house an angle, but it is simultaneously the Lord of the 11th house which is not good. So Saturn being a Lord of angle is afflicted with negative qualities. In the same manner for Leo rising people Jupiter is the ruler of the 5th and 8th houses, as such it is a Lord of a trine but is not pure because of the ownership of the 8th as well.

In this Sloka it has been explained that even though they are afflicted yet if there is a relationship between the Lord of an angle or and Lord of a trine, then they gain strength and they create a Yoga.

त्रिकोणाधिपयोर्मध्ये सम्बन्धो येन केनचित्।
केन्द्रनाथस्य बलिनो भवेद्यदि स योगकृत्॥४६॥

Out of both the trines *i.e.* 5th and 9th, if the Lord of any one has a relationship with the Lord of an angle who is also strong then this relationship creates a Rajyoga. Here one word also should be explained why 'strong'? The meaning is that it should be endowed with certain strength. Another thing is that the Lord of an angle which is the strong sometimes is Synonym with the Lord of 10th because out of the four angles. 1st, 4th, 7th and 10th. The 10th is supposed to be the strongest. If we take the 2nd meaning then it means that if the Lord of the 5th and 9th, out of these any one is related to the Lord of the 10th house then it creates Yoga. But other people take the meaning of strong and apply it only to the Lords of all the angles. According to this view if the Lord of any angle is strong and has relationship with any of the trine Lord then it creates a Raja Yoga.

केन्द्रत्रिकोणाधिपयोरैक्ये तौ योगकारकौ।
अन्यत्रिकोणपतिनां संबन्धो यदि किं पुनः॥४७॥

If the Lord of any angle is related to the Lord of any trine then due to this relationship between the Lord of an angle and trine, they become Yoga Karak. If the Lord of a angle is related to one of the Lord of the trine and simultaneously also gets related to the Lord of the 2nd trine then it is an excellent relationship and result in a very big Raj Yog *i.e.* the Lord of any angle when related to the both of the Lord of trine 5th and 9th then is a Magnanimous Yoga.

It is also necessary to explain here that if one planet is simultaneously the Lord of an angle and trine then the planet itself become a Yoga Karak.

For example— for the Cancer rising people and the Leo rising people Mars is a Yoga Karak. For Capricorn and Aquarius rising people Venus is a Yoga Karak for Taurus and Libra rising people Saturn is a Yoga Karak. This Yoga Karak brings in good fortunes during its minor periodic influence.*

---

*In the original Sloka the word 'Aaikya' has come i.e. when they are together. But our opinion is that if they are related in any of the four manners described in Chapter—15, then it is a relationship.

योगकारकसम्बन्धात्पापिनोऽपि ग्रहाः स्वतः ।
तत्तद्भक्त्यानुसारेण दिशेयुर्यौगिकं फलम् ॥४८ ॥

We have explained previously that the relationship between the Lord of an angle and a trine results in Raj Yoga. During the major period of any one of these planets if the minor period is that of a benefic even if it is not related to the Lord whose major period is in the offing, then the minor period will give benefic results.

Now we explain that if any planet is a natural malefic viz. Mars, Saturn etc. and even though they are malefic yet if they are related to the planets creating the Yoga then what is the effect? If the Papa *i.e.* malefic planets are related to the planets creating the Yoga then in their minor periodic influence, they give good results. For details consideration see the book 'Sugam Jyotish Paraveshika' (page- 121 and page 136).

स्वदशायां त्रिकोणेशो भुक्तौ केन्द्रपतेः शुभम् ।
दिशेत्सोऽपि तथा नो चेदसंबन्धेऽपि पापकृत् ॥४९ ॥

If the Lord of an angle is related to the Lord of a trine then in the minor period of the Lord of the trine in its own major period, benefic results will come. Similarly the Lord of the trine in its Dasha and in the minor period of the Lord of the angle gives benefic results. If the Lord of the angle and the Lord of a trine are not related in any manner then in the major period of one and in the minor period of another benefic result will not be realised.

If both the planets whose major and minor period is running are benefic and even though they may not have any relationship yet the major period of one and the minor period of another will give benefic results. Our opinion is that if the Lord of an angle and trine have no relationship and in the major period of one and the minor period of the 2nd, one more thing should be considered. Both the planets besides being the Lord of angle and trine what other rulership they have? Where are they posited? If they in the 6th, 8th or 12th from each other? If they are strong or weak? And then proper conclusion should be drawn. If there is no relationship between the Lord of angle and the Lord of trine and the Lord of angle is a malefic then it should be noted that there will be ill effects.

केन्द्राधिपत्यदोषस्तु बलवान् गुरुशुक्रयोः।
मारकत्वेऽपि च तयोर्मारकस्थानसंस्थितिः ॥५०॥

We have mentioned before that if a benefic is the Lord of angle then it is not a good factor.

Now we tell another things that if Jupiter and Venus own an angle then it is bad. If besides this, they are also posited in the Marak Sthan *i.e.* in the 2nd or 7th house then they become strong Markesh. We make it more clear that if Jupiter and Venus own an angle and are simultaneously placed in the 2nd or 7th house then they are strong Markesh. Markesh means one which kills.

बुधस्तदनु चंद्रोऽपि भवेत्तदनु तद्विधः।
पापाश्चेत्केन्द्रपतयः शुभदाश्चोत्तरोत्तरम् ॥५१॥

The way the ownership and placement of Jupiter and Venus in a Marksthan is supposed to be not good. Similarly the same should hold true for Mercury and Moon *i.e.* if Mercury is the ruler of angle then it is not a benefic and if simultaneously not only it own an angle but is also posited in a Marksthan then it is supposed to be worst. Similarly if Moon is the ruler of an angle it is bad and if simultaneously it is placed in a Maraksthan then worst. But if malefic are owners of angles then they bestow benefic effect. If Sun is the owner of angle then it gives excellent results. Mars if it owns an angle then it gives a still better effect and if Saturn is the owner of an angle then it is very good.

यदि केन्द्र त्रिकोणे वा निवसेतां तमोग्रहौ।
नाथेनान्यतरस्यैव संबन्धाद्योगकारकौ ॥५२॥

If Rahu or Ketu are posited in an angle and have a relationship with a Lord of a trine then it is a Yoga Karak situation. Or if Rahu or Ketu are posited in a trine and are related to the Lord of an angle, then also it is a rajayoga.

तमोग्रहौ शुभारूढौऽसंबद्धौ येन केनचित्।
अन्तर्दशानुरूपेण भवेतां योगकारकौ ॥५३॥

If Rahu or Ketu are posited in the sign of a benefic in a good place and are not conjoined with any other planet then in their minor periods they give benefic results.

If Rahu or Ketu are not related to any planet and are placed in good houses (in an angle or trine) then during their major period when the minor period of a Yoga creating planets comes, then benefic results will ensue.

आरम्भो राजयोगस्य भवेन्मारकभुक्तिषु ।
प्रथमयन्ति तमारभ्य क्रमशः पापभुक्तयः ॥५४॥

If in the minor period of any Marak planet the Raj Yoga commences then during that minor period only the realisation of fame related to the high position comes, but there is no concrete enjoyment of that position.

रन्ध्रस्थरन्ध्रेक्षकरन्ध्रनाथ-
रन्ध्रत्रिभागाधिपमान्दिभेषाः ।
दुःखप्रदास्तेष्वपि दुर्बलो यः
स नाशकारी स्वदशापहारे ॥५५॥

The following planets give much sorrow and sufferings-

1. The planet posited in the 8th house.
2. The planet which aspects the 8th house.
3. The Lord of the 8th house.
4. The Lord of the 22nd decanet from the ascendant.
5. The Lord of the sign were 'Mandi' is posited.

The purpose of mentioning this is that the above mentioned planets in their major and minor periods give much suffering and the one which is the weakest out of the above, during its major and minor period, death can take place.

भ्रष्टस्य तुङ्गादवरोहिसंज्ञा
मध्या भवेत्सा सुहृदुच्चभागे ।

आरोहिणी निम्नपरिच्युतस्य
नीचारिभांशेष्वधमा भवेत्सा ॥५६ ॥

It has been mentioned before as to which planet, in which sign and degree, is at its highest degree of exaltation or which planet is at the lowest in which degree and sign.

For example— In Aries - 10 degrees of Sun is at the highest degrees of exaltation and in Libra 10 degrees is the maximum debilitation point. Therefore when Sun after crossing 10 degrees of Libra, is moving towards Aries 10 degrees then it is called 'Aarohee' *i.e.* going upward towards its sign of exaltation and when it reaches 10 degrees of Aries and after crossing the 10 degrees of Aries moves towards the 10 degrees of Libra, then that portion is called 'Avrohi' *i.e.* going down. Because it is moving towards the sign of debilitation so it is called going down.

The periodic influence of a planet which is Avrohi is not good and the periodic influence of a planet which is Aarohi is very good. Whatever may be the Dasha even if it is Avrohi, if the planet whose Dasha is in the offing is in the Navansha of a friend or is exalted in the Navansha, then the periodic influence is not that bad, but in general it is quite good.

Against this if a planet is Aarohi but is in the sign of his debilitation or in the sign of an enemy or is debilitated in the Navansha or in a Navansha owned by an enemy, then its period is worse and the entire period goes bad.

In the following paragraph A, B, and C if a planet is good in all the three and then the dasha will be very good. If it is bad in all the three A, B and C then the dasha will be very bad. And if out of A, B and C in one it is good and in others not good, then logical conclusion should be drawn because it will be a mixed period.

(A) 1. Aarohi (good)

2. Avrohi (bad)

(B) 1. In sign of exaltation, in the sign of a great friend, in the sign of a friend (good)

2. Debilitated sign in the sign of great enemy, in the sign of an enemy (bad)

(C) 1. Exhalted in Navansha, Vargottam in Navansha or in the Navansha of a great friend or in the Navansha of a friend (excellent).

2. Debilitated in Navansha in the Navansha of a great enemy or in the Navansha of enemy (bad).

In the 8th Chapter of Brihat Jaatak, this has been explained in detail—

(A) If any planet is very strong or is in the highest degree of exaltation then the entire period of that planet generates wealth and good health.

(B) If any planet is in its sign of exaltation and is some what strong also then its period is called Poorna. This planet's major and minor period gives increase of wealth.

(C) If any planet is weak then its period is called Rikta. In Rikta period there is lack of wealth and health is not good. There is disease and poverty to a great extend.

(D) If any planet is debilitated in Navansha or in the Navansha of enemy then the period is called Anishta. In this period there is physical sufferings and lack of wealth creates problems.

(E) If a planet is Avrohi *i.e.* moving downwards but is posited in the Navansha of a friend or a great friend then the period is called a 'Madhya' and in this period there is some wealth.

शस्तगृहे शस्तांशे नीचे रिपुभेऽस्तसंस्थिते वाऽपि।
तस्य दशा मिश्रफला दशापरार्धे फलप्रदा ज्ञेया॥५७॥

Even if a planet is debilitated, in the sign of an enemy, or combust but if it is posited in a good house and good Navansha, then its period will be mixed *i.e.* will give some good or some bad results.

According to Varahmihir the planetary period of that planet is called a mixture which is in a good sign (exalted or own sign) but is debilitated in the Navansha, or in the Navansha of an enemy. The periodic influence of that planet is mixed. At times good health, at times wealth but at other times sickness and poverty. According to Mantreshwar Maharaj the mixed result will be in the first half, and benefic results will be felt in the second half.

तत्तद्भावात्व्ययस्थस्य तद्भावव्ययपस्य।
वीर्यहीनस्य खेटस्य पाके मृत्युमवाप्नुयात्॥५८॥

Death can occur in the major and minor period of a planet which is devoid of strength. The question is death of 'Whom'? If a weak planet is in the 12th house from a sign then from that sign whoever is considered or the person indicated by the house from which the 12th sign is ruled by the weak planet.

An example will make it clear. Suppose a weak planet is the Lord of the 2nd house and is posited in the 9th house then in the periodic influence (major or minor) of that planet the native's brother and father can expire Why? The answer is that it is Lord of the 2nd house *i.e.* the 12th from the 3rd and from the 3rd house the 12th is the 2nd house from the Ascendant so the Lord of the 2nd is the one which causes the destruction of the 3rd house. This has been explained above that the Lord of the 12th house if weak then the house is destroyed.

From the 3rd house brother is considered so if the Lord of the 2nd house is devoid of strength then in its period trouble to brother should be predicted. The second thing that has been explained in the Sloka is that— The placement of planet itself in the 12th from a house then the weak planet will also destroy the house. In the above example it is in the 12th from the 10th house. Consideration of father is done from the 10th house and because a weak planet is posited in the 9th house and the 9th is the 12th from the 10th, so it causes suffering to father. The result is that a weak planet destroys whichever house it is the 12th Lord of, as well as the 2nd house from where it is placed.

Now we talk of the result of the transit of a planet whose periodic influence is running and what are the different results of its transit in various houses.

दशापतिर्लग्नगतो यदि स्यात्
त्रिषट्दशैकादशगश्च लग्नात्।
तत्सप्तवर्गेऽप्यथ तत्सुहृद्वा
लग्ने शुभो वा शुभदा दशा स्यात्॥५९॥

The planet whose Dasha is invoke when it is in the 1st house or in the 3rd, 6th, 10th or 11th from the ascendant then its period shows good results. If the planet whose dasha is running is in the 7th house from the ascendant then also its period is good. If the planet whose dasha is running and its friend or any other benefic in transit comes to the 1st house, then good results ensue.

यावन्ति वर्षाणि दशा च सा स्यात्-
चारक्रमात्तत्र दशापतिः सः।
यत्र स्थितस्तद्भवनाद्विधोस्तु
स्थितेः प्रकल्प्यं सदसत्फलं हि ॥६०॥

Look to house in which a planet whose major or minor period is invoke, is passing through in transit. If the planet whose dasha or Antardasha is running is passing through good houses from the Moon at birth, then it shows good results. But when it passes through negative houses from the Moon then the result will be bad.

दशाधिनाथस्य सुहृद्गृहस्थ-
स्तदुच्चगो वाऽथ दशाधिनाथात्।
स्मरत्रिकोणोपचयोपगश्च
ददाति चन्द्रः खलु सत्फलानि ॥६१॥

When Moon in transit passes through any of the following places then it shows benefic effect.

(A) In the sign of a friend of the planet whose dasha is running.

(B) In the sign where the planet who's dasha is running is placed in the birth chart.

(C) In the 3rd, 5th, 6th, 7th, 9th, 10th and 11th houses from the planet whose dasha is running.

उक्तेषु राशिषु गतस्य विधोः स राशिः
स्याज्जन्मकालभवमूर्तिधनादिभावः।
तत्तद्विवृद्धिकृदसौ कथितो नराणां
तद्भावहानिकृदथेतरराशिसंस्थः ॥६२॥

In the above Sloka it has been mentioned, in which houses Moon is benefic. In other houses show malefic effect. If the benefic house also synchronises with the ascendant, 2nd, 11th houses etc. then it increases the efficacy of those houses. In the same manner if Moon is malefic viz., - 6th, 8th and 12th etc. and they also coincides with the negative signs in the birth chart, then loss of matters related to that house will be there.

For example— If Aries is the rising sign and the Lord of the dasha is Jupiter which is posited in sagittarius then the exalted sign of Jupiter is Cancer. So Moon will be well placed in Cancer and good result when it is transiting through it and will improve the 4th house.

In the 61st Sloka Cancer is a benefic place and Capricorn is a negative place for Moon to transit. Therefore Cancer is the 4th from the ascendant so the transit of Moon in that will increase the efficacy of that house. Capricorn which is the 10th house from the ascendant and Moon in Capricorn will show negative results related to the 10th house.

सारावलीमुडुदशां च वराहहोरा-
मालोक्य जातकफलं प्रवदेन्नराणाम्।
प्रश्नोदयग्रहवशादथ वा स्वजन्म-
राश्यादिना वदतु नास्त्यनयोर्विशेषः ॥६३॥

In Saravali a book of a predictive Astrology in Sanskrit, written by Sh. Kalyan Verma, is a famous Book, Udoo dasha (Udai Pradeep Udoo dasha or constellation dasha is also a predictive Book of Astrology) as well as in Hora Shastra written by Varaha Mihir, the horoscope of a native is in consideration from Ascendant or Moon sign or when an Horary Chart is erected and prediction is done, then there is not much difference between them. We repeat according to these three books mentioned above whether the prediction is done from Horary Chart or from the birth chart or from the Moon sign it does not make much difference. According to Mantreshwar Maharaj— the systematic manner which is applicable to prediction from nativity, the same can be applied and easily used when predicting from the Moon used as the Ascendant or from the Horary Astrology. We give now some combinations from 'Bhavarta Ratnakar'.

DHAN YOG VICHAR- CONSIDERATION FOR WEALTH

1. If the Lord of the 2nd house is in the 5th and the 5th Lord is in the 2nd, or the Lord of the 2nd in the 11th and the Lord of the 11th is in the 2nd, or Lord of the 5th is in the 5th and the Lord of 9th is in the 9th then it indicates special combination for wealth.

2. If the Lord of any other house is posited with the Lord of the 2nd or 11th then it does not give that much wealth which is when the Lord of the 2nd is related to the Lord of 11th.

   Here we mention that logical conclusion should be drawn as to what other house or houses the other planet owns. Who is that planet? If it is the Lord of the 1st then it will be an indication of good results. If it is the Lord of the 4th then it is excellent but if the Lord of the 6th, 8th or 12th are with the Lord of 2nd or 11th then it will destroy the combination. The effect will be mala-fide. Side by side it should also be considered, that if the Lord of the 5th house or the 9th house are also posited where the Lord of the 2nd and 11th are then they will increase the efficacy of that combination they will not cause limitations to it.

3. If the Lord of the 2nd and 11th house get related to Lord of 5th or 9th then it is a special combination for wealth. But if the Lords of the 6th, 8th and 12th which are the Dusthan they are related to the Lord of the 2nd or the 11th or with the Lord of 5th and 9th then the Yoga is destroyed.

4. If the Lord of the 2nd and 11th are posited with the Lord of the 12th house or are related to the Lord of 12th house then the Yoga for wealth is destroyed.

5. If the significator of wealth Jupiter is related to the Lord of the 2nd house or if Jupiter is related to Mercury then also a wealth giving combination occurs.

6. If the Lord of the ascendant is in the ascendant, the Lord of the 2nd is in the 2nd, and Lord of the 11th is in the 11th, then it is also a special wealth giving combination.

7. If the Lord of 2nd and 11th are both in the 1st house then wealth is attained easily.

8. If the significator of a house is posited in the house itself then the good effect of the house is reduced.*

सर्वेषु भावस्थानेषु तत्तद्भावादिकारकः ।
विद्यते तस्यभावस्य फलम् स्वल्पमुदीरितम् ॥

9. If Moon as the ruler of the 7th house is posited in the 2nd house and there is no other planet with Moon, then the lost money or money which has been stolen is recovered.

'NIRDHAN YOG VICHAR'- CONSIDERATION OF COMBINATIONS FOR POVERTY

1. If the Lords of the 1st, 4th and 9th house is posited in the 8th house then the native will be poor from birth.
2. If the Lord of the 2nd house is in the 12th and the Lord of the 12th house goes to the 2nd.
3. If the Lord of the 2nd house is in the 12th house and the Lord of 12th is in the 1st and a Markesh aspect them.
4. The Lord of the 5th is posited in the 6th, the Lord of the 9th is in the 8th house and both of them receive the aspect of Markesh.

   In all the above four Yogas the native will be devoid of wealth.

'VIDYA VICHAR'- CONSIDERATION FOR EDUCATION

1. Venus in the 4th house makes one an expert in singing.
2. If Mercury is in the 4th house then one is an expert in Astrology.
3. If Sun is in the 5th house or Rahu and Mercury are in the 5th house then the native is expert in Astrology or is a doctor who is expert in curing disease connected with poison.
4. (a) If Sun is in the 2nd house and Mercury is also there, then a person is expert in Astrology,

*Which planet is the significator of which house has been given in Chapter-15, Sloka-17.

(b) If these two receive an aspect of Saturn then he is excellent in mathematics.

5. If Sun and Mars are in the 2nd house then the native is expert in logic and arguments.

6. Sun, Mercury and Saturn in the 5th house make one an expert in 'Vedanta'.

7. Sun and Mercury together in an angle or in a trine or in the 11th house then it is a good Yoga for excellence in mathematics. In the original Sloka the the word 'Ganak' has come and the second meaning of this is that he can be an Astrologer.

8. If Venus is placed in the 2nd house then it makes one a poet or one who loves poetry.

9. If Rahu is in the 5th house then the person has deep knowledge of such subjects which are very difficult and so difficult that general people can not understand its deeper meanings.

10. If Rahu is posited in the 10th house then the mother is long lived.

11. If Jupiter is in the 2nd house then the native is a knowledgeable person of Veda and Vedant. If Jupiter is in Cancer, Sagittarius or Pisces then definitely one is honoured in society, meetings and big gatherings due to his learnings.

12. If Jupiter as the ruler of the 2nd house is posited in an angle or trine then the native is a person who is a scholar of various subjects.

13. Mars in the 2nd house makes one expert in logic and discussion.

14. If with the above mentioned Mars, Moon is also posited then the native knows 'Sutras'.

15. If Saturn is in the 2nd house then the native is dull headed and bad by temperament.

VAANI (VOICE) SPEECH

1. If Saturn is posited in the 2nd house then the native's speech is not clear and even his manner of speaking is not sophisticated.

2. Jupiter or Ketu in the 2nd house makes one clever and expert in speech. All these are related with speech.
3. If Sun and Mars are in the 2nd house then the native's speech is always against others *i.e.* he criticises others and can be sarcastic.
4. Moon in the 2nd house makes one speak very much.
5. Mercury in the 2nd house endow the native with logical speech *i.e.* his speech is full of cleverness and to the point.
6. Rahu in the 2nd house makes one utter words in a very humble and sickly manner.

TEESRE BHAVA KA VICHAR- CONSIDERATION FOR THE 3RD HOUSE

1. The consideration for brother and sisters is done with the Lord of the 3rd house the significators of brothers Mars, or with planets placed with Mars.
2. If Sun, Mars and the Lord of the 3rd are in the 3rd the native is courageous and patient.
3. Rahu, Ketu in the 3rd makes the natives courageous.
4. Mercury in the 3rd house makes one lack patience.
5. If the 3rd house is weak but Jupiter and Mars aspect the 3rd house then the native will have brothers.
6. If Jupiter is in the 11th house then the native suffers on account of elder brothers.*
7. If Mars is in the 11th house and it receives aspect from Saturn then there will be no elder brothers.
8. If the Lord of the 3rd house is posited in the 6th or 8th then the brother will die prematurely or they will have a short span of life.
9. In the horoscope of Kshatriya's if the Lord of the 10th house is posited in the 3rd then the rajayoga gets downgraded. In the

*The difference of opinion exists with elder brother or the elder brother causes, loss to the native or the elder brother is short lived. All these are called sufferings on account of elder brother.

horoscope of the Pt. Jawahar Lal Nehru the first Prime Minister of Independent India, the Lord of 10th house was Mars, and it was posited in the 3rd. If it would be in an angle or trine then he would have got a high position earlier in life. Mr. Nehru was a Brahmin. In the past Kshatriyas used to be the kings so the word Kshatriya has been used.

10. If the Lord of the 2nd and 3rd are together then the native is generous.
11. If Saturn is related to the Lord of the 2nd and 3rd then the native is very greedy.
12. If the lord of the 3rd is in the 6th, 8th or 12th houses then the brothers die. They have short life. If benefic are also with the Lord of the 3rd then it will give death to brothers but after they have good longevity.

CONSIDERATION FOR 4TH HOUSE (VEHICLES)

1. If the Lord of 4th and 9th are in the ascendant then it gives increase in fortunes and yoga for vehicles.*
2. If Jupiter is in the 4th house or throws an aspect to the 4th then the native gets lot of happiness.
3. If the Lord of the 4th house and Jupiter are together in an angle or trine then the native has a lot of happiness.
4. If Venus is placed in the 4th house together with the Lord of the 4th house then the native will have very few Cars.
5. If Venus, with the Lord of the 4th is posited in the 9th, 10th or 11th house then it does give a native a number of vehicles.
6. If Cancer is the ascendant and Mercury and Venus are in the 4th house then in the major period of Mercury and the minor period of Venus many vehicles are gained.
7. Venus in the 7th house makes the native extremely romantic by nature *i.e.* all the time he desires to indulge in love.

---

*In the past vehicles used to mean elephants, horses, planquein, carriers etc. Now in the present context these are scooters, cars, aeroplanes, helicopters etc.

8. The Saturn is in the 4th house then the native is very hard hearted. He does not live in a new house and lives away from home in other place.

9. If the Lord of the 4th house is in the 9th house and the Lord of the 9th house is in the 4th house then it indicates good fortunes and combination for vehicles.

10. If the Lord of 4th house is in the 11th and the Lord of the 11th in the 4th house then also the results as indicated in 9th will take place.

11. The lord of the 4th in the 5th and the 5th Lord in the 4th then also it is a special combination for fortunes and number of vehicles.

12. If the Lord of 4th is in the ascendant and the ascendant Lord is in the 4th then also benefic result should be understood.

13. If the Lord of the 5th house is in the 9th and the Lord of the 9th is in the 5th then also the same are realised.

14. If the Lord of the 4th is in 4th and the Lord of 5th is in the 5th then it is a combination for vehicles.

15. If the Lord of the 5th house is in the 11th and the Lord of the 11th is in the 5th then it brings in fortunes. The 11th house is called the house of gains.

16. If the Lord of the 1st is in the 1st and the Lord of the 9th is in the 9th then the benefic Yoga mentioned above takes place.

17. If the Lord of the 5th house is in the 9th house and the Lord of 9th is in the 10th, then also the Yoga mentioned in 15th above takes place.

CONSIDERATION FOR SON

1. If the Lord of the 5th house and Jupiter are related then it is a good combination for sons *i.e.* the native will have sons and will have happiness from them.

2. If the Lord of 1st, 5th and Jupiter are in an angle or in trine then the native gets happiness from sons.

SHATRU - CONSIDERATION OF ENEMIES AND DISEASE

From the horoscope disease and enemies are taken into account from the 6th house. Therefore in Bhavarth Ratnakar in the heading of 'Shatru Rogadi Tarang'. The following combinations have been given:-

The name of the Book is Bhavarth Ratnakar. Why? Ratnakar is sea and instead of writing different Chapters as Chapters or divisions it has been named as 'Tarang'. Tarang or different ideas. Tarang is Sanskrit word, (Hindi word) meaning waves. So the Book Ratnakar is the name of the sea and the waves in the sea *i.e.* 'Tarang'.

1. If the Lord of the 1st house is in the 8th house then generally the person has disease. He is sickly.
2. If the Lord of the 6th house in the 1st house then a person from own caste and community causes harm. The native's own people become his enemies and develop enmity with him. The native also suffers from disease.
3. If Lord of the 1st and Lord of 6th are placed with Sun then the person suffers from fever (high temperature).
4. If the Lord of the 1st and 6th are with Moon, then there is fear of water.
5. If the Lord of the 1st and 6th are related to Mars then possibility exist of having hurt wounds, injury from weapons and such type of problems where there will be knots in the body like plague etc.
6. If Lords of the 1st and the 6th house are with Mercury then the natives suffers from access of biles disorder of pitta.
7. The lord of the 1st and 6th are with Jupiter then the health is good and there will be no disease.
8. The lord of the 1st and 6th are with Venus then it is not good for the health of the native's wife.
9. If Lord of 1st and 6th are with Saturn then there is fear from thieves and persons of low caste.
10. Lord of 1st and 6th are with Rahu or Ketu then there is danger from snakes, tigers etc.

11. If the Lord of the 6th is in the 12th house with a debilitated planet and the Lord of 1st is strong, then the disease is destroyed *i.e.* the health improves.
12. If the lord of 6th house is weak comparatively to the lord of the 1st and the Lord of the 6th house is also related to benefic then the natives enemies will become his friends.

PATNI VICHAR

In this wave consideration of wife is given.

If in the horoscope of a woman consideration of the following principles are taken into account then husband is considered from the 7 th house and in this logic should be used. Where the combination for plurality of marriage is given for many wives, then to have more then one husband will depend upon the type of Society, the woman comes from.

For Example– In such places where women come from hill areas, a woman have many husbands or where there are widow marriages then this will apply.

In the horoscope of a Hindu in India— now a person cannot have a second wife if his first wife is living and they are not legally divorced. So many of these Yogas will not apply and in many places where yogas for many wifes are given, then instead of marriages there will be relationship or connection with *i.e.* emotional connection with more then one woman. This can always take place. The Yogas given in ancient books undergo a change and Astrology also takes into account, when doing the prediction, the country, the person and the times prevailing.

1. If the Lord of 7th house is with Venus and does not have a relationship with malefic.

   Relationship are of four types. The placement of two planets together in one signs, exchange of sign between two planets, aspecting each other with full aspect, one planet is placed in the sign of another and receives an aspect from the other planet, then there will be only one wife.
2. If the Lord of the 7th house has any relationship with a malefic

or malefic are placed in the 2nd or 7th house or Venus is in the 11th house which is the house of gains or Venus is debilitated or the Lord of the 7th house is posited in the 6th or 12th house then there will be a second marriage.

3. If a malefic is in the ascendant then second marriage takes place *i.e.* the 1st marriage does not last.
4. Mars and Venus together in the 2nd, 4th, 7th, 8th or 12th house and Venus is weak then there will be a 2nd marriage.
5. Mars in the 2nd, 4th 7th, 8th or 12th then also it causes two marriages. In other texts this has been called a Manglik Dosh or Kuja Dosh. Therefore if the wife of the native also has a manglik Dosh then she will live and there will be no second marriage. This is a general principle that negative cancel each other. We would like to point out that in North India instead of the 2nd house Mars in the first house creates Kuja Dosh and not in the 2nd house. So Mars in the 1st, 4th, 7th, 8th or 12th creates manglik and Kuja Dosh.
6. If Jupiter is in the 2nd house and there is an indication of more then one marriage in the horoscope then the 2nd marriage takes place is in the later years of life.
7. If Saturn is placed in the 2nd house and Rahu is in the 7th house* then two marriages take place.
8. If the Lords of the 2nd and 7th house or Venus is in the 2nd or 7th house and the 2nd and 7th houses receive an aspect from benefic, then the number of benefic aspect will indicate the number of wives that one will have or the native will have happiness from that number of women. However if malefic are also posited in the houses mentioned above or Venus is conjoined with malefic then this Yoga will not take place *i.e.* will be nullified.
9. If Saturn and Venus are in the 7th house then the native is devoted and is in love with his own wife.
10. Mercury in the 7th house makes one affecionate towards other's wives.

---

*Rahu in general in the 7th house gives clandestine relationships.

11. Jupiter in the 7th house gives a spiritual and devoted wife to the native.
12. Lords of the 2nd, 7th and 10th houses if they are in the 4th house then the native is attracted to other women (wives of other persons).
13. Rahu in the 7th house makes once an expert (in love).
14. Ketu in the 7th house gives a very cunning wife.

AAYU, AROGYA, TARANG (AGE AND HEALTH WAVES)

1. Jupiter is the significator of wealth, physical health and sons.
2. If Jupiter is with the Lord of the 1st house then there is long life.
3. If Saturn the significator of the age is related to the Lord of the 8th house then there will be long life.
4. Saturn in the 8th house gives longevity.
5. If the Lord of the 8th house together with Ketu is posited in the Ascendant then there is a short life.
6. If the Lord of the 9th house and the significator of father, sons are related then the father of the native will have long life.
7. Sun in the 9th house reduces the longevity of the father.*
8. Moon in the 4th house gives short life to mother.
9. Sun and the Lord of the 9th house if both of them are posited in the 9th house then the father is short lived. However if the Lord of the 9th house is in the 11th house then the father will have long life.
10. Mars in the 3rd house reduce the longevity of brothers. Jupiter in the 3rd house gives problems to brothers.
11. If Jupiter is in the 3rd house which coincides with Sagittarius or Pisces, then the native will have only one brother.

---

*In South of India father is considered from the 9th house. Sun is the significator of father so the significator if the posited in the house it signifies then it destroys the house.

12. Jupiter in the 5th house reduce the age of Sons.

13. Venus in the 7th house reduce the longevity of wife.

    Note: The conclusion of the above mentioned combination is that if the significator of a house is posited in that house then it reduces the benefic effects. Only in the case of Saturn it does not apply because it is the significator of age and in the 8th house it increases the longevity. We think that the significator being posited in the house it signifies reduce the living things but it increases the nonliving things.

    For Example– Age is non-living does not have a formation or a body so it increases but the living things are brother, father, mother, wife and so it reduces their longevity.

14. If Moon and the Lord of the 4th house are in the 5th, 9th, 10th or 11th in any one of these houses, it is not necessary that they should be only in one house, then the mother of the native has long life. If the Lord of the 4th house is related to Moon then also the mother will have long life.

15. If in their Moola Trikona, Sun in Leo, Mars in Aries, Mercury in Virgo, Jupiter in Sagittarius, Venus in Libra or Saturn in Aquarius are in the 4th house then the mother will have long life. If the Lord of the 4th house is also in the 4th house then also it is a good indication for mother and if the Lord of the 4th house is in the Moola Trikona then much better. In which degrees it is in Moola Trikona and in which degrees it is in own sign has been mentioned in the commentary in Chapter—1, Sloka No. 7.

17. If the Lord of the 4th house and Moon are posited in a strong place but Moon is waning, weak from the 10th day of the dark half to the 5th day of the bright half then it is considered weak, and Saturn also aspects them then the mother is short lived.*

BHAGYA YOGA TARANG- FORTUNES

Now some Yogas according to Bhawarth Ratnakar are given below:— These are related to fortunes-

*According to one opinion Moon is weak on the 14th day of the dark half and on amavasya.

1. If the Lord of the 9th house is in the 11th house and the Lord of the 11th house is in the 9th or there is a relationship between the Lord of the 9th and 11th house.
2. If two planets are together in each sign so that in four signs eight planets are posited (in each sign 2 planets).
3. If six planets are posited in three signs and each sign contains two planets.
4. If all the four benefic planets (Mercury, Jupiter, Venus and Moon) of the bright half receive an aspect from malefic then the native is not very fortunate but it does give Yoga for wealth.
5. Malefic in the 3rd, 6th and 11th houses.
6. If any planet is in the 12th house from the Ascendant then it brings to enlighten that house of which it is the significator of. Which planet signifies what houses has been mentioned earlier in the book.
7. If the Lord of the 4th house, Venus, the Lord of the 7th and 9th houses are posited in the 9th or 11th houses or in both houses whether all the four of them are together or some are in the 9th and the remaining are in the 11th house and they also are related to Saturn then during the major and minor period of Saturn good gains are realised and acquisition of a Vehicle also takes place.
8. If the Lord of the 1st, 4th, 9th and 10th houses are placed in the the 1st, 7th or 10th houses. All the four should be in the any of the three angles but they should be placed together. Then during their major and minor period, great fortunes are the results.
9. If any planet in its sign of exaltation is posited in the 5th or 9th then the native's fortunes improves *i.e.* he is very fortunate.
10. If Sun, Mercury and Venus are posited in the 5th house and Jupiter is in the 11th house, then during the period of Mercury much wealth is acquired.
11. If the Lord of the 9th house and Sun are together in the 12th house from the ascendant then the native's fortune rise on account of his father or with the help of the father.
12. If Sun is in Aries then it gives fortunes to father.

13. If Sun is in Libra then luck of the father diminishes.
14. If the ascendant is Sagittarius then the natives fortunes rise on account of his father or the father's fortune will be on account of the Son. Even if Sun is posited in Libra this Yoga will take effect.
15. (i) If Sun and the Lord of 9th house and the Lord of the 12th house the three of them are posited in the 12th house or
    (ii) Jupiter and the Lord of the 12th are posited in the 12th house then also the native's father's luck will shine.
16. If Venus is in the 12th house then wife brings luck or on account of wife the native's fortune will shine.
17. Moon in the 12th house gives betterment and fortunate time due to mother.
18. Mars in the 12th house gives good luck and rise of fortunes on account of brothers or native is fortunate in the context of brothers.
19. If the Lord of the 9th house is in the 12th house, then the fortunes of father will improve or the native's own fortunes will rise due to the father.
20. If the Lord of the 9th house is in the 7th house and the Lord of the 7th is in the 9th then there will be fortunes on account of wife.
21. If the Lord of the 2nd house and Mercury are posited in the 6th house, then acquisition of wealth will be on account of relatives *i.e.* from cousins etc.
22. Even if Mercury is posited all alone in the 6th house then also the above mentioned effects take place.
23. If the Lord of the 5th house and Jupiter, both of them are in their sign of exaltation then the native's children will be fortunate in life.

RAJ YOGTARANG- RAJ YOGAS

We give below certain Raj Yoga.

1. If (i) the small Lord of the 2nd house is in the 2nd house and Lord of the 5th house is in the 5th house or

(ii) The Lord of the 2nd house, is in the 9th house and the Lord of the 5th is in the 10th, then it is a Raj Yoga.

2. If the Lords of the 2nd and 11th house are posited together in the 10th house and are devoid of any negative factors, then during their dashas Raj Yoga takes place.

   Negative factors or Dosh are of two types.

   (a) One is relationship with the Lord of the 6th, 8th and 12th houses, the Lords of Dusthana.

   (b) Secondly if posited in a debilitation sign or in the sign owned by an enemy or being combust.

3. If Rahu is posited in the 4th, 5th, 10th or 11th house, then in its own Dasha and Antardasha *i.e.* in the major and minor period confers Rajyoga.

4. If Ketu is in the 3rd house then defiantly it gives a Yoga.

5. Ketu if posited in the 5th and 9th house then it is not a benefic placement. This is endowed with negative effects.

6. If Moon and Venus are posited together in the third then Venus shows defiantly Yoga effect and particularly in the periods of Venus special benefic results will ensue.

7. If the Lord of the 3rd house is posited in the 3rd or 11th house then there will be no Raj Yoga throughout life and if at any time there is a Raj Yog then it does not show good effect. However with our experience we found that the Lord of the 10th house was posited in the 3rd which was Mars in the Horoscope of Pt. Jawahar Lal Nehru who was the first Prime Minister of India and this law was not applicable.

8. If the Lord of the 9th house is posited in the 8th house then during its Dasha the Yoga does not take place.

9. If the Lord of the 9th house is Jupiter and if it is the 8th house then there is fortunate time during the dasha of Jupiter.

10. If there is a relationship between the Lords of the 8th and 9th houses then there is Yoga in the periodic influence of the Lord of the 8th house. Relationship are of four types, the placement of two planets together in one house, aspecting each other with

full aspect etc. These have been mentioned at other places.

11. If there is a relationship between the Lord of 8th and the Lord of the 9th house then there is no Yoga in the major period of the Lord of the 9th house, but in the minor period of the Lord of the 8th there is a Yoga.
12. If there is a relationship between the Lord of the 10th and 11th houses then in the period of the Lord of 11th there will be a Raj Yoga.
13. If the Lord of the 10th and 11th are related then in the period of the Lord of the 10th only ordinary conditions will prevail *i.e.* neither very good nor very bad.
14. If Venus is posited in the 10th house then during its period there is no Yoga.
15. If Saturn is in the 7th house then in its period there is a Raj Yoga.
16. If Rahu is in the 7th house then its period definitely gives a Yoga.
17. If Saturn is in the 3rd or the 9th house then it does give a Yoga.
18. If Jupiter is in the 3rd, 8th or 9th house then it gives a Yoga.
19. If Jupiter is posited in the 12th house then the native after death *i.e.* after life attains Heaven.
20. If the Lord of the house of fortunes *i.e.* 9th and the Lord of Karma *i.e.* 10th are posited in the 9th or 10th house then it is an excellent Raj Yoga and results in much fame.
21. If the Lord of the 9th is posited in 10th house and the Lord of the 10th house occupies the 9th house then the same results which has been mentioned in 20 above will take place.
22. If the Lord of 10th house is posited in the 10th and the Lord of the 9th is in 9th then also the same effects which has been mentioned in 20 above take place.
23. If Lord of 10th and 5th houses are together or separately are in 10th or 5th house then it is a Raj Yog and the natives attains fame.
24. If the Lord of 9th and 10th houses are in the 7th and 1st house then it is a Raj Yog and fame comes.

25. If the Lords of 5th, 7th and 10th houses are in angles or trine then the native enjoys Raj Yoga and attains fame.

MAHADASHA PHAL TARANG (EFFECT OF MAHADASHA WAVES)

Now we give some Yogas related to the major periods of planets.

1. In the major period of Venus and the minor period of Saturn or in the major period of Saturn and the minor period of Venus the native is devoid of Yoga *i.e.* this minor period is full of sufferings.
2. Those persons who are born with Sagittarius or Pisces ascendant, in their life the minor period of Venus in the major period of Saturn, shows good effect and in the minor period of Saturn in major period of Venus also good result will ensue.
3. If the Lord of the 8th house is in the 6th, 8th or 12th house then in its major period the minor period of the Lords of 6th, 8th or 12th houses will give ' Marak' results, Maarkesh *i.e.* this will be fatal.
4. If the Lords of the 3rd and 10th houses are related then in the period of the Lord of the 10th there is no Yoga but is Avayoga *i.e.* negative things happen. However in the period of the Lord of the 3rd house it is an excellent Yoga when benefic result come.
5. If (i) any planet is in the 1st and the 7th house or (ii) the Lord of the 9th is in 7th then the native earns wealth due to his own efforts.
6. If the major period of Rahu is running then in the minor periods of Rahu, Ketu, Saturn or Sun the death of father can take place.
7. If the major period is that of Ketu then in the minor period of Mars, Saturn, Sun or Rahu death of father can take place.
8. If the major period is that of Mars then the minor period of Rahu, Ketu or Saturn can cause death of father.
9. In the major period of Saturn the minor period of Rahu, Sun, Ketu or Mars can caused death of father.
10. During the ending of the major period of Mars and the beginning

of the major period of Rahu death of father can take place i.e. one dasha is about to be completed and the next dasha is about to commence.

11. If the major period is of a malefic then the minor period of Rahu in that major period, can cause the death of father.
12. If both Jupiter and Venus are in Scorpio then in the major period of Venus there will be Raja Yoga. There is no doubt about this.
13. If Sun and Mercury are together in a house or Sun is Virgo, Mercury is in Leo, then the Mahadasha *i.e.* the major period of the Mercury is very strong and beneficial and the period of Sun is of medium intensity.
14. If Moon and Mars are related then the major period of Moon gives many Yogas and the period of Mars is medium.
15. If Jupiter and Saturn are related then the period of Saturn gives many Yogas and the period of Jupiter is medium.
16. If Mars and Jupiter are related then the period of Mars is excellent and the period of Jupiter is medium.
17. If Moon and Jupiter are related then the period of Moon gives extra ordinary Yogas but the period of Jupiter is medium.
18. If Rahu is in an angle or a trine then in itself it is a Raj Yog, the natives attains big fame.
19. If Mercury, Jupiter and Venus are related then it is a special Yoga for wealth. The native is fortunate and well known.
20. If Venus is related to Mercury or Jupiter then in the period of Venus wealth is gained. In the major period of Jupiter the native becomes poor and the periodic influence of Mercury gives mixed results *i.e.* at times wealth and at other times loss of wealth.
21. If Sun is with any planet then in the period of Sun wealth is gained but in the period of the other planets which are with Sun the results are medium.
22. In case of Rahu if it is related with many planets then Rahu will give the effect of the strongest planet.
23. If Rahu, Sun and Saturn are together in the 3rd house then in the major or minor period of Rahu the natives fortunate times commences and his valour increases.

24. If Mercury is in the 3rd house then in the Mahadasha of Rahu the native loses his patience. He becomes confused, depressed and fearful.

GRAH SAMANYA YOG TARANG (GENERAL PLANETARY CONFIGURATIONS)

1. If the Lord of any house conjoins with the significator of that house then the efficacy of the house increases many folds *i.e.* the house becomes strong. Which planet is the significator of which house has been mentioned in Chapter—15, Sloka No. 17.

   Example— If the Lord of the 5th house is placed with Jupiter or Lord of the 7th house is with Venus, then the 5th house or the 7th house, they are endowed with strength.

2. It is not good if a planet is the Lord of the 3rd house, 8th house or 11th house. But if a planet is the Lord of the 9th or the Lord of the 5th house then becomes benefic.

3. If Jupiter is the Lord of the 3rd, 6th or 8th house then it takes in negatives qualities. However even with the lordship of the 8th house, it is capable of giving Yoga.

4. If Venus is in the 6th house then it gives Yoga and same effect Venus shows in the 12th house.

5. If Rahu is in the 4th, 5th, 10th or 11th house then gives Yoga. This is the opinion of Astrologers of the highest category.

6. If benefic are the owners of the angles then they do not confirm Yogas. If malefic own the angles and are posited in them then they give Yogas.

7. If Saturn is posited in a house or aspect a house then the efficacy of the house is reduced. But if Saturn aspects the 3rd or the 9th house then the house gains in strength.

8. If a weak (waning) Moon is in the 1st house then the native has a low I.Q. and he is brought up by other people. If the full Moon is in the 1st house then the native is endowed with good traits and is fortunate.

9. If Moon and Mars are in the ascendant or Moon and Mars are in the 8th house, then the native is fortunate.

10. Mars if posited with the Lord of the 4th house then definitely it indicates immovable properties (agricultural lands, houses etc.).
11. If the Lord of the 4th house is with Jupiter and is posited in the 4th house then the native becomes the owner of cattles.
12. The house or the Lord of a house or the significator of a house if it is hemmed in between malefic then that house, the Lord or the significator causes sorrows and sufferings.
13. If the Lord of the 11th and 12th houses are related then it causes Yoga.
14. If the Lord of the 11th house is in the 3rd house or 12th house then these are Yoga giving placements.
15. In any ascendant if the Lord of the 9th house is in the 8th house then there is no Yoga. The native lives in ordinary circumstances.
16. If Moon is in the 6th house then the native is intelligent. If Moon is in the 2nd house then his eyes are expressive.

GRAHA MAALIKA YOG (NECKLACE OF PLANETS)

1. If the nine planets are in the nine houses starting from ascendant to the ninth, only one planet in one house then it called 'Maalika Yoga'. The Yoga of Necklace.
2. If all the planets are from the ascendant to the 6th house then this is called 'Sashtakhet' Maalika Yoga.
3. If all the seven houses from ascendant to the 7th contain all the seven planet *i.e.* no house should be empty then it is called Maalika Yoga.
4. If all the planets are in between the ascendant and the 8th house and every house has a planet, then it is called 'Ashta Khechar Malayoga'.
5. Many Astrologers are of the opinion that begining from Sun, Maalika Yog takes place. Other Astrologer are of the opinion that it is the ascendant from where Maalika Yog commences.
6. If all the planets are in the 6th, 7th, 8th and 9th houses then it is a fortune giving Yoga.

7. If all the planets are in the five houses beginning from the ascendant to the 5th and no house should be empty then this is a Bhagya Yoga.

THE ORDER IN WHICH THE OWNERS OF TWO HOUSES SHOW THEIR EFFECTS

1. The planets which are posited in even signs they first show the results of their Mool Tirikona Sign in the beginning and then the effect of the 2nd sign that they own.

   For example— If Saturn is posited in an even sign like— Taurus, Cancer, Virgo, Scorpio, Capricorn or Pisces then in its major or minor period it will show the effect of its Moola Trikon Sign which is Acquarius in the 1st half of its major and minor periods. In the 2nd half it will show the effect of the second sign which is Capricorn.

   The major and minor period is divided in two sections.

   For example— If a native has Gemini as the ascendant then Saturn is the ruler of the 8th and 9th houses. The 8th house is Capricorn, the 9th house is Aquarius and suppose Saturn is in the sign Virgo see the horoscope of Seth Ram Krishna Dalmiya on the next page Date of Birth 7th April, 1893. Saturn in Virgo is in an even sign so in the period of Saturn it will show.

*'Maalika Yoga' is an Excellent Yoga.

Horoscope (7th April 1893)

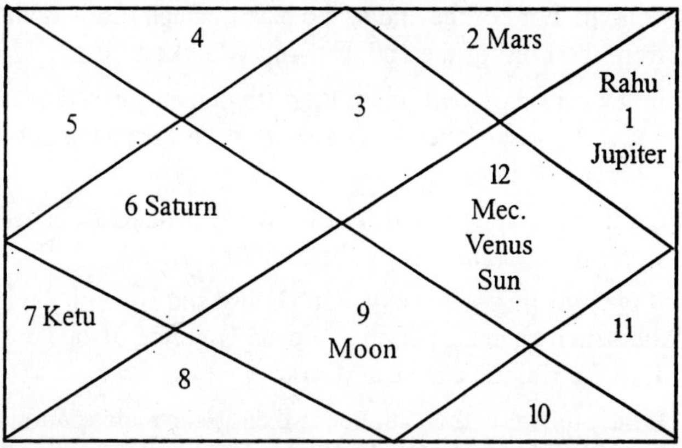

The result of its Moola Trikona Sign which is Acquarius in the 1st half and in the 2nd half it will show the effect of the ownership of Capricorn.

2. If a planet is in an odd sign then it will show the effect of the Moola Trikona Sign in the 2nd half and the effect of the ownership of the other sign in the 1st half.

   For example— In the example Horoscope given over here, Jupiter is in Aries, Aries is an odd sign so, the ownership of the Moola Trikona Sign which is Sagittarius will be felt in the 2nd half and in the 1st half the ownership of the sign Pisces will be felt. Mars, Mercury, Venus, Jupiter and Saturn all five of them own two signs each but in order to explain in a proper manner one sign is called the Moola Trikona Sign and other sign is its own sign. The Horoscope is given with Gemini rising, Saturn is in the 4th house, Ketu in the 5th , Moon is in the 7th, Sun, Venus, Mercury are in Pisces, Jupiter and Rahu are in Aries in the 11th, Mars is in the 12th house.

MARAK TARANG (THE FATAL PLANETS IN A HOROSCOPE)

1. In the periodic influence of the Lord of the 12th house the Lord of the 2nd is a Markesh. In the period of the Lord of the 2nd, the Lord of the 12th can be a Markesh.

2. In the period of the Lord of 12th the planet which is posited with the Lord of the 2nd or the planet which receives an aspect from the Lord of the 2nd, can be a Maarkesh.
3. In the period of the Lord of the 12th planets posited in the 12th house or those planet which receive aspect from the Lord of the 12th can be fatal.
4. In the major period of the Lord of the 12th malefic posited in the 12th house can be fatal in their minor periods.
5. If malefic are posited in the 2nd house and are with the Lord of the 12th then in the period of the major period of the Lord of the 12th the malefic can be a Maarkesh.
6. If malefic are in the 12th house then in the major period of that malefic, other malefic which are related to the Lord of the 2nd can be Maarkesh.
7. In the major dasha of the Lord of the 8th house its own minor period can be fatal.
8. In the major period of the Lord of the 8th a malefic if posited in the 6th house can be Maarkesh in its minor period.
9. In the major period the Lord of the 6th the minor period of the planet situated in the 8th house can be a Maarkesh.
10. In the major period of the Lord of the 8th the planet which receives an aspect from the Lord of the 8th can be a Maarkesh in its minor period.
11. In the major period of the Lord of the 8th the planets which are posited with the Lord of 6th can cause death in their minor period.
12. If malefic are posited in the 8th house then the minor period of the Lord of the 6th can be a Maarkesh.
13. In the major period of the Lord of the 6th house the minor period of the Lord of the 8th can be a Maarkesh.
14. If malefic are posited in the 6th house then in its major period the minor period of the planet posited in the 8th house can be a 'Marak'.
15. In the major period of the Lord of 6th the minor period of the Lord of 8th can be fatal.

16. If malefic are situated in the 8th house then during its major period the minor period of planets which are posited in the 6th house can be fatal.

    These principles which have been enunciated due to the Lordships of the 6th, 8th or 12th houses or the planets posited in the 6th, 8th and 12th houses these can be easily understood in the following manners.

    1. In order to decide the planets which are Marak and whose major and minor period can be fatal the above conditions which has been enunciated can be expressed in the following manner.

       (1) During the major period of the Lord of the 8th house.

       (A) The minor period of the Lord of the 8th house.

       (B) The minor period of the planet posited in the 6th house.

       (C) The planet which conjoins with the Lord of the 6th house.

       (D) The planet which receives an aspect of the Lord of 8th house.

    2. The planets posited in the 8th house and if they are malefic then during their major period—

       (A) The minor period of the Lord of the 6th house.

       (B) The planet posited in the 6th house and if it is malefic then its minor period can be fatal.

    3. In the major period the Lord of the 6th house—

       (A) The minor period of the Lord of the 8th house.

       (B) The planet posited in the 8th house its minor period.

    4. A malefic if posited in the 6th house then during its major period—

       (A) The Antardasha of the Lord of the 8th house. Even if the Lord of 8th is in the 8th house even then its minor period.

    5. In the major period of the Lord of the 12th house.

       (A) The minor period of the Lord of the 2nd house.

(B) The planet which is posited with the Lord of the 2nd house its minor period.

(C) The minor period of the planet which receives an aspect from the Lord of the 2nd.

(D) The malefic situated in the 12th house its minor period.

(E) The malefic which is posited with the Lord of the 12th house in the 2nd house its minor period.

6. If malefic are in the 12th house then during their major period.

(A) The malefic which are related to the Lord of the 2nd house their minor periods.

7. In the major period the Lord of the 2nd house—

(A) The minor period of the Lord of the 12th house.

(B) The planet situated in the 12th house or the planet which are receiving an aspect from the Lord of the 12th, their minor period.

In order to decide which planet will be a Maarkesh or fatal there are other combinations which we state below:-

17. If Mercury and Venus are together in the 5th house then they could be fatal in the major period of one and the minor period of the other *i.e.* Mercury in Venus, and Venus in Mercury. Here due consideration should also be given to the Lordship of Mercury and Venus.

18. If Mars is the ruler of the Marak places *i.e.* the 2nd or the 7th or is the ruler of the negative houses (in the original Sloka it is written that if Mars has malefic Lordship) then the period of Mars is fatal.

19. Even if Saturn is the ruler of good houses but if it is placed with fatal planet then it a strong Marak.

20. If Lord of the 8th house is in the 1st house then it is fatal during its major period.

21. If two or three sons of a person are undergoing the major period of Rahu, then the native dies.

Besides the above mentioned major and minor periods of planets, it should also be considered whether the person is endowed with long life, medium life or short life, and only then due waitage should be given to the periodical influences. Otherwise the major and minor periods of the planets posited in the 6th, 8th and 12th or the Lords of these houses will always be present at times. Death does not takes place. At times wealth is reduced or the native suffers during these periods from disease and enemies. The writer Sh. Ramanuj indicates that the purpose of mentioning that the 6th, 8th and 12th houses are dusthana and the Lords of these houses or the planets posited in these houses are capable of giving sufferings. According to 'Jatak Chandrika' a well known treatise on Astrology, the following planets are endowed with fatal qualities:

1. The Lord of the 2nd house.
2. The malefic posited in the 2nd house.
3. The Lord of 7th house.
4. Malefic posited in the 7th house.
5. The malefic which are posited with the Lord of the 2nd house.
6. The malefic posited with the Lord of the 7th house.
7. Lord of the 8th house.
8. The lord of 3rd or 8th house if posited with the Lord of the 2nd or the Lord of the 7th house.
9. Saturn if posited with a Markesh.
10. Lord of the 6th house.
11. The planet which is very weak in a horoscope.

The 2nd house is the house of mouth, 7th house is the house of private parts. It is a well known saying that the regularity of eating food. (That's the Mukh) and relationship with women if it is controlled, then the longevity will increase. The native will shorten his life, if he spoils his 2nd or 7th house by irregular actions.

Refers to the Rules mentioned in the predictive Astrology related to 'Bhavarth Ratnakar'. These are 225 principles and has been mentioned over here so that the readers benefit from them.

21

Pratyantar Dasha Phal (Sub Period in the Minor Period of Planets)

अपहारविभागलक्षणं तत्पंक्ति क्रमशः स्फुटं प्रवच्मि।
यदुदीरितमत्र तत्समस्तं कथयेत्स्वदशान्तरान्तरादौ ॥१॥

पाकेशाब्दहता दशेश्वरसमा नेत्राङ्कभक्ताः समाः
शिष्टा रूपहता नराङ्कविहृता मासा नगैर्वासराः।
छिद्रादिष्वपि चैवमेव कलयेत्पाकक्रमाच्चेद्देशा-
नाथाद्या पुनरन्तरान्तरदशास्तत्पाकनाथक्रमाः ॥२॥

In this Chapter we explain the method of minor and sub-period of planets. One major period of a planet consists of the minor periods of all the nine planets. For example, the major period of Sun is of the duration of six years and this six years of Sun will be divided into nine parts which will be the minor periods of Nine Planets. The first minor period belongs to the same planet, whose major period is divided.

For example— In the major period of Jupiter the order of the minor periods will be Jupiter, in the beginning, and then Saturn, Mercury, Ketu, Venus, Sun, Moon, Mars and Rahu. In the major period of the Venus the order of the minor periods will be Venus, Sun, Moon, Mars, Rahu, Jupiter, Saturn, Mercury and Ketu.

In one Mahadasha there are nine minor dashas. Similarly in one minor dashas, there are nine sub-periods. (pratyantar dasha).

The first sub-period will be of the same planet whose minor period is running. The order of the planetary cycles in the sub-periods will be the same as has been mentioned for the major and minor periods. The duration of the minor period in the major period of any planet should be calculated by the rule of three. (by proportion).

For example— If we have to calculate the minor period of Sun in the major period of Venus then we follow the method given below-

In 120 years the period of Sun is	6 years
In 1 year the period of Sun is	6/120
In 20 years the period of Sun is	6/120 × 20 = 1 year.

The period of Sun is 6 years and the full period of Venus is 20 years. So the number—20 and 6 has been taken above. The method which is used to calculate the minor period in the major period of a planet, the same method is used to calculate the sub-period in the minor period of any planet. We have mentioned that the minor period of Sun is 1 year in the major period of Venus.

Now in the minor period of Sun what will be the sub-period of Sun itself. In 120 years it is 6/120= 1/20 and in 360 days it give us 1/20 × 360 = 18 days. So in the major period of Venus the minor period of Sun is 1 year and the sub-period comes to only 18 days. The tables of major periods, minor periods and sub-periods of planets are given in the ephemeris, so it has not been reproduced over here.

महीश्वरादुपलभतेऽधिकं यशो
वनाचलस्थलवसतिं धनागमम्।
ज्वरोष्णरुग्जनकवियोगजं भयं
निजां दशां प्रविशति तीक्ष्णदीधितौ ॥३॥

रिपुक्ष्योऽ व्यसनशमो धनागमः
कृषिक्रिया गृहकरणं सुहृद्युतिः।
क्षयानलप्रतिहतिर्कदायकं
शशी यदा हरति जलोद्भवा रुजः ॥४॥

रुजागमः पदविरहोऽरिपीडनं
व्रणोद्भवः स्वकुलजनैर्विरोधिता।

महीभृतो भवति भयं धनच्युति-
    र्यदा कुजो हरति तदाऽर्कवत्सरम् ॥५॥

रिपूदयो धनहृतिरापदुद्गमो
    विषाद्भयं विषयविमूढता पुनः।
शिरोदृशोरधिकरुगेव देहिनाम्
    अहौ अवेदहिमकरायुरन्तरे ॥६॥

रिपुक्ष्यो विविधधनाप्तिरन्वहं
    सुरार्चनं द्विजगुरुबन्धुपूजनम्।
श्रवःश्रमो भवति च यक्ष्मरोगिता
    सुरार्चिते प्रविशति गोपतेर्दशाम् ॥७॥

धनाहतिः सुतविरहः स्त्रिया रुजो
    गुरुव्यः सपदि परिच्छदच्युतिः।
मलिष्ठता भवति कफप्रपीडनं
    शनैश्चरे सवितृदशान्तरं गते ॥८॥

विचर्चिका पिटकसकुष्ठकामिला
    विशर्धनं जठरकटिप्रपीडनम्।
महीक्षयः त्रिगदभयं भवेत्तदा
    विधोः सुते चरति रवेरथाब्दकम् ॥९॥

सुहृव्द्ययः स्वजनकुटुम्बविग्रहो
    रिपोर्भयं धनहरणं पदच्युतिः।
गुरोर्गदश्चरणशिरोरुगुच्चकैः
    शिखी यदा विशति दशां विवश्वतः ॥१०॥

शिरोरुजा जठरगुदार्तिपीडनं
कृषिक्रिया गृहधनधान्यविच्युतिः ।
सुतस्त्रियोरसुखमतीव देहिनां
भृगोः सुते चरति रवेरथाब्दकम् ॥११॥

Minor Periods in the Major Period of Sun

The minor periods in the major period of Sun are given below:

1. During the minor period of Sun in its major period, one gets more fame than a king, acquisition of wealth, likely to live in forest and hills, fever and disease related to Pitta in the body, separation from father. If Sun is good then good result should be understood. If Sun is weak or posited in the dusthana then ill-effects should be predicted.

2. *Moon*

When the minor period Moon runs in the major period of Sun, then the native overcomes and annihiliates his enemies, his sufferings, subside; gain of wealth, work related to agriculture, construction of house, meeting with friends. If Moon is in dusthana *i.e.* in the 6th, 8th or 12th then the results are negative and the native suffers from T.B. or disease connected with water as well as danger and loss from fire.

3. *Mars*

When the minor period of Mars is in the major period of Sun, then the native falls sick, has a downfall in his status or loses his job, and troubles from enemies. He will be opposed by his own family people. The native has fear from the ruler and loses wealth. The native thinks that he has danger of getting wounds and boils. Our opinion is that if both the Sun and Mars are well placed and are in good signs related to each other then the minor period of Mars is good.

4. *Rahu*

In the minor period of Rahu in the major period of Sun the

enemies rise, enmity increases, loss of wealth and loss due to theft; Calamities come, the native suffers from poison, the native has problem in the head, eye disease but his emotions and desires to enjoy the luxuries of life is very intense.

5. *Jupiter*

During the minor period of Jupiter in the major period of Sun, the enemies are destroyed. Money comes in various ways, everyday worship of Gods, Brahmins, Gurus and relatives are honoured and respected. But one may suffer from pains in the ears or disease related to T.B. Our opinion is that the negative effect in the minor period of Jupiter will be when Jupiter is a strong Markesh and is posited in the dusthana.

6. *Saturn*

The minor period of Saturn in the major period of Sun, then loss of wealth, separation from son; the wife suffers from disease, some elderly person like- Guru, father, uncle may die. Expenses increases much. The loss of clothes and other things in the house, dirtiness prevails (house, clothes, body are not clean) and the native suffers from phlegm and disease.

Disease related to phlegm. Although in the above Slokas the disease related to phlegm has been mentioned, yet Sun being the ruler of the biles and Saturn of vata so during the period of Saturn there will be disease connected or on account of excess of Vata and Pitta.

7. *Mercury*

In the minor period of Mercury and the major period of Sun, there is a possibility of Jaundice, Boils, Skin disease, Leprosy etc. Pain in stomach, waist, backache and due to disorder of the vata, pitta and cough, various disease occur. Mercury is the ruler of all the three doshas, vata, pitta and cough so imbalance may cause disease. Therefore disease related to two or three, has been mentioned.

8. Ketu

When there is the minor period of Ketu in the major period of Sun, then loss of a friend or the death of a friend should be interpreted. There is opposition from own people and family members. Danger from enemies, loss of wealth due to theft or in other manner. Sickness to elderly people in the family. The native's feet and head may have lot of pains, headache. Sun and Ketu are mutual enemies. Therefore the minor period of Ketu in the major period of Sun, creates lot of negative and ill effects.

9. Venus

When the minor period of Venus comes in the major period of Sun, then headache or pain in stomach, disease connected with stomach, private parts, loss in agriculture, houses, loss and reduction in the quantity of grains and wealth, children falls sick, and disease comes to wife as well.

Different Minor Periods in the Major Period of Moon

स्त्रीप्रजाप्तिरमलांशुकागमो
भूसुरोत्तमसमागमो भवेत्।
मातुरिष्टफलमङ्गनासुखं
स्वां दशां विशति शीतदीधितौ ॥१२ ॥

पित्तवह्निरुधिरोद्भवा रुजः
क्लेशदुःखरिपुचोरपीडनम्।
वित्तमानविहतिर्भवेत्कुजे
शीतदीधितिदशान्तरं गते ॥१३ ॥

---

*The ill effect which has been described in the Sloka from 5 to 11 will take place only when the lord of the major period or the lord of the minor period, or the lord of the minor period and the lord of the sub-period are both malefic or are badly posited.

तीव्रदोषरिपुवृद्धिबन्धुरुङ् मारुताशनिभयार्तिरुद्भवेत्।
अन्नपानजनितज्वरोदयाश्चन्द्रवत्सरविहारके ह्यहौ ॥१४॥

दानधर्मनिरतिः सुखोदयो वस्त्रभूषणसुहृत्समागमः।
राजसत्कृतिरतीव जायते कैरवप्रियवयोहरे गुरौ ॥१५॥

नैकरोगविहतिः सुहृत्सुत-
स्त्रीरुजा व्यसनसंभवो महान्।
प्राणहानिरथवा भवेच्छनौ
मारबन्धुवयसो गतेऽन्तरम् ॥१६॥

सर्वदा धनगजाश्वगोकुल-
प्राप्तिराभरणसौख्यसम्पदः।
चित्तबोध इति जायते विधो-
रायुषि प्रविशति प्रबोधने ॥१७॥

चित्तहानिरपि सम्पदशच्युति-
र्बन्धुहानिरपि तोयजं भयम्।
दासभृत्यहतिरस्ति देहिनां
केतुके हरति चान्द्रमब्दकम् ॥१८॥

तोययानवसुभूषणाङ्गनाविक्रयक्रयकृषिक्रियादयः।
पुत्रमित्रपशुधान्यसंयुतिश्चन्द्रदायहरणोन्मुखे भृगौ ॥१९॥

राजमाननमतीव शूरता
रोगशान्तिररिपक्षविच्युतिः।
पित्तवातरुगिने गते तदा
स्याच्छशाङ्कपरिवत्सरान्तरम् ॥२०॥

1. When the minor period of Moon runs in the major period of Moon then there is a possibility of birth of a daughter. One receives white and bright clothes. Meeting with excellent and high class learned Brahmins. The mother is happy due to things going as per desires and the native has happiness from his own wife.

   *The effect of the minor period in the major period of planets has been given in this Chapter. In the same way the effects of the sub-periods in the minor periods should be understood.

2. When the minor period of Mars comes in the major period of Moon then there is disorder of the biles, danger of fire and due to impurity of blood various disease. Problems created by enemies and thieves; sufferings and sorrow; loss of prestige and wealth. (The body temperature is always more than normal changes in food habits and extra vitamins will help).

3. In the minor period of Rahu and the major period of Moon there is intense and sudden events which cause mental anguish *i.e.* certain events of so much intensity which cause mental and emotional disturbances, or possibility of physical sickness. Increase of enemies, relatives fall sick, danger of getting hurt from thunder storms and storms and lightenings and suffering. Due to disorder of the food habits or impure food, fever occurs and other physical ailments. (like typhoid, stomachache etc.)

4. When the minor period of Jupiter runs in the major period of Moon, then the native's desire is to give donations and to be very spiritual. He gains honour from the kings, visit from friends. Gain of new clothes and ornaments and beginning of happiness of all kinds.

5. During the minor period of Saturn in the major period of Moon, there are various disease, the native's friends, sons and wife has sickness. There is some big calamity and loss of life. The purpose of mentioning is that the minor period of Saturn in the major period of Moon is not good at all and causes all type of sufferings.

6. When the minor period of Mercury runs in the major period of Moon then there is acquisition of elephants, horses, cows and all type of wealth. Gain of ornaments and property. The native is

happy and his inner self is desirous of gaining knowledge, intellectual learnings and wisdom.

7. When there is the minor period of Ketu in the major period of Moon then certain events happen which cause uneasiness and tension to the native. Danger from water, loss of wealth and loss of relatives *i.e.* some relative suffers or difference of opinion with them. The native also suffers on account of slaves, servants and lower class of people. In short the period of Ketu in that of Moon, causes various problems.

8. During the period of Venus in that of Moon the results to be expected are good, happiness connected with shipping, vehicles, wealth, ornaments and all type of work related to water and women. The native also benefits from agriculture. If he is a business person then money comes in the trading. During this minor period realization of friends, animals, grains, sons and happiness from them.

9. When there is the minor period of Sun in the major period of Moon then honour from kings. The native does courageous work. If he has some type of disease then he overcomes disease and gets well *i.e.* the health is very good. However he may suffer from excess of biles and vata disorder, some type of new disease may take place but the native is victorious and his enemies are defeated.

पित्तोष्णरुग्व्रणभयं सहजैर्वियोग:
क्षेत्रप्रवादजनितार्थविभूतिसिद्धि: ।
ज्ञात्यग्निशत्रु नृपचोरजनैर्विरोधो
धात्रीसुतो हरति चेच्छरदं स्वकीयाम् ॥२१ ॥

शास्त्रग्निचोररिपुभूपभयं विषार्ति:
कुक्ष्यक्षिशीर्षजगदो गुरुबन्धुहानि: ।
प्राणव्ययोऽथ यदिवा विपुलापदो वा
वक्रायुरन्तरगते भुजगाधिनाथे ॥२२ ॥

द्विजविबुधसमर्चा तीर्थपुण्यानुसेवा
सततमतिथिपूजा पुत्रमित्रादिवृद्धिः ।
श्रवणरुगतिमात्रं श्लेष्मरोगोद्भवो वा
भवति कुजदशान्तः संगते वागधीशे ॥२३॥

उपर्युपरिविनाशः स्वात्मजस्त्रीगुरुणा-
मगणितविपदन्तर्दुःखमर्थोपहानिः ।
वसुहरणमरिभ्यो भीतिरुष्णनिलाग्नि-
र्भवति कुजादशायामर्कजे सम्प्रयाते ॥२४॥

अरिभयमुरुचोरोपद्रवोऽथार्थहानिः
पशुगजतुरगाणां विप्लवोऽमित्रयोगः ।
नृपकृतपरिपीडा शूद्रवैरोद्भवो वा
विशति शशितनूजे विश्वधात्रीसुतायुः ॥२५॥

अशनिभयमकस्मादग्निशस्त्रप्रपीडा
विगमनमथ देशाद्वित्तनाशोऽथवा स्यात् ।
अपगमनमसुभ्यो योषितो वा विनाशः ।
प्रविशति यदि केतुः क्रुरनेत्रायुरन्तम् ॥२६॥

युधि जनितविमानं विप्रवासः स्वदेशा-
द्वसुहृतिरपि चौरैर्वामनेत्रोपरोधः ।
परिजनपरिहानिर्जायते मानवाना-
मपहरति यदायुर्भौमिजं भार्गवेन्द्रः ॥२७॥

नृपकृतपरिपूजा युद्धलब्धप्रभावः
परिजनधनधान्यश्रीमदन्तःपुरं च ।
अतिविलासितवृत्तिः साहसादाप्तलक्ष्मी-
स्तिमिरभिदि कुजायुर्दायसंहारिणीति ॥२८॥

विविधधनसुताप्तिर्विप्रयोगोऽरिवर्गै-
र्वसनशयनभूषारत्नसम्पत्प्रसूतिः ।
भवति गुरुजनार्तिर्गुल्मपित्तप्रपीडा
धरणितनयवर्षे शीतगौ सम्प्रयाते ॥२९ ॥

1. During the minor period of Mars, in the major period of Mars comes then possibility of Pitta disorder, disease related to heat in the body like Sun stroke, fever etc. Danger of getting wounds and getting hurt, separation or loss of brothers, troubles caused by relatives and people of own community. Opposition from enemies, kings and thieves. There is danger of trouble and loss through fire. But the native will get money from agricultural lands, products and legal disputes. Our experience is that if Mars is Yoga Karak then during its dasha.it shows good results. If Mars is strong then inspite of enmity and opposition the natives is victorious. However if Mars is not strong then the native's enemy cause him losses and defeat and various other kinds of problems creep up.

2. The Rahu's minor period in the major period of Mars. Fear from weapons, fire, thieves, enemies, king. Due to poison, suffering and sickness; loss of an older person or relative. The native has disease connected with flanks, eyes and head. The native can die or he suffers from some type of calamity.

3. During the minor period of Jupiter in the major period of Mars.

   During this minor period the results are beneficial. The negative effect is that one may have pains in ears or due to disorder of the Phlegm disease occurs in the body. The other things are good in the sense that there is increase in the number of friends, birth of sons. The native is devoted to Gods and Brahmins and busy in worshiping them. All the time guests visit his house and he does good to them. He is busy in doing Punya Karmas and will travel to holy places.

4. The minor period of Saturn in the major period of Mars is a very difficult and stressful period. The native's children, sons, elderly people and respected person, they pass through difficulties one after the other. The native himself is surrounded by various

problems. The enemy take away his wealth. Danger from fire and wind - loss of property or due to the disorders of the biles and wind, physical disease comes. Loss of health, emotional distress and certain events happen to cause him unhappiness.

5. In the minor period of Mercury in the major period of Mars there is trouble from the governments or kings. Due to enmity with a person of low cast or community, sufferings come, fear from enemies, thieves cause problems and loss of wealth. There is loss of cattle, elephants and horses and fight with enemies. These days people do not keep cattles or elephants and horses the general meaning is that because in the original text these words are used and these day it could be interpreted as loss of vehicles, car, property *i.e.* negative results ensue.

6. In the minor period of Ketu in that of Mars, sudden thunder bolts, loss, fears, danger from fire and weapons, loss of ones own country. He may have to leave it due to problems. Loss of wealth or the native himself may die or his wife may die.

7. In the minor period of Venus and the major period of Mars, defeat in war or fight or legal matters. One may have to leave ones country or residence and one goes to a forgien country, trouble in the left eyes and the thieves take away his wealth, loss of servants *i.e.* either the natives suffers from the servants or the number of servants may be reduced due to financial stress.

8. In the minor period of Sun and the major period of Mars, the native is honoured by the king. The native's valour and fame increases due to victory in war. Increase of servants, wealth, gains, prosperity and increase in the number of women and he enjoys life— *i.e.* he will have a luxurious life and his prosperity will increase. The native earns wealth due to his courage.

9. In the minor period of Moon in the major period of Mars, wealth comes in different manners and from various sources. Birth of a son, gain of clothes, beds, ornaments, gems, and property. Separation from enemies *i.e.* the enemies will not be able to cause sufferings or loss. But possibility of death to some older person or the native himself may have tumours and certain disease related to disorder of pitta.

The Interpretation of Various Minor Periods in the Major period of Rahu

विषाम्बुरुग्दुष्टभुजङ्गदर्शनं
परावलासंयुतिरिष्टविच्युतिः।
अरिष्टवाग्दुष्टजनव्यथा
भवेद्विधुंतुदेनापहृते स्ववत्सरे ॥३०॥

सुखोपनीतिः सुरविप्रपूजनं
विरोगता वामदृशां समागमः।
सुपुण्यशास्त्रार्थविचारसम्भवः
सुरारिदायान्तरगे बृहस्पतौ ॥३१॥

समीरपित्तप्रगदक्षतिस्तनौ
तनूजयोषितसहजैश्च विग्रहः।
स्वभृत्यनाशश्च पदच्युतिर्भवेत्-
दितिप्रजायुः प्रविशत्यथार्कजे ॥३२॥

सुतस्वसिद्धिः सुहृदां समागमो
मनोविनिन्द्यत्वमतीव जायते।
पटुक्रियाभूषणकौशलादयो
भुजङ्गसंवत्सरहारिणीन्दुजे ॥३३॥

ज्वराग्निशस्त्रारिभयं शिरोरुजा
शरीरकम्पः स्वसुहृद्गुरुव्यथा।
विषव्रणार्तिः कलहः सुहृज्जनै-
रहीन्द्रदायान्तरगे शिखाधरे ॥३४॥

कलत्रलब्धिः शयनोपचारता
तुरङ्गमातङ्गमहीसमागमः ।
कफानिलाप्तिः स्वजनैर्विरोधिता
भवेद्भुजङ्गयुरपाहृतौ भृगोः ॥३५ ॥

अरिव्यथा स्यादतिपीडनं
दृशोर्विषाग्निशस्त्राहतिरापदुद्गमः ।
वधूसुतार्तिर्नृपतेर्महद्भयं
भुजङ्गवर्षे तितिरारिणा हृते ॥३६ ॥

वधूविनाशः कलहो मनोरुजा
कृषिक्रियावित्तपशुप्रजाक्षयः ।
सुहृद्विपत्तिः सलिलाद्भयं भवे-
द्वधौ दशाभक्तरि देवविद्विषः ॥३७ ॥

नृपाग्निचोरास्त्रभयं शरारिणां
शरीरनाशो यदि वा महारुजः ।
पदभ्रमो हृन्नयनप्रपीडनं
यदात्र सर्पायुषि संचरेत्कुजः ॥३८ ॥

1. During the minor period of Rahu in the major period of Rahu itself, disease due to poison and water. The native can get snake bite. He gets involved with others wife, loss of some one close to him. The native utters harsh speech and he suffers due to rogues.
2. The minor period of Jupiter in the major period of Rahu, gives happiness, worship of Gods and Brahmins; the health is good, no disease left in the body; the native comes in contact with women who have beautiful eyes, engaged in religious debates and thinking and analysing.
3. During the minor period of Saturn in the major period of Rahu,

quarrels with ones own wife, sons and brothers, the native is displaced and his servants are destroyed. He gets hurt physically and has disease related to imbalance of wind and biles.

4. In the minor period of Mercury and the major period of Rahu gain of wealth and sons, meeting with friends, happiness in the mind.*

   The native works with attention and cleverness, gains ornaments and learning and expertness. In short Mercury and Rahu are friend and in the period of Mercury expertness, cleverness etc. in trade and business is considered. Therefore in the minor period of Mercury which comes in the major period of Rahu, the native attains success in attributes which are indicated by Mercury. This period brings increase in the good qualities of Mercury.

5. In the minor period of Ketu and the major period of Rahu, there is bad results. Fear of fevers, fire, weapons and enemies; disease in the head, tremblings in the body. The native suffers due to poison and wounds. Quarrels with friends and the native's friend and elderly people pass through anguish.

6. In the minor period of Venus and the major period of Rahu gain of women, company of women, attainment of elephants, horses and lands, or the native enjoys these. But there is opposition from own people and the native suffers from disease due to imbalance of wind and phlegm.

7. During the minor period of Sun in the major period of Rahu, trouble created by enemies. Many calamities, danger from poison and fire, injuries from weapons. The native suffers from disease related to eyes. The native has great fear from king and governments; His wife and sons also suffers and have sorrow. Rahu and Sun are enemies and during this period many negative things have been indicated.

8. In the minor period of Moon during in the majoir period of Rahu, loss of wife or death comes to her, quarrels with others,

---

*One Commentator has interpreted that the native will have cheap thoughts in the mind. But if we look to the other good factors mentioned in this minor period it does not match.

emotional distress, danger for own friends, fear from water and loss of agriculture, wealth, cattles and children.*

9. During the minor period of Mars in the major period of Rahu there is danger from kings, fires, thieves and arms or the native dies and suffers from mental problems. Disease and pains in eyes, heart problems and his status is lost *i.e.* loss of place or set back in position. Generally the minor period of Mars in Rahu does not show good effect.

Interpretation of the Minor Periods in the Major Period of Jupiter

सौभाग्यकान्तिबहुमानगुणोदयः
स्यात्सत्पुत्रसिद्धिरवनीपतिपूजनं च।
आचार्यसाधुजनसंयुंतिरिष्टसिद्धिः
सवत्सरं हरति देवगुरौ स्वकीयम्॥३९॥

वेश्याङ्गनामदकृदासवदोषसङ्ग
उत्कर्षसौख्यसकुटुम्बपशुप्रपीडा।
अर्थव्ययोरुभयमक्षिजरुक्सुतार्ति
जैवीं दशां विशति दैनकरे नराणाम्॥४०॥

स्त्रीद्यूतमद्यजमहाव्यसनं त्रिदोषैः
केचिद्वदन्त्यपि च केवलमङ्गलाप्तिः।
देवद्विजार्चनसुतार्थसुखप्रयोगै-
र्गीर्वाणपूजितदशां हरतीन्दुसूनौ॥४१॥

*When the lord of the minor period and the lord of the major period are posited in the 6th, 8th from each other or lord of the minor period is in the 12th from the lord of the major period, then generally ill effect comes. If any planet is posited in a dusthan then also it causes troubles. If the lord of one of the major or minor period own an angle and the other one a trine and they are not related then the minor period of one in the major period of the other will be bad.

शस्त्रव्रणं भवति भृत्यजनैर्विरोध-
श्चित्तव्यथा तनययोषिदुपद्रवश्च।
प्राणच्युतिर्गुरुसुहृज्जनविप्रयोगः
सौरेड्यमायुरपहृत्य ददाति केतुः ॥४२॥

नानाविधार्थपशुधान्यपरिच्छदस्त्री-
पुत्रान्नपानशयनाम्बरभूषणाप्तिः।
देवद्विजार्चनमुपासनतत्परत्व-
मायुर्यदा हरति जैवमथासुरेड्यः ॥४३॥

शत्रोर्जयः क्षितिपमाननकीर्तिलाभः
स्याच्चण्डता नरतुरङ्गमवाहनाप्तिः।
श्रेण्यग्रहारपुरराष्ट्रसमस्तसंपद
दुच्चैरुचथ्यसहजायुरपाहृतेऽर्के ॥४४॥

योषिद्बहुत्वमरनाशनमर्थलाभः
कृष्यर्थवस्तुपरमोन्नतकीर्तिलाभः।
देवद्विजार्चनपरत्वमतीव पुंसां
संजायते गुरुदशाहृति शर्वरीशे ॥४५॥

बन्धूपतोषणमरिव्रजतोऽर्थलाभः
सुक्षेत्रसत्कृतिरिह प्रथितप्रभावः।
ईषद्गुरूपहतिरीक्षणसुक्षतिर्वा
क्षित्यात्मजे हरति वत्सरमार्यजातम् ॥४६॥

बन्धूपतप्तिरुरुमानसरुग्गदार्ति-
श्चोराद्भयं गुरुगदो जठरोद्भवो वा।

राजेन्द्रपीडनमरिव्यसनं स्वनाशः ।
सम्पद्यते हरति सूरिदशां सुरारौ ॥४७ ॥

1. During the minor period of Jupiter in the major period of Jupiter itself, the results are increase of fortunes, luster increases, honour from all sides, birth of a son, the native's good qualities comes to be re-recognised and he is honoured in the court. He is the good company of teachers and good people. His desires are fulfilled.

2. The minor period of Saturn in the major period of Jupiter, company of prostitutes, increase in the habits of drinking, prosperity, happiness comes. But the native's family and cattles suffer. Heavy expenses; there is constant fear in the natives mind; eye sight problems and problem to sons.

3. The minor period of Mercury in the major period of Jupiter, there are two opinion about this.
   (i) opinion is that the minor period of Mercury shows ill effects— like company of women, excess drinking, bad habits and traits, gambling etc. He falls sick due to the imbalance of Vata, Pitta and Phlegm.
   (ii) the second opinion is that the minor period of Mercury in the major period of Jupiter shows good effect. The native is engaged in the worship of Gods and Brahmins. Gains of sons, wealth and happiness.

4. The minor period of Ketu in the major period of Jupiter causes injuries due to weapons. Opposition from servants, mental anguish. The native's wife and children suffer. Separation from elderly people and people dear to him and danger that the native himself might lose his life.

5. During the minor period of Venus in the major period of Jupiter, the native gains and acquires wealth, cattles, grains, clothes, wife, women, sons, food, liquids, (which are used for drinking), ornaments and happiness from these. He constantly worships Brahmins and Gods.

6. In the minor period of Sun during the major period of Jupiter, success over enemies, honour from the kings, increase of fame,

gains, the native gets horses and palanquin. The native's valour and courage increases. The native lives in a big city and enjoys his property and prosperity.

7. In the minor period of Moon during the major period of Jupiter, gain of many women, gain of wealth, worship of Gods and Brahmins. The native's fame increases, benefit from agriculture. Gains in buying and selling of goods and the enemies are destroyed.

8. In the minor period of Mars during the major period of Jupiter, the native's relatives are happy with the work of the native. The native gains from his enemies, realisation of high class lands. The native does good deeds and his influence increases. Some elderly person in the family is injured or he himself may have eye sight problems.

9. In the minor period of Rahu during the major period of Jupiter the relatives suffer and are unhappy or they cause sufferings to the native. The mind is worried due to problems and anguish, sickness and fear of thieves. Some respected person in the family is sick or the native himself suffers from stomach problems. Problems and suffering created by kings. The enemies cause problems, loss of wealth. Jupiter is the Guru of the Gods and Rahu is the enemy of Gods. Therefore Rahu in Jupiter shows ill effect.

Various Minor Periods in the Major Period of Saturn

कृषिवृद्धिभृत्यमहिषाभ्युदयः
पवनामयो वृषलजातिधनम् ।
स्थाविराङ्गनाप्तिरलसत्वमघो
निजवत्सरान्तरगते रविजे ॥४८ ॥

सुभगत्वमस्ति सुखिता वनिता
नृपलालनं विजयमित्रयुतिः ।
त्रिगदोद्भवः सहजपुत्ररुजा
शनिदायहारिणि शशङ्कसुते ॥४९ ॥

मरुदग्निपीडनमरव्यिसनं
सुतदारविग्रहमतिः सततम्॥
अशुभावलोकनमहेश्च भयं
मृदवत्सरं हरति केतुपतौ॥५०॥

सुहृदङ्गनातनयसौख्युतः
कृषितोययानजनितार्थचयः।
शुभकीर्तिरुद्भवति देहभृतां
यमदायहारिणि भृगोस्तनये॥५१॥

मरणं तु वा रिपुभयं सततं
गुरुवर्गरुग्जठरनेत्ररुजा।
धनधान्यविच्युतिरिह प्रभवेत्-
रविजायुराविशति तीव्रकरे॥५२॥

वनिताहतिर्मरणमेव नृणां
सुहृदां विपत्तिरथ रोगभयम्।
जलवातजं भयमतीव भवेत्-
रविजायुराविशति रात्रिकरे॥५३॥

स्वपदच्युतिः स्वजनविग्रहरुक्-
ज्वरवाह्नशस्त्रविषभीरथ वा।
अरिवृद्धिरान्तररुगक्षिभयं
रविजायुराविशति भूमिसुते॥५४॥

अपमार्गयानमसुभिर्विरहस्तु
अथ वा प्रमेहगुरुगुल्मभयम्।

ज्वररुक्क्षतिः सततमेव नृणा-
मसितान्तरं विशति भोगिपतौ ॥५५ ॥

अमरार्चनद्विजगणभिरुचि-
गृहपुत्रदारविहृतिस्तु भवेत्।
धनधान्यवृद्धिरधिका हि नृणां
गतवत्यथार्किवयसीन्द्रगुरौ ॥५६ ॥

1. The minor period of Saturn in the major period of Saturn itself gives increase in agriculture, increase in the number of servants and buffalo *i.e.* the native will keep more servants and more buffalo, suffer from vata roga, disease of the vata. Gain from someone who is of a low caste or low social background. Relationship with a women who is older; laziness and sins increase.
2. In the minor period of Mercury during the major period of Saturn, increase of fortunes, honour from governments and kings. Success, victory, friends cooperate and help in uplifting fortunes. Woman is gained and happiness comes. But the native is likely to suffer from the excess of vata, pita and cough either three or from one of them. There is sickness to the native's brothers, sisters and sons.
3. In the minor period of Ketu and the major period of Saturn, pains related to wind and fire or due to wind and heat in the body, sickness comes to the native. His enemies cause problems, constant quarrels with wife and sons. He has to see unhappy events and fear from the snakes.
4. In the minor period of Venus in the major period of Saturn, wealth is collected from work connected with agriculture and import-export; happiness from wife, sons and friends. In the original Sloka it is mentioned that goods which are brought from across the seas in ships, those goods give gains. During this minor period the fame increases.
5. In the minor period of Sun and the major period of Saturn, the native can die or has constant fear of enemies. Older and

respected people in the family have sickness. The native himself suffers from stomach problems and disease connected with eyes. Loss of wealth and grains.

6. In the minor period of Moon and the major period of Saturn, the native's wife or mother might die or he himself might die. His friends have various types of problems, danger from air and water, strong fears of disease.

7. In the minor period of Mars and the major period of Saturn, the native is displaced and has a fall in the status *i.e.* he might lose his job or the position he occupies. He will be removed from his position. He has fight with his own people or disease, fever, fire, weapons and poison cause danger. The enemies increase in numbers. He suffers from Hernia or eye sight problems.

8. During the minor period of Rahu and in the major period of Saturn, the native chooses a wrong path for himself *i.e.* does wrong things. There is danger to his life. He suffers from high temperature, spleen, injury etc. Saturn and Rahu are both malefic and so the minor period of one malefic in the major period of another malefic is bad.

9. The minor period of Jupiter in the major period of Saturn, this is a benefic minor period, the native is specially interested in the workshop of Brahmins and Gods. He enjoys life lives happily with his wife and sons in his own house. Much increase of wealth and grains.

Various Minor Periods in the Major Period of Mercury

धर्ममार्गनिरतिर्विपश्चितां
सङ्गमो विमलधीर्धनं द्विजात्।
विद्यया बहुयशः सुखं सदा
चन्द्रजे हरति वत्सरं स्वकम्॥५७॥

दुःखशोककलहाकुलात्मता
गात्रकम्पनममित्रसंयुतिः।

क्षेत्रयानवियुतिर्यदा भवेत्-
सोममसूनुशरदं गतः शिखी ॥५८॥

देवविप्रगुरुपूजनक्रिया दानधर्मपरतासमागमः।
वस्त्रभूषणसुहृद्युतिर्भवेद्बोधनायुषि समागते सिते ॥५९॥

हेमविद्रु मतुरङ्गवारणप्रावृतं भवनमन्नपानयुक्।
भूपतेरपि च पूजनं भवेद्भानुमालिनि बुधाब्दकं गते ॥६०॥

मस्तकव्यसनमक्षिपीडनं कुष्ठदद्रु बहुकण्ठपीडनम्।
प्राणसंशययुतिर्नृणां भवेज्ज्ञायुषं व्रजति शीतदीधितौ ॥६१॥

अग्निभतिरपि नेत्रजा रुजा
चोरजं भयमतीव दुःखिता।
स्थानहानिरथ वातरोगिता
ज्ञायुषं हरति मेदिनीसुते ॥६२॥

मानहानिरथवाश्रयच्युतिः
स्वक्षयोऽग्निविषतोयजं भयम्।
मस्तकाक्षिजठरप्रपीडनं
शीतरश्मिजदशां गतेऽसुरे ॥६३॥

व्याधिशत्रु भयविच्युतिर्भवे-
द्ब्रह्मसिद्धिरवनीशसत्कृतिः।
धर्मसिद्धितपसां समुद्गमो
देवमन्त्रिणि विदो दशां गते ॥६४॥

अर्थधर्मपरिलुप्तिरुच्चकैः
सर्वकार्यविफलत्वमङ्गिनाम्।

श्लेष्मवातजनिता रुगुद्भवे-
द्वोधनायुषि समागतेऽसिते ॥६५ ॥

1. The minor period of the Mercury in the major period of Mercury itself, the native is on the path of religion. He meets with learned people. His mind is pure and he gains wealth from Brahmins. Due to high education he attains fame and constant happiness.

2. The minor period of Ketu in the major period of Mercury causes tensions due to sorrows, sufferings and quarrels. The native's body trembles or he has some type of sickness like parkinson's disease. He has to face his enemies, and his vehicles and agriculture, products are destroyed.

3. During the minor period of Venus in the major period of Mercury, Gods, Brahmins and spiritual master are worshipped. The native is engaged in work of religion and gives donations. Gain of clothes and ornaments; meeting with friends.

4. The minor period of Sun in the major period of Mercury the native gains gold, corals, horses and elephants and big house. The native has happiness and gets good food and drinks. Honour from the king.

5. The minor period of Moon in the major period of Mercury gives pain in the heads and throat. The native suffers from eye disease, leprosy, itching etc. There is danger to life or possibility exists that he may die. Certain things happens to create danger of life. Our opinion is that if both Mercury and Moon are Markesh *i.e.* fatal, only then this negative result will happen otherwise not.

6. The minor period of Mars in the major period of Mercury, danger from fire, disease of the eyes, fear of thieves and the native is constantly unhappy. He has loss of place *i.e.* either he loses his house, loses his status, and suffers from disorder of vata. All these result will be when the minor period of Mars comes in the major period of Mercury.

7. The minor period of Rahu in the major period of Mercury, causes pains in stomach, eyes and head, loss of weight *i.e* due to disease the native's physical strength is reduced or the native's wealth

is lost. Danger from fire, poison and water. The native's prestige suffers or the status and position is lost.

8. The minor period of Jupiter in the major period of Mercury, the enemies are defeated. The native overcomes disease. Realisation of truth and spiritual life. Honour from the king, due to good deeds and hardwork. His interest in spirituality, increases.

9. The minor period of Saturn in the major period of Mercury, the native's religion and wealth is destroyed. He has failure in all works, suffers from vata and cough disorders.

Various Minor Periods in the Major Period of Ketu

रिपुजनकलहं सुहृद्विरोधं
त्वशुभवचः श्रवणं ज्वराङ्गदाहम्।
गमनपरधाम्नि वित्तनाशं
शिखिनि लभेत दशां गते स्वकीयम् ॥६६॥

द्विजवरकलहः स्त्रिया विरोधः
स्वकुलजनैरपि कन्यकाप्रसूतिः।
परिभवजननं परोपतापो
भवति सिते शिखिवत्सरान्तराले ॥६७॥

गुरुजनमरणं ज्वरावतारः
स्वजनविरोधविदेशयानलाभः।
नृपकृतकलहः कफानिलार्ति-
र्विशति रवौ शिखिवत्सरान्तरालम् ॥६८॥

सुलभबहुधनं तथैव हानिः
सुतविरहो बहुदुःखभाक्प्रसूतिः।
परिजनयुवतिप्रजाप्रलाभः
शशिनि यदा शिखिदायमभ्युपेते ॥६९॥

स्वकुलजकलहं स्वबन्धुनाशं
भयमपि पन्नगजं वदन्ति चोरात्।
हुतवहभयशत्रु पीडनं च
व्रजति कुजे ध्वजनामखेचरायुः ॥७०॥

अरिकृतकलहं नृपाग्निचौरै-
र्भयमपि पन्नगजं वदन्ति तज्ज्ञाः।
खलजनवचनं दुरिष्टचेष्टा
तमसि गतेऽत्र शिखीन्द्रदायमाहुः ॥७१॥

सुतवरजननं सुरेन्द्रपूजा
धरणिधनाप्तिरुपायनार्थसिद्धिः।
धनचयजननं महशमानो
भवति गतेऽत्र गुरौ शिखीन्द्रदायम् ॥७२॥

परिजनविहतिं परोपतापं
रिपुजनविग्रहमङ्गभङ्गतां च
धनपदवियुतिं तथाहुरार्या
गतवति सूर्यसुते शिखाधरायुः ॥७३॥

सुतवरजननं प्रभुप्रशस्तिः
क्षितिधनसिद्धिररीश्वरप्रपीडा।
पशुकृषिविहतिर्भवेत्तु पुंसां
विशति बुधे शिखिवत्सरान्तरालम् ॥७४॥

1. The minor period of Ketu in the major period of Ketu itself, quarrels with enemies, opposition from friends. The native has to listen to sarcastic and unhappy remarks. Fever in the body or in some part of body burning sensations. The native may have to live in others place and loss of wealth. We have found that

during the period of Ketu theft takes place and loss due to fire.

2. The minor period of Venus in the major period of Ketu, quarrels with a high class Brahmin; opposition from ones wife and family members but the native is blessed with a daughter. The native loses his prestige or he may have to bow down to others. He suffers on account of others.

3. During the minor period of Sun in the major period of Ketu, some respected 'Gurujan' viz., older person* in the family dies. Opposition from own people. Fevers and sufferings; Problems and quarrels with king and government. The native suffers from vata and cough disorders. But he gains wealth by travelling to foreign countries.

4. During the minor period of Moon in the major period of Ketu, sudden gain of big money and sudden losses of wealth as well. Separation from sons. A child is born in the house due to which lot of sufferings come. Sometimes we have seen a deformed child is born. However during this period support from servants and birth of a daughter is possible.

5. During the minor period of Mars in the major period of Ketu, the native has quarrels with elderly people in the family. His relatives are destroyed; danger from snakes, thieves and fire. Troubles caused by enemies.

6. The minor period of Rahu in the major period of Ketu quarrels due to enemies, troubles comes from kings, danger from fire and thieves. The native may have to listen to bad people and he himself is engaged in work which cause loss to others.

7. The minor period of Jupiter in the major period of Ketu birth of a good son who brings in fortunes. Worship of Gods, gain of wealth and property. Otherwise wealth comes from property. Income increases, presents from various places. Honour from

---

*In Sanskrit the word Gurujan i.e. older person does not mean only Guru or Acharya. But it also includes father, uncles, older brothers, maternal uncles, father's elder brother, mother's brother- in-law, ones own father-in-law or teachers. All these come under Gurujan. The mother, grandmother and grandfather should also be considered under Gurujan.

king or government. The minor period shows good results.

8. The minor period of Saturn in the major period of Ketu, loss of servants, troubles from others, quarrels with enemies. The native may lose some part of his body, loss of wealth, loss of house or job. This minor period is full of ill effects.

9. Minor period of Mercury in the major period of Ketu, gain of a good son. The native receives praise from his masters. Gain of wealth and property. But the native has trouble and is put under pressure by a strong enemy. Loss of cattles and agriculture. The effect of this minor period is mixed.

Various Minor Periods in the Major Periods of Venus

वसनभूषणवाहनचन्दना-
द्यनुभवः प्रमदासुखसंपदः ।
द्युतियुतिः क्षितिपाद्धनलब्धयो
भृगुसुते स्वदशां प्रविशत्यपि ॥७५ ॥

नयनकुक्षिकपोलगदोद्भवः
क्षितिभृतो भयमस्ति शरीरिणाम् ।
गुरुकुलोद्भवबान्धवपीडनं
भृगुसुतायुषि भानुमति स्थिते ॥७६ ॥

नखशिरोरदनक्षतिरुच्चिकैः
पवनपित्तरुगर्थविनाशनम् ।
ग्रहणिगुल्मकयक्ष्मकपीडनं
सितवयोहृति तत्र हिमत्विषि ॥७७ ॥

रुधिरपित्तदागर्तिसमाश्रयः
कनकताम्रचयावनिसंग्रहः ।
युवतिदूषणमुद्यमविच्युति-
र्वृषभवल्लभवत्सरगे कुजे ॥७८ ॥

निधिभवः सुतलब्धिरभीष्टवाक्
स्वजनपूजनमप्यरिबन्धनम्।
दहनचोरविषोद्भवपीडनं
तुलधरेश्वरवत्सगेऽसुरे॥७९॥

विविधधर्मसुरेशनमस्क्रिया
भवति चात्मजवामदृगागमः।
विविधराज्यसुखं च शरीरिणां
कविदशाहति कार्मुकनायके॥८०॥

नगरयोधनृपोद्भवपूजनं
प्रवरयोषिदवाप्तिरथास्ति वा।
विविधवित्तपरिच्छदसंयुति-
र्दितिपूजितदायगते शनौ॥८१॥

तनसौख्यसमागमसम्पदां
निचयलब्धिरतिप्रभुता यशः।
पवनपित्तकफार्तिररिच्युति
र्दनुजमन्त्रिदशाहति चन्द्रजे॥८२॥

सुतसुखादिबहिः स्थितिरनिग्जं
भयमतीव विनाशमङ्गरुक्।
अपि च वारवधूजनसंयुतिः
शिखिनि यात्यलमौशनसीं दशाम्॥८३॥

1. In the minor period of Venus and the major period of Venus itself, gain of clothes, ornaments, vehicles, sandal wood and other scented materials and goods. Enjoyment of women, happiness and property. The native's body is full of luster and gain of much wealth from the king.

2. The minor period of Sun in the major period of Venus, eyes, flanks, cheeks related sickness, fear from king *i.e.* some type of legal disputes and problems created by the ruler or on account of changes in the law. Some respected elder person and family members suffers relatives pass through bad time. The result of this minor period is not good.
3. In the minor period of Moon and the major period of Venus, there is danger of injuries to teeth, head and nails. There are disease related to vatta and pitta disorders. Loss of wealth, dysentery, T. B. or sufferings from Tumorous, Spleen enlargement.
4. The minor period of Mars in the major period of Venus, sickness due to blood disorders and access of biles, collection of gold, copper and lands. The native may leave the work. He is engaged in before this period ends. He has illicit connection with a young woman.
5. The minor period of Rahu in the major period of Venus, gain of wealth, birth of a son etc. benefic results follow. The native speak nicely and such word which are dear to others. His family people honour him. He is victorious over his enemies. Possibility is that his enemies may have go to prison. But the native himself suffers to some extent. There is danger from poison, fire and thieves.
6. During minor period of Jupiter in the major period of Venus, there are different types of religious activities, worship of Gods; Good relations with own wife and sons. Different and various types of happiness. Rise in status and more powers, the native gets happiness due to high status.
7. Minor period of Saturn in the major period of Venus, honour from government, from the army and general public. Gain of a good wife; wealth comes in various manners and the native receives luxurious goods and other items.
8. Minor period of Mercury in the major period of Venus, happiness from sons. Gain of prosperity wealth and property; gain of fame, authority and happiness. The native's enemies are defeated. But he himself might suffer from the disorder of vata, pitta and

cough from all the three doshas or from one of them. The health is a cause of concern.

9. The minor period of Ketu in the major period of Venus, danger from fire, some part of the body suffers. Wealth is destroyed, lack of happiness, company of prostitutes, separation from ones sons.

दशापहारेषु फलं यदुक्तं
वर्णाधिकारानुगुणं वदन्तु ।
छिद्रेषु सूक्ष्मेष्वपि तत्फलाप्तिः
छायाङ्कवार्ताश्रवणानि वा स्युः ॥८४॥

The results which have been described for the major and minor period of planets, should be interpreted after the native's conditions, caste, his status, what work he does and all these matters. In the above Slokas the results of only the major and minor periods have been explained. But the principles given when the major period is of a planet 'A' and the minor period of the planet 'B' should also be applied if the minor period is of 'A' and the sub period is of 'B'. Logic should be used when interpreting the sub-period and 'Sooksham' (very small) dashas.

Varamihir has written that the native gets the shadow of the planet on to him depending whose dasha he is running. By looking at that person it can be deducted as to planetary influence he is in. The Elements of Sun and Mars is fire. The element of Moon and Venus is water. The element of Mercury is earth and that of Jupiter is the Akash Tatwa *i.e.* the Ether and Vayu is the element of Saturn.

In the 2nd Chapter various attributes of planets have been given. The native receives the traits of the planets whose major and minor period he is passing through. His physical appearance and manner of speech also changes according to the planetary influence. The basic manners will be the same but the secondary manner will change.

The conclusion from all this is that it depends upon the major and minor period one is undergoing and what type of influence is on the native, and only after logically examining all the factors about the planet, about his status, his position conclusion should be drawn.

One whose horoscope does not exist or can not be found as his time of birth or date of birth was not recorded, then from the hue of his body, his shadow, his behaviour, his speech, his manner of acting, his efforts etc. should be taken into account and then conclusion should be drawn as to the planet whose major period or the planet whose minor period or the sub-period he is passing through. But one who has his accurate horoscope then no speculation is needed.

22

Mixed Periods

दस्रादितः पादवशेन मेषान्-
मीनांशकान्तं क्रमशोऽपसव्यम्।
कीटाद्धयान्तं गणयेच्च सव्य-
मार्गेण पादक्रमशोऽजतारात् ॥१ ॥

(i) Ashwini, Bharani, Krittika- the three constellations have 12 quarters (Charan viz pada).

(a) Aries, Taurus, Gemini, Cancer- the four navansha constitute the four quarters of Ashwini.

(b) Leo, Virgo, Libra, Scorpio- the four Navansha are in Bharani.

(c) Sagittarius, Capricorn, Aquarius, Pisces fall in Krittika, this way divide the three constellation into these 12 navanshas.

(ii) From Rohini the three constellations are Rohini, Mrigsiras, Ardra- these three have 12 navanshas. Counting them in the reverse order from Scorpio- *i.e.* Scorpio, Libra, Virgo, Leo, Cancer, Gemini, Taurus, Aries, Pisces, Aquarius, Capricorn, Sagittarius divide them in 12 navanshas. Rohini's first quarter will be Scorpio, second quarter will be Libra and so on. In this order Ardra's fourth quarter will be Sagittarius Navansha.

एवं भूयाच्चापसव्यं च सव्यं
भानि त्रीणि विद्यात्क्रमेण।
तद्राशीशप्रोक्तवर्षैर्दशास्य
देवं प्राहुः कालचक्रे महान्तः ॥२ ॥

In the manner mentioned above in (i) the order of counting is kept for the constellations of Punarvasu, Pusya, Aslesa and the order in (ii) should be adhered for Magha, Porvaphalguni, Uttaraphalguni, again the order of (i) is followed for Hasta, Chitra, Swati and (ii) is followed for Vishkha, Anuradha, Jyestha; the same order used in (i) is kept for Moola, Purvashada, Uttavashada and the order used in (ii) is followed for Shravana, Dhamishta and Shatbhisa and the same order used in (i) above be kept for Porvabhadrapada, Uttarabhadrapada and Revati.

The years of a sign is the same as the years of its lord. This has been given in the next Sloka.

मनुः परः सनिर्धनिर्नृपस्तपो वने क्रमात्।
दिवाकरादिवत्सराः शुभाशुभाप्तिहेतवः ॥३ ॥

Sun has 5 years (the sign of Sun is Leo- therefore the period of Leo is of 5 years.

Moon has 21 years (Cancer is ruled by Moon and so the period of Cancer will be of 21 years). The years of other planets, which are also of their signs, are given below:-

Mars,- Aries- Scorpio-	7 years for each
Mercury-Gemini-Virgo-	9 years for each
Jupiter-Sagittarius-Pisces-	10 years for each
Venus-Taurus-Libra-	16 years for each
Saturn-Capricorn-Aquarius-	4 years for each

The rule is to predict the effect of the periods of signs in Kalchakra Dasha is according to the (i) sign and (ii) its lord. Therefore in Kalachakra Dasha it is not said that the dasha is of Mars or Aries but that the Dasha (period) is of Aries-Mars. In the same manner of Scorpio-Mars.

The influence and effect of Mars will be the same in both its signs of Aries and Scorpio but suppose Mars is in Aries and Jupiter etc. benefic planets are also placed in Aries; and in Scorpio, Saturn, Rahu etc. malefic planets are position then the period of Aries-Mars will be good. But Scorpio-Mars will show ill effects.

दशापहारादिककालचक्रे
वाक्यानि दस्रादिपदादिजानि।
वक्ष्यामि वर्णैर्नभिर्भमानै
राशीशवर्षैः परमायुरत्र ॥४॥

Which periods come in what orders of the Kalachakra Dashas according to the quarter of the constellation of birth?

Depending upon the quarter of the birth star- the periods which have been given below- The total of these periods is the longevity of the native. The order of the signs are mentioned according to the Sanskrit alphabetical orders. In the ancient system of Sanskrit the numbers were coded into alphabets. This is called the order of the 'Katpayadi' *i.e.* 'a, b, c, d, etc. :

Table of Katpayadi*

1	क	Ka	1	ट	Ta
2	ख	Kha	2	ठ	Tha
3	ग	Ga	3	ड	Da
4	घ	Gha	4	ढ	Dha
5	ङ	Ng	5	ण	Na
6	च	Cha	6	त	Ta
7	छ	Chha	7	थ	Tha
8	ज	Ja	8	द	Da
9	झ	Jha	9	ध	Dha
10	ञ	Ny	10	न	Na
1	प	Pa	1	य	Ya
2	फ	Pha	2	र	Ra
3	ब	Ba	3	ल	La
4	भ	Bha	4	व	Va or Wa
5	म	Ma	5	श	Sha
6	ष	Sha	3+1	ज्ञ	Gya
7	स	Sa	(=4)	(ग+ज्ञ)	
8	ह	Ha			
11	क्ष	Ksha			
12	त्र	Tra			

The following are the 36 consonants. Those serially numbered 5 and 10 below are not used independently but are compounded with other consonants. Those serially numbered 34, 35 and 36 are syllables representing the combined sound of more than one letter, but have, for certain phonetic reasons, been included as consonants.

1	क	Ka	13	ड	Da	25	e	Ma
2	ख	Kha	14	ढ़	Dha	26	;	Ya
3	ग	Ga	15	ण	Na	27	j	Ra
4	घ	Gha	16	त	Ta	28	y	La
5	ङ	Ng	17	थ	Tha	29	o	Va or Wa
6	च	Cha	18	द	Da	30	"k	Sha
7	छ	Chha	19	ध	Dha	31	'k	Sha
8	ज	Ja	20	न	Na	32	1	Sa
9	झ	Jha	21	प	Pa	33	g	Ha
10	ञ	Ny	22	फ	Pha	34	{k	Ksha
11	ट	Ta	23	c	ब	35	=	Tra
12	ठ	Tha	24	Hk	भ	36	K	Gya

Note : ण is also written as .k

As some of the English letters are used to convey more than one sound, we are explaining the pronunciation indicated by the English letters used above.

1. k - sound of k as in keep, kite, kernel.
2. kha- this is the compound sound of k and h as in khan, khud etc.
3. g- as pronounced in get, go, give.
4. gha- this is the compound sound of gh. In English we write ghetto, ghost etc. but when pronouncing them we omit the sound of h, but in Hindi gha represents a sound in which the sound of g and h are combined as in Ghosh (a Bengali surname).

*In order to indicate the method of pronouncing we have added appendix-I here itself from our book 'Hindi- English Teacher (by Ashutosh Ojha)

5. ng- this has the faint sound of ng as in sing.
6. cha- as pronounced in chat, chair, chalk.
7. chha- this is the compound sound of ch and h. This is absent in English.
8. j- as in jug, jail, just.
9. jha- this is the compound sound of j and h as in Jha (a Bihari surname).
10. ny- this has the nasal sound of ny. This letter is never used independently.
11. t- this has the hard consonant sound of t as in tea, taste, talk.
12. tha- this is the compound hard sound if t and h as pronounced in Thakur (a surname in India).
13. d- has the sound of d as in do, deed, day.
14. dha- this is the compound sound of hard d and h as in adhere.
15. n- this is the hard sound of n. If we raise the tip of the tongue towards the throat we can emit this sound.
16. t- soft sound of t as in French.
17. th- as in thorn, truth, thumb, thence.
18. d-has the sound of th as pronounced in then, that, the.
19. dha- this is the compound sound of soft d and h as in Gandhi, dharma (Sanskrit word meaning religion).
20. n-sound of n as in then, needle, nib.
21. p- as pronounced in paper, pure, purse.
22. pha- there is no corresponding sound in English because in English words, wherever ph occurs as in philosophy, philology etc. we use the consonant sound of ' f '. If we eliminate the aspirate sound from ' f ' it will be nearer to the sound of the Hindi consonant indicated by pha.
23. b- as pronounced in book, bun, Bible.
24. bha- this is the compound sound of b and h as spoken in Bharat (India).
25. m- as in me, mother, may.

26. y-as in your, yellow.
27. r- as in rat, raw, rub.
28. l- as in lame, like, lie.
29. v- as in van, very, vehicle. In Hindi there is no distinction between the sound of v and w and for the Hindi consonant sound of o] we may use v or w.
30. sh- as in she, sheep, show, shove.
31. sha- the distinction between the sounds of "k] and 'k] in Hindi is very subtle. Linguists would understand that "k] is palatal while 'k] is cerebral. We have used sha for this cerebral sound of sh. The beginners may omit the distinction for the cerebral sound of sh is very rarely used.
32. s- as in say, seat, sell.
33. h-as in him, her, haste.
34, 35, 36- These are syllables, having compound sound of more than one consonant.

पौरं गावो मित सन्दिग्धं
नक्षत्रेन्दुः स तु भूशूलम्।
रूपेत्रक्षत्रिधयोरङ्गे
वाणी चस्थं दक्षि नक्षत्रम्॥५॥

One who is born in the first quarter of Ashwini, he will have (i) Aries-Mars (ii) Taurus- Venus (iii) Gemini-Mercury (iv) Cancer-Moon (v) Leo-Sun (vi) Virgo- Mercury (vii) Libra- Venus (viii) Scorpio-Mars (ix) Sagittarius- Jupiter- these nine periods.

One who is born in the second quarter of Ashwini, he will have

(i) Capricorn- Saturn

(ii) 11- *Saturn

(iii) 12- Jupiter

*Instead of writing the names of signs we have used their numbers viz. '11' for Aquarius, 12 for Pisces and so on.

(iv) 8- Mars

(v) 7- Venus

(vi) 6- Mercury

(vii) 4- Moon

(viii) 5- Sun

(ix) 3- Mercury - These nine periods.

One who is born in the (iii) quarter of Ashwini, he will have—

(i) 2- Venus

(ii) 1- Mars

(iii) 12- Jupiter

(iv) 11- Saturn

(v) 10- Saturn

(vi) 9 - Jupiter

(vii) 1 - Mercury

(viii) 2- Venus

(ix) 3- Mercury

These nine periods.

One who is born in the iv pada of Ashwini, he will have —

(i) Cancer- Mars

(ii) Leo- Sun

(iii) Virgo-Mercury

(iv) Libra- Venus

(v) Scorpio- Mars

(vi) Sagittarius- Jupiter

(vii) Capricorn- Saturn

(viii) Aquarius- Saturn

(ix) Pisces - Jupiter

These nine periods.

दासतवेशो गौरीपुत्रं
क्षन्निधकारो गोभूशेषम् ।
सौदधिनक्षेत्रहासन्तो
भौमगुरुः पुत्राक्षोनाधिः ॥६ ॥

One who is born in Bharani- I pada, he will have—

(i) Scorpio- Mars
(ii) Libra- Venus
(iii) 6- Mercury
(iv) 4- Moon
(v) 5- Sun
(vi) 3- Mercury
(vii) 2- Venus
(viii) 1- Mars
(ix) 12- Jupiter

These nine periods.

One who is born in the second pada of Bharani will have—

(i) Aquarius - Saturn
(ii) 10 - Saturn
(iii) 9- Jupiter
(iv) Aries- Mars
(v) 2- Venus
(vi) 3- Mercury
(vii) 4- Moon
(viii) Leo- Sun
(ix) 6- Mercury

These nine periods.

One who is born Bharani-III pada will have the following-

(i) 7- Venus
(ii) 8- Mars

(iii) 9- Jupiter

(iv) Capricorn- Saturn

(v) Aquarius- Saturn

(vi) Pisces- Jupiter

(vii) Scorpio- Mars

(viii) Libra - Venus

(ix) Virgo- Mercury

These nine periods.

One who is born in Bharni- 4th quarter will have the following-

(i) Cancer- Moon

(ii) Leo- Sun

(iii) Gemini- Mercury

(iv) Taurus- Venus

(v) Aries- Mars

(vi) Pisces- Jupiter

(vii) Aquarius- Saturn

(viii) Capricorn- Saturn

(ix) Sagittarius- Jupiter

These nine periods.

वाक्यान्येतान्यश्वियाम्यर्क्षयोर्या-
न्यश्विन्याद्यान्यग्निभस्यापसव्ये ।
सव्येऽजेन्द्वोर्वक्ष्यमाणेषु वाक्ये-
ष्विन्दोर्वाक्यान्येव रौद्रस्य भूयः ॥७॥

The period and the order in which they influence the native born in the various quarters of Ashwini and Bharani, has been mentioned in the above slokas.

The above order which has been indicated for the first, second, third and fourth quarters of Ashwini, these will also apply respectively for the first, second, third and fourth quarters of Krittika- *i.e.* the order of periods for the first quarters of Ashwini will be applicable for the first quarters of Krittika. The order of the second quarter of Ashwini to the second quarter of Krittika and so on.

When the birth is in the different padas of Rohini, Mrigsiras, then what will be the sequence of the period has been mentioned in the slokas given below—

The order which will be mentioned for the four quarters of Mrigsiras will also be applicable to the four padas of Ardra. Mrigsiras first pada order to the first pada of Ardra; the order of the second pada of Mrigsiras to the second pada of Ardra.......and so on.

धेनुः क्षेत्रे पुरगो शुंभु-
स्तासां जत्रु क्षन्निधि दासी।
चर्मभोगी रायधिनाक्ष-
स्त्रीपौराङ्गी शिवतीर्थाब्जे ॥८ ॥

One who is born in the first pada of Rohini he will have—

(i) Sagittarius - Jupiter

(ii) Capricorn - Saturn

(iii) Aquarius- Saturn

(iv) Pisces- Jupiter

(v) Aries- Mars

(vi) Taurus- Venus

(vii) Gemini- Mercury

(viii) Leo- Sun

(ix) Caner- Moon

These nine periods.

One who is born in the second quarter of Rohini he will have—

(i) Virgo- Mercury

(ii) Libra- Venus

(iii) Scorpio- Mars

(iv) Pisces- Jupiter

(v) Aquarius- Saturn

(vi) Capricorn- Saturn

(vii) Sagittarius- Jupiter

(viii) Scorpio- Mars

(ix) Libra- Venus

These nine periods.

One who is born in the third quarter of Rohini he will have—

(i) Virgo- Mercury

(ii) Leo- Sun

(iii) Cancer- Moon

(iv) Gemini- Mercury

(v) Taurus- Venus

(vi) Aries- Mars

(vii) Sagittarius- Jupiter

(viii) Capricorn- Saturn and

(ix) Aquarius- Saturn

These nine periods.

One who is born in the 4th pada of Rohini he will have—

(i) Pisces- Jupiter

(ii) Aries- Mars

(iii) Taurus- Venus

(iv) Gemini- Mercury

(v) Leo- Sun

(vi) Cancer- Moon

(vii) Virgo- Mercury

(viii) Libra- Venus

(ix) Scorpio- Mars

त्रक्षनिधिर्दा सूचीशंभो
गौरयधी नक्षत्रं पारम्।

गोशिवतीर्थे दात्रीक्षन्नो
धीहसितांशुर्भोगी रम्या ॥९ ॥

One who is born in the first quarter of Mrigsiras constellation he will have—

(i) Pisces- Jupiter

(ii) Aquarius- Saturn

(iii) Capricorn- Saturn

(iv) Sagittarius- Jupiter

(v) Scorpio- Mars

(vi) Libra- Venus

(vii) Virgo- Mercury

(viii) Leo- Sun

(ix) Cancer- Moon

These nine periods.

One who is born in the second quarter of Mrigsiras, he will have—

(i) Gemini- Mercury

(ii) Taurus- Venus

(iii) Aries- Mars

(iv) Sagittarius- Jupiter

(v) Capricorn- Saturn

(vi) Aquarius- Saturn

(vii) Pisces- Jupiter

(viii) Aries- Mars

(ix) Taurus- Venus

These nine periods.

One who is born in the third quarter of Mrigsiras he will have—

(i) Gemini- Mercury

(ii) Leo- Sun

(iii) Cancer- Moon

(iv) Virgo- Mercury

(v) Libra- Venus

(vi) Scorpio- Mars

(vii) Pisces- Jupiter

(viii) Aquarius- Saturn and

(ix) Capricorn- Saturn

These nine periods.

One who is born in the 4th pada of Mrigsiras, he will have—

(i) Sagittarius- Jupiter

(ii) Scorpio- Mars

(iii) Libra- Venus

(iv) Virgo- Mercury

(v) Leo- Sun

(vi) Cancer- Mars

(vii) Gemini- Mercury

(viii) Taurus- Venus

(ix) Aries- Mars

These nine periods.

We have mentioned above the order of the dasha for Ashwini, Bharani, Rohini and Mrigsiras— These four constellation according to their different quarters viz. first, second, third and fourth. In all we have 27 constellations. Each remaining Nakshatra out of 23 have four charans each and their dasha sequence is according to the 4 Nakhatras that have been given above.

(i) Krittika, Punarvasu, Aslesa, Hasta, Swati, Moola, Uttarashada, Porvavabhadra pada, Revati-the sequence of the padas of these constellation will be according to that of Ashwini.

(ii) Pushya, Chitra, Porvashada, Uttarabhadrapada- the order of the different padas of the above will be as per that of Bharani.

(iii) Magha, Vishakha, Shravana- according to that of the various padas of Rohini.

(iv) Ardra, Porvaphalguni, Uttaraphalguni, Anuradha, Jyestha, Dhanishta, Shatbhisaj- The sequence of the different quarter of the above constellation will be as per the four quarters of Mrigsiras.

नक्षत्रपादैष्यघटी समुत्था
पूर्वा दशा तत्पतिवर्षजाता।
पूर्वोक्तपादक्रमशोऽत्र विद्यात्-
केषांचिदेवं मतमाहुरार्या ॥१०॥

We have now indicate the method of finding out the elapsed period and the balance period of the major periods in Kala Chakra Dashas. Only one fourth duration of a constellation is taken as each nakshatra consists of four equal quarters.

The method of proportion is used to find out the balance of Dasha and for this (a) the degree, minutes etc. covered in the quarter of a nakshatra and (b) the balance left to be covered. (c) The total duration of the signs and then we can calculate the balance of Dasha.

For example in Mrigsira— I quarter the first Dasha is Sagittarius-Jupiter. The number of years of Sagittarius should be multiplied by (b) and divided by one fourth of the duration of the nakshatra then the balance of dasha will be the result.

The other dashas will follow the sequence. This is the opinion of some scholars.

दस्रादिपादप्रभृतीनि भानां
वाक्यानि यान्यक्षरपंक्तिजानि।
तेषां क्रमेणैव दशा प्रकल्प्या
वाक्यक्रमं साध्विति केचिदाहु: ॥११॥

According to other scholars the full duration of the period of that nakshatra should be taken. These are 100 years or 85 years, 83 years or 86 years for different quarters.

The duration of the entire period is taken to calculate the elapsed and balanced periods according to the longitude covered and the longitudes to be covered in the quarter of the nakshatra. (for example in the first quarter of Ashwini, if half the portion has elapsed then out of 100 years, 50 years are over and the balance left is 50 years).

वाक्यक्रमे कर्क्यलिमीनसन्धौ
मण्डूकगत्यश्वरप्लुतिश्च।
सिंहावलोकस्त्रिविधा तदानीं
दशान्तरं दुःखफलप्रदं स्यात् ॥१२॥

When the period of other signs follows that of the period of Cancer (Moon) then the motion is called Manduk- (Manduk is a Sanskrit word and it means a frog) *i.e.* frog leaps and so a forward - backward movement. When the period of other signs follow that of Scorpio (Mars) then it is called 'Turag' motion Turag means horse. When the period of other signs follow that of Pisces- Jupiter then it is called 'Singhavalokan'. This joint period (the ending of Cancer, Scorpio or Pisces) is the period of sufferings. (N.B. this is due to the 'Moola' Nakshatras at birth for which propitiation of planets is done for a child born in them).

तद्वाक्यवर्णक्रमाशोपहार-
वर्षाहते तत्परमायुराप्ते।
तदा दशायामपहारवर्ष-
संख्याश्च मासान्दिवसान्वदेयुः ॥१३॥

How to calculate the minor periods in the major period of signs? This is given below—

The period of the first quarter of Ashwini are- Aries-Mars 7 years, Taurus- Venus 16 years etc........of the 9 signs.

Now the minor periods of all the 9 signs will be proportionately divided according to the total duration of each sign out of the 7 years of Aries Mars.

Steps—

1. The total duration of Ashwini- Ist quarter is 100 years.
2. The duration of Taurus- Venus is 16 years.
3. The duration of Aries- Mars is 7 years.

4. So the duration of Taurus- Venus in that of Aries -Mars will be (say-x)

   100: 16: : 7: x

   or x = 16×7/100 = 112/100 years.

Converting these into years, months, days, we get 1 year 1 month and 13 days approximately. The ready reckoner of these minor periods are also available which saves the time of doing mathematical calculation.

वाक्येषु यावच्छरदां प्रमाणं
वदन्ति तावत्परमायुरत्र।
मेषादनीकं मदनं गजेन
तुन्दः पुनश्चैवमुदीरितं तत् ॥१४॥

In the previous slokas the Sum of the major periods of the four quarters of Ashwini, Bharani-Krittika has been given respectively as 100, 85, 83 and 86 years.

Table

Nakshatra	Quarters	Years	Nakshatra	Quarters	Years
Ashwini	I	100	Rohini	I	86
Ashwini	II	85	Rohini	II	83
Ashwini	III	83	Rohini	III	85
Ashwini	IV	86	Rohini	IV	100
Bharani	I	100	Mrigsira	I	86
Bharani	II	85	Mrigsira	II	83
Bharani	III	83	Mrigsira	III	85
Bharani	IV	86	Mrigsira	IV	100
Krittika	I	100	Ardra	I	86
Krittika	II	85	Ardra	II	85
Krittika	III	83	Ardra	III	83
Krittika	IV	86	Ardra	IV	100

Similarly the total duration of the major period of the four quarters Rohini, Mrigsiras, Ardra are 86, 83, 85 and 100 years respectively (shown in the table above).

In this manner Mantreshwar Maharaj had initiated the entire 'Kala Chakra Dasha'......both its mathematical as well as the predictive part in the 14 slokas. When 40 years* ago, we tried to learn the mathematical and predictive parts from these slokas then we could understand a little bit but not that much that we can do the correct calculations and apply them in horoscopes and reach to correct interpretations.

Then we studied 'Jatka Parijata', 'Brihat Parashar Horashatra' etc. in order to completely understand (mathematical and predictive parts) the subject matter of Kalachakra Dasha.

In the past 40 years we had the opportunity to teach the mathematical and predictive parts to many persons but some readers who wanted to either not understand it due to lack of intellectual abilities or on account of incapability of working hard, avoided learning this topic. Now we explain the Kalachakra Dasha independently in our own manner. So that the lovers of Astrology can benefit from its predictive advantages.

We talked to hundreds of Astrologers but we regret to say that even those who used to cast gorgeous horoscopes and were supposed to be scholars of the subject of Astrology, even their knowledge of Kalachakra dasha was negligible. Out of hundred - two hundred astrologers only one could do the mathematical part of Kalachakradasha and do the interpretation on that basis.

We had the opportunity to go through few thousand horoscopes but not even in one, the calculation of Kalachakra Dasha was present. The reason of all this is that the mathematical method of Kalachakra Dashas has not been explained elaborately. In Sanskrit it has been initiated in symbolic basis in a few slokas.

We had tried to explain and comment in Hindi about the 14 Slokas given above. By reading these highly learned scholars will be able to calculate the Dasha but general readers may not be able to take the full advantage of these. Therefore we are now explaining the

---

*Written in the year of 1969

calculation part of Kalachakra Dasha in Tabular forms. (This will make it much easier like a child's play to follow it).

1. Look to Table 'A' in order to know the longevity for various quarters of constellation.

2. In Table 'B' the different dasha of signs have been given. In various ephemeris like Raphael's or Lahari's, Logarithms method has been given to calculate the exact longitudes of Moon and therefore we have also given in brackets the longitudes of different quarters of constellations in the above tables.

3. In the Table 'A' in the first row in brackets- a, c, e, g, i has been given from top to bottom. Under these the sequence of constellation and their quarters viz. I, II, III, IV have been given. In the next column the duration (*i.e.* the sum total) of the dashas falling in that quarter) has been mentioned. In the next two columns the Dashadhip (the lord of the Dasha sign) and Jeevadhip (the lord of the Jeeva sign) has been mentioned.

   The sign which comes in the beginning is called 'Deha' and the sign whose dasha comes in the end is called 'Jeeva'.

4. In the table 'A' the constellation (in brackets a, d, f, h from bottom to top) from IV, III, II, I quarters are given. In this the first dasha of the sign is Jeeva and the lord of this sign is called Jeevadhip. The dasha of the sign in the end is called Deha and the lord of that sign is called Dehadhip. These Jeeva and Deha signs will be needed in the predicting part subsequently so these should be kept in mind.

   Moon has been given in the Tables at the end of the book.

---

*To calculate the elapsed and balance periods from the longitude.

Table- 'A'

Constellation Pada (a)	Constellation Pada (b)	Constellation Pada (c)	Full Age	Dehadhip	Jeevadhip
1. Ashwini -I	24. Ardra - I	25. Punavuasu - I	100	Mars	Jupiter
2. Ashwini -II	25. Ardra- II	26. Punavuasu - II	85	Saturn	Mercury
3. Ashwini -III	26. Ardra - III	27. Punavuasu -III	83	Venus	Mercury
4. Ashwini -IV	27. Ardra- IV	28. Punavuasu -IV	86	Moon	Jupiter
5. Bharani -I	28. Mrigsira - I	29. Pushya - I	100	Mars	Jupiter
6. Bharani -II	29. Mrigsira- II	30. Pushya - II	85	Saturn	Mercury
7. Bharani -III	30. Mrigsira -III	31. Pushya - III	83	Venus	Mercury
8. Bharani-IV	31. Mrigsira -IV	32. Pushya - IV	86	Moon	Jupiter
9. Krittika-I	32. Rohini- I	33. Ardra - I	100	Mars	Jupiter
10. Krittika -II	33. Rohini- II	34. Ardra - II	85	Saturn	Mercury
11. Krittika -III	34. Rohini- III	35. Ardra - III	83	Venus	Mercury
12. Krittika-IV	35. Rohini - IV	36. Ardra - IV	86	Moon	Jupiter

Constellation Pada (d)	Constellation Pada (e)	Constellation Pada (f)	Full Age	Dehadhip	Jeevadhip
48. Uttraphalguni -I	49. Hasta-I	Jyestha-I	100	Mars	Jupiter
47. Uttraphalguni -II	50. Hasta-II	Jyestha-II	85	Saturn	Mercury
46. Uttraphalguni -III	51. Hasta-III	Jyestha-III	83	Venus	Mercury
45. Uttraphalguni -IV	52. Hasta-IV	Jyestha-IV	86	Moon	Jupiter
44. Porvaphalguni-I	53. Chitra-I	Anuradha-I	100	Mars	Jupiter
43. Porvaphalguni-II	54. Chitra-II	Anuradha-II	85	Saturn	Mercury
42. Porvaphalguni-III	55. Chitra-III	Anuradha-III	83	Venus	Mercury
41. Porvaphalguni-IV	56. Chitra-IV	Anuradha-IV	86	Moon	Jupiter
40. Magha-I	57. Swati-I	Vishaka-I	100	Mars	Jupiter
39. Magha-II	58. Swati-II	Vishaka-II	85	Saturn	Mercury
38. Magha-III	59. Swati-III	Vishaka-III	83	Venus	Mercury
37. Magha-IV	60. Swati-IV	Vishaka-IV	86	Moon	Jupiter

Constellation Pada (g)	Constellation Pada (h)	Constellation Pada (i)	Full Age	Dehadhip	Jeevadhip
73. Moola -I	96. Shatbhisa-I	97. Porvabhapada-I	100	Mars	Jupiter
74. Moola -II	95. Shatbhisa-II	98. Porvabhapada-II	85	Saturn	Mercury
75. Moola -III	94. Shatbhisa-III	99.Porvabhapada-III	83	Venus	Mercury
76. Moola -IV	93. Shatbhisa-IV	100. Porvabhapada-IV	86	Moon	Jupiter
77.Porvashada-I	92. Dhanishta-I	101. Uttarabhapada-I	100	Mars	Jupiter
78.Porvashada-II	91. Dhanishta-II	102.Uttarabhapada-II	85	Saturn	Mercury
79.Porvashada-III	90. Dhanishta-III	103.Uttarabhapada-III	83	Venus	Mercury
80. Porvashada-IV	89. Dhanishta-IV	104.Uttarabhapada-IV	86	Moon	Jupiter
81. Uttarashada-I	88. Shravana-I	105. Revati- I	100	Mars	Jupiter
82. Uttarashada-II	87. Shravana-II	106. Revati- II	85	Saturn	Mercury
83. Uttarashada-III	86. Shravana-III	107. Revati- III	83	Venus	Mercury
84. Uttarashada-IV	85. Shravana-IV	108. Revati- IV	86	Moon	Jupiter

KALACHAKRA DASHA SEQUENCE (TABLE B)

There are 27 Constellations - Ashwini, Bharani, etc. In each of these, there are four quarters of 3 degrees and 20 minutes. What is the sequence (order) of the major Periods (Maha Dashas) in each quarter of a constellation is given below :-

Name of Nakshtra:

Ashwini

1. First Quarter (0-0-0 to 0-3-20)

   Aries, Taurus, Gemini, Cancer, Leo, Virgo, Libra, Scorpio, Sagittarius,

2. Second Quarter (0-30-20 to 0-60-40)

   Capricorn, Aquarius, Pisces, Scorpio, Libra, Virgo, Cancer, Leo, Gemini,

3. Third Quarter (0-60-40 to 0-10-0)

   Taurus, Aries, Pisces, Aquarius, Capricorn, Sagittarius, Aries, Taurus, Gemini,

4. Fourth Quarter (0-10-0 to 0-13-20)

   Cancer, Leo, Virgo, Libra, Scorpio, Sagittarius, Capricorn, Aquarius, Pisces,

Bharani

5. First Quarter (0-13-20 to 0-16-40)

   Scorpio, Libra, Virgo, Cancer, Leo, Gemini, Taurus Aries, Pisces,

6. Second Quarter (0-16-40 to 0-20-0)

   Auqarius, Capricorn, Sagittarius, Aries, Taurus, Gemini Cancer, Leo, Virgo,

7. Third Quarter (0-20-0 to 0-23-20)

   Libra, Scorpio, Sagittarius, Capricorn, Aquarius, Pisces, Scorpio, Libra, Virgo,

8. Fourth Quarter (0-23-20 to 0-26-40)

Cancer, Leo, Gemini, Taurus, Aries, Pisces, Aquarius, Capricorn, Sagittarius,

Krittika

9. First Quarter (0-26-40 to 1-0-0)

   Aries, Taurus, Gemini, Cancer, Leo, Virgo, Libra, Scorpio, Sagittarius,

10. Second Quarter (1-0-0 to 1-3-20)

    Capricorn, Aquarius, Pisces, Scorpio, Libra, Virgo, Cancer, Leo, Gemini,

11. Third Quarter (1-3-20 to 1-6-40)

    Taurus, Aries, Pisces, Aquarius, Capricorn, Sagittarius, Aries, Taurus, Gemini,

12. Fourth Quarter (1-6-40 to 1-10-0)

    Cancer, Leo, Virgo, Libra, Scorpio, Sagittarius, Capricorn, Aquarius, Pisces,

Rohini

13. First Quarter (1-10-0 to 1-13-20)

    Sagittarius, Capricorn, Aquarius, Pisces, Aries, Taurus, Gemini, Leo, Cancer,

14. Second Quarter (1-13-20 to 1-16-40)

    Virgo, Libra, Scorpio, Pisces, Aquarius, Capricorn, Sagittarius, Scorpio, Libra,

15. Third Quarter (1-16-40 to 1-20-0)

    Virgo, Leo, Cancer, Gemini, Taurus, Aries, Sagittarius, Capricorn, Aquarius,

16. Fourth Quarter (1-20-0 to 1-23-20)

    Pisces, Aries, Taurus, Gemini, Leo, Cancer, Virgo, Libra, Scorpio,

Mrigsiras

17. First Quarter (1-23-20 to 1-26-40)

Pisces, Aquarius, Capricorn, Sagittarius, Scorpio, Libra, Virgo, Leo, Cancer,

18. Second Quarter (1-26-40 to 2-0-0)

    Gemini, Taurus, Aries, Sagittarius, Capricorn, Aquarius, Pisces, Aries, Taurus,

19. Third Quarter (2-0-0 to 2-3-20)

    Gemini, Leo, Cancer, Virgo, Libra, Scorpio, Pisces, Aquarius, Capricorn,

20. Fourth Quarter (2-3-20 to 2-6-40)

    Sagittarius, Scorpio, Libra, Virgo, Leo, Cancer, Gemini, Taurus, Aries,

Arda

21. First Quarter (2-6-40 to 2-10-0)

    Pisces, Aquarius, Capricorn, Sagittarius, Scorpio, Libra, Virgo, Leo, Cancer,

22. Second Quarter (2-10-0 to 2-13-20)

    Gemini, Taurus, Aries, Sagittarius, Capricorn, Aquarius, Pisces, Aries, Taurus,

23. Third Quarter (2-13-20 to 2-16-40)

    Gemini, Leo, Cancer, Virgo, Libra, Scorpio, Pisces, Aquarius, Capricorn,

24. Fourth Quarter (2-16-40 to 2-20-0)

    Sagittarius, Scorpio, Libra, Virgo, Leo, Cancer, Gemini, Taurus Aries,

Punarvasu

25. First Quarter (2-20-0 to 2-23-20)

    Aries, Taurus, Gemini, Cancer, Leo, Virgo, Libra, Scorpio, Sagittarius,

26. Second Quarter (2-23-20 to 2-26-40)

    Capricorn, Aquarius, Pisces, Scorpio, Libra, Virgo, Cancer, Leo, Gemini,

27. Third Quarter (2-26-40 to 3-0-0)

    Taurus, Aries, Pisces, Aquarius, Capricorn, Sagittarius, Aries, Taurus, Gemini,

28. Fourth Quarter (3-0-0 to 3-20-0)

    Cancer, Leo, Virgo, Libra, Scorpio, Sagittarius, Capricorn, Aquarius, Pisces.

Pusya

29. First Quarter (3-3-20 to 3-6-40)

    Scorpio, Libra, Virgo, Cancer, Leo, Gemini, Taurus Aries, Pisces

30. Second Quarter (3-6-40 to 3-10-0)

    Auqarius, Capricorn, Sagittarius, Aries, Taurus, Gemini Cancer, Leo, Virgo

31. Third Quarter (3-10-0 to 3-13-20)

    Libra, Scorpio, Sagittarius, Capricorn, Auqrius, Pisces, Scorpio, Libra, Virgo,

32. Fourth Quarter (3-13-20 to 3-16-40)

    Cancer, Leo, Gemini, Taurus, Aries, Pisces, Aquarius, Capricorn, Sagittarius

Aslesha

33. First Quarter (3-16-40 to 3-20-0)

    Aries, Taurus, Gemini, Cancer, Leo, Virgo, Libra, Scorpio, Sagittarius,

34. Second Quarter (3-20-0 to 3-23-20)

    Capricorn, Aquarius, Pisces, Scorpio, Libra, Virgo, Cancer, Leo, Gemini,

35. Third Quarter (3-23-20 to 3-26-40)

    Taurus, Aries, Pisces, Aquarius, Capricorn, Sagittarius, Aries, Taurus, Gemini,

36. Fourth Quarter (3-26-40 to 4-0-0)

    Cancer, Leo, Virgo, Libra, Scorpio, Sagittarius, Capricorn, Aquarius, Pisces,

Magha

37. First Quarter (4-0-0 to 4-3-20)

    Sagittarius, Capricorn, Aquarius, Pisces, Aries, Taurus, Gemini, Leo, Cancer,

38. Second Quarter (4-3-20 to 4-6-40)

    Virgo, Libra, Scorpio, Pisces, Aquarius, Capricorn, Sagittarius, Scorpio, Libra,

39. Third Quarter (4-6-40 to 4-10-0)

    Virgo, Leo, Cancer, Gemini, Taurus, Aries, Sagittarius, Capricorn, Auqarius,

40. Fourth Quarter (4-10-0 to 4-13-20)

    Pisces, Aries, Taurus, Gemini, Leo, Cancer, Virgo, Libra, Scorpio,

Purvaphalguni

41. First Quarter (4-13-20 to 4-16-40)

    Pisces, Aquarius, Capricorn, Sagittarius, Scorpio, Libra, Virgo, Leo, Cancer,

42. Second Quarter (4-16-40 to 4-20-0)

    Gemini, Taurus Aries, Sagittarius, Capricorn, Aquarius, Pisces, Aries, Taurus,

43. Third Quarter (4-20-0 to 4-23-20)

    Gemini, Leo, Cancer, Virgo, Libra, Scorpio, Pisces, Aquarius, Capricorn,

44. Fourth Quarter (4-23-20 to 4-26-40)

    Sagittarius, Scorpio, Libra, Virgo, Leo, Cancer, Gemini, Taurus Aries,

Uttaraphalguni

45. First Quarter (4-26-40 to 5-0-0)

    Pisces, Aquarius, Capricorn, Sagittarius, Scorpio, Libra, Virgo, Leo, Cancer

46. Second Quarter (5-0-0 to 5-3-20)

    Gemini, Taurus Aries, Sagittarius, Capricorn, Aquarius, Pisces, Aries, Taurus,

47. Third Quarter (5-3-20 to 5-6-40)

    Gemini, Leo, Cancer, Virgo, Libra, Scorpio, Pisces, Aquarius, Capricorn,

48. Fourth Quarter (5-6-40 to 5-10-0)

    Sagittarius, Scorpio, Libra, Virgo, Leo, Cancer, Gemini, Taurus Aries,

Hasta

49. First Quarter (5-10-0 to 5-13-20)

    Aries, Taurus, Gemini, Cancer, Leo, Virgo, Libra, Scorpio, Sagittarius,

50. Second Quarter (5-13-20 to 5-16-40)

    Capricorn, Aquarius, Pisces, Scorpio, Libra, Virgo, Cancer, Leo, Gemini,

51. Third Quarter (5-16-40 to 5-20-0)

    Taurus, Aries, Pisces, Aquarius, Capricorn, Sagittarius, Aries, Taurus, Gemini,

52. Fourth Quarter (5-20-0 to 5-23-20)

    Cancer, Leo, Virgo, Libra, Scorpio, Sagittarius, Capricorn, Aquarius, Pises,

Chitra

53. First Quarter (5-23-20 to 5-26-40)

    Scorpio, Libra, Virgo, Cancer, Leo, Gemini, Taurus Aries, Pisces,

54. Second Quarter (5-26-40 to 6-0-0)

    Aquarius, Capricorn, Sagittarius, Aries, Taurus, Gemini Cancer, Leo, Virgo.

55. Third Quarter (6-0-0 to 6-3-20)

    Libra, Scorpio, Sagittarius, Capricorn, Aquarius, Pisces, Scorpio, Libra, Virgo,

56. Fourth Quarter (6-3-20 to 6-6-40)

    Cancer, Leo, Gemini, Taurus, Aries, Pisces, Aquarius, Capricorn, Sagittarius,

Swati

57. First Quarter (6-6-40 to 6-10-0)

    Aries, Taurus, Gemini, Cancer, Leo, Virgo, Libra, Scorpio, Sagittarius,

58. Second Quarter (6-10-0 to 6-13-20)

    Capricorn, Aquarius, Pisces, Scorpio, Libra, Virgo, Cancer, Leo, Gemini

59. Third Quarter (6-13-20 to 6-16-40)

    Taurus, Aries, Pisces, Aquarius, Capricorn, Sagittarius, Aries, Taurus, Gemini,

60. Fourth Quarter (6-16-40 to 6-20-0)

    Cancer, Leo, Virgo, Libra, Scorpio, Sagittarius, Capricorn, Aquarius, Pisces,

Visakha

61. First Quarter (6-20-0 to 6-23-20)

    Sagittarius, Capricorn, Aquarius, Pisces, Aries, Taurus, Gemini, Leo, Cancer,

62. Second Quarter (6-23-20 to 6-26-40)

    Virgo, Libra, Scorpio, Pisces, Aquarius, Capricorn, Sagittarius. Scorpio, Libra,

63. Third Quarter (6-26-40 to 7-0-0)

    Virgo, Leo, Cancer, Gemini, Taurus, Aries, Sagittarius, Capricorn, Aquarius,

64. Fourth Quarter (7-0-0 to 7-3-20)

    Pisces, Aries, Taurus, Gemini, Leo, Cancer, Virgo, Libra, Scorpio,

Anuradha

65. First Quarter (7-3-20 to 7-6-40)

    Pisces, Aquarius, Capricorn, Sagittarius, Scorpio, Libra, Virgo, Leo, Cancer,

66. Second Quarter (7-6-40 to 7-10-0)

    Gemini, Taurus Aries, Sagittarius, Capricorn, Aquarius, Pisces, Aries, Taurus,

67. Third Quarter (7-10-0 to 7-13-20)

    Gemini, Leo, Cancer, Virgo, Libra, Scorpio, Pisces, Aquarius, Capricorn,

68. Fourth Quarter (7-13-20 to 7-16-40)

    Sagittarius, Scorpio, Libra, Virgo, Leo, Cancer, Gemini, Taurus Aries,

Jyestha

69. First Quarter (7-16-40 to 7-20-0)

    Pisces, Aquarius, Capricorn, Sagittarius, Scorpio, Libra, Virgo, Leo, Cancer,

70. Second Quarter (7-20-0 to 7-23-20)

    Gemini, Taurus Aries, Sagittarius,Capricorn, Aquarius, Pisces, Aries, Taurus,

71. Third Quarter (7-23-20 to 7-26-40)

    Gemini, Leo, Cancer, Virgo, Libra, Scorpio, Pisces, Aquarius, Capricorn,

72. Fourth Quarter (7-26-40 to 8-0-0)

    Sagittarius, Scorpio, Libra, Virgo, Leo, Cancer, Gemini, Taurus Aries,

Mula

73. First Quarter (8-0-0 to 8-3-20)

    Aries, Taurus, Gemini, Cancer, Leo, Virgo, Libra, Scorpio, Sagittarius,

74. Second Quarter (8-3-20 to 8-6-40)

    Capricorn, Aquarius, Pisces, Scorpio, Libra, Virgo, Cancer, Leo, Gemini,

75. Third Quarter (8-6-40 to 8-10-0)

    Taurus, Aries, Pisces, Aquarius, Capricorn, Sagittarius, Aries, Taurus, Gemini,

76. Fourth Quarter (8-10-0 to 8-13-20)

    Cancer, Leo, Virgo, Libra, Scorpio, Sagittarius, Capricorn, Aquarius, Pisces,

Purvasadha

77. First Quarter (8-13-20 to 8-16-40)

    Scorpio, Libra, Virgo, Cancer, Leo, Gemini, Taurus Aries, Pisces,

78. Second Quarter (8-16-40 to 8-20-0)

    Aquarius, Capricorn, Sagittarius, Aries, Taurus, Gemini Cancer, Leo, Virgo,

79. Third Quarter (8-20-0 to 8-23-20)

    Libra, Scorpio, Sagittarius, Capricorn, Aquarius, Pisces, Scorpio, Libra, Virgo,

80. Fourth Quarter (8-23-20 to 8-26-40)

    Cancer, Leo, Gemini, Taurus, Aries, Pisces, Aquarius, Capricorn, Sagittarius,

Uttarasadha

81. First Quarter (8-26-40 to 9-0-0)

    Aries, Taurus, Gemini, Cancer, Leo, Virgo, Libra, Scorpio, Sagittarius,

82. Second Quarter (9-0-0 to 9-3-20)

    Capricorn, Aquarius, Pisces,Scorpio, Libra, Virgo, Cancer, Leo, Gemini,

83. Third Quarter (9-3-20 to 9-6-40)

    Taurus, Aries, Pisces, Aquarius, Capricorn, Sagittarius, Aries, Taurus, Gemini,

84. Fourth Quarter (9-6-40 to 9-10-0)

Cancer, Leo, Virgo, Libra, Scorpio, Sagittarius, Capricorn, Aquarius, Pisces,

Sravana

85. First Quarter (9-10-0 to 9-13-20)

Sagittarius, Capricorn, Aquarius, Pisces, Aries, Taurus, Gemini, Leo, Cancer,

86. Second Quarter (9-13-20 to 9-16-40)

Virgo, Libra, Scorpio, Pisces, Aquarius, Capricorn, Sagittarius, Scorpio, Libra,

87. Third Quarter (9-16-40 to 9-20-0)

Virgo, Leo, Cancer, Gemini, Taurus, Aries, Sagittarius,Capricorn, Aquarius,

88. Fourth Quarter (9-20-0 to 9-23-20)

Pisces, Aries, Taurus, Gemini, Leo, Cancer, Virgo, Libra, Scorpio,

Dhanistha

89. First Quarter (9-23-20 to 9-26-40)

Pisces, Aquarius, Capricorn, Sagittarius, Scorpio, Libra, Virgo, Leo, Cancer,

90. Second Quarter (9-26-40 to 10-0-0)

Gemini, Leo, Cancer, Virgo, Libra, Scorpio, Pisces, Aquarius, Capricorn,

91. Third Quarter (10-0-0 to 10-3-20)

Gemini, Leo, Cancer, Virgo, Libra, Scorpio, Pisces, Aquarius, Capricorn,

92. Fourth Quarter (10-3-20 to 10-6-40)

Sagittarius, Scorpio, Libra, Virgo, Leo, Cancer, Gemini, Taurus Aries,

Satabhisaj

93. First Quarter (10-6-40 to 10-10-0)

    Pisces, Aquarius, Capricorn, Sagittarius, Scorpio, Libra, Virgo, Leo, Cancer,

94. Second Quarter (10-10-0 to 10-13-20)

    Gemini, Taurus Aries, Sagittarius, Capricorn, Aquarius, Pisces, Aries, Taurus,

95. Third Quarter (10-13-20 to 10-16-40)

    Gemini, Leo, Cancer, Virgo, Libra, Scorpio, Pisces, Aquarius, Capricorn,

96. Fourth Quarter (10-16-40 to 10-20-0)

    Sagittarius, Scorpio, Libra, Virgo, Leo, Cancer, Gemini, Taurus Aries,

Purvabhadrapada

97. First Quarter (10-20-0 to 10-23-20).

    Aries, Taurus, Gemini, Cancer, Leo, Virgo, Libra, Scorpio, Sagittarius,

98. Second Quarter (10-23-20 to 10-26-40)

    Capricorn, Aquarius, Pisces, Scorpio, Libra, Virgo, Cancer, Leo, Gemini,

99. Third Quarter (10-26-40 to 11-0-0)

    Taurus, Aries, Pisces, Aquarius, Capricorn, Sagittarius, Aries, Taurus, Gemini,

100. Fourth Quarter (11-0-0 to 11-3-20)

    Cancer, Leo, Virgo, Libra, Scorpio, Sagittarius, Capricorn, Aquarius, Pisces

Uttarbhadrapada

101. First Quarter (11-3-20 to 11-6-40)

    Scorpio, Libra, Virgo, Cancer, Leo, Gemini, Taurus Aries, Pisces

102. Second Quarter (11-6-40 to 11-10-0)

Aquarius, Capricorn, Sagittarius, Aries, Taurus, Gemini, Cancer, Leo, Virgo,

103. Third Quarter (11-10-0 to 11-13-20)

Libra, Scorpio, Sagittarius, Capricorn, Aquarius, Pisces, Scorpio, Libra, Virgo,

104. Fourth Quarter (11-13-20 to 11-16-40)

Cancer, Leo, Gemini, Taurus, Aries, Pisces, Aquarius, Capricorn, Sagittarius

Revati

105. First Quarter (11-16-40 to 11-20-0)

Aries, Taurus, Gemini, Cancer, Leo, Virgo, Libra, Scorpio, Sagittarius,

106. Second Quarter (11-20-0 to 11-23-20)

Capricorn, Aquarius, Pisces, Scorpio, Libra, Virgo, Cancer, Leo, Gemini,

107. Third Quarter (11-23-20 to 11-26-40)

Taurus, Aries, Pisces, Aquarius, Capricorn, Sagittarius, Aries, Taurus, Gemini,

108. Fourth Quarter (11-26-40 to 12-0-0)

Cancer, Leo, Virgo, Libra, Scorpio, Sagittarius, Capricorn, Aquarius, Pisces

What is the duration of the major period in any particular quarters of a constellation? This has been given in the pages (499-501). Without even that the readers can decipher from the details given above as to the total years of a dasha in a particular quarter of a constellation. For example if a native is born in the first quarter of Revati then he will have the periods of 100 years (given below):

Aries, Taurus, Gemini, Cancer, Leo, Virgo

7 + 16 + 9 + 21 + 5 + 9

Libra, Scorpio, Sagittarius

+ 16 + 7 +10 = 100 years.

We have mentioned before the Dashas of every sign viz., 7 years for Aries, 16 years for Taurus etc. Therefore for each sign these number of years are written below them and then when added they give 100 years. Now suppose that on the date of birth (by adding the first day or second day). The total duration of Revati is 56 Ghatis (1 Ghatis=24 minutes). Then the one pada of Revati will be the one fourth of 56 ghatis *i.e.* will be of 14 ghatis. Out of this 7 ghatis have elapsed and the balance ghatis left are 7 Ghatis. Then the question arises as to what is the duration of the elapsed dasha?

There are two opinions for this.

1. One opinion is that in the first quarters of Revati, first of all the period of Aries comes. It has 7 years. Half of the Ist pada is elapsed so we will take half of 7 years or 3 and a half years as the elapsed dasha and the balance left (which will run after birth) is also 3 and a half years. After that 16 years of Taurus, 9 years of Gemini etc. will follow in the sequence. We do not side with this opinion. It is so because when the total duration of the dasha is 100 years and when half of the Nakshatra- Quarter has elapsed then why only three and half years will elapse and the balance left will be 96 years and 6 months. This does not look so logical. Still some astrologers follow it.
2. The second opinion which from our view is more authentic is that when one quarter has 100 years then as half of it has elapsed— So 50 years should be taken as the elapsed years and the balance lift is also 50 years.

Now count-

Aries	-	7 years
Taurus	-	16 years
Gemini	-	9 years
and Cancer	-	21 years
The total is	-	53 years

Out of these 50 years have elapsed therefore the balance (53-50) = 3 years.

The dasha of the native at birth in the first quarter of Revati will start with :

Cancer- Moon	-	3 years
Leo-Sun	-	5 years
Virgo- Mercury	-	9 years
Libra- Venus	-	16 years
Scorpio-Mars	-	7 years
Sagittarius- Jupiter	-	10 years
		50 years

When the native completes 50 years of age then what will be his dasha? After Revati first quarter, the second quarter commences—So the native will enter (after 50 years) into the

Capricorn -Saturn	-	4 years
Aquaries - Saturn	-	4 years
Pisces - Jupiter	-	10 years
Scorpio - Mars	-	7 years and the sequence of dasha will be kept.

If the birth is in the last quarter of Revati—IV quarter and in that suppose the balance is only 40 years, then the native after 40 years will enter into the Dashas given for the first quarter of Ashwini and their sequence (order) will be maintained.

In the end of the book we have given Table 1,2,3, 4— From these Tables the major periods of signs elapsed as well as the balanced dashas, will be known (from the longitudes of Moon).

Table No. 5
Duration of Minutes

Minutes of Moon	Full age 100 Years Y-M-D	85 Years Y-M-D	83 Years Y-M-D	86 Years Y-M-D
1.	0-6-0	0-5-3	0-4-29	0-5-5
2.	1-0-0	0-10-6	0-9-29	0-10-10
3.	1-6-0	1-3-9	1-2-28	1-3-14
4.	2-0-0	1-8-12	1-7-28	1-8-19
5.	2-6-0	2-1-15	2-0-27	2-1-24
6.	3-0-0	2-6-18	2-5-26	2-6-29
7.	3-6-0	2-11-21	2-10-26	3-0-4
8.	4-0-0	3-4-24	3-3-25	3-5-8
9.	4-6-0	3-9-27	3-8-25	3-10-13
10.	5-0-0	4-3-0	4-1-24	4-3-8
11.	5-6-0	4-8-3	4-6-23	4-8-23
12.	6-0-0	5-1-6	4-11-23	5-1-28
13.	6-6-0	5-6-9	5-4-22	5-7-2
14.	7-0-0	5-11-12	5-9-22	6-0-7
15.	7-6-0	6-11-15	6-2-21	6-5-12
16.	8-0-0	6-9-18	6-7-20	6-10-17
17.	8-6-0	7-2-21	7-0-20	7-3-22
18.	9-0-0	7-7-24	7-5-19	7-8-26
19.	9-6-0	8-0-27	7-10-19	8-2-1
20.	10-0-0	8-6-0	8-3-18	8-7-6
21.	10-6-0	8-11-3	8-8-17	9-0-11
22.	11-0-0	9-4-6	9-1-17	9-5-16
23.	11-6-0	9-9-9	9-6-16	9-10-20
24.	12-0-0	10-2-12	9-11-16	10-3-25
25.	12-6-0	10-7-15	10-4-15	10-9-

Note : Where more than half a day covers in the calculation, we have taken it to be 1 day and where less than half a day (less than 30 Ghatis) then we have left them out.

Example: Suppose the longitude of Moon in one case is 11 signs 20 degree and 39 minutes *i.e.* at birth Moon is posited in Pisces at 20 degree and 39 minutes. This position gives the constellation of Revati second quarter. Now look to Table 'A'. The longevity of Revati second pada is 85 years. Then in the table 2 of 85 years (these have been given in the end of the book).

	Y - M - D
11^s-20^0-25', period is	74 - 4 - 15
11^s-20^0-50' period is	63- 9 - 0

We have to find the balance for - 11^s-20^0-39'

Now from 11^s-20^0-25' deduct (39-25=14) motion of 14 minutes or from 11-20-50 add (50-39=11) add the motion of 11 minutes. The balance period will come out—

			Y - M - D
	11-20-25	=	74 - 4 -15
Subtract motion of	0-0-14	=	5 - 11-12*
	The balance period	=	68- 5 -3
Second method			Y - M - D
	10-20-50 (Table no. 2)	=	63 - 9 - 0
Add motion of 11' (in Table No. 5, below 85 in the row of '11' page...)		=	4 - 8 - 3
With this method the same balance period comes		=	68 - 5 - 3

Now see Table 'B'

The duration of Revati second quarter is 85 years.

In these, there are 9 different periods viz.,

Capricorn- Saturn (4 years), Aquarius- Saturn (4 Years)
Pisces- Jupiter (10 Years), Scorpio- Mars (7 years)
Libra-Venus (16 years), Virgo- Mercury (9 years)
Cancer- Moon (21 years), Leo- Sun (5 Years)
Gemini- Mercury (9 years)

The total of these are 4+4+10+7+16+9+21+5+9= 85 Years.

The balance period to run is-	68 Years, 5 Months, 3 Days
The total period is -	85 Years.

So the period which finished when the child was born were 16 Years, 6 Months, 27 Days.

The periods which passed before birth took place were-

Capricorn- Saturn-	4 Years
Aquarius- Saturn-	4 Years
and Pisces- Jupiter's	8 Years - 6 Months -27 Days
Total	16 Years - 6 Months -27 Days

Pisces- Jupiter's total duration is 10 years. Out of these we subtract 8 Years- 6 Months- 27 Days (The period already passed) then the balance is -

Pisces- Jupiter 1 Years - 5 Months - 3 Days

This balance is at birth to be enjoyed by the native.

The Table of Periods of the native will be -

Deha Rashi- Capricorn	Kalachakra	Jeeva Rashi- Gemini
Dehadhip- Saturn	Mahadasha	Jeevadhip- Mercury

Sign and its Lord	Duration Y-M-D	Until the age of, Y-M-D
Pisces- Jupiter	1-5-3	1-5-3
Scorpio- Mars	7-0-0	8-5-3
Libra - Venus	16-0-0	24-5-3
Virgo- Mercury	9-0-0	33-5-3
Cancer- Moon	21-0-0	54-5-3
Leo - Sun	5-0-0	59-5-3
Gemini- Mercury	9-0-0	68-5-3
Total		68-5-3

After 68 years, 5 months, 3 days, the Table given for Revati, 3rd quarter will run. See Table 'B'- Rohini 3rd quarter where the periods starts from Taurus— Venus. As the period commences with Taurus- Venus - So the Deha Rashi is Taurus and the Dehadhip is Venus.

The periods of Rohini 3rd quarter ends at Gemini- Mercury so the Jeeva Rashi will be Gemini and the Jeevadhip will be Mercury. This will be after the natives completes 68 years, 5 months and 3 days.

		Y - M - D	
Until		68 - 5 - 3	
Deha Rahi - Taurus			Jeeva Rashi - Gemini
Dehadhip - Venus			Jeevadhip - Mercury
Taurus - Venus	+	16 - 0 - 0	
Aries - Mars	+	7 - 0 - 0	
		91 - 5- 3	

This is the order of the periods.

Minor periods (Antardashas)

Suppose we have to find the minor periods in the Major period of Mars. Mars commences from 1 year, 5 months and 3 days.

Cycle of Minor periods-

Sign and its Lord	Duration Y-M-D	Until the age of, Y-M-D
Pisces- Jupiter	1-5-3	1-5-3
Scorpio- Mars in Scorpio- Mars	0-6-27	2-0-0
Libra - Venus in Scorpio- Mars	1-3-24	3-3-24
Virgo- Mercury in Scorpio- Mars	0-8-27	4-0-21
Cancer- Moon in Scorpio- Mars	1-8-23	5-9-14
Leo - Sun in Scorpio- Mars	0-4-28	6-2-12
Gemini- Mercury in Scorpio- Mars	0-8-27	6-11-9
Capricorn- Saturn in Scorpio- Mars	0-3-29	7-3-8
Aquarius- Saturn in Scorpio-Mars	0-3-29	7-7-7
Pisces - Jupiter in Scorpio-Mars	0-9-26	8-5-3

In the same manner other minor periods should be calculated.

Now the mathematical portion of the Kala Chakra Dasha *i.e.* the period of Kalachakra, is complete (page-518). We hope that with the tables dealing with the balance and elapsed periods and which period follows which dasha is clear to the readers. The tables are given at the end of the Book.

PREDICTIVE PART

Now in order to decipher the good or ill effect of the signs in the Kala Chakra period, certain principles are enunciated.

1. The sign whose dasha is to be considered. If that sign is strong and benefic are posited in that sign....... The lord of that sign is in it, the other sign receives the aspect of benefic and that sign is in a good place from the ascendant or the lord of that sign is strong is also getting associated with benefic, is also posited in a good house from the ascendant, then the period of that sign about which we are considering is good.

   By example— we make it more clear. If we have talk of Taurus then—

   (i) If Taurus is strong and benefic are posited in it. The lord of Taurus is Venus and let us say Venus is in Cancer, then Cancer should receive aspect of benefic; Cancer should also be in a good place. Let us say in the 4th house from the ascendant. The lord of Cancer is Moon *i.e.* Moon should be strong and Moon should be associated with benefic. So in this case Moon should get a full aspect from Jupiter and should also be well placed. Let us say in the 9th house *i.e.* a good place to be in for a planet, then the period of Taurus will be very good.

2. If the sign is weak and malefic are posited in it the lord of the sign is in the sign of a enemy or in a sign owned by a malefic, and the sign also receives the aspect of malefic, is also in a bad house from the ascendant. The lord of that sign is also weak (*i.e.* combust, debilitated and in the Navansha also debilitated or in the sign of enemy etc.); Malefic also aspect that lord or it may be posited with malefic. The dispositer of the lord of that sign is

placed in bad house (6, 8 or 12) from the ascendant, then the period of that sign will show ill effects.

Now we give the interpretation of how the period of a sign will be based upon its placement from the ascendant.

1. If it is in the ascendant then there will be good health related to body, happiness, fame, ornaments, high position, wealth, sons and happiness from women (wife).

   If the Lord of this sign is a benefic then, benefic result will ensue.

   If it is a sign owned by a malefic then there will be no good effect.

   If malefic and benefic both are posited in the sign *i.e.* (the ascendant) then it will show mixed results.

   If malefic are more then more sufferings.

   If benefic are more then more good results.

   This is the meaning of mixed results.

   In the coming matter wherever we talk of the mixed results, this should be interpreted as given above.

   If a planet who is exalted in own sign, or in the sign of a friend, is posited in the ascendant, then attainment of a high status, honour from the king or the government.

   If a planet is debilitated, in the sign of an enemy, or is combust, and is posited in the sign of the ascendant, then sufferings related to sons, wife etc. The ill effect will be severe.

2. The sign under consideration if it is in the 2nd house from the ascendant, then there will be increase of wealth and grains, good food, happiness from wife and sons, gain of lands, honour from the king, acquisition of education, expertness in speech, company of good people etc. will be the benefic results. This depends upon if the sign is benefic. If it is a malefic sign then the reverse will be the results.

3. If the sign is in the 3rd from the ascendant, then extraordinary happiness, excellent and good food, increase of patience and valour, great enthusiasm, control on the senses—these are the

benefic result if it is a benefic sign. If the sign is malefic or does not possess strength then results will always be the opposite to the one described above.

4. If the sign is in the 4th from the ascendant, then gain of ornaments, vehicles, lands, houses, holy trips, company of rich and well known people. Mind is pure, increase in enthusiasm, special agricultural success, happiness from wife and sons. Increase in the number of relatives, gain of new property, good health and gains. These are realised if the sign is benefic. If a malefic sign is in the 4th house, then various types of sufferings and destructions related to the 4th house matters.

5. If the sign is in the 5th house from the ascendant, then honour from the kings, high status will be realized. Happiness from wife and sons, patience, good health, ability to support relatives, donation of food, grains, fame, enthusiasm and happiness. Opportunity for celebrations, gain of wealth and the native is able to do good to others. These are the benefic results. If benefic sign is in the 5th house then all these benefic results are there. If it is a malefic sign then ill effects simultaneously besides being a malefic sign if it is also a movable sign then there is loss of status, (loss of job) for the native.

6. If the sign is in the 6th house from the ascendant and is a Papa Raṣhi (owned by a malefic) then in the period of that sign, there will be danger from fire, thieves, enemies, poison. Suffering from kings, loss of status (house), great fear, health problems, tumours, dysentery, T. B. etc. various disease. Bad name, imprisonment or debts, poverty suffering of various types. Mostly negative things happen. If the sign is benefic then the results are mixed.

7. If the sign under consideration is in the 7th house from the ascendant, then marriage. (If the native is of a marriageable age and is unmarried), happiness from wife. In the horoscope of women it indicates happiness from husband, happiness from children or birth of a child, good food, agricultural gains, new business in partnership, fame, honour from the king. All these good results will happen. If it is a benefic sign or if it is also associated with benefic planets.

8. If the sign under consideration is in the 8th house from the ascendant then loss of wealth, unhappiness of the highest intensity, loss of position and status, loss of relatives. Problem in the stomach or private parts, fear of enemies, poverty, lack of food, difficulties and no interest in eating. All these will be if the sign is malefic and a malefic is posited in that sign then all these negative results will definitely happen.
9. If the sign under consideration is in the 9th house then, good times. Happiness from friends, wife, sons, gain of wealth, success in good work, spiritual celebrations. Contact with high class people and if benefic sign is there then success in all work will be the good results. If it is a malefic sign then the results will be just the reverse.
10. If the sign under consideration is in the 10th house from the ascendant then realisation of high status and position, favour from the king, fame, company of wife, sons and relatives, great celebrations, Authority, good health and the native is able to spend time in good company, luxuries, success in good and big work etc. will be the good results.
11. If the sign falls in the 11th house from the ascendant then realisation of wealth, good health, new and extraordinary things are gained. Furniture, carpets, cousins, sofa etc. realized. Happiness comes from wife, sons, relatives. The money if given as loan to others will be regained. love from the king. Company and contact with well known people etc. are the benefic results if the sign is benefic.
12. If the sign falls in the 12th house from the ascendant then there will be pains in the body, loss of job or status. Danger from thieves, fire, anger of kings and sufferings caused by king. Sickness and problem to wife, tension regarding sons. Laziness and failure in whatever efforts are put in (*i.e.* whatever work is undertaken that is lost and nothing is accomplished, tensions as a result of failure. These are the bad results if the sign is a malefic and is also teneted by a malefic.
13. As counted from the ascendant, the place where the sign falls, all the results which have been predicted according to this

position, in that one thing should be kept in mind and that is how strong the lord of the sign is? If the lord of the sign is strong, is posited in its sign of exaltation, sign of a friend and also in own Navansha and Vargas etc., well placed, is posited with a friend, and is also receiving aspect from benefic then the result is benefic. If the lord of the sign is weak, debilitated, or in the sign of an enemy, is combust, is associated with malefic, or receives aspect from malefic, is posited in the 6th, 8th or 12th house from the ascendant, then there will be sufferings *i.e.* in this bad position of the lord of such a sign in the horoscope, the result in the period of that sign will be negative.

If the result of a sign is bad, still if its lord is specially strong then comparatively it gives benefic resutls. If both the sign and the lord are benefic and strong then the benefic results will be much better. If both are associated with malefic and weak, then it will show the worst effect. If the sign is strong but the lord thereof is weak then it will show bad effect. Out of the sign and the lord of that sign the lord of the sign has been given more priority. But suppose Gemini is teneted by malefic or is receiving aspect from malefic and Virgo is associated with benefic or receives an aspect from benefic, the lord of both the signs is Mercury, then the period of Gemini - Mercury will be bad and the period of Virgo - Mercury will be good.

14. Whatever sign is under consideration if it is movable, the lord thereof is also posited in a movable sign and in a movable Navansha, then the native will go to a foreign country far away from birth place. The three movable indication which have been mentioned above- (movable sign, the lord of the sign in a movable house and the lord of the sign in a movable Navansha). If out of all these three, one is in a moveable and other is in a fixed sign then logical conclusion should be drawn.

15. The period of a sign will, during its the period show the effect of different matters and attributes which have been mentioned about them viz., the type of earnings or the effect of different planets in different houses and signs or Rajyoga or as counted from the Moon wherever a planet is posited what is its effect? What is the effect of the combination of two or three and more

planets. All these should be considered when describing the prediction and the periods of the Kala Chakra. If it is so because all the Yogas and their effects will be realized during this period of the sign.

DEHA - JEEV - PHAL

We have mentioned above how the dasha of a sign will be depending upon the place it occupies from the Ascendant.

Now if there are different planets in the 'Deha and Jeev' signs, then what results will the period of Deha sings and what will be the results of the Jeev signs? This is mentioned below :

1. If Mars, Sun, Saturn, Rahu are posited in the Deha and Jeev signs, then even with one malefic, there is a possibility of death. If there are many malefic in the Deha or Jeev signs then there is no doubt in death.

2. If malefic are only in the Deha sign then incurable disease can take place. If malefic are in the Jeev Rashi, then great fears. If both have malefic then death should be judged.

3. If two malefic are in 1 or 2 mentioned above then the intensity of disease increases very much. If three planets are there in the above mentioned 1 and 2 then untimely death. If all the four malefic are in the Deha and Jeev signs then definite death should be predicted.

4. If simultaneously the Jeev signs and the Deha signs are afflicted by malefic then there will be fear from the government, thieves, and other intense fears. If Sun indicates problems then there will be danger from fire. If Moon then troubles on account of water. If Mars then injury from weapons. If Mercury then problem due to wind; If Jupiter then disease of stomach. If Venus then fear from fire; If Saturn then tumorous etc. and Rahu indicates problems and disease related to poison. All these Yogas are related to the nativity, (the birth chart). But if in the Jeev- Deha signs benefic are passing through (in transit) then benefic results and if malefic are transiting then ill effects is to predicted, *i.e.* transit should be considered.

5. If Jupiter is in the third, Mars is posited in seventh, Saturn is in the ascendant, Rahu in the 9th house, Moon in the 8th house, Sun in the 12th house, Mercury in the 7th house, Venus in the 6th house, are with malefic, or weak or debilitated, or posited in the sign of an enemy and malefic are aspecting them, then the native gets unhappiness. These are position of planets and it does not mean that they should all be in this position. The more the number of planets the more will be the intensity.

POSITION IN THE DEHA OR JEEV SIGNS

Interpretation of the periods according to the nature and attributes.

Benefic planets show good effects. Malefic or planet receiving aspect from malefic show bad results.

1. Sun— destroys wealth, calamities, suffering, fear, fear from enemies, loss of status or place. Disease related to biles, tumours, dysentery, T. B. disease of the ears, death of cattles, and relatives, destroys brothers and sisters.
2. Moon - brings meeting with relatives, birth of a daughter, good health, ornaments, happiness, clothes, honour from the king. Donations, worship of Gods and Brahmins, holy trips like visiting temples, place of worship, bathing in the sea and Ganges, eating excellent food etc. are the beneficial results.
3. Mars— fever, sickness, fire, fears, danger from thieves, quarrels with kinsmen, brothers and sisters are destroyed, loss of agriculture lands and grains; fighting, war, loss of status, tumours, piles, leprosy, poison and obstacles created by enemies. Fevers, boils in the body, trouble due to biles. malignant tumours, danger from poision, danger from fire, loss due to weapons and thieves, fear from kings. These are the things which takes place during the period of Mars.
4. Mercury— gives meeting with friends and relatives, patronage of high class people, increase of education and intellectual abilities, studies, increase of knowledge, education of scriptures. Happiness from wife, sons, kings; ornaments, cow, horses, goats etc. are gained. Intellectual knowledge, discrimination, wealth, intelligence and fame, increases.

5. Jupiter- increases importance; various types of happiness, honour from king, happiness from wife and sons or birth or a son or gain of wife, gain of wealth, ornaments, happiness, rich food, good health, fame and help to others etc. are the good results.

6. Venus— gives intimate relationship with woman, gain, happiness various varieties of beautiful clothes, ornaments, cattles, vehicles, gems; Happiness from woman, enjoyment. Music, singing and society of friends. Increase of name and valour; Good fame etc. all benefic results.

7. Saturn— causes quarrels, physical sickness, death, problems and suffering to relatives, likely to have danger from relatives, fear of fire, enemies, ghosts and other entities in the fourth dimensions. Sufferings due to poison, loss of prestige, loss of wealth, problem to wife, unhappiness to sons, destruction of agriculture, business, cow, cattles etc. and due to own arrogance one is unhappy.

8. Rahu— causes health problems, roaming about for no reason; Problem to or from relatives. Paralytic stroke and danger from king.

9. Ketu— causes loss due to theft and fire, blood loss, poverty, destruction of relatives, loss of place etc. the negative results.

These are the natural traits of planets. The stronger the horoscope and the sign in consideration, its strength, and the lord of the sign under consideration, a benefic, the strength of that lord will give so much better and benefic results. The weaker the horoscope and more the number of bad combinations in that, the weaker the sign in consideration, the more the malefic posited in that sign, or aspect that sign, the weaker the lord of that sign, the more will be the ill effect in the period of the malefic.

VARIOUS SPEEDS

Now we speak of one more subject of the Kala Chakra Dasha and then complete this section. In this the period of all the signs are not in order—

1. From Pisces to Scorpio
2. From Virgo to Cancer

3. From Leo to Gemini
4. From Sagittarius to Aries
5. From Scorpio to Pisces
6. From Aries to Sagittarius.

These are the six positions or Gaties which jump the sequence of Dashas. Aries, Taurus, Gemini— This way the sign are counted or they may be counted in the reverse orders like - Pisces, Aquarius, Capricorn, then there is nothing special. But jumping from Aries and going to Sagittarius or jumping from Sagittarius to Aries or jumping from Scorpio to Pisces or Pisces to Scorpio or to jump over one sign from Gemini to Leo or Cancer to Virgo or from Leo to Gemini, then in the beginning of such a period generally sufferings and problems occurs.

The period of the Kal Chakra Dasha has been thoroughly discussed above. Now after the 14 Slokas we shall mention different types of other periods: For how many years they prevail and what are there traits? So we start with the commentary on Sloka No. 15.

UTPANNA, SHEMA AND ADHAN MAHA DASHAS

महादशासु यत्फलं प्रकीर्तितं मया पुरा।
तदेव योजयेद् दशासुं चैवमादिषु ॥१५ ॥

The matters which have been mentioned for other periodic influences of planet should also be applied to the following three dashas and these are -

1. Utpanna Mahadasha
2. Shema Maha Dasha
3. Adhan Maha Dasha.

जन्मर्क्षात्परतस्तु पञ्चमभवाऽथोत्पन्नसंज्ञा दशा
स्यादाधानदशाऽप्यतोऽष्टमभवात् क्षेमान्महाख्या दशा।
आसामेव दशावसानसमये मृत्युप्रदा स्यान्नृणां
स्वल्पानल्पसमायुषां त्रिवधपञ्चर्क्षेदायान्तिमे ॥१६ ॥

1. Which is the 5th constellation from the birth star. Birth star is the constellation where the Moon was posited at birth. Counting from this 5th constellation, whatever periodic influence commences, is called Utpanna Mahadasha.

2. From birth constellation count the 8th constellation (both are included) *i.e.* birth will be one the next one will be two that way to eighth. Whatever Mahadasha commences from this 8th constellation is called Adhan Dasha. Similarly the Mahadasha which starts from the 4th constellation from the birth Nakshatra is called the Shema Mahadasha. Utpanna, Adhan and Shema are Sanskrit words. Utpanna in English means born. Adhan is related to the time when the conception of a child takes place and Shema Mahadasha is not very clearly mentioned.

If all the three periodic influences mentioned above, terminates at the same time *i.e.* one period is over and the next one commences in all the three then that is the time, when there will be death- this is a Marak Period. In the case of a person who has a short span of life 'Alpayu', the third period; in the case of one which has medium life span; Madhyayu is the 5th Dasha; and in the case of one with long life *i.e* 'Dheergayu', the 7th Dasha is fatal. (causes death).

एवं द्वे नव विंशतिर्धृतिकृतिः पञ्चाशदेषां क्रमात्
चन्द्रारेन्दुजशुक्रजीवदिनकृद्दैवाकरीणां समाः ।
स्वै स्वैः पुष्टफला निसर्गजनितैः पक्तिर्दशाया क्रमा-
दन्ते लग्नदशा शुभेति यवना नेच्छन्ति केचित्तथा ॥१७॥

NISARGA DASHA

1 year for Moon, 2 years for Mars, 9 years for Mercury, 20 years of Venus, 18 years of Jupiter, 20 years of Sun, 50 years of Saturn are the Nisarga or the Naisargik periods. Naisargik means natural. According to Yavanacharya* the 50 years of Saturn also includes the period of the ascendant. But other people do not agree with this

*The Persian Master - a great Astrologer who brought to light the system of the Solar Returns (Annual horoscopes).

view. A planet which is well placed in the nativity - that is a benefic and a planet which is not well placed *i.e.* badly placed becomes a malefic. After calculating the Shada Bala, the six type of strength of planets, the natural dasha which is used for that the learned readers should look into the Keshaviya Jatak Paddhati and the Shreepati Paddhati.

लिप्तीकृत्य भजेद् ग्रहं खखजिनैस्तच्छिष्टमायुष्कला
आशाखाश्विहृताब्दमासदिवसाः सत्योदितेंऽशायुषि।
वक्रिण्युच्चगते त्रिसङ्गुणमिदं स्वांशत्रिभागोत्तमे
द्विघ्नं नीचगतेऽर्धमप्यथ दलं मौढ्ये सितार्कौ बिना॥१८॥

ANSH DASHA

1. Each planet should be converted into minutes *i.e.* the sign, the degree, the minute should be converted into minutes and then it should be divided by 2400. The balance will be the age depicted in minute that the planet will bestow. These balance should be divided by 200. The dividend will be the year. The remaining should be multiplied by 12 and again reminded by 200 will give the month and the balance now should be multiplied by 30 and divided by 200 will give the days. This is the opinion of Satyacharya. The planet which is exalted in sign or is retrograde then the age indicated by them in years, months and days should be increased three times.
2. If a planet is in own Navansha, own Decanet or Vargottam then the period indicated by them, should be doubled *i.e.* multiplied by 2.
3. If a planet is debilitated or combust then the period of that planet should be reduced by half *i.e.* divide by 2. The rule of reduction of the dasha of a combust planet by half does not apply to Venus and Saturn *i.e.* it will apply only to all the other planets but not to Venus and Saturn.

सर्वार्द्धत्रिकृतेषुषण्मितलवह्रसोऽसतामुत्क्रमा-
द्रि:फात्सत्सु दलं तदा हरति बल्येको बहुष्वेकभे।

त्र्यंशोनं रिपुभे विना क्षितिसुतं सत्योपदेशे दशा
लग्नस्यांशसमा बलिन्युदयभेऽस्यात्रापि तुल्यापि च ॥१९ ॥

If a malefic is posited in the 12th house then the period indicated by that is totally reduced and it would not have any participation in the periodic influence; if a planet is in the 11th house then its period is reduced by half; If a planet is in the 10th house then the period is reduced by one third; If a planet is in the 9th house then its period is reduced by one fourth; If a planet is in the 8th house then its period is reduced by one fifth; and in the 7th house it is reduced by one sixth.

If benefic are in the 12th, 11th, 10th, 9th, 8th or 7th house then their periods which are reduced are only half of the reduction done for malefic. For example- instead of 1/2 only 1/4; instead of 1/3 only 1/6 and so on. If there are more then one planet, posited in a house in the nativity, from the 7th house to the 12th house, then out of these six houses, the planet which is the strongest and posited in sign with other planet, only the age given by that planet is reduced and the balance given by other planets is left as it is. If any planet, except Mars, is in the sign of an enemy then the age indicated by them is reduced by one third.

सत्योंपदेशो वरमत्र किन्तु
कुर्वन्त्योग्यं बहुवर्गणाभिः ।
आचार्यकं त्वत्र बहुघ्नतायाम्
सके तु यद्भूरि तदेव कार्यम् ॥२० ॥

According to Satyacharya the number of Navansha which has risen in the ascendant, the same is the age of ascendant. It is a universal application whether the ascendant is strong or weak. The opinion and rules indicated by Satyacharya are not that fine then the ones which has been given by Maya or Jeev Sharma. But the question is that the rules of reduction which has been mentioned above when many rules apply simultaneously to a planet then should we apply all of them? In this matter it has been mentioned that :-

1. When there is a possibility of reduction due to many reasons applicable to a planet posited in (from 12th to 7th houses) *i.e.* 12th, 11th, 10th, 9th, 8th, 7th due to debilitation, posited in the

sign of enemy and combust etc. then in this case the maximum reduction which is applicable, only that should be applied.

For example- Suppose in one place it has to be reduced by one third or by half then only one half should be reduced as if it is more than one third.

2. Similarly in exalted or retrograde planets when there is an increase and many rules may apply, then only the one where the maximum increase of age can be given, should be applied and not the other ones.

PINDAYU DASHA

धेयं शूर शके श्रियं स्मय परे निद्राः समा भास्करात्
पिण्डाख्यायुषि पूर्ववच्च हरणं सर्वं विदध्यादिह।
लग्ने पापिनि भं विनोदयलवैर्निघ्नं तनाङ्गैर्हृतं
त्याज्यं सौम्यनिरीक्षितेऽर्धमृणामत्रायुष्यभिज्ञा विदुः ॥२१॥

If Sun etc. the planets are in their highest degree of exaltation then each planet has the following years-

Sun- 19 years, Moon- 25 years, Mars- 15 years, Mercury- 12 years, Jupiter- 15 years, Venus - 21 years and Saturn - 20 years.

If the planets are in their lowest debilitation degree, then they get - 0. Any where in between should be used and calculated proportionately. The rules which has been mentioned for increase or decrease of the period for Anshayu should also be applied to this Pindayu Dasha.

If a malefic is in the ascendant, then the degree and minute of the ascendant, should be converted into minutes. The sign is not used in this only the degree and minute are reduced to minutes. The age which comes from the total of the others should be multiplied and then it should be divided 360. The dividend which comes should be reduced from the 'Purnaya' - Full Age.

If there are benefic in the ascendant then the deduction which is done for malefic, only half of that deduction should be done. This is the opinion of the scholars.

लग्नादशामंशसमां बलवत्यंशे वदन्ति पैण्डाख्ये।
बलयुक्तं यदि लग्नं राशिसमैवात्र नांशेत्था॥२२॥

In Pindayurdai - if the Navansha of ascendant is stronger than the Ascendant then,

1. The age is according to the number of Navansha which has risen.
2. If the sign of the ascendant is comparatively stronger then the years are according to the natural number of the ascendant *i.e.* for Aries ascendant, 1 year for Taurus ascendant 2 years, for Gemini ascendant 3 years, and so on.

हरणं नीचेऽर्द्धमृणं स्यात्पूर्णं प्रोक्तवर्षमुच्चगृहे।
पैण्डादौ व्यन्तरगे प्राज्ञैस्त्रैराशिकं चिन्त्यम्॥२३॥

पैण्डाख्यमायुर्ब्रवते प्रधानं
मणित्थचाणक्यमयादयश्च।
एतन्न साध्वित्यवदद्धदन्तो
वराहसूर्यस्य तथैव वाक्यम्॥२४॥

Manithya, Chanakya, Maya and other scholars has indicated that Pindayu is the best manner to estimate or calculate the longevity. But according to Satyacharya's opinion this is not the best. According to Varamihir this Pindayu is also not the best. So difference of opinion exits among great scholars of Astrology.

सूर्यादिकानां स्वमतेन जीव-
शर्मा स्वरांशं परमायुषोऽत्र।
अस्यापि सर्वं हरणं विधेयं
पूर्वोक्तवल्लग्नदशामपीह॥२५॥

According to Jeev Sharma 120 years and 5 days should be divided by 7, then we get 17 years, 73 days or each planet gives 17 years, 2 months and 13 days. In this period which is given by each planet, the same type of reduction should be applied as has been discussed before.

As mentioned before the age given by the ascendant should also be added to this.

नृणां द्वादशवत्सरा दशहता ह्यायुःप्रमाणं परै-
राख्यातं परमं शनेस्त्रिभगणं यावत्परैरीरितम्।
कैश्चिच्चन्द्रसहस्रदर्शनमिह प्रोक्तं कलौ किन्तु यत्
वेदोक्तं शरदः शतं हि परमायुर्दायमाचक्ष्महे ॥२६॥

Some persons have mentioned that the full age of a man is 120 years others are of the opinion that the time taken by Saturn to complete three circles of 360 degrees that should be the maximum age of a person. The third opinion is that the time taken by Moon in completing 100 cycles is the maximum age. Our opinion is that in Kalyug (we are living in it), according to veda the full age is 100 years.

Shruti - Speaks - "शतायुवै पुरूष" i.e. 100 years is the age.

लग्नादित्येन्दुकानामधिकबलवतः स्याद्दशादौ ततोऽन्या
तत्केन्द्रादिस्थितानामिह बहुषु पुनर्वीर्यतो वीर्यसाम्ये।
बह्वायुर्वर्षदातुः प्रथममिनावशाच्चोदितस्याब्दसाम्ये
वीर्यं किन्त्वत्र सन्धिग्रहविवरहतं भावसन्ध्यन्तराप्तम्॥२७॥

Out of the ascendant, Sun and Moon whichever is stronger, the period of that will come in the beginning *i.e.* the period will start from that planet. Then the periods of those planets will come which are in angles from the strongest of the three *i.e.* Sun, Moon or Ascendant; then of those planet which are in the succeedent houses from the strongest and in the end of the planet which are in cadent houses. Suppose more then one planet is in an angle, then the question is of whose dasha will come first of all? The answer is that the dasha of that planet which is the strongest of all the planet in angular position will come first of all and this order will follow. If two planets are of the equal strength then the planet which is bestowing more years then its dasha will come first.

In any event the years given by two planets are the same, then the first period will be of that planet which after getting combust rises first of all. This order in general is as follows—

1. Ascendant - Sun, Moon, Mars, Mercury, Jupiter, Venus, Saturn. Here the strength of a planet is calculated in the following manner. The difference between the longitude of a planet. (The longitude compromises, degree, minute and second) from the cusp of the house then that difference should be divided by the difference between cusp and the midpoint, to know the real strength of the planet. The planet which is nearer to the cusp is stronger.

अंशोद्भवं लग्नबलात्प्रसाध्य-
मायुश्च पिण्डोद्भवमर्कवीर्यात्।
नैसर्गिकं चन्द्रबलात्प्रसाध्यं
ब्रूमस्त्रयाणामपि वीर्यसाम्ये ॥२८॥

If the ascendant is the stronger then use Anshayurdaya if Sun is stronger then Pindayu should be used. If Moon is strongest then Nisargayu *i.e* the natural period should be used. If all the three are strong then what? This is discussed in the next Sloka.

तेषां त्रयाणमिह संयुतिस्तु
त्रिभिर्हता सैव दशा प्रकल्प्या।
वीर्ये द्वयोरैक्यदलं तयोः स्यात्
चेज्जीवशर्मायुरमी बलोनाः ॥२९॥

If all the three are equally strong then the age which come from all the three add them together and divide it by three. If two are strong then add the two of them and divide by 2. If all the three are weak then the age should be calculated according to the method which Jeev Sharma has mentioned.

कालचक्रदाशा ज्ञेया चन्द्रांशेशे बलान्विते।
सदा नक्षत्रमार्गेण दशा बलवती स्मृता ॥३०॥

If the lord of the Navansha occupied by Moon is strong then Kala Chakra Dasha should be used. Vimshotari Dasha is always strong and can be used in all cases.

समाः षष्टिर्द्विघ्ना मनुजकरिणां पञ्च च निशा
हयानां द्वात्रिंशत्खरकरभयोः पञ्चककृतिः ।
विरूपा साप्यायुर्वृषमहिषयोर्द्वादश शुनां
स्मृतं छागादीनां दशकसहिताः षट् च परमम् ॥३१ ॥

Manushya - *i.e.* human beings (Male - Female) and Elephants has a life span of 120 years, Horses have 32 years. Camel and Donkeys have the longevity of 25 years. Bulls and Buffalo 24 years, Dogs 12 years and Sheep etc. have 16 years of total age.

ये धर्मकर्मनिरता विजितेन्द्रिया ये
ये पथ्यभोजनजुषो द्विजदेवभक्ताः ।
लोके नरा दधति ये कुलशीललीलां
तेषामिदं कथितमायुरुदारधीभिः ॥३२ ॥

Those who are engaged in religion and do their work as dictated by scriptures those who have control on senses and eat only healthy and proper and fresh food and only the number of time which is necessary. Those who worship Brahmins and Gods, those who always take care of themselves in traditional manner their life span is as per the rules mentioned above.

23

Ashtak Vargas

What are the benefic or ill effects on a particular person due to the movements of planets through various signs of the Zodiac ?. The effect of this transits of planets is considered in this Chapter. Generally the transit is considered from the sign occupied by Moon at birth (Radical Moon). For example when Jupiter in transit passes through the 4th house from the Moon (at birth) then it indicates bad results. Jupiter's movement through one sign takes one year. After a year when Jupiter moves over to the 5th house (from Moon) then the results are very good— and when it comes to the 6th house then ill effects manifest themselves again although on different planets - all these are called the effect of transit.

In considering transits, the planetary position at birth has a status quo *i.e.* they will be taken as where they were when a native was born and then an ephemeris is consulted to see where the planets to be considered are at a particular time (date). The transit of planet in various houses from the Moon is taken in a general manner. But those who consider the transits in a pin point manner are of the opinion that agreed that Jupiter at a particular time is in transit in a place which it shows ill effects but from other radical planets it is in good houses then will we call Jupiter bad, or take the reverse example— that Jupiter is transiting through a good house from the radical Moon but it is at the same time not in good places from Sun, Mars, Mercury, Jupiter (at birth) itself, Venus, Saturn and the Ascendant then would we call the transit of Jupiter as a benefic transit? The purpose of stating all this so elaborately is to point out that as the transit is considered from the radical Moon so also it should be considered from other planets and the Ascendant— This is called 'Ashtakvarga method'.

'Ashtak', the Sanskrit word means 'eight'- which are these eight? These are the Seven Planets and the Ascendant. Consideration of the transit of a planet from the eight will mathematically indicate if the transit is good, medium or bad. If it is benefic from many planets then the effect is benefic. If it is not so then the results will not be good all this analysis of transit is called Ashtak Varga method or in short 'Ashtakvarga'.

गोचरग्रहवशान्मनुजानां यच्छुभाशुभफलाभ्य पलब्ध्यै।
अष्टवर्ग इति यो महदुक्तस्तत्प्रसाधनमिहाभिदधेऽहम् ॥१॥

What are the good or bad effects of the transit of planets through various signs (houses)? To understand it thoroughly the Ashtakvarga has been highly recommended. Therefore now I unfold the method to calculate it.

आलिख्य सम्यग्भुवि राशिचक्रं ग्रहस्थितिं तज्जननप्रवृत्ताम्।
तत्तद्‌ग्रहर्क्षात्क्रमशोऽष्टवर्गं प्रोक्तं करोत्यक्षविधानमत्र ॥२॥

In the past when paper, tampatra etc. were not in use then the system of making figures (of any type) on earth were prevalent. When the counting or any other type of symbol was to be used then a rudraksha bead* or any other seed of a fruit or something round were used to make it easier. But now we use paper and Rudraksha beads have been replaced by the sign of Zero '0'. Although in the Sanskrit Slokas the placement of an 'Aksha' (circular-spherical figure) has been stated yet in our commentary we will explain this subject in the modern method:

1. Make a horoscope on paper.
2. The Ascendant and the planets should be carefully placed in their proper places.

---

*Rudraksha is a fruit and its beads are the kernels of it. The strings of these are used to do the Japas. Mostly these trees are found in Nepal in the Himalyan Valleys.

3. In the following slokas eight chakras** have been mentioned to be created- the Seven for the 7 planets (Sun, Moon, Mars, Mercury, Jupiter, Venus, Saturn) and the 8th Chakra to be used collectively for the 7th planets.

(1) In the South India '0' or Bindu is used for benefic places and 'Rekha' or line to indicate malefic strength. In North India it is the other way round the purpose is the same - call it a Rekha or Bindu.

Example Horoscope

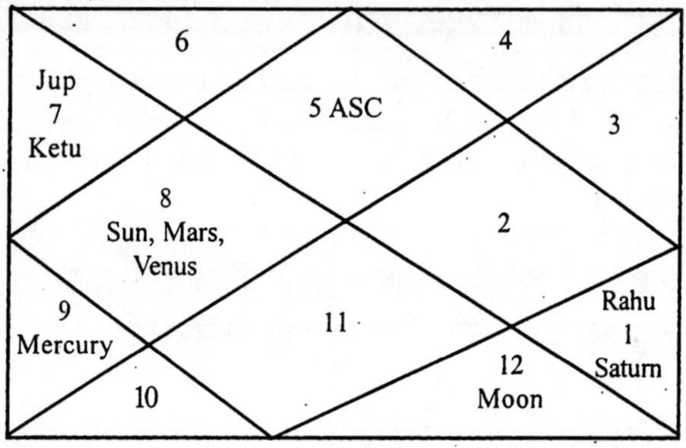

Suppose we have to make the Ashtakvarga Chakra for the above mentioned example horoscope. Here the Ashtakvargas mentioned are for the 7 planets and the Ascendant. These do not include Rahu and Ketu. No doubts these two are planets but they are only shadow planets- these two do not have any material substance. These are only mathematically proved positions (points). First of all, the Sun's Astakvarga is calculated.

पुत्रीवंसाहिधनिकेऽर्ककुजार्कजेभ्यो
मुक्ताळके सुरगुरोर्भृगुजात्तथाश्रीः ।
ज्ञाद्गोमतीधनपरा रविरिष्टदोब्जात्–
गीतोन्नयेप्युदयभाल्लघुतान्नपात्रे ॥३ ॥

Sun from its position, is benefic in the following places:-

**Circular diagrams or according to the Northern system rectangular diagrams divided into 12 parts for the 12 signs.

1, 2, 4, 7, 8, 9, 10, 11. So in the horoscope look to the sign in which Sun is at birth in the diagram for Sun's Ashtakvarga place Zero '0' or Bindu in the 1-2-4-7-8-9-10-11 places from it.

Similarly Sun in transit is beneficial from Moon in the 3,6,10,11- So place Bindus on these places. From Mars and Saturn, it is beneficial in the - 1-2-4-7-8-9-10-11 from Jupiter in the 5-6-9-11 places. From Venus in the 6-7-12, Sun is beneficial. In the 3-5-6-9-10-11 and 12 places from Mercury. The other houses which have not been indicated as beneficial should be taken to be malefic. From the Ascendant, the 3, 4, 6, 10, 11, 12 are beneficial and so place Bindus in them.

After compiling and placing all the Bindus for the 7 planets and Ascendant, the following figure (given below) will emerge and this is the Sun's Ashtakvarga.

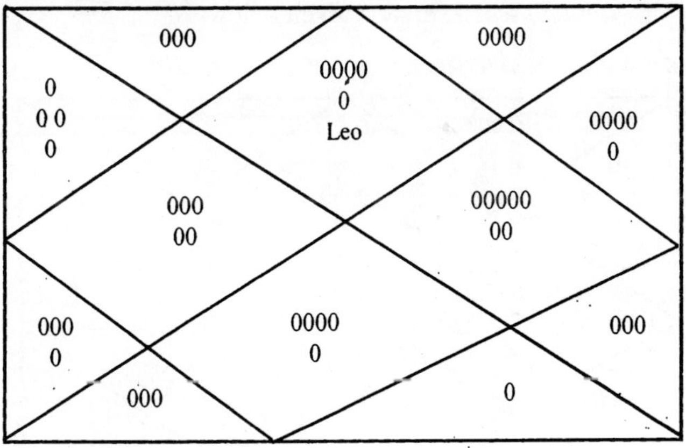

This has in all 48 Bindus which are as follows-

From Sun-8, Moon-4, Mars-8
Mercury-7, Jupiter-4, Venus-3
Saturn-8, Ascendant-6

गीतासौ जनके रवेः कलितसान्निष्के तुषारद्युतेः
भौमाच्छ्रीगुणिते धनस्य युगवन्मासाब्दनित्ये बुधात्।
जीवात्कौरवसज्जनस्य भृगुजाद्गूढात्मसिद्धाज्ञया
मन्दाद्व्रणचये तनोर्गतिनये चन्द्रः शुभो गोचरे ॥४॥

How to calculate the Ashtakvarga of Moon has been indicated in this sloka-

Sun is benefic in transit from Moon in 3-6-7-8-10-11. Moon is benefic in transit from the radical Moon (Moon at birth) in the 1-3-6-7-10-11. In the same manner Moon is good in the 2-3-5-6-9-10-11 from Mars.

From Mercury in the 1-3-4-5-7-8-10-11.
From Jupiter in the 1-2-4-7-8-10-11
From Venus in the 3-4-5-7-9-10-11
From Saturn in the the 3-5-6-11 and
From Ascendant in the 3-6-10-11.

Benefic Bindus should be placed in these places.

The example horoscope given above in the Chapter on (page 506), its Moon's Ashtakvarga is given below-

Moon's Ashtakvarga

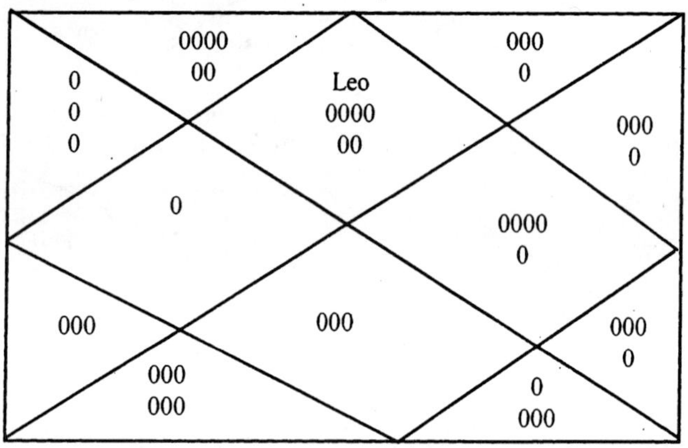

In this the total benefic Bindus are 49. Six from Sun, 6 from the radical Moon, 7 from Mars, 8 from Mercury, 7 from Jupiter, 7 from Venus, 4 from Saturn and 4 also from Ascendant has been placed.

तीक्ष्णांशोर्गणितानके शिशिरगोर्लाक्षाय भूमेः सुतात्
पुत्रीवासजनाय चन्द्रतनयाद्गोमेतके गीष्पतेः।
तन्नाकारि सितात्तदा कुरुशनेः कोवासदाधेनुको
लग्नात्स्वात्कलितं नयेत् क्षितिसुतः क्षेमप्रदो गोचरे ॥५॥

Now we speak about the Ashtakvarga of Mars. In Mars Ashtakvarga the following houses are benefic.

From Sun in the	3-5-6-10-11
From Moon in the	3-6-11
From Mars in the	1-2-4-7-8-10-11
From Mercury in the	3-5-6-11
From Jupiter in the	6-10-11-12
From Venus in the	6-8-11-12
From Saturn in the	1-4-7-8-9-10-11
From Ascendant	1-3-6-10-11

By placing Bindus from the place occupied by Mars in the Birth Chart. The Ashtakvarga of Mars will be erected.

Mars's, Ashtakvarga

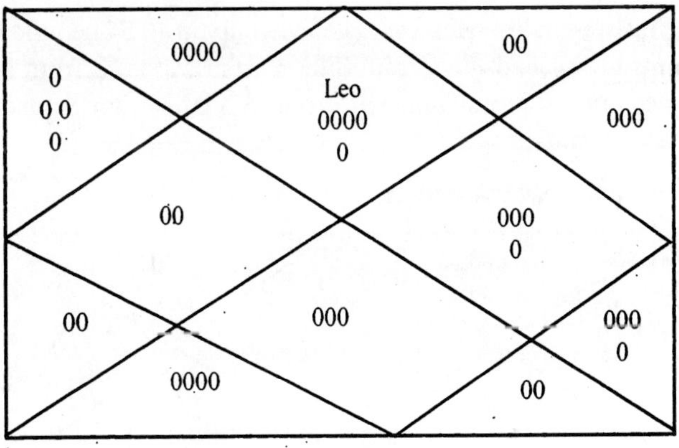

In the Ashtakvarga of Mars, the total number of benefic Bindus are 39. The details of these are as follows-

From Sun-5,	Moon-3,	Mars-7,	Mercury-4,
Jupiter-4,	Venus- 4,	Saturn-7 and	From Ascendant-5

सौम्याद्योगशतं धनैः कुरुवेर्मोषाधिकश्रीगुरोः

तेजो यत्र यमारयोः पुरवसन्दिग्धेनये भार्गवात्।

पुत्रो गर्भमहान्धके परभृतां दानाय लग्नात्सुधा-
मूर्तेः प्रावृषि जानकी शशिसुतस्त्वत्र स्थितश्चेच्छुभः ॥६ ॥

Now we undertake the Ashtakvarga of Mercury. In order to make Mercury's Ashtakvarga at which places the benefic Bindus of different planets are placed? This is given below-

From Sun	5-6-9-11-12
Moon	2-4-6-8-10-11
Mars	1-3-5-6-9-10-11-12
Mercury	1-3-5-6-9-10-11-12
Jupiter	3-8-11-12
Venus	1-2-3-4-5-8-9-11
Saturn	1-2-4-7-8-9-10-11
Ascendant	1-2-4-6-8-10-11

This way in the Ashtakvarga of Mercury in all 54 benefic Bindus or points are placed. Five from Sun, 6 from Moon, 8 from Mars, 8 from Mercury, 4 from Jupiter, 8 from Venus, 8 from Saturn and 7 from an Ascendant.

Mercury's Ashtakvarga

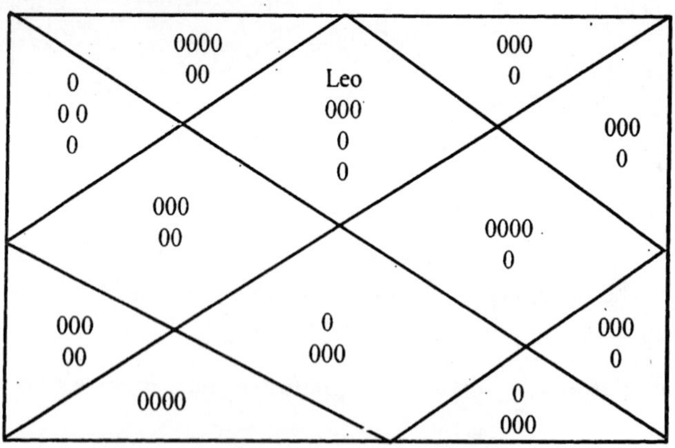

मार्ताझडात्करलाभसज्जधनिके चन्द्राद्रु मैसाळिके
भौमात्किं प्रभुसूदनाय कुरवः शिक्षाधनाढ्ये बुधात्।

पुत्री गर्भसदानके सुरगुरोः स्वल्लक्ष्मिमचन्द्रे शनेः
श्रीमन्तो धनिकाः सितात्करिविशेष सिद्धिनित्यं तनोः ॥७॥

In which places benefic points should be placed has been given below and then the Ashtakvarga of Jupiter is given below-

From Sun	1-2-3-4-7-8-9-10-11
Moon	2-5-7-9-11
Mars	1-2-4-7-8-10-11
Mercury	1-2-4-5-6-9-10-11
Jupiter	1-2-3-4-7-8-10-11
Venus	2-5-6-9-10-11
Saturn	3-5-6-12
Ascendant	1-2-4-5-6-7-9-10-11

Jupiter's Ashtakvarga

This way in Jupiter's Ashtakvarga these are 56 benefic points which are as follows-

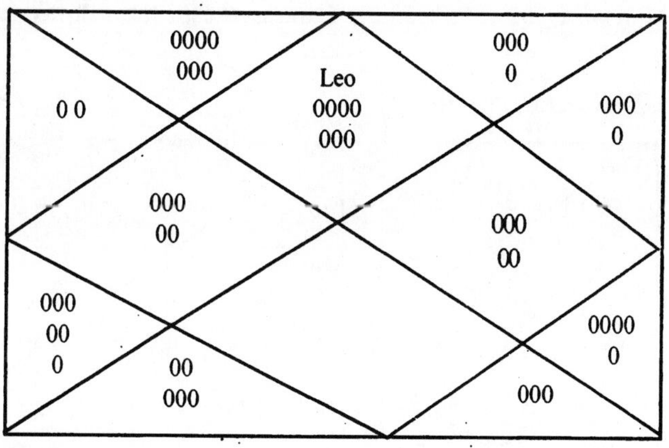

From-	Sun-9,	Moon-5,	Mars-7,
Mercury- 8,	Jupiter-8,	Venus-6	Saturn-4 and
Ascendant-9			

Now we give the Ashtakvarga of Venus.

जात्यां श्रीस्तु रवेर्विधोः पुरगवामन्दोळ्पुत्रे तनोः
पौरे लाभमदळिके कुरुलवं मोहे धनेढ्ये भृगोः।
लोभस्ताळिपरे कुजाद्रविसुतान्नार्भ महाब्धौ नये
ज्ञाळक्ष्मीचुळके गुरोर्मदधताढ्योऽसौ भृगुः सौख्यदः ॥८॥

In order to cast the Ashtakvarga of Venus, from which planets at what points the benefic Bindus are to be placed- has been given below-

From Sun	8-10-11
Moon	1-2-3-4-5-8-9-11-12
*Mars	3-4-6-9-11-12
Mercury	3-5-6-9-11
Jupiter	5-8-9-10-11
Venus	1-2-3-4-5-8-9-10-11
Saturn	3-4-5-8-9-10-11
Ascendant	1-2-3-4-5-8-9-11

This way 52 total benefic Bindus are in the Ashtakvarga of Venus.

Venus' Ashtakvarga

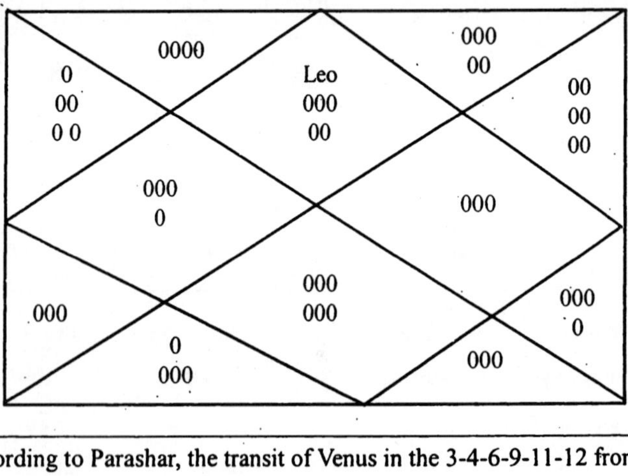

*According to Parashar, the transit of Venus in the 3-4-6-9-11-12 from Mars is beneficial.

From Sun- 3, Moon-9, Mars-6, Mercury-5, Jupiter-5, Venus-9, Saturn-7, Ascendant-8.

Now we construct the Ashtakvarga of Saturn.

रवेर्यात्रावीथीजनय शशिनो लक्षय शनेः
　　गुणेस्तत्यो भौमाद्गणितनिकरोऽसौ शुभकरः ।
शताकारे जीवात्तदधनपरे ज्ञादुदयभात्
　　कलाभूतानम्ये भृगुज चयखे सूर्यतनयः ॥९ ॥

In order to cast the Ashtakvarga of Saturn, place benefic points in the following signs from the signs occupied by various planets:-

From	Sun	1-2-4-7-8-10-11
	Moon	3-6-1
	Mars	3-5-6-10-11-12
	Mercury	6-8-9-10-11-12
	Jupiter	5-6-11-12
	Venus	6-11-12
	Saturn	3-5-6-11
	Ascendant	1-3-4-6-10-11

Saturn's Ashtakvarga

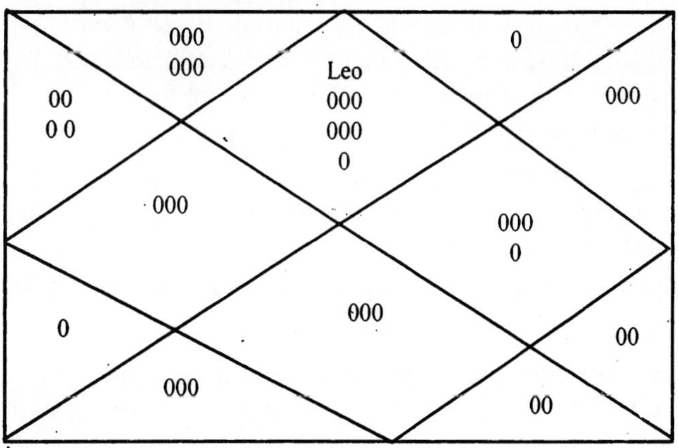

This way there are 39 benefic points in Saturn's Ashtakvarga,

7 from Sun, 3 from Moon; 6 from Mars, 6 from Mercury, 4 from Jupiter, 3 from Venus, 4 from Saturn, 6 from Ascendant.

इति निगदितमिष्टं नेष्टमन्यद्विशेषा-
दधिकफलविपाकं जन्मिनां वत्र दद्युः ।
उपचयगृहमित्रस्वोच्चगैः पुष्टमिष्टं
त्वपचयगृहनीचारातिगैर्नेष्टसम्पत् ॥१० ॥

When planets in transit pass through the houses where benefic Bindus are placed in the Ashtakvargas given above then they will give benefic results. The places which have not been indicated the transit of planets in those house will show evil results. For example Saturn in 1-2-4-7-8-10-11 places from Sun, shows good results. (This is mentioned above in Sloka No. 9). For example (see horoscope on page 513). Sun is in Scorpio so from Sun when Saturn transits in Scorpio, Sagittarius, Aquarius, Taurus, Gemini, Leo and Virgo as these are in the 1,2,4,7,8, 10 and 11 signs from Scorpio where Sun is posited at birth, then it will show beneficial results.

In the remaining signs *i.e.* Aries, Cancer, Libra, Capricorn, Pisces, the transit of Saturn will not be good. Therefore as has been illustrated with the transit of Saturn from Sun, in similar manner when the other planets and Ascendant (7+1) *i.e.* 8 in all are considered then it is called 'Ashtakvarga'. This should be observed as to how many benefic points are placed. If in one house (sign), there are 8 benefic points then it should be concluded that the transit of planet will give full good effects and if there are no benefic point then the transit will show enormous ill effects.

If there are four benefic points then it should be understood that from the angle of 4 planets it will be beneficial and from the angle of the other 4 it will be evil*.

In Saturn's Ashtakvarga made above, there are 7 benefic Bindus in Leo. Only the transit of Venus in that sign is not benefic.

See horoscope (on page 513) Venus is in Scorpio and from it only the 6-11-12 houses from it, in Saturn's Ashtakvarga can get

---

*Seven planet and the Ascendant make it eight.

benefic Bindus. (see page 513). Leo is the 10th house from Scorpio and therefore there would be no benefic point for Venus. It has only 7 points of other planets and the Ascendant. It is a benefic place from Sun, Moon, Mars, Mercury, Jupiter, Saturn and the Ascendant for the transit of Saturn.

Due to 7 Bindus the transit will be quite positive and effective. Where there is only one benefic point then Saturn when it transits that house than it will show much ill effects.

When there are 4 Bindus, the result will be medium. The more the benefic points than 4, the more the benefic effect. Less than 4 indicates ill effects. This is a general rule. Besides this two extra things should be kept in mind:

A. If a planet in transit is in own sign or exalted sign or in the sign of a friend and is also in an Upachayas* then the ill effects are reduced and good effects are increased. The meaning of this is that suppose there are three benefic points. But the planet is transiting in its own sign and also is in an Upchay Sthan then the results will not be that bad. If five points are there and it is also in Upchay Sthan and in the sign of a friend then the benefic results that comes due to having five benefic points will be much more.

B. If a planet is debilitated or in the sign of an enemy and also in places which are Unupchay** in transit then if there are very less benefic points and the planet is supposed to show ill effect then the ill effect will increase in intensity. If in the Unupchay sign it also co-insides with the debilitated sign of a planet in transit then inspite of having more benefic points it will not be able to show that much better results* as it would otherwise show. Rather the benefic results are be reduced. Here one doubt comes that if a planet is in the sign of a friend but it is not in, Unupchay sign or if it is in the sign of an enemy but is in Upchayy sign then what will be the effect? The answer to this is that;

---

*The 3rd, 6th, 10th and 11th houses from the ascendant are called Upchay places.

**The 1, 2, 4, 5, 7, 8, 9 and 12 places from the ascendant are called Unupchayasthana.

Benefics	Malefics
(i) To have more bindus	(iv) To have less bindus
(ii) To be in own sign, excalted sign, sign of a great friend or sign of a friend.	(v) To be in sign of debilitation, great enemy or enemy.
(iii) To be in Upachaya Sthana.	(vi) To be in Unupchaya Sthana.

(i), (ii) and (iii) indicate benefic results. (iv), ((v) and (vi) indicates ill effects. If some indications are of benefic results and some signs of ill effects then mixed results should be concluded.

कृत्वाष्टवर्गं द्युसदां क्रियादि-
ष्वक्षैर्विहीने मृतिरेकबिन्दोः ।
नाशो व्ययो भीतिभयार्थनारी-
श्रीराज्यसिद्धिः क्रमशः फलानि ॥११ ॥

When Ashtak Vargas are cast then it should be seen as to which sign contains how many bindus. If in a sign there are no benefic bindus then when a planet comes to that sign then there is sufferings equal to death. Here the doubt aries that suppose in the Ashtakvarga of Sun there are no points, and Sun in transit goes to that sign every year for one month. Will that month every year give suffering equal to death? Here one thing should be kept in mind that one planet alone does not cause that much sufferings. When many planets are malefic and indicate ill-effects and the major and minor periods and transits are all bad then death can take place. And in transit when many planet are bad only then the intensity of sufferings increase. If eight planets are favourable and only one is unfavourable then how can one glass of hot water reduce the coldness of eight glasses of cold water? In general malefic planets do not show that much ill effect during transit. Secondly when the death has been mentioned it does not mean actual death but it should be interpreted that it is time of sufferings, sorrows and problems equal to death *i.e.* disease, loss of wealth etc.

When there is only one benefic point then there is loss. If there are two points then expenses, three points fear, four points then also fear should be concluded. Although Mantreshwar Maharaj has said that three points or four points they show almost the same type of effect but we are of the opinion that in the sign which has four points, the transit over there will not show ill effect. If five points are there then attainment of the desired object or wealth. Six points indicate gain of women. Seven indicates gain of laxmi and eight indicates attainment of kingdom *i.e.* honour and prestige increases in the king's court.

तत्तद्ग्रहाधिष्ठितसर्वराशीं-
स्तत्संज्ञितं लग्नमिति प्रकल्प्य।
तेभ्यः फलान्यष्टविधान्यभूवं-
स्तत्तद्गृहाद्धा ववशाद्वदन्तु ॥१२॥

In India two type of Ashtakvarga Charts are cast-

1. Like the one we have done for the Sun's Ashtak Varga on (Page 517) i.e. the ascendant is Leo in the nativity and in the Ashtak Varga of Sun Leo is taken as the ascendant.
2. The second system is that the number of bindus in signs will be kept as it is. But instead of using the common ascendant (Leo) it will vary according to the planet whose Ashtak Varga has to be cast *i.e.* if Sun is in Scorpio then Scorpio will be placed in the ascendant. On page 517 the Sun's Ashtakvarga will be written as follows *i.e.* the Ashtakvarga of whichever planet has to be cast then the sign where the planet is, will be used as the ascendant.

Ashtakvarga of Sun

Now see in this lagna as to how many benefic points are in various houses. From this ascendant the house which has more benefic points that house will show good effect when Sun in transit passes through that house.

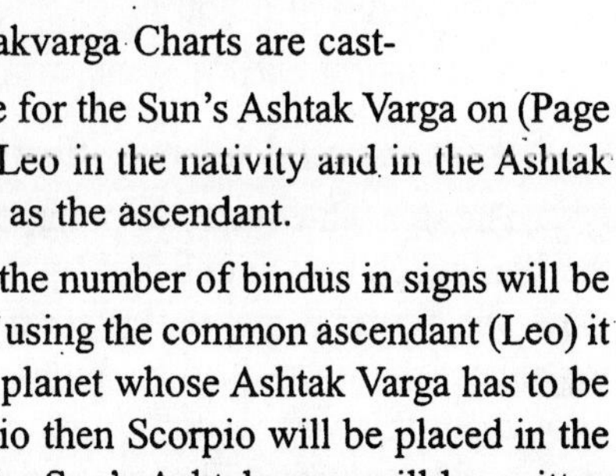

For example— Sun is in Scorpio and the 7th from this is Taurus. In Taurus we have 7 benefic points. So when Sun goes in transit to Taurus there will be excellent result related to wife or related to the 7th house matters. In the chart above with Scorpio as the ascendant in the Sun's Ashtak Varga. There is only one point in the 5th (from the Scorpio ascendant) *i.e.* in Pisces in the 5th house. So when Sun will transit Pisces it will cause mental tension, anguish, problem to children, stomach problem etc. The essence of this Sloka is that use the sign where a planet is posited as Ascendant and then count from that place different houses to know the effect of the transit of that planet.

तत्तद्ग्रहर्क्षांशकतुल्यभांश
स्थिता ग्रहाश्चारवशादिदानीम्।
तथैव तद्भावसमुत्थितानि
फलानि कुर्वन्ति शुभाशुभानि ॥१३॥

When the good and bad effect of the transit will be felt?

The sign which has few points the ill effect will be felt there and the sign which has more benefic points good results will be realized. However Jupiter is in one sign for one year and Saturn is in one sign for almost two years and six month; then how can it be decided if throughout this year or for a long period of two and half years, the transit of the planet will show good or bad effects. We explain this now.

Suppose in the example horoscope on page 517, Jupiter has covered 14 degrees and in the 2nd house in Virgo, which is the 2nd house from the ascendant, Jupiter has 7 benefic points. So when in transit Jupiter will enter into Virgo *i.e.* the 2nd house and by transit it will proceed to 14 degrees then it will show the full benefic effect. In different horoscope, different planets have different degrees. So a planet in transit will show good or ill effects at different times because it will go to separate degrees in different nativities *i.e.* suppose three persons viz. Yagyadatta, Devdatta and Bhavadatta. All the three has a favourable Jupiter in transit in Sagittarius then in the horoscope of Yagyadatta if Jupiter has 7 degrees, in the horoscope of Devdatta, 14 degrees, and in the horoscope of Bhavadatta, 21 degrees, then when Jupiter traverses to 7 degrees of Sagittarius then Yagyadatta will feel the good effect. When Jupiter will go to 14 degrees then Devdatta will realise good effects and when in the same Sagittarius when it will attain 21 degrees in transit then Bhavadatta will get beneficial results.

कृतेऽष्टवर्गे सति कारकर्क्षात्-
यद्भावमुक्ताङ्कमुपैति खेटः ।
तद्भावपुष्टिं सशुभोऽशुभो वा
करोत्यनुक्ते विपरीतमेव ॥१४॥

In this Sloka the same thing have been repeated which has been mentioned in the Sloka 12 above that the planet whose transit is under consideration its position in the nativity, and from that house in which house it is transiting. It will show the good or bad effect of the house where it is in transit. If there are more benefic points then the effect will be good.

If there are very few benefic points then it will show ill effect. The same thing is explained by example. In Sloka No. 13, see the example about the transit of Jupiter in Sagittarius for three persons viz. Yagyadatta, Devdatta and Bhavadatta. Will they be able to realize the same type of effect with the same intensity? The answer is No. If in the birth chart of Yagyadatta. Jupiter is posited in Aries then Sagittarius being the 9th house from Aries he will get the happiness of the 9th house *i.e.* his fortunes will smile. In the horoscope of Devdatta Jupiter is in Gemini and from Gemini, Sagittarius is in the 7th house so Devdatta will have happiness related to 7th house *i.e.* may get married or happiness related to wife may come and in the horoscope of Bhavadatta Jupiter is in Leo at birth so Sagittarius being the 5th from Leo. He will have happiness related to sons or education depending upon his age.

एकत्र भावे बहवो यदानी-
मुक्ताङ्कगाश्चारवशाद्व्रजन्ति ।
पुष्णन्ति तद्भावफलानि सम्यक्
तत्कारकात्तत्तनुपूर्वभावे ॥१५॥

We have explained above the principle that when the effect of a house will be felt. In order to consider this it should be seen as to the planet whose transit is under consideration, where that planet is posited, in the birth chart.

Suppose Jupiter is transiting in the 10th house from the radical position it occupies at birth and in the Ashtak Varga of Jupiter there are more points; Saturn is transiting the 10th house from its radical position at birth and in the Ashtak Varga of Saturn, there are more bindus. Sun is transiting the 10th from the radical position it occupies at birth and in the Sun's Ashtak Varga there are more points in that place and so on this way when many planets are transiting from their radical positions the same houses simultaneously then the houses, they are passing through where there are more points then special good results are realized related to that house. As we have mentioned above about Sun, Jupiter and Saturn are transiting the 10th house from their radical positions in their respective AshtakVargas and that house has more points, then the full effect related to the 10th will be realized.

बिन्दौ स्थिते तत्फलसिद्धिकाल
विनिर्णयाय प्रहितेऽष्टवर्गे।
भान्यष्टधा तत्र विभज्य कक्षा
क्रमेण तेषां फलमाहुरन्ये ॥१६ ॥

आलिख्य चक्रं नव पूर्वरेखाः
याम्योत्तरस्था दश च त्रिरेखाः ।
प्रस्तारकं षणणवतिप्रकोष्ठं
पङ्क्त्यष्टकं चाष्टकवर्गजं स्यात् ॥१७ ॥

होराशशीबोधनशुक्रसूर्य-
भौमामरेन्द्रार्चितभानुपुत्राः ।
याम्यादिपङ् क्त्यष्टकराशिनाथाः
क्रमेण तद्बिन्दुफलप्रदाः स्युः ॥१८ ॥

Ashtakvarga of Saturn

	Aries	Taurus	Gemini	Cancer	Leo	Virgo	Libra	Scorpio	Sag.	Cap.	Aquarius	Pisces
Sat			0		0	0					0	
Jup					0	0					0	0
Mars	0				0	0	0			0		0
Sun		0	0		0	0		0	0		0	
Ven	0					0	0					
Mer		0		0	0	0	0	0				
Moon		0			0					0		
Asc.		0	0		0		0	0		0		
	2	4	3	1	7	6	4	3	1	3	3	2

राश्यष्टभागप्रथमांशकाले
शनिर्द्वितीये तु गुरुः फलाय।
कक्षाक्रमेणैवमिहान्त्यभाग-
काले विलग्नं फलदं प्रदिष्टम्॥१९॥

In this Sloka-16 it has been mentioned when the effect of the transit will take place. In the next page the detailed Ashtak Varga of Saturn has been given.

The Ashtak Varga of Saturn

Saturn is in one sign for two and half years. When will it show benefic result and what other time it will show ill effects? We have already pointed out in Sloka No. 13 above one method to decide about it. Now we tell another method, (on Page 521).

Make a chart of 96 squares - and suppose we have to consider the transit of Saturn then the Ashtak Varga of Saturn which has been erected on page 513, in the same manner make the Ashtak Varga of Saturn. It has been mentioned that in order to make the Ashtak Varga of Saturn. Then from the Sun benefic points are placed in the 1,2,4,7,8,10,11 house and so from Sun being in Scorpio and then from the Scorpio the 1, 2, 4, 7, 8, 10, 11 are Scorpio, Sagittarius, Aquarius, Taurus, Gemini, Leo and Virgo place benefic points. Similarly the benefic points from other planets should be placed. Where the benefic points will be placed is given in the previous page and we will get the Ashtak Varga of Saturn.

In Aries above Saturn has two points— four in Taurus and three in Gemini, one in Cancer, seven in Leo, six in Virgo, 4 in Libra, three in Scorpio; one in Sagittarius, three in Capricorn, three in Aquarius and two in Pisces.

Now look at page 513 where the Ashtak Varga of Saturn is cast. In the ascendant in Leo, there are seven points. In the second from ascendant in Virgo six points, in the 3rd from the ascendant *i.e.* Libra four points etc. on Page 513 and Page 521, in both places is Saturn's Ashtak Varga of the same horoscope. Why did we cast another Ashtak Varga for Saturn on page 521 the reason is that on page 521 the Ashtak Varga that we have, indicates as to which planet has contributed a positive points to which sign. What is the purpose of all this? We explain the same here as under.

Divide each sign into 8 parts. We know that each sign has 30 degrees. When this 30 degrees are divided by 8 then we gets 3 degrees and 45 minutes. So there are 8 parts and each part has 3 degrees and 45 minutes. Whichever sign it may be the first part out of the 8, will come under the jurisdiction of Saturn. So beginning from the first 3 degrees and 45 minutes it will be called the portion of Saturn. On the 2nd part of this 8th division Jupiter will have its control. Therefore from 3 degrees, 45 minutes to 7 degrees, 30 minutes will be the portion of Jupiter. After Jupiter, the 3rd portion of 7 degrees, 30 minutes to 11 degrees, 15 minutes will be the portion of Mars. After Mars the portion of Sun, it will be followed by that of Venus. After that will be Mercury and after Mercury will be Moon. The last portion between 26 degrees, 15 minutes to 30 degrees will be the portion of the ascendant. Therefore in the table of the Ashtak Varga Chakra of Saturn on Page 521, the order will be Saturn, Jupiter, Mars, Sun, Venus, Mercury, Moon and ascendant.

Now look to the sign Leo - Saturn, Jupiter, Mars, Sun, Mercury, Moon and ascendant has contributed their benefic points. Therefore when Saturn will go in the portions of these planets during transit then it will show good effect. But when it will transit the portion of Venus *i.e.* the 5th portion between 15 degrees to 18°.45', then it will not show any benefic results but will show ill results. It is so because in the Ashtak Varga of Saturn, Venus has not been able to contribute any benefic points. This is a Microscopic analysis of transits.

सर्वग्रहाणां प्रहितेऽष्टवर्गे
तत्कालराशिस्थितबिन्दुयोगे।
अष्टाक्षसंख्याधिकविन्दवश्वेत्
शुभं तदूने व्यसनं क्रमेण॥२०॥

Now we mention how to cast Sarvashtak Varga. Construct the Sarvashtak Varga in the following manner—

First of all take into account the benefic points—

1. In which Ashtak Varga, which sign and how many bindus are there write it down.

2. Then make a new chart of the Ashtak Varga and then total the benefic points in different Ashtak Vargas in each sign.

For example- In Leo- In the 7 Ashtak Vargas, we have benefic points viz., 5, 6, 5, 5, 7, 5, 7 respectively. These benefic points are in the Ashtak Vargas of the 7 planets- Sun, Moon, Mars, etc. The total of is this is 40. So in the Sarwashtak Varga Chart write 40 in the sign Leo. Similarly the points in each sign of the bindus of different Ashtak Vargas should be added and placed in the Sarvashtak Varga Chart.

We now give below the Chart of Sun, Moon, Mars, Mercury, Jupiter, Venus, Saturn and the next one is Sarvashtak Varga. In each sign the number of benefic points are written in different Ashtak Vargas and the sum total separately of each sign is filled in the Sarvashtak Vargas.

Sun's Ashtakvarga

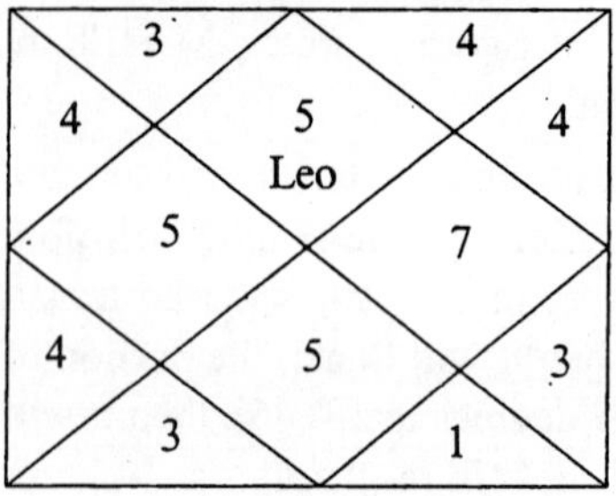

Moon's Ashtakvarga

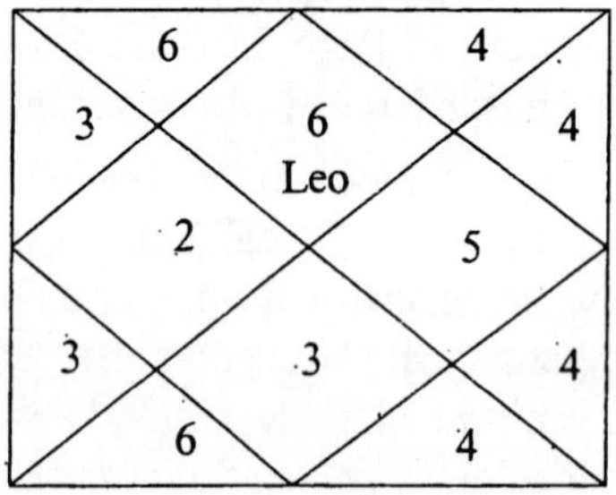

Mars'sAshtakvarga

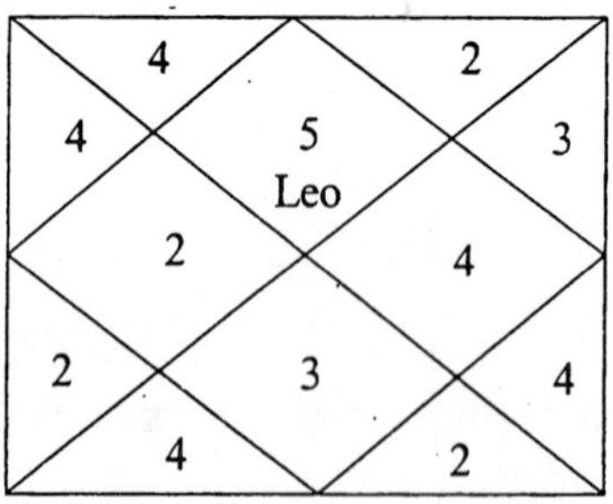

Mercury's Ashtakvarga

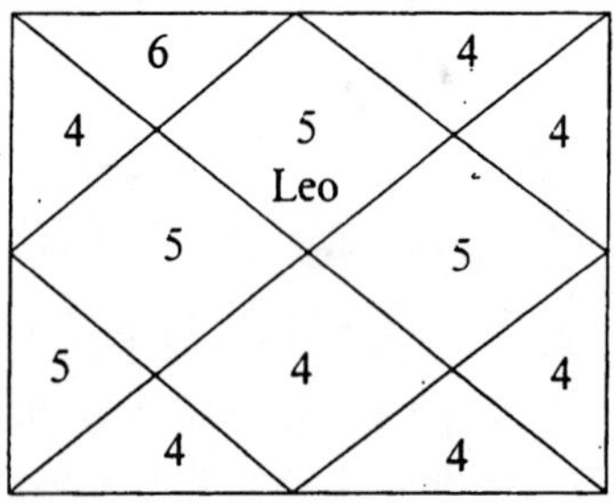

Jupiter's Ashtakvarga

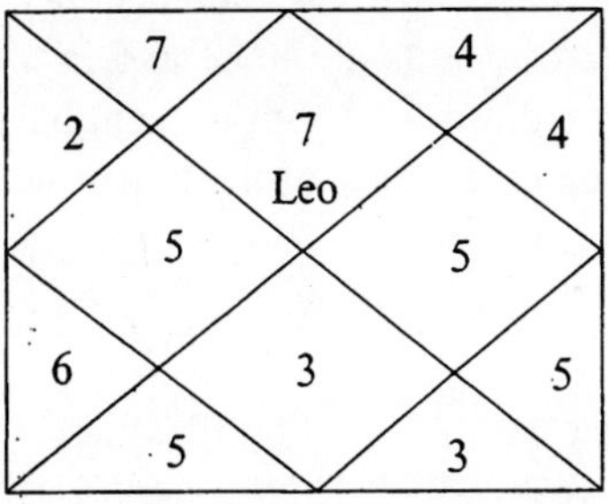

Venus's Ashtakvarga

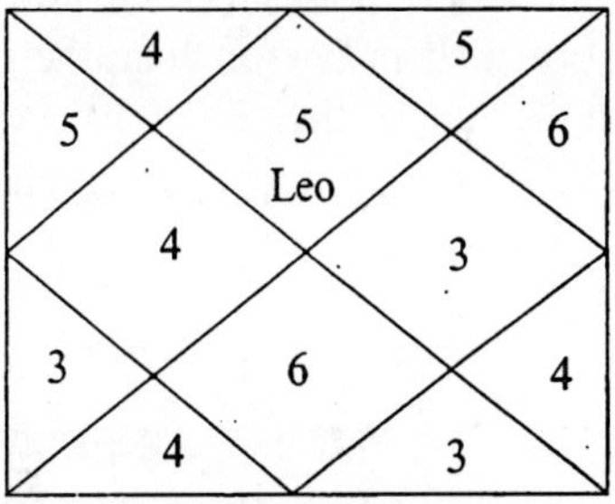

Saturn's Ashtakvarga

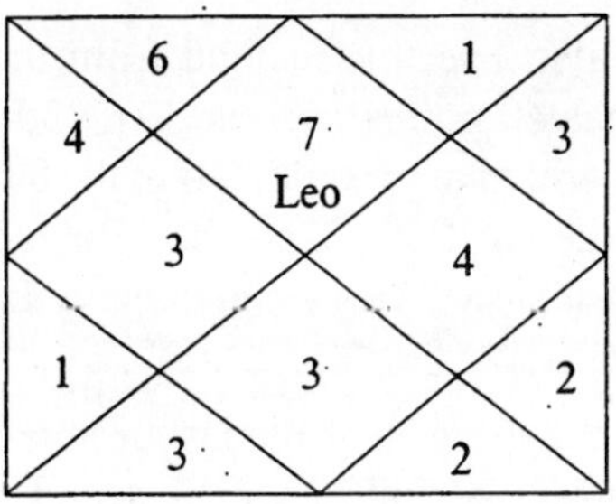

Sarvashtakvarga

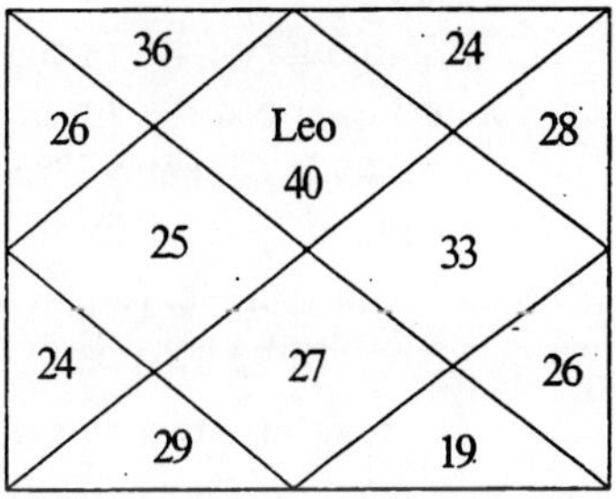

After creating the Sarvashtak Varga we should see as to how many benefic points are in different signs. Where the number of total points are 28 and more then when a planet in transit goes to that sign then it shows good effects. If the number is less then 28 then the transit of a planet in that sign will be negative. The lesser the number from 28, the more will be the malefic effects. Here one doubt comes to mind that suppose we have to consider the transit of Saturn in the Sarvashtak Varga where there are 30 points in a sign, but in the Saturn's Ashtak Varga there are only two benefic points in that sign, then whether it will show beneficial effect? Or suppose that in the Saturn's Ashtak Varga there are six benefic points, but in the Sarvashtak Varga there are 22 points only, then will the transit of Saturn in that sign will show malefic effect?

The answer to this is that in the Ashtak Varga of each planet whatever are the benefic points and side by side in the Sarvashtak Varga the number of points in that sign both of these should be examined and then logical conclusion be drawn. If both of them have good number of points then the transit of a planet will show full beneficial effect. If in one of them the number of points are more and in the other not so then the transit will be medium or if both of them have very little points, then completely negative effect of the transit will take place.

यावन्तुस्तुहिनरुचे: शुभाङ्कसंस्था
यावन्त: शुभभवने हिमद्युतेर्वा।
इत्थं तद्विदितमिहाधिके च तेभ्य:
स्तस्त्यूने विपदिति सूचितं परेषाम्॥२१॥

Commentary- Many persons also use this method from the ascendant: Suppose the 1st house, has 40 points, then the 1st, 13th, 25th, 37th, 49th, 61st and 73rd years will give rise in life. If in the 8th house there are 19 total points, then the 8th, 20th, 32nd, the 44th, the 56th and 68th years there will be physical suffering *i.e.* after every 12 years, there will be a repeat.

This way in whichever house the number of bindus are more than that year, and every 12th years after that will be beneficial and if there are less points in a house then that year and every 12 years subsequently, there will be sufferings. For special reference to this please see— 'Janma Patrika Vidhnam' by Sh. Jeev Nath Sharma, pages 36 to page 41.

Generally the three houses the 6th, the 8th, and the 12th - All these three are not good houses and the remaining houses are good houses. It is nice to have more benefic points in benefic houses. In the same manner consideration should also be done from the radical Moon *i.e.* using Moon at birth as ascendant.

a. If from the Moon ascendant in the benefic houses there are 28 or more bindus then it indicates efficacy and good effect of that house. If it is less then 28 then losses and negative results related to those houses will be felt.

b. See also the placement of benefic planets from the radical Moon. If in these signs where the benefic planets are posited, there are 28 or more points then it will increase the good effects of that house. If there are 28 or less points then ill effects related to these houses should be concluded.

कुर्तः स्वजन्मसमयावसथग्रहणां
कृत्वाष्टवर्गकथिताक्षविधानमत्र।
बह्वक्षयोगवशतः शुभराशिमास-
भावग्रहस्थितिषु कर्मशुभं विदध्यात्॥२२॥

The system of how to make Sarvashtak Varga has been mentioned above. It can also be used in another manner. The ascendant and the 7 planet all these 8, are in the Sarvashtak Varga which has been cast. Based on this Varga whichever sign has more points then good work should be undertaken in that sign. This will result in special success.

For example— If it is Leo ascendant and in this Leo sign, in the Sarvashtak Varga there are 40 benefic points. Then when Sun is in Leo or Moon is in Leo or Jupiter is in Leo or when Leo is rising in the Eastern horizon, then the person whose nativity is being considered above, whatever work he will undertake that will result in special success. For a person— which year, which month and which day will be favourable for success? The answer is that this system of Sarvashtak Varga is very authentic and mathematical to arrive at a conclusion.

पापोऽपि स्वगृहस्थश्चेद्भाववृद्धिं करोत्यलम्।
नीचारातिगृहस्थचेत्कुर्याद्भावक्षयं ध्रुवम्॥२३॥

Now we speak of one more method of how to take the transit into account. If a malefic goes by transit in it own sign then it increases the efficacy of that sign *i.e.* the effect is beneficial. But if a planet in transit, in its sign of debilitation or sign belonging to its enemy then it spoils the effect of that house.

स्वोच्चस्थोऽपि शुभो भावहानिं दुःस्थानपो यदि।
सुस्थानपश्चेत् स्वोच्चस्थः पापी भावानुकूल्यकृत॥२४॥

If a planet is the ruler of dusthan *i.e.* 6th, 8th or 12th house then even if it is a benefic planet is and even if it is in its sign of exaltation it will spoil the house it is posited in. However if it is the lord of a good house and is exalted then it will increase the efficacy of that house.

Comments— In the Sloka No. 23 and 24 above the principles which have been mentioned in the context of the transit should also be used in both the nativity and transit, with equal importance.

24

Ashtak Varga Phala (Interpretations of the Ashtak Varga)

अर्कस्थितस्य नवमो राशिः पितृगृहः स्मृतः।
तद्राशिफलसंख्याभिर्वर्द्धयेच्छोध्यपिण्डकम् ॥१॥

Now we speak of the interpretation which have been given in 'Horasar'. Count from the sign where Sun is placed. The 9th sign from that Sun sign is called the house of father *i.e.* consideration about father is done from that house. In the Sun's Ashtakvarga see how many benefic points are there in the house of father. Multiply those points by 'Shodhya Pind'. How to make Shodhya Pind is explained subsequently.

सप्तविंशहृताल्लब्धं नक्षत्र याति भानुजे।
तस्मिन् काले पितृक्लेशो भविष्यति न संशयः ॥२॥

The number that comes according to the method explained above, divide this by 27. The balance which comes after this division that will be counted as one for Ashwini, two as Bharani, three as Krittika etc., When Saturn in transit comes to that Nakshatra then there is definitely sufferings for the father.

तत्त्रिकोणगते वाऽपि पितृतुल्यस्य वा मृतिः।
संयोगः शोध्यशोषाणां शोध्यपिण्ड इति स्मृतः ॥३॥

Otherwise when Saturn transits a trine from the constellation which has been mentioned in Sloka No. 2, then there is death to Uncle or people as good as father. The number of Ashwini is one and the trine from Ashwini is 'Magha' and 'Mool'. In the trine from Bharani are Poorva Phalguni and Poorvashad. Similarly the trine from other constellation should be followed. After doing the Trikon Sodhan and Ekadhipadtya Sodhan, whatever the benefic points are left, they are called the Shodhya Pind. We shall explain how to do the Trikon Shodhan and Ekadhipadtya Shodhan.

लग्नात्सुखेश्वरांशेशदशायां च पितृक्षयः।
सुखनाथदशायां वा पितृतुल्यमृतिं वदेत् ॥४॥

The death of father can take place in the periodic influence of the lord of the Navansha occupied by the lord of the 4th house from the ascendant. In the periodic influences of the lord of the 4th house there is death of Uncle or people equivalent to father.

संशोध्य पिण्डं सूर्यस्य रन्ध्रामानेन वर्द्धयेत्।
द्वादशेन हताच्छेषराशिं याते दिवाकरे ॥५॥

तत्त्रिकोणगते वाऽपि मरणं तस्य निर्दिशेत्।
एवं ग्रहाणां सर्वेषां चिन्तयेन्मतिमान्नरः ॥६॥

In the Suryashtakvarga, whatever Shodhya Pind comes, add 8 and whatever comes out of adding 8 divide that number by 12. The remainder will give the signs viz. if it left, then Aries, 2 is left then Taurus etc. 12th. When Sun in transits comes to that sign or in the 5th or 9th signs from that signs, then the possibility of the death of father exists. Although Sun comes in those signs every year yet the real meaning is that at that time the major and minor periodic influences, and the transit of Saturn should also indicate the death of father. Only then the transit of Sun should be taken into account to judge the month of death and that is why the transit of Sun has to be explained. As the timing of the death of father has been mentioned in the Sun's Ashtakvarga in the above Slokas, in the same manner, decision about the mother's death from the Moon's Ashtakvarga and from the Mars' Ashtakvarga about brother etc. should be considered by the intelligent persons.

चन्द्रात्सुखाष्टमेशांशत्रिकोणे दिवसाधिपे।
मातुर्वियोगं तन्मासे निर्दिशेल्लग्नतः पितुः॥८॥

Multiply the benefic points in the 4th sign in the Moon's Ashtakvarga by the Shodhya Pind in the Ashtakvarga of Moon. The product so realised should be divided by 27. The balance or the trine from it will indicate the number of the constellation in which when Saturn comes in transit then the death of mother should be surmised.

चन्द्रात्सुखफलैः पिण्डं हत्वा सारावशेषितम्।
शनौ याते मातृहानिः त्रिकोणर्क्षगतेऽपि वा ॥७॥

Look to the Navanshas where the lords of the 4th and 8th house from the Moon sign are placed. When Sun transits the Navansha or transit a sign in trine to this Navansha then the death of mother should be judged. As the Navansha of the lords of the 4th and 8th houses from the Moon has been judged in the same manner the Navanshas of the lords of the 4th and 8th houses from the ascendant should be considered when Sun in transit comes to these Navanshas or to a Navansha in trine to these then the death of father can take place.

भौमात्तृतीयराशिस्थफलर्भ्रातृगणं वदेत्।
बुधात्सुखफलैर्बन्धुगणं वा मातुलस्य च ॥९॥

See the number of the benefic point in the 3rd house from the sign Mars is placed in its own Ashtakvarga. The native will have the same number of brothers as indicated by the benefic points. In the Ashtakvarga of Mercury the benefic points in the 4th sign from the sign occupied by Mercury should be observed. The number of benefic points will indicate the number of maternal uncles or relatives from the mother's side.

गुरुस्थितसुतस्थाने यावतां विद्यते फलम्।
शत्रुनीचग्रहं त्यक्त्वा शेषास्तस्यात्मजाः स्मृताः ॥१०॥

Look to the sign occupied by Jupiter in its Ashtakvarga. The benefic points in the 5th sign from the sign occupied by Jupiter will indicate the number of sons. But if some enemy or debilitated planet has contributed a point in this place then that number given by the enemy or debilitated planet, should be reduced from the total number of benefic points.

गुरोरष्टकवर्गे तु शोध्यशिष्टफलानि वै।
क्रूरराशिफलं त्यक्त्वा शेषास्तस्यात्मजाः स्मृताः ॥११॥

In the Ashtakvarga of Jupiter after doing the Trikon Sodhan and Ekadhipadtya Sodhan whichever number comes, from that number we should subtract the points contributed by malefic planets. The balance will indicate the number of sons.

फलाधिकं भृगोर्यत्र तत्र भार्याजनिर्यदि।
तस्यां वंशाभिवृद्धिः स्यादल्पे क्षीणार्थसंततिः ॥१२॥

In the Ashtakvarga of Venus the signs which have more benefic points and if marriage takes place with a girl whose ascendant or Moon sign is that sign where the number of benefic are more then there children will be born and the family continues. If in the horoscope of the native in the Ashtakvarga of Venus the signs which have very little benefic points and then marriage takes place with a girl whose ascendant or Moon signs falls in those signs then there will be few issues. Same Commentators have translated this Sloka in the manner given below—

A girl born in the periodic influence of that sign which contains more benefic points in the Venus Ashtakvarga of Venus in a native's chart, then marriage with that girl is fruitful. Marriage with a girl who is born in the periodic influence of that sign where the number of benefic points in a native's horoscope in the Ashtakvarga of Venus are few then there will be less children. Therefore association and marriage with a girl sign where born in a sign where benefic points are more auspicious.

शोध्यपिण्डं श्लेर्लग्नाद्धत्वा रन्ध्रफलैः सुखैः।
हत्वावशेषभं याते मन्दे जीवेऽपि वा मृतिः ॥१३॥

In the Ashtakvarga of Saturn multiply the total benefic points between the ascendant and the 8th sign from the lagna with Shodhya Pind. Divide this product by 27. The remainder will give the number of the constellation where when Jupiter or Saturn in transit passes through then the death of the native can take place. This is possible if the native is also at the same time passing through the major or minor periodic influence of a Markesh.

लग्नादिमन्दान्तफलैक्यसंख्या-
वर्षे विपत्तिस्तु तथार्कपुत्रात्।
यावद्विलग्गान्तफलानि तस्मिन्-
नाशो हि तद्योगसमानवर्षे ॥१४॥

Count from the ascendant to the sign in which Saturn is placed in the birth chart. Add together the benefic points in the Ashtakvarga of Saturn. Both the ascendant and the sign occupied by Saturn are included. The total number will indicate the year in which calamities will come. Similarly count from the sign occupied by Saturn to the ascendant (all the signs including the ascendant and the sign occupied by Saturn are included). Add together the benefic points in all these signs. The sum total will indicate the number of the year in which sufferings will come.

For example - If the total comes to 15 then the 15th year will be a difficult year of life.

अष्टमस्थफलैर्लग्नात्पिण्डं हत्वा सुखैर्भजेत्।
फलमायुर्विजानीयात्प्राग्वद्वेलां तु कल्पयेत्॥१५॥

In the Ashtakvarga of Saturn multiply the total of the benefic points in between the ascendant and the 8th house. This product is now divided by 27. The Dividend will indicate the age *i.e.* the longevity of the native. Besides the timing of death should be decided with the principles given before.

त्रिकोणेषु तु यन्नयूनं तत्तुल्यं त्रिषु शोधयेत्।
एकस्मिन् भवने शून्ये तत्त्रिकोणं न शोधयेत्॥१६॥

भवनद्वयशून्ये तु शोधयेदन्यमन्दिरम्।
समत्वे सर्वगेहेषु सर्वं संशोधयेत्तदा॥१७॥

Trikonsodhan

Now we will speak of the Trikon Sodhan and Ekadhipatya Sodhan. This is an important part of the Ashtakvarga. Before going into what Mantreshwar has to say in this regard, it is necessary to introduce this subject to some extent, so that the readers will find it easy to understand the Slokas.

1. Aries, Leo and Sagittarius together make a trine because Leo is the 5th from Aries and Sagittarius is the 5th sign from Leo and Aries is the 5th sign from Sagittarius. The Sanskrit word 'Trikona' in English means trine.
2. Similarly Taurus, Virgo and Capricorn is another trine.
3. Gemini, Libra and Aquarius is the 3rd trine.
4. Cancer, Scorpio and Pisces is the 4th trine.

We have first introduced the method to cast an Ashtakvarga.

Sun, Moon, Mars, Mercury, Jupiter, Venus and Saturn for all these seven planets, seven Ashtakvargas are made. The Trikon Sodhan of all the Ashtakvarga is done separately.

For example— Suppose we have to do the Trikon Sodhan of Sun's Ashtakvarga then observe as to how many benefic points are in Aries, Leo and Sagittarius.

Here Aries has 3, Leo has 5 and Sagittarius has 4 benefic points.

Now among the Scholars of Sanskrit and famous Astrologer as well as between different well known learned people there are differences as to how to perform the Trikon Sodhan. The various opinions are :

1. The first opinion is that in the three sign of a trine whichever is the minimum number that number should be subtracted from the numbers in all the signs of the Trikon.

Sarvashtak Varga

PL/Sign	Aries	Taurus	Gemini	Cancer	Leo	Virgo	Libra	Scorpio	Sagittarius	Capricorn	Aquarius	Pisces	Total
Sun	3	7	4	4	5	3	4	5	4	3	5	1	48
Moon	4	5	4	4	6	6	3	1	3	6	3	4	49
Mars	4	4	3	2	5	4	4	2	2	4	3	2	39
Mercury	4	5	4	4	5	6	4	5	5	4	4	4	54
Jupiter	5	5	4	4	7	7	2	5	6	5	3	3	36
Venus	4	3	6	5	5	4	5	4	3	4	6	3	52
Saturn	2	4	3	1	7	6	4	3	1	3	3	2	39
Total	26	33	28	24	40	36	26	25	24	29	27	19	337

For example— If in the Sun's Asthakvarga, Aries has 3, Leo 5 and Sagittarius 4, then out of these the minimum number is 3. So 3 should be subtracted from the number 5 in Leo like 5-3=2 as balance. Similarly 3 should also be subtracted in the number 4 in Sagittarius i.e. 4 -3 = 1 as balance. From Aries 3 should be subtracted, so 3-3 = 0 is the balance. Similarly in the Sun's Ashtakvarga the other trine Taurus, Virgo and Capricorn the three signs of the trine; in Taurus we have 7 number, in Virgo 3 and in Capricorn 3. Out of these 3, 7 and 3 we should subtract 3 as it is the smallest number, so the balance left in Taurus is 4, in Virgo 3 - 3 = 0, and Capricorn 3 -3 = 0. This should be the ordinary rule. Now in the 3rd trine of Gemini, Libra and Acquarius in the Sun's Ashtakvarga see how many Bindus are there. In Gemini 4, in Libra 4, and in Acquarius 5. According to the above rule the minimum number is 4. So this 4 should be subtracted from the numbers in each of the 3 signs. In Gemini 4 - 4 = 0, in Libra 4 - 4 = 0 and in Aquarius 5 - 4 = 1. These should be plotted. This is the ordinary rule. Now take the 4th trine in Sun's Ashtakvarga which compromises Cancer, Scorpio and Pisces. In Cancer the number is 4, in Scorpio is 5 and Pisces 1. The minimum here is 1 in Pisces. So this 1 should be subtracted from the number 4 in Cancer and so in Cancer we get 4 - 1 = 3 as the balance; in Scorpio we get 5 - 1 = 4 and in Pisces 1-1=0.

The rule that we have explained as the first opinion can be written out in the following manner—

a. In the three signs of a trine—whichever is the minimum number in any one of the sign that minimum number should be subtracted from the two signs of the trine separately. And whatever is the balance that balance should be written down below these three signs.

b. If there is a 0 in one sign of a trine then if we subtract 0 from the other two signs then there will no change and the remaining two signs of the trine will keep the same number in those places which has been before the process was done.

c. If there is the same number in all the three signs of the trine then if we subtract the same number from all the signs then there will be 0 at all places. For example in the Ashtakvarga of Mars we have to do the Trikon Sodhan and in this we have Taurus, Virgo and Capricorn then see that in the Ashtakvarga of Mars, Taurus has 4, Virgo has 4 and Capricorn has 4. Now this 4 when subtracted from 4 of Taurus then we have 4-4=0. Similarly in Virgo 4-4=0 and in Capricorn 4-4=0. This is one opinion and this is the opinion of Maharishi Parashar.

Second Opinion

Now we give the second opinion in the matter of Trikon Sodhan.

Suppose in the Sun's Ashtakvarga we have to do the Trikon Sodhan and in Aries we have 3, Leo 5 and in Sagittarius 4. The minimum number out of these is 3. So we will put 3 at all places *i.e.* Aries 3, Leo 3 and also in Sagittarius 3.

In Taurus 7, Virgo 3 and Capricorn 3 the minimum is 3. So we will place 3 in Taurus, 3 in Virgo and 3 in Capricorn. In the 3rd trine of Sun's Ashtakvarga Gemini has 4, Libra has 4 and Aquarius has 5. The minimum is 4 so we will place 4 in Aquarius and Gemini and Libra will also have 4.

In Cancer we have 4, Scorpio 5 and Pisces 1. The minimum is 1. So in Sun's Ashtakvarga in this trine after doing the Trikon Sodhan, 1 in Cancer, 1 in Scorpio and 1 in Pisces will be kept. This 2nd opinion is by the author of Hora Ratna, Sh. Bal Bhadra Ji. The opinion of Parashar prevails much more in the North of India and in South India more authoritative is the method of Bal Bhadra Ji. In the original Sanskrit text the part of the Sloka is as follow—

त्रिकोणेषुतु यन्यूनं तत्तुल्यं त्रिषु शोधयेत्।

That is in the trines whichever is the minimum the same should be kept after Trikon Sodhan. The other opinion has translated the Sloka in the manner that the minimum should be reduced from all the three of signs of the trine. So there are two opinions of the translation.

1. Keep the minimum number in all the three signs of a trine.
2. Reduce the minimum number from all the three.

Mantreshwar's Opinion

Mantreshwar Maharaj in Phal Deepika has written the same Sloka in Sanskrit which is available in the treatise of Parashar or Bal Bhadra *i.e.* Sloka 16 and 17.

The interpretation is-

1. If trikon sodhan is required in the Ashtakvarga of Sun or of any other planet, then the minimum number should be processed from all the three sings of a trine. The question is whether the number should be subtracted from all the three and then the balance should be written under every sign or the minimum number should be kept in all the signs *i.e.* the minimum number should be written under the three signs. The sloka given above has two meanings. The Commentators of Parashar has translated it in the manner that we have given as the first opinion and the opinion expressed in Hora Ratna (of Bal Bhadra Ji) we have used as the 2nd opinion, and it is more prevalent in the South of India.
2. If in two signs of a trine there is 0 then in the 3rd signs also we should do the processing *i.e.* in the 3rd sign we should place - 0. (with this opinion the authenticity of Bal Bhadra is proved because the commentators of Parashar has translated it that the minimum number should be reduced and the balance to be kept in the signs. If we subtract 0 from the sign then the number will remain as it was before the process of subtracting was done. But the commentators of Phal Deepika writes that the processing should be done here also and 0 should be placed.
3. If in all the three signs the same number exist then the processing for all 3 should be done and 0 should be kept in all places. "This is the opinion of Jatak Parijat an authentic classical treatise of Astrology that—
    1. In the 3 signs of a trine the 1 which has minimum number that minimum number should also be placed under the remaining 2 signs,
    2. If there is 0 in one sign of the trine then no processing for the remaining 2 signs should be done.
    3. If all the 3 signs of a trine has the same number then 0 should be kept for all the signs.

Prashnamarga another authentic classical work states:-

भूचक्रे निहतेऽष्टवर्गजफले भेषु त्रिकोणेषु यन्नूनं
तेन संम त्यतेत्रिषु च यद्येकत्र न स्यात् फलम्।
जह्यात् सर्वमथान्ययोर्यदि फलोन्येकत्र चेत्केवलं
ह्यात्तानि यदा समं त्रिषु तदा सर्वं विशोध्यं ततः ॥

According to this opinion if in or 2 signs of a trine there is no number then in all the 3 signs of the trine 0 should be placed. If all the 3 signs has the same number then also in the 3 signs 0 should be placed.

त्रिकोणशोधनां कृत्वा पश्चादेकाधिपत्यकम्।
क्षेत्रद्वये फलानि स्युस्तदा संशोधयेत्सुधीः ॥१८।

ग्रहयुक्ते फलैर्हीने ग्रहाभावे फलाधिके।
ऊनेन सदृशन्त्वस्मिन् शोधयेद्ग्रहवर्जिते ॥१९ ॥

फलाधिके ग्रहैर्युक्ते चान्यस्मिन् सर्वमुत्सृजेत्।
सग्रहाग्रहतुल्यत्वे सर्वं संशोध्यमग्रहात् ॥२० ॥

उभाभ्यां ग्रहहीनाभ्यां समत्वे सकलं त्यजेत्।
उभयोर्ग्रहसंयुक्ते न संशोध्यं कदाचन ॥२१ ॥

एकस्मिन् भवने शून्ये न संशोध्य कदाचन।
द्वावग्रहौ चेद्यन्नयूनं तत्तुल्यं शोधयेद्द्वयोः ॥२२ ॥

शोध्यावशिष्टं संस्थाप्य राशिमानेन वर्द्धयेत्।
ग्रहयुक्तेऽपि तद्राशी ग्रहमानेन वर्द्धयेत् ॥२३ ॥

---

*"See Jatak Parijat, Chapter-10, Sloka- 38.

Sun's Ashtakvarga (Trikonashodhan)

	Aries	Taurus	Gemini	Cancer	Leo	Virgo	Libra	Scorpio	Sagittarius	Capricorn	Aquarius	Pisces	Total
	3	7	4	4	5	3	4	5	4	3	5	1	48
Subtract	3	3	4	1	3	3	4	1	3	3	4	1	33
Balance	0	4	0	3	2	0	0	4	1	0	1	0	15

Aries, Leo, Sagittarius is one trine. The minimum is 3 in Aries so 3 is deducted from these signs. Taurus, Virgo, Capricorn is second trine - here the minimum is 3 in Virgo. Therefore 3 is deducted from these signs. Gemini, Libra, Aquarius is the third trine - here 4 is the minimum in Gemini so 4 is deducted from each sign. Cancer, Scorpio, Pisces is the fourth trine. Here the minimum here is 1 in cancer so 1 is deducted from each.

Now we give the Trikona Shodhan of other Ashtak Vargas.

Moon's Ashtakvarga (Trikonashodhan)

	Aries	Taurus	Gemini	Cancer	Leo	Virgo	Libra	Scorpio	Sagittarius	Capricorn	Aquarius	Pisces	Total
	4	5	4	4	6	6	3	3	3	6	3	4	49
Subtract	3	5	3	1	3	5	3	1	3	5	3	1	36
Balance	1	0	1	3	3	1	0	0	0	1	0	3	13

Mars's Ashtakvarga (Trikonashodhan)

	Aries	Taurus	Gemini	Cancer	Leo	Virgo	Libra	Scorpio	Sagittarius	Capricorn	Aquarius	Pisces	Total
	4	4	3	2	5	4	4	2	2	4	3	2	39
Subtract	2	4	3	2	2	4	3	2	2	4	3	2	33
Balance	2	0	0	0	3	0	1	0	0	0	0	0	6

Mercury's Ashtakvarga (Trikonashodhan)

	Aries	Taurus	Gemini	Cancer	Leo	Virgo	Libra	Scorpio	Sagittarius	Capricorn	Aquarius	Pisces	Total
	4	5	4	4	5	6	4	5	5	4	4	4	54
Subtract	4	4	4	4	4	4	4	4	4	4	4	4	48
Balance	0	1	0	0	1	2	0	1	1	0	0	0	6

Jupiter's Ashtakvarga (Trikonashodhan)

	Aries	Taurus	Gemini	Cancer	Leo	Virgo	Libra	Scorpio	Sagittarius	Capricorn	Aquarius	Pisces	Total
	5	5	4	4	7	7	2	5	6	5	3	3	56
Subtract	5	5	2	3	5	5	2	3	5	5	2	3	45
Balance	0	0	2	1	2	2	0	2	1	0	1	0	11

Venus's Ashtakvarga (Trikonashodhan)

	Aries	Taurus	Gemini	Cancer	Leo	Virgo	Libra	Scorpio	Sagittarius	Capricorn	Aquarius	Pisces	Total
	4	3	6	5	5	4	5	4	3	4	6	3	52
Subtract	3	3	5	3	3	3	5	3	3	3	5	3	42
Balance	1	0	1	2	2	1	0	1	0	1	1	0	10

Saturn's Ashtakvarga (Trikonashodhan)

	Aries	Taurus	Gemini	Cancer	Leo	Virgo	Libra	Scorpio	Sagittarius	Capricorn	Aquarius	Pisces	Total
	2	4	3	1	7	6	4	3	1	3	3	2	39
Subtract	1	3	3	1	1	3	3	1	1	3	3	1	24
Balance	1	1	0	0	6	3	1	2	0	0	0	1	15

After the Trikona Shodhan Aries, Scorpio: Taurus, Libra: Sagittarius, Pisces: Capricorn, Aquarius: in these pairs of signs, the following 14 types of condition can exist.

	Old Sign	**Second Sign**
	With Planet	**Without Planet**
1.	similar points	similar points
2.	more points	less points
3.	more points	zero points
4.	zero points	zero points
	With Planet	**Without Planet**
5.	similar points	similar points
6.	more points	less points
7.	more points	zero points
8.	less points	more points
9.	zero points	more points
10.	zero points	zero points
	With Planet	**Without Planet**
11.	similar points	similar points
12.	more points	less points
13.	more points	zero points
14.	zero points	zero points

0 means there is no point. Now we give the rules of the Ekadhipatya Sodhan. Sodhan means processing for, Ekadhipatya means for the lordship or the superiority of 1.

(a) We have shown that 14 types of conditions can exist between the 2 signs owned by a planet. In the conditions that 1, 2, 3, 4, then 7, 9, 10 then 13, 14 there is no correction or processing. The number of points will be allowed to be as it is before *i.e.* the same points will be kept and there is *statusquo*.

(b) In the conditions of 5 or 6 given above remove all the points from the 2nd sign which does not have any planet in it. In the sign where a planet is posited the number will remain as it was.

(c) If the condition is as mentioned in no. 8 then look to the sign which has a planet posited in it. In the 2nd sign which does not have a planet reduce the number to that of the 1st sign. In the sign which has a planet the number will remain as it was before processing.

(d) If the condition of the 11 prevails then from both the signs the number should be removed and 0 should be placed for both of them.

(e) If the condition is as in 12, then the lesser bindus should be kept in both the signs. We would like to clarify here that the original Slokas of Sanskrit, the language is such that sometimes two different inferences can be drawn from each Slokas and the meaning can be different. In that matter we have accepted those translations and meanings which has been supported by Parashar. But where there is a difference with the opinion of Parashar we have then stated the opinion of Mantreshwar. This is not philosophy when many principles are discussed but then no results are drawn and the subject matter is left wide open.

For example in Bhagwat Geeta the Chapter of Sanyas, the Chapter of unattachment, Niskam Karma, Bhakti, Sayankya, Yoga etc, different principles has been propogated and great learned scholars have translated and commented on it in various manners. No learned person was less than the other ones. But then whatever is one's disposition or whatever you like then those principles can be interpreted as it suits. But in 'Jyotish', Astrology it is a subject matter of mathematics where accuracy has to be maintained one principle has to be decided, whether in this place in this square, 2 should be there or 3 or 4 etc. Those learned people who want to do a comparative study, should turn to the original books read them from beginning to end. But the purpose of this commentary in (Hindi) (now in English) is to make the new readers, familiar with the subject, so that they can follow one method and rules mentioned and apply them in a horoscope when doing the Trikon Sodhan or Ekadipatya Sodhan.

Sun's Ekadhipatya Shodhan
Sun's processing of single rulership

	Aries	Taurus	Gemini	Cancer	Leo	Virgo	Libra	Scorpio	Sagittarius	Capricorn	Aquarius	Pisces	Total
	0	4	0	3	2	0	0	4	1	0	1	0	
after the sodhan	0	4	0	3	2	0	0	4	1	0	1	0	15

Moon's Ekadhipatya Shodhan
Sun's processing of single rulership

	Aries	Taurus	Gemini	Cancer	Leo	Virgo	Libra	Scorpio	Sagittarius	Capricorn	Aquarius	Pisces	Total
	1	0	1	3	3	1	0	0	0	1	0	3	
after the sodhan	1	0	0	3	3	0	0	0	0	1	0	3	11

Mars's Ekadhipatya Shodhan
Sun's processing of single rulership

	Aries	Taurus	Gemini	Cancer	Leo	Virgo	Libra	Scorpio	Sagittarius	Capricorn	Aquarius	Pisces	Total
	2	0	0	0	3	0	1	0	0	0	0	0	
after the sodhan	2	0	0	0	3	0	1	0	0	0	0	0	15

Mercury's Ekadhipatya Shodhan
Sun's processing of single rulership

	Aries	Taurus	Gemini	Cancer	Leo	Virgo	Libra	Scorpio	Sagittarius	Capricorn	Aquarius	Pisces	Total
	0	1	0	0	1	2	0	1	1	0	0	0	
after the sodhan	0	1	0	0	1	2	0	1	1	0	0	0	6

Jupiter's Ekadhipatya Shodhan
Sun's processing of single rulership

	Aries	Taurus	Gemini	Cancer	Leo	Virgo	Libra	Scorpio	Sagittarius	Capricorn	Aquarius	Pisces	Total
	0	0	2	1	2	2	0	2	1	1	1	0	
after the sodhan	0	0	0	1	2	0	0	2	1	0	0	0	7

Venus's Ekadhipatya Shodhan
Sun's processing of single rulership

	Aries	Taurus	Gemini	Cancer	Leo	Virgo	Libra	Scorpio	Sagittarius	Capricorn	Aquarius	Pisces	Total
	1	0	1	2	2	1	0	1	0	1	1	0	
after the	0	0	0	1	2	0	0	2	1	0	0	0	7

For example— The Ekadipatya Sodhan of the example horoscope is given below—

गोसिंहौ दशगुणितौ वसुभिर्मिथुनालिभे।
वणिङ्मेषौ च मुनिभिः कन्यकामकरे शरैः ॥२४॥

शेषाः स्वमानगुणिताः कर्किचापघटीझषाः।
एते राशिगुणाः प्रोक्ताः पृथग्ग्रहगुणाः पृथक्कार्यः ॥२५॥

जीवारशुक्रसौम्यानां दशवसुसप्तेन्द्रियैः क्रमाद्गुणिता।
बुधसंख्या शेषाणां राशिगुणाद्ग्रहगुणः पृथक्कार्यः ॥२६॥

Shodhyapinda

The Shodhyapinda is the total which comes after the processing of Ekadipatya in the Ashtakvarga of each planet. We write it in the following manner—

Sun,	Moon,	Mars,	Mercury,	Jupiter,	Venus,	Saturn
15	11	6	6	7	5	14

This is the Shodhyapinda of the example horoscope. In different horoscope the Shodhyapinda will be different. Mantreshwar has enunciated the principle of Shodhyapinda in the Sloka above is that after both the processing. Trikon Sodhan and Ekadipatya Sodhan, the balance should be added together and this total is called the Shodyapind. According to Parashar the products (i) which comes after multiplying with the sign multiplier and (ii) the planet multiplier when added together is the Shodyapind.

Venus's Ekadhipatya Shodhan

Sun's processing of single rulership

	Aries	Taurus	Gemini	Cancer	Leo	Virgo	Libra	Scorpio	Sagittarius	Capricorn	Aquarius	Pisces	Total
	1	1	0	0	6	3	1	2	0	0	0	1	
after the sodhan	1	0	0	0	6	3	1	2	0	0	0	1	14

Sign-Multiplier Table

Sign	Aries	Taurus	Gemini	Cancer	Leo	Virgo	Libra	Scorpio	Sagittarius	Capricorn	Aquarius	Pisces
Multiplier	7	10	8	4	10	5	7	8	9	5	11	12

Planet Multiplier Table

Planet	Sun	Moon	Mars	Mercury	Jupiter	Venus	Saturn
Multiplier	5	5	8	5	10	7	5

Sun's Ashtakvarga (Sign-multiplier and planet - multiplier)

	Aries	Taurus	Gemini	Cancer	Leo	Virgo	Libra	Scorpio	Sagittarius	Capricorn	Aquarius	Pisces	Total
A.S.	0	4	0	3	2	0	0	4	1	0	1	0	
S.M.		40		12	20			32	9		11		124
P.M.								80	5				85

Moon's Ashtakvarga (Sign-multiplier and planet - multiplier)

	Aries	Taurus	Gemini	Cancer	Leo	Virgo	Libra	Scorpio	Sagittarius	Capricorn	Aquarius	Pisces	Total
	Sat.						Jup.	M. Ve Sun.	Merc.			Moon	
A.S.	1	0	0	3	3	0	0	0	0	1	0	3	
S.M.	7			12	30					5		36	90
P.M.	5											15	20

Mar's Ashtakvarga (Sign-multiplier and planet - multiplier)

	Aries	Taurus	Gemini	Cancer	Leo	Virgo	Libra	Scorpio	Sagittarius	Capricorn	Aquarius	Pisces	Total
A.S.	2	0	0	0	3	0	1	0	0	0	0	0	
S.M.	14				30		7						51
P.M.	10						10						20

Note: As. stands for Ekadhipatya shodhan, S.M. for sign multiplier and P.M. for planet multiplier.

Mercury's Ashtakvarga (Sign-multiplier and planet - multiplier)

	Aries	Taurus	Gemini	Cancer	Leo	Virgo	Libra	Scorpio	Sagittarius	Capricorn	Aquarius	Pisces	Total
A.S.	0	1	0	0	1	2	0	1	1	0	0	0	
S.M.		10			10	10		8	9				47
P.M.								20	5				25

Jupiter's Ashtakvarga (Sign-multiplier and planet - multiplier)

	Aries	Taurus	Gemini	Cancer	Leo	Virgo	Libra	Scorpio	Sagittarius	Capricorn	Aquarius	Pisces	Total
A.S.	0	0	0	1	2	0	0	2	1	0	1	0	
S.M.				4	20			16	9		11		60
P.M.								40	5				45

Venus's Ashtakvarga (Sign-multiplier and planet - multiplier)

	Aries	Taurus	Gemini	Cancer	Leo	Virgo	Libra	Scorpio	Sagittarius	Capricorn	Aquarius	Pisces	Total
A.S.	1	0	0	2	2	0	0	1	0	1	0	0	6
S.M.	7			8	20			8		5			48
P.M.	5							20					25

Saturn's Ashtakvarga (Sign-multiplier and planet - multiplier)

	Aries	Taurus	Gemini	Cancer	Leo	Virgo	Libra	Scorpio	Sagittarius	Capricorn	Aquarius	Pisces	Total
A.S.	1	0	0	0	6	3	1	2	0	0	0	1	
S.M.	7				60	15	7	16				12	117
P.M.	5						10	40				5	60

Multiply as shown above and then add together the Sign-multiplier and the Planet-multiplier.

	Sun	Moon	Mars	Mercury	Jupiter	Venus	Saturn
Product of Sign multiplier	124	90	51	47	60	43	117
Product of planet multiplier	85	20	20	25	45	25	60
Yoga Pinda (Total)	209	110	71	72	105	68	177

Sign Multiplier and Planet Multiplier

After the Ekadipatya processing the number which is obtained under each sign *i.e.* called the sign multiplier *i.e.* Rashi Gunak. Under every sign a number is given which should be used for multiplying. Similarly the balance after Ekadipatya Sodhan has been done those should also be multiplied with the number which has been given for different planets. These numbers are different for different planets and they are called the Graha Gunak. Graha means— Planet, Gunak means— the number by which we multiply. Every sign has different numbers, every planet also has different numbers.

Sun etc. the 7 planets has sign multipliers and planet multipliers will be written out in the format. First we look to the Ekadipatya Sodhan table of Sun. In the table Aries has 0 and when this is multiplied by 7 then we get 0 as the balance. So under sign Aries we will not write any thing. In Taurus it has 4 and the multiplier number of Taurus is 10. So 4 × 10 = to 40, so 40 will be written. In Cancer the multiplier number is 4. So we write 3×4=12.

Now take the planet multiplier in Aries, Saturn is there and the multiplier number of Saturn is 5. But because the points in Aries is 0. So 0x5=0. So we write 0. In Scorpio 4 is there and there are three planets in Scorpio. The multiplier number of Sun is 5, of Mars is 8 and of Venus is 7. So in the sign Taurus we have 4x5=20, 4x8 for Mars is 32, 4x7 for Venus is 28 and the total of all this is 80. So we write 80 for Scorpio. So in Scorpio we write 80. In Sagittarius 1 is there and Mercury is in Sagittarius. The multiplier of Mercury is 5. So we write 1x5=5 which is written under Sagittarius. In the same manner we do the processing of the Moon's Ashtakvarga, Ashtakvargas of Mars, Mercury, Jupiter, Venus, Saturn etc. and we write down the number separately in all the Ashtakvargas.

एवं गुणित्वा संयोज्य सप्तभिर्गुणयेत्पुनः ।
सप्तविंशहृताल्लब्धवर्षाण्यत्र भवन्ति हि ॥२७॥

द्वादशाद्गुणयेल्लब्धा मासाहर्घटिकाः क्रमात् ।
सप्तविंशति वर्षाणि मण्डलं शोधयेत्पुनः ॥२८॥

Now multiply this total of 209 by 7 and divide the product by 27. The dividend will be the years. Multiplying the remainder by 12 and then divide it by 27. The dividend are the months. The balance should be multiplied by 30 and divided by 27 and the dividend are the days. Similarly multiplying it by 60 and dividing it by 27- gives the Ghatis.

Add all of them. One Mandal is of 27 years. So if the years are more than 27 then deduct 27 from the number- the balance will be the years of the periodic influence of that planet. The periodic influence (Dasha) of planets in the example horoscope is worked out below.

1. In the Sun's Ashtak Varga the total of signs and planets are 209. When 209 is multiplied by 7, we get 1463. Divide it by 27 and we get 1463/27 (= 54 years). The balance is 5. Multiply it by 12 and we get 60. This 60 when divided by 27 the dividend is 2 so 2 months. The balance 6 is multiplied by 30 and divided by 27— (6×30/27) = 7 app.- so 7 days.

   Now we have 54 years 2 months 7 days which being more than 27 years. So we subtract 27 from the years and the remainder viz., 27 years, 2 months and 7 days is the Dasha of Sun.

2. Similarly in the Moon's Ashtak Varga the Sum Table is 110. When this is multiplied by 7 then we get 770. Dividing this by 27 we get 28 years 6 months and 7 days. Reducing by 27 years which is one mandal we get 1 year 6 months and 7 days as the Moon's Dasha.

3. The sum total of Mars is 71. Multiplying it by 7 and then dividing the product by 27 we have— 71×7 = (497/27)= 18 yrs, 6 months and 4 days - is the period of Mars.

   In all there calculations we have stopped at days and not gone upto the Ghatis. (one Ghati= 24 minutes).

4. The sum total of Mercury is 72. When multiplied by 7 we get = 504. Divide this by 27 and we have 18 years, 8 months and 1 day *i.e.* the Dasha of Mercury.

5. The Jupiter's Sum Total is 105. Multiply this by 7. We get= 735. Dividing this by 27 we get 27 years, 2 months and 20 days. Subtracting 27 years, we have 0 yr. 2 months 20 days— is the period of Jupiter.

6. The total of Venus is 68. This when multiplied by 7 results in 476. Divide 476/27=17 years, 7 months and 17 days.

7. Saturn's Sum Total is 177. Multiply this by 7= 1239. Divide now 1239 by 27=45 years, 10 months and 20 days. Subtract 27 years and we get 18 years, 10 months and 20 days as the Dasha of Saturn.

In 'Jataka Parijata' and Shambhu Hora Prakash, there is a different manner to calculate the periodic influences from the Ashtak Varga method. We have not gone into it here as it would need a lengthy procedure.

'Haran' (Reduction in the Dashas) or Technical Corrections

अन्योऽन्यमर्द्धहरणं ग्रहयुक्ते तु कारयेत्।
नीचेऽर्द्धमस्तगेऽप्यर्द्धहरणं तेषु कारयेत्॥२९॥

1. If one planet is posited in the same sign with another planet then its Dasha should be reduced by 50% *i.e.* halved.

2. If a planet is combust or is posited in its sign of debilitation then also the dasha should be reduced by 50%.

शत्रुक्षेत्रे त्रिभागोनं दृश्यार्द्धहरणं तथा।
त्र्यंशोनहरणं भङ्गे सूर्येन्द्वोः पातसंश्रयात्॥३०॥

1. If a planet is in the sign of an enemy then its period should be reduced by one third.

2. If a planet is in the visible half (*i.e.* in the 12th, 11th, 10th and 9th house— the portion above earth) then also reduce the dasha by one third.

3. The planet which is defeated in war due to being in the same sign, degree and minute with a planet or is in the Pata (orb of) Sun or Moon then also the dasha of such a planet is reduced by one third.

बहुत्वे हरणे प्राप्ते कारयेद्दलवत्तरम्।
पश्चात्तान् सकलान कृत्वा वराङ्गेण विवर्द्धयेत्॥३१॥

मातङ्गलब्धं शुद्धायुर्भवतीति न संशयः ।
पूर्ववदिदमासाब्दान् कृत्वा तस्य दशा भवेत् ॥३२ ॥

If many of the conditions for reduction which have been mentioned above prevail, then apply only the one in which the maximum reduction of the Dasha takes place and leave the other reductions.

This way whatever age comes then multiply it by 324 and divide the product by 365— that will be the years, months and days of the Dasha.

एवं ग्रहाणां सर्वेषां दशां कुर्यात् पृथक् पृथक् ।
अष्टवर्गदशामार्गः सर्वेषामुत्तमोत्तमः ॥३३ ॥

In this manner, the dasha of each planet should be calculated from their Ashtak Vargas. Predictions based on the dashas calculated from the Ashtak Varga are the best, compared to the different types of dashas that prevail.

बालो बलिष्ठो लवणागमोसुरो
रागी मुरारिः शिखरीन्द्रगाथया ।
भौमो गणेन्द्रो लघुभावतासुरो
गोकर्णरक्ता तु पुराणमैथिली ॥३४ ॥

रुद्रः परं गह्वरभैरवस्थली
रागी वली भास्वरगीर्भगाचलाः ।
गिरौ विवस्वान्बलवद्विवक्षया
शूली मम प्रीतिकरोऽत्र तीर्थकृत् ॥३५ ॥

In Ashtakvarga which planet is in what sign and as counted from that sign how many benefic points it contributes to each sign is given here under.

	Sat.				Asc.		Jup.	Su. Ma. Venus	Mercury			Moon	
PL/Sign	Aries	Taurus	Gemini	Cancer	Leo	Virgo	Libra	Scorpio	Sagittarius	Capricorn	Aquarius	Pisces	Total
Sun	3	4	5	3	5	7	2	3*	3	3	3	2	43
Moon	3	5	2	2	5	2	2	2	3	7	1	2*	36
Mars	3	4	4	4	6	7	2	4*	5	3	5	2	49
Mercury	6	6	1	2	5	5	7	3	3*	1	5	2	46
Jupiter	2	4	2	4	7	3	2	2	1	2	3	4	36
Venus	4	2	3	4	3	6	3	2*	3	3	3	4	40
Saturn	3*	2	4	4	4	3	3	4	4	4	6	1	42
Asc.	2	6	7	1	5	3	5*	5	2	6	1	2	45
Total	26	33	28	24	40	36	26	25	24	29	27	19	337

Sun	3,3,3,3	2,3,4,5	3,5,7,2	=43
Moon	2,3,5,2	2,5,2,2	2,3,7,1	=36
Mars	4,5,3,5	2,3,4,4	4,6,7,2	=49
Mercury	3,1,5,2	6,6,1,2	5,5,7,3	=46
Jupiter	2,2,1,2	3,4,2,4	2,4,7,3	=36
Venus	2,3,3,3	4,4,2,3	4,3,6,3	=40
Saturn	3,2,4,4	4,3,3,4	4,4,6,1	=42
Ascendant	5,3,5,5	2,6,1,2	2,6,7,1	=45
Total of Sarvashtak varga				=337

Sun contributes in its own Ashtakvarga a point in the first sign; In Jupiter's Ashtakvarga it contributes a point in the first sign (where it is posited); in Saturn's Ashtakvarga it contributes a point in the first. In this manner Sun contributed 3 points in the first sign. In the same manner Sun contributes in the second place (In own Ashtakvarga 1, in Jupiter's Ashtakvarga 1, in Saturn's Ashtavarga 1)- so in all 3 points. Similarly the number of benefic points contributed by Sun etc. The seven planets and also by the Ascendant come to be as given in the table below.

Sarvashtakvarga Yoga

Varahmihir's system of contributing benefic points for each planet at different places, slightly differs from the system given above. Now according to the above method, Sarvashtakvarga has been calculated (see page 556- table).

For Sun the numbers mentioned above 3, 3, 3, 3, 2, 3, etc. As Sun is in Scorpio so we will begin from Scorpio and write the numbers from Scorpio onwards. We have placed an * in Scorpio in the Sun's column to indicate the position of a planet in that sign. Similarly place the numbers of every planet. Moon is in Pisces so 2, 3, 5, 2, 2, 5, 2, 2 etc. has been written down Pisces. An * sign to indicate the place of the Moon is also put up at Pisces.

सर्वकर्मफलोपेतमष्टवर्गकमुच्यते ।
अन्यथा बलविज्ञानं दुर्ज्ञेयं गुणदोषजम् ॥३६ ॥

Examination of the predictive side of Astrology from Ashtakvarga method is very good. There is no other way to know besides it, if a house, sign or planet is strong or weak.

त्रिंशाधिकफला ये स्यू राशयस्ते शुभप्रदाः।
पञ्चविंशात्परं मध्यं कष्टं तस्मादधः फलम्॥३७॥

The signs which has 30 points are good. Those which contain 25 to 30 are medium and the ones which has less than 25 are no good at all *i.e.* they give bad result.

मध्यात्फलाधिकं लाभे लाभात् क्षीणतरे व्यये।
यस्य व्ययाधिके लग्ने भोगवानर्थवान् भवेत्॥३८॥

If the 11th house has more points compared to the 10th house, the 12th house has less than those in the 11th house and the first house (Ascendant) has more than that in the 12th house then that native roles in worldly luxurious, commodities and is wealthy.

मूर्त्यादि व्ययभावन्तं दृष्ट्वा भावफलानि वै।
अधिके शोभनं विद्याद्धीने दोषं विनिर्दिशेत्॥३९॥

The prediction should be done after examining the benefic points in the Ascendant and all the other houses, as well as the Sarvashtakvarga. If more benefic points are in the Ascendant than the health will be good; in the 2nd house - the more the points so much will be the preservation and accumulations of money, in the 7th house, happiness from wife, in the 9th house (fortunes) and the native will be fortunate. The results are bad if the points are less.

षष्ठाष्ठमव्ययांस्त्यक्त्वा शेषेष्वेव प्रकल्पयेत्।
श्रेष्ठशिषु सर्वाणि शुभकार्याणि कारयेत्॥४०॥

The rule enunciated above that more the benefic points so much better will be the results— This rule does not apply to the 6th, 8th and 12th houses.

Those signs which are strong - *i.e.* have more benefic points then when Sun, Moon and other planets come in transit in that

Ascendant and signs than one should take up new and benefic work. Success comes and upliftment takes place easily.

लग्नात्प्रभूति मन्दान्तमेकीकृत्य फलानि वै।
सप्तभिर्गुणयेत्पश्चात्ससप्तविंशहृतात्फलम् ॥४१ ॥

तत्समानगते वर्षे दुःखं वा रोगमाप्नुयात्।
एवं मन्दानि लग्नान्तं भौमाराह्वोस्तथा फलम् ॥४२ ॥

Add together the points in each of the signs of Sarvashtakvarga from Ascendant to the sign in which Saturn is posited. Multiply the sum total by 7 and divide the product by 27. The number of the dividend is the year in which sufferings— sorrow or disease takes place.

Similarly count the points in the Sarvashtakvarga from the sign Saturn is into the Ascendant (both included). Multiply this by 7 and then divide the product by 27. The number which comes is the year when suffering, sorrow or disease occurs.

Similarly (1) from Ascendant to Mars (2) Mars to Ascendant (3) Ascendant to Rahu and (4) Rahu to Ascendant— process similarly as has been indicated for Saturn - viz., add then multiply by 7 and divide by 27, should be done. The numbers so realised are the years during which negative results will be felt.

शुभग्रहाणां संयोगसमानाब्दे शुभं भवेत्।
पुत्रवित्तसुखादीनि लभते नात्र संशयः ॥४३ ॥

As the years of sufferings are calculated from Saturn, Mars, Rahu etc. malefic to Ascendant and from Ascendant to the signs occupied by malefic from the points in the Sarvashtakvarga similarly (1) From Ascendant to where benefic planets are placed (2) from benefic planets up to the Ascendant- count the total points in those sign in the Sarvashtakvarga and multiply the total by 7 and divide the product by 27 to know the years (age) when good and benefic events will take place. Strong Moon endowed with much pakshabala and not posited with a malefic; Mercury (which is not with a malefic), Venus and Jupiter are benefic planets. During these benefic years birth of a son, gain of money etc. good events take place.

संग्रहेण मया प्रोक्तमष्टवर्गफलं त्विह ।
तज्ज्ञैर्विस्तरतः प्रोक्तमन्यत्र पटुबुद्धिभिः ॥४४॥

I have described here the results of the Ashtakvarga in short. In other works, scholars have discussed these in details.

25

Gullikadi Upagrahas

CALCULATION OF GULLIKADI AND THEIR INFLUENCE

नमामि मान्दिं यमकण्टकाख्य-
मर्द्धप्रहारं भुवि कालसंज्ञम्।
धूमव्यतीपातपरिध्यभिख्यान्-
उपग्रहानिन्द्रधनुश्च केतून् ॥१॥

चरं रुद्रदास्यं घटं नित्यतानं
खनिर्मान्दिनाड्यः क्रमेणार्कवारात्।
अहर्मानवृद्धिक्षयौ तत्र कार्यौ
निशायां तु वारेश्वरात्पञ्चमाद्याः ॥२॥

दिव्या घटी नित्यतनुः खनीनां
चन्दे रुरुः स्याद्यमकण्टकस्य।
अर्द्धप्रहारस्य भटो नटेन
स्तनौ खनी चन्द्रखरौ जयज्ञः ॥३॥

कालस्य फेनं तनुरुद्रदिव्यं
वन्द्यो नटस्तैरनुसूर्यवारात्।
एषां समं मान्दिवदेव तत्त
न्नाड्या स्फुट लग्नवदत्र साध्यम् ॥४॥

धूमो वेदगृहैस्त्रयोदशभिरप्यंशैः समेते रवौ
स्यात्तस्मिन् व्यतिपातको विलगते चक्रदथास्मि न्युते।
षड्भिभैः परिवेश इन्द्रधनुरित्यस्मिश्च्युते मण्डला-
दत्यष्टयंशयुतेऽत्र केतुरथ तत्रैकर्क्षयुक्तो रविः ॥५॥

1. Mandi
2. Yama Kantak
3. Ardha Prahar
4. Kala
5. Dhoom
6. Vyatipata
7. Paridhi
8. Indra Dhanu and
9. Upketu-I pay homage to the nine upagrahas.

If Dinman (the duration of day) is of 30 Ghatikas then Mandi will be after certain Ghatikas after Sunrise which will be different due to the day of the week.

Mandi (During the day births)

Week day	Ghatis after Sunrise
Sunday	26
Monday	22
Tuesday	18
Wednesday	14
Thursday	10
Friday	6
Saturday	2

If the Dinman is not completely of 30 Ghatikas then there should be proportionate increase /decrease in the calculation of Mandi in the same proportion of 26th, 22nd, 18th, 14th, 10th 6th and 2nd. This way calculation for the day time is done.

Now we give below the position (status) of Mandi on different week days after how many Ghatikas after the commencement of night (*i.e.* when Dinman ends and the Ratriman viz. duration of the night begins)- in the table below:

Weekday	After Sunset
Sunday	10
Monday	6
Tuesday	2
Wednesday	26
Thursday	22
Friday	18
Saturday	14

The above are the Ghatis if the duration of night is 30 Ghatis in all. If the duration of night is other than 30 then proportionate increase or decrease should be done.

We give another method to calculate mandi—other than the one given in the original Sloka in Sanskrit.

Mandi and Gulika is one and the same thing. Divide the duration of the day into 8 parts. The seven parts are ruled by the lord of the week day. There is no lord or owner of the 8th part. The part which is the portion of Saturn is called Mandi or Gulika. 'Manda' is the name of Saturn in Sanskrit. Manda means slow. The meaning of the Sanskrit word 'Shaneshchar' *i.e.* Saturn is also one who walks slowly. The portion of Mandi or the part of Saturn is called Mandi; *i.e.* the son of Manda (Saturn).

Suppose you have to calculate the Mandi on a Sunday. Then divide the duration of day by 8th. The 7th portion when it ends will be the Ghatis and Palas of Mandi. Why? The answer is that the first part is of Sun, 2nd of Moon, 3rd of Mars, 4th is of Mercury, 5th of Jupiter, 6th of Venus, 7th is of Saturn so in this order the seventh portion is of Saturn.

If the Mandi is calculated on a Wednesday then the first portion belongs to Mercury, the 2nd to Jupiter, the 3rd to Venus with 4th to Saturn - So this is Mandi.

Suppose 32 Ghatis is the duration of day and when divided by 8 we get each portion of 4 Ghatis. So the 4th part of Saturn ends at 16

Ghatis - so whatever longitude of Ascendant comes at that time will be the calculation of Mandi (sign, degree, minutes etc.).

The first portion always belongs to the lord of that week day on which the calculation is done and then the others follow in order. This is during the day time.

At night it is a different order. Divide the duration of night by 8. Then observe as to when the portion of Saturn is ending. Mandi is over at that time.

At night the counting is done from the 5th - as counted from the lord of the weekday. Example: Suppose that calculation of Mandi is to be done on a Sunday night. Then divide the duration of night by 8. The first portion will be ruled by Jupiter as it is the 5th one after the Sun (as has been mentioned above - Sun, Moon, Mars, Mercury and then Jupiter)- this way Jupiter is the 5th from Sun- so the counting is commenced with Jupiter. The second one is of Venus, the third on is of Saturn and so on.

Suppose that the duration of the night is 32 Ghatis then each portion will be of 4 ghatis.

Saturn's portion ends at 4×3=12 ghatis. Therefore whatever will be the sign, degree, minute etc. of the Ascendant after 12 ghatis from Sunset-will also be the sign, degree, minutes etc. of Mandi.

Yamakantaka, Ardhaprahar and Kal

Now we proceed with the calculation of Yamakantaka, Ardhaprahar and Kal.

Weekday	Yamakantaka After Ghatis	Ardhaprahar After Ghatis	Kal After Ghatis
Sunday	18	14	2
Monday	14	10	26
Tuesday	10	6	22
Wednesday	6	2	18
Thursday	2	26	14
Friday	26	22	10
Saturday	22	18	6

The Ghatikans given above are with the assumption that the duration of the day is of 30 ghatis. If the Dinman (duration of day) is different then proportionate changes should be done in the ghatis.

Dhoom, Vyatipata, Parivesh (Paridhi), Indrachap, Upketu.

1. In the sign, degree, minute of Sun add 4 signs 13 degree and 20 minutes and we will get the position of Dhoom.
2. By deducting the position of Dhoom from 12 signs we get Vyatipata.
3. By adding 6 signs in Vyatipatak we get Paridhi. Paridhi is also called Parivesh.
4. If Paridhi is subtracted from 12 signs then the position of Indrachap comes.
5. By adding 16 degrees 40 minutes to the position of Indrachap we get Upketu. Upketu is also in short called Ketu- It is different from Rahu-Ketu.
6. By adding 1 sign the Sun's position - sign - degree - minutes etc comes back.

Example- Suppose the Sun's position in one case works out to be Scorpio 26 degree. Then we will calculate in the following way:-

		Signs	Degree	Minutes	
(i)	Sun =	7-	26-	0	
	Add	+4	13-	20	
		12 (0)	9-	20	(Dhoom)
(ii)	From 12 signs	12-	0-	0	
	Deduct	0-	9-	20	
		11-	20-	40	(Vyatipate)
(iii)	Vyatipate	11-	20-	40	
	(Add 6 signs)	6-	0-	0	
		5-	20-	40	(Parivesh)

(iv)	From 12 signs	12-	0-	0	
	Subtract Parivesh	-5 -	20-	40	
		6	-9 -	20	(Indrachap)
(v)	In Indrachap	6 -	9 -	20	
	Add +	0	-16-	40	
		6-	26-	0	(Ketu or Upketu)
(vi)	Ketu or Upketu	6-	26-	0	
	Add	1-	0-	0	
		7-	26-	0	(Sun's position)

When the total comes to be more than 12 signs then 12 should be subtracted. As is the case in the position of Dhoom which will be 0 sign-9 degree, 20 minutes.

भावाध्याये पूर्वमेव मया प्रोक्तं समुच्चयम्।
मुक्तानां यत्तदेवात्र वाच्यं भावफलं दृढम् ॥६ ॥

तथापि गुलिकादीनां विशेषोऽत्र निगद्यते।
पूर्वाचार्यैर्यदाख्यातं तत्संगृह्य मयोदितम् ॥७ ॥

We have stated before the reasons by which a house is destroyed and also the reasons how a house improves. In the previous chapters general consideration of houses has been discussed. Now we speak of the Gulik etc. and their effect in different houses. Whatever influence of Gulik etc., that has been stated by the Masters (in the past) have been collected and presented here.

चोरः क्रूरो विनयरहितो वेदशास्त्रहीनो
नातिस्थलो नयनविकृतो नातिधीर्नातिपुत्रः।
नाल्पाहारी सुखविरहितो लम्पटो नातिजीवी
शूरो न स्यादपि जडमतिः कोपनो मान्दिलग्ने ॥८ ॥

*This Ketu - is not the one of Rahu-Ketu but it is a satellite named Ketu (or upketu).

न चाटुवाक्यं कलहायमानो
न वित्तधान्यं परदेशवासी।
न वाङ्न सूक्ष्मार्थविवादवाक्यो
दिनेशपौत्रे धनराशिसंस्थे ॥९ ॥

विरहगर्वमदादिगुणैर्यतः
प्रचुरकोपधनार्जनसंभ्रमः।
र्विगतशोकभयश्च विसोदरः
सहजधामनि मन्दसुतो यदा ॥१० ॥

सुहृदि शनिसुते स्याद्बन्धुयानार्थहीन-
श्चलमतिरवबुद्धिस्त्वल्पजीवी च पुत्रे।
बहुरिपुगणहन्ता भूतविद्याविनोदी
रिपुगतगुलिके सच्छ्रेष्ठपुत्रः स शूरः ॥११ ॥

कलत्रसंस्थे गुलिको कलही वहुभार्यफः।
लोकद्वेष्ज्ञी कृतघ्नश्च स्वल्पज्ञः स्वल्पकोपनः ॥१२ ॥

विकलनयनवक्त्रो ह्रस्वदेहोऽष्टमस्थे
गुरुसुतवियुतोऽभूद्धर्मसंस्थेऽर्कपौत्रे।
न शुभफलकर्मा कर्मसंस्थे विदानः
सुखसुतमतितेजः कान्तिमाँल्लाभसंस्थें ॥१३ ॥

विषयविरहितो दीनो बहुव्ययः
स्याद्व्यये गुलिकसंस्थे।
गुलिकत्रिकोणभे वा
जन्म ब्रूयान्नवांशे वा ॥१४ ॥

1. If Gulik is in the Ascendant then the native is a thief, cruel,

without humility. He is not very fat. He has disease of the eyes. Not many sons and the intellectual ability is very little. Such a person does not study the Vedas and Scriptures. The native eats much food but is unhappy and does not live for a long time. Such a person is angry by temperament, a fool and a coward. He is engaged in lustful deeds and he is a fickle minded low character.

2. If Gulik is in the 2nd house then the native does not use pleasing speech for others. Such a person is mostly engaged in quarrels with others. He lacks money and grains (*i.e.* not rich), he lives most times away from home. He does not keep his words and he is inefficient to discuss subjects, which require keen intellect. The meaning is that the native's I.Q. is low and the subject matters which require high intellectual ability are beyond his capacity.

3. If Gulik is in the 3rd house then the native is arrogant, intolerant and has a lust for money. Such a person wants to live alone. Generally he is intoxicated by nature or he is fond of drinking (wine). He gets very little happiness from brothers/sisters. The native himself is fearless and does not grieve. He adopts high and showing methods to earn money.

4. If Gulik is in the 4th house then the native has no kinsmen and lacks wealth. He does not possess vehicles.

5. In the 5th house Gulik makes the native a person of shameful and bad mentality. He is fickle in the mind. He also does not live long.

6. If Gulik is in the 6th house then the native is fond of witchcraft and black magic. Those people who are engaged in the worship of ghosts, evil spirits and use them to get their work achieved are called the lovers of witchcraft. Woo-doo comes to them easily. Gulik in the 6th house endows one with courage and he is able to defeat his enemies. The son born to such a native is of a very high level (class) and successful.

7. If Gulik is placed in the 7th house then the native is quarrelsome and hates people. Such a person has low comprehension, very little anger and unfaithful. He has many wives (or mistresses).

8. If Gulik is in the 8th house then the native has a small build up. The face and eyes lack symmetry *i.e.* either there is some deficiency in the body or some dosha (defect) in speech.
9. If Gulik is in the 9th house then the native has no Guru (Guru, father, etc.) *i.e.* does not get along well with them. He does not beget a son (or his son is a source of problem).
10. If Gulik is in the 10th house then it deprives the native from doing good deeds. He does not donate.
11. In the 11th house the native is happy, has a very aristocratic and bright appearance and is lustrous. He gets happiness from his son.
12. In the 12th house the native is deprived of luxuries and pleasures of the bed, he spends too much and presents a faded appearance.

Now we take up a different subject. The natives Ascendant at birth or Moon sign will be (1) The signs in trine to the sign occupied by Gulik or (2) The Navansha of Mandi is the Ascendant.

रवियुक्ते पितृहन्ता मातृक्लेशी निशापसंयुक्ते ।
भ्रातृवियोगः सकुजे बुधयुक्ते मन्दजे च सोन्मादी ॥१५ ॥

गुरुयुक्ते पाषण्डी शुक्रयुते नीचकामिनीसङ्गः ।
शनियुक्ते शनिपुत्रे कुष्ठव्याध्यर्दितश्च सोऽपल्पायुः ॥१६ ॥

विषरेगी राहुयुते शिखियुक्ते वह्निपीडितो मान्दौ ।
गुलिकस्त्याज्ययुतश्वेत्तस्मिञ्जातो नृपोऽपि भिक्षाशी ॥१७ ॥

गुलिकस्य तु संयोगे दोषान्सर्वत्र निर्दिशेत् ।
यमकण्टकसंयोगे सर्वत्र कथयेच्छुभम् ॥१८ ॥

Now we take up the subject if Gulik is posited with other planets. The planet with which Gulik is conjoined with generally takes over the negative effects (ill-effects). Sun is the significator of father and if Gulik is with Sun in a nativity then it shortens the life of father *i.e.* the father dies; Moon signifies mother so Gulik if posited with Moon then the native's mother is destroyed; Mars signifies brothers so Gulik with Mars causes separation with brothers. Mercury rules intelligence and the association of Mercury and Gulik in one sign causes mental derangement, lunacy etc.

Jupiter is the significator of religion and here Gulik's association will make the native a Hippocrat. Venus signifies women (wife) so Gulik with Venus brings the native in close contact with low caste and worthless females. Gulik and Saturn together causes sufferings from leprosy, severe disease etc. and shortens the life span.

If Rahu and Gulik are together then disease related to poison takes place (viz. septic, impurities in the system etc.). Ketu and Gulik causes sufferings and losses from fire. If the birth of the native is on such a day when Gulik is in a 'Tyaja Kala' then even if he is born in a royal family, he loses everything and begs for food *i.e.* becomes poor.

Note : The original Sanskrit Sloka mentions 'Tyajute' *i.e.* a time which is to be discarded- none of the commentators has tried to explain or discuss it as to what does it mean?

According to our opinion the following is the 'Tyajyakala'.

(a) Vishghatis - Suppose that every constellation has 60 ghatis (=24 hrs.) then

Constellation	Ghatis from	To Ghatis
Ashwini	50	54
Bharani	24	28
Kritika	30	34
Rohini	40	44
Mrigsiras	4	18
Ardra	21	25
Punarvasu	30	34
Pushya	20	24
Aslesa	32	36
Magha	30	34
Porva Phalguni	20	24

Uttara Phalguni	18	22
Hasta	21	25
Chitra	20	24
Swati	14	18
Vishakha	14	18
Anuradha	10	14
Jyestha	14	18
Moola	56	60
Purvashada	24	28
Uttarashada	20	24
Shravana	10	14
Dhanishtha	10	14
Shatbhisa	18	22
Porvabhadrapada	16	20
Uttarabhadrapada	24	28
Revati	30	34

दोषप्रदाने गुलिको बलीयान्
शुभप्रदाने यमकष्टकः स्यात्।
अन्ये च सर्वे व्यसनप्रदाने
मान्द्युक्तवीर्यर्द्धबलान्विताः स्युः ॥१९॥

शनिवद्गुलिके प्रोक्तं गुरुवद्यमकण्टके।
अर्धप्रहारे बुधवत्फलं काले तु राहुवत्॥२०॥

(b) Vyatipatu and Vadhriti Yoga are also Tyajaya (discarded).

(c) Bhadra Karan is discarded.

(d) The lost thithi (the day where lunar thithi is lost)

(e) The increased thithi. (the day a lunar thithi increases)

(f) Kulik, Ardhyam, patayoga, vishkumbha and vajra.

(g) (i) The first half of parigha Yoga.

(ii) Gand Yoga- 6 ghatis.

(iii) Vyaghat- 9 ghatis.

All these are tyajaya kala but in this context the tyajaya kala of constellation (ghatis) should be applied.

कालस्तु राहुर्गुलिकस्तु मृत्यु-
जींवातुकः स्याद्यमकण्टकोपि।
अर्द्धप्रहारः शुभदः शुभाङ्क-
युक्तोऽन्यथा चेदशुभं विदध्यात्॥२१॥

आत्मादयोऽधिपैर्युक्ता धूमादिग्रहसंयुताः।
ते भावा नाशतां यान्ति वदतीति पराशरः॥२२॥

धूमे सन्ततमुष्णं स्यादग्निभीतिर्मनोव्यथा।
व्यतीपते मृगभयं चतुष्पान्मरणं तु वा॥२३॥

परिवेषे जले भीरुर्जलरोगश्च बन्धनम्।
इन्द्रचापे शिलाघातः क्षतं शस्त्रैरपि च्युतिः॥२४॥

केतौ पतनघाताद्यं कार्यनाशोऽशनेर्भयम्।
एते यद्भावसहितास्तद्दशायां फलं वदेत्॥२५॥

1. The association with Gulik creates ill-effects at all places. We have mentioned above that except in the 6th and 11th houses, wherever Gulik is posited then it destroys the benefic effects- and increases the ill-effects.

2. The result of Yama -Kantak is that with whichever planet Yama-Kantak is, then it increases the good effect of the planet- in whichever house it is placed then the efficacy and beneficial results increase.

3. In increasing the negative effects, Gulik is strong. Yama Kantak is strong in improving the good effect. The other upagrahas (Satellites) give bad effects. However there ill-effect is only half

as compared to the ill-effects given by Mandi. Suppose Mandi gives 16 annas (unit of counting currency in India in the past) of bad effects then Kala, Ketu etc. will give ill effects only to the extent of 8 annas.

4. The influence of Gulik is like that of Saturn. Yama Kantak's effect is like that of Jupiter.

   Ardhaprahar shows effect like Mercury and Kala like Rahu.

5. Kala's effect is similar to that of Rahu. So if, Kala is in any house then the effect of Kala in that house will be the same as Rahu, if posited, in that house will give Gulik is Death incarnate. Yama Kantak is endowed with the life giving substance as Jupiter does. Jupiter is called 'Jeeva' in Sanskrit.

   In whatever house these are more benefic points then 'Ardha Prahar' shows good results if posited in that houses. But if Ardh Prahar is posited in such a house where there are not many benefic points in the 'Sarvashtak Varga' then it will show bad results.

6. Parashar Rishi states that Ascendant and other houses and the lords of those house if they conjoin with Dhoom and other Upagrahas than they are destroyed. All of them give bad effects except Yama Kantak, and it shows benefic results. This should be remembered.

7. Dhoom creates fears from burning, heat and fire. Causes mental anguish. Vyatipata causes fear of animals with horns and is instrumental in giving death from a four legged animal (cattle).

8. Parivesh or Paridhi creates fear of water (drowning) *i.e.* one who has Parivesh (or Paridhi as it is also called) in the Ascendant then such a person is afraid to bathe in a river, tank. The person is also likely to suffer from water getting accumulated in some part of the body (stomach, legs, lungs etc). The native is also liable to be imprisoned (or kidnapped). Indra chap gives injury from a stone or weapon or the native falls from a house, vehicle or tree.

9. 'Upketu' causes falling down or hurt. Danger of lightening. This is a planet which destroys the work.

10. The results which has been mentioned above when and in which Dasha they will be effective? The upgrahas does not have their periods so their effect will be felt during the period of the lord of sign in which they are posited *i.e.* suppose an upagraha is in the 8th house then in the dasha of the lord of the 8th house, its effect will take place.

अल्पायु: कुमुख: पराक्रमगुणो दु:खी च नष्टात्मज:
प्रत्यर्थिक्षुभितो विशीर्णमदनो दुर्मार्गमृत्युं गतं।
धर्मादिप्रतिकूलताटनरुचिर्लाभान्वितो दोषवा-
नित्येवं क्रमशो विलग्नभवनात्केतो: फलं कीर्ययेत्॥२६॥

If Upketu is in the Ascendant etc. any of the 12th houses then its result is as given below in the 12th houses respectively:-

1. Short life
2. Bad face (mouth)
3. Courageous
4. Unhappy
5. Children are destroyed
6. Sufferings caused by enemies
7. Insufficiency or impotancy
8. Death due to misfortunes
9. Against the established principles of religion (I CONOCLAST)
10. Fond of travelling
11. Gains
12. Full of defect.

अप्रकाशा: संचरन्ति धूमाद्या: पंच खेचरा:।
क्वचित्कदाचिद्दृश्यन्ते लोकोपद्रवहेतवे॥२७॥

Dhoom etc. the five Upgrahas viz., Dhoom, Vyatipata, Parivesh, Indrachap, Upketu- transit in the sky even if they are not visible *i.e.* as Sun, Moon etc. the 7 planets are visible to the eyes. These five Upgrahas are not visible. These Upagrahas (Dhoom etc.) at times are suddenly visible at some places.

When they are visible then conclude that some bad happening will take place in the country or the state they are seen.

(N.B. they cause economic disasters, earthquakes, fires, upheavals, changes in the Govt. etc.)

धूमस्तु धूमपटलः पुच्छर्क्षमिति केचन।
उल्कापातो व्यतीपातः परिवेषस्तु दृश्यते ॥२८ ॥

Some people are of the opinion that 'Dhoom' is a cluster of smoke but others are of the opinion that it is a star with a tail. (not a shooting star). At times it is visible in the East or West for many weeks.

'Vyatipat' is like a thunderbolt.

'Parivesh' is like a round circular disc around Sun or Moon.

लोके प्रसिद्धं यद्दृष्टं तदेवेन्द्रघनुः स्मृतम।
केतुश्च धूमकेतुः स्याल्लोकोपद्रवकारकः ॥२९ ॥

After the rains during the day (when the rains stops in the afternoon) a bow of seven colours called in India as 'Indra Dhanush'- the bow of Lord Indira, is visible- this is the same - 'Indra Chap'.

'Dhoom Ketu' in short in called Ketu.*

गुलिकभवनाथे केन्द्रगे वा त्रिकोणे
बलिनि निजगृहस्थे स्वोच्चमित्रस्थिते वा।
रथगजतुरगाणां नायको मारतुल्यो
महितपृथुयशास्स्यान्मेदिनीमण्डलकेन्द्रः ॥३० ॥

The Lord of the sign in which Gulik is placed— if strong, in own sign or exalted sign, house of a friend then the native is very handsome, famous and the ruler of the Earth.

*N. B. This Ketu is different from the ones Rahu and Ketu - the shadow.

26

The Effect of Transit

सर्वेषु लग्नेष्वपि सत्सु चन्द्र-
लग्नं प्रधानं खलु गोचरेषु।
तस्मात्तदृक्षादपि वर्तमान-
ग्रहेन्द्रचारैः कथयेत्फलानि ॥१ ॥

1. In a horoscope, the ascendant, or the Sun sign or the sign of any planet can be taken as the first house to make judgement about the transits. But the main importance is given to the sign where Moon is placed *i.e.* the radical Moon.

The sign occupied by Moon should always be considered as the Ascendant when we have to take the transit in consideration. We should see where other planets are going in transit and whether this will give benefic or malefic results.

In Chapter—23 the effect of transit from each planet and the ascendant has been discussed in Ashtakvarga. 'Ashtak' is the Sanskrit word which means— Eight. Lagna is one, and the Seven Planets— Sun, Moon, Mars, Mercury, Jupiter, Venus and Saturn. From all these eight planets one dot is used to see if in transit how much benefic results will come and how much will be the negative effect. If the lines or some people call them benefic dots are more then it will show good effect. If it is less then it will not be good. The result will be benefic if more planets are in good transit from the sign occupied by Moon at birth and the Sum total of transit of all planets and their aspects are taken in consideration. If malefic predominate and the benefics are less then the result will be malefic.

From the 9th sign *i.e.* the sign occupied by Sun in the birth chart, consideration about father should be done; the 4th house from the Moon should be taken to consider about mother. The 3rd sign from Mars tells about brothers or sisters. Therefore by using Sun as the ascendant, or Moon as the ascendant, or Mars as the ascendant, we should take into account the transits through the 9th, 4th and the 3rd respectively. All this has been mentioned in Chapter—24.

Why then in Chapter - 26 the sign occupied by the Moon has been given prime importance and the transits are considered from that Moon sign? The question is why is it so? The reason given is that Moon is the 'Mana', 'The emotional nature'. In the Vedas it is written that Moon is born out of the Mana of the 'Virat Purush' - The Supreme Lord. The 'Parbrahma Parmeshwar' *i.e.* Moon is the ruler of the Mana. Mana is the emotion. In Greek Moon is called Luna. Lunacy comes from Lunas– it makes one means madness. "चन्द्रमा मनसो जात: " ।

When the mind is imbalanced then madness comes due to loss of control on mind. The good and bad is felt by the mind*. The effect of all planets is felt by a human being by his mind. So Varahamihir, the noted Astrologer in his बृहद् जातक Chapter—2, Sloka No. 1 has written 'मनस्तुहितग: ' *i.e.* Moon as Mana. This is the reason why Moon sign has been given the prime importance when taking the transits in consideration. In the horoscope of many people if Moon sign is comparatively much stronger then the ascendant, then the interpretation of the chart should be done by making Moon sign as the ascendant and then much better results will come.

For example see the horoscope below—

Birth Chart

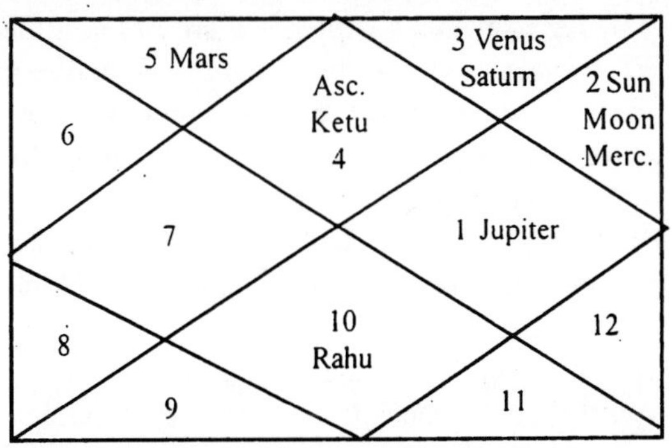

---

i.e. the emotions - it does not stand here for intellect (which comes under Mercury).

Moon Chart

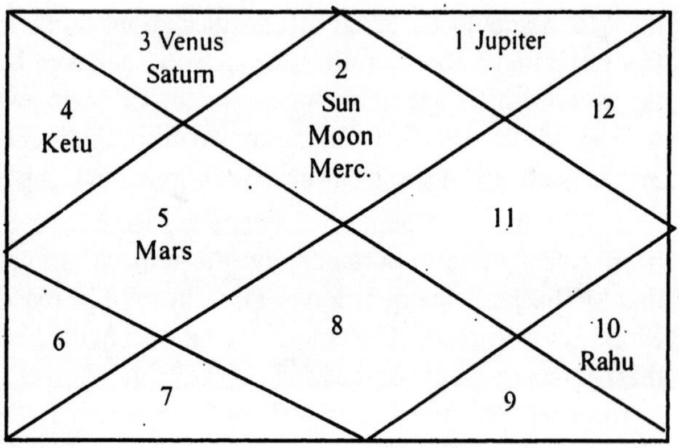

The Ascendant starts with No. 4 it will be the 1st house and Ketu in it; Mars is the 2nd, Venus and Saturn in the 12th, Sun, Moon, Mercury in the 11th, Rahu in the 7th, Jupiter in the 10th. In the Chandra Lagna when we make the same horoscope Sun, Moon, Mercury, comes in the 1st house, Venus and Saturn in the 2nd, Ketu in the 3rd, Mars in the 4th, Jupiter in the 12th, Rahu in the 9th, Moon is exalted in sign. When the Saturn Mahadasha started, due to the Cancer rising Saturn is the ruler of the 7th and 8th house and is a Markesh. But as Taurus the sign occupied by Moon is more prominent and as such Saturn is the ruler of the 9th and 10th house from it and becomes a Yoga Karak so it caused good effects. The native went to England during the beginning of the Saturn period and started to make much better money and a big improvement in his career.

Here, in this Chapter, we are not considering any horoscope. We are talking about the transits. The above matter has only been mentioned to explain the effect is not only in transit but also when doing general predictions for a horoscope. Moon ascendant i.e. the sign in which Moon is placed has been attached importance. Varahamihir etc. the great propagators of Astrology has stated that the same importance should be given to the Moon ascendant as to the ascendant at birth. The manner in which we consider different houses from the ascendant, in the same manner we should consider the houses from Moon. In the 9th Chapter- The ascendant, if Aries or Taurus etc. what will be the results of this has been explained. Mantreshwar in the 13th Sloka of 9th Chapter has mentioned that the results which have been mentioned for Aries, Taurus etc. should also be applied if Moon is in these sign. The same results, which has been mentioned from the ascendant at birth, should also be applicable from the radical Moon (as Ascendant).

For example— If someone has Leo ascendant and Moon is in Aries then the result of the ascendant in Leo will take place and side by side the results which has been mentioned for Aries will also apply. Chapter—9, Sloka No. 1. So both these things will be applicable because the Aries is the ascendant from the Moon *i.e.* Moon was placed in the sign of Aries.

All these things has been explained in detail over here that when considering a horoscope Moon ascendant should be attached the same importance as we give to the ascendant. In Western Astrology most of the things are judged from the ascendant. (or Sun sign).

For example— If a malefic is transiting the 12th house from the ascendant then there will be a heavy expenses, loss of wealth etc. Dr. Tuckar* who was a great scholar of Astrology in the West, has mentioned that by making the Sun sign as the ascendant and then consider the transit from the Sun sign.

For example— If Sun is in Leo then Virgo will be the 2nd house, Libra will be the 3rd house etc. The speciality in his transit method is that besides the 27 constellations, the fixed star, the other big stars are also considered. He takes into account the conjuctions of various planets and big stars at birth.

Here we are considering the method from the Indian Astrological point of view. The horoscope which has been mentioned above on page 577, in that horoscope, the Moon chart is also given. Most of the time Astrologers in India they give a horoscope, with an ascendant rising and all also with Moon rising as the ascendant. In this Chapter the transit has been mentioned from the Moon.

For example— If Saturn is transiting in Pisces then from the birth ascendant which is Cancer in the example horoscope it is in the 9th house. However from the Moon ascendant, Taurus the Pisces is

---

*See the 'fixed stars and your horoscope' by Dr. W. J. Tuckar.

the 11th house so the transiting Saturn, will be in the 11th from the Moon. The counting should be done from the sign occupied by the Moon and not from the ascendant. (All the time this will not be mentioned that the transit should be taken from the Moon. So we have pointed out this matter that wherever we used the transit word here in this Chapter it means transiting from the sign occupied by Moon).

सूर्यः षटत्रिदशस्थितस्त्रिदशषट्सप्ताद्यगश्चन्द्रमाः
जीवस्त्वस्ततपोद्विपंचमगतो वक्रार्कजौ षटत्रिगौ ।
सौम्यः षट्स्वचतुर्दशाष्टमगतः सर्वेऽप्युपान्तस्थिताः
शुक्रः खास्तरिपून्विहाय शुभदस्तिग्मांशुवद्भोगिनौ ॥२॥

When we are considering the benefic or malefic effects in transit then we should look into an Ephemeris to see which planets are in which signs. The planets transiting the sign mentioned below from the Moon ascendant are considered as auspicious—

Sun when transiting the 3rd, 6th, 10th and 11 th houses is good. Moon when transiting from its own position at birth which is the radical position of the Moon.

Moon-	In the 1st, 3rd, 6th, 7th, 10th, 11th.
Mars -	3rd, 6th, 11th.
Mercury-	2nd, 4th, 6th, 8th, 10th, 11th.
Jupiter-	2nd, 5th, 7th, 9th, 11th.
Venus-	1st, 2nd, 3rd, 4th, 5th, 8th, 9th, 11th, 12th.
Saturn-	3rd, 6th, 11th.
Rahu -	3rd, 6th, 10th.
Ketu-	3rd, 6th, 10th, 11th.

For example the chart given before on page 578, with the Moon ascendant. The Moon is in Taurus. So consideration should be given from Taurus and that should be taken as the 1st house. When Sun is in Cancer then it will be taken as transiting the 3rd house *i.e.* from Taurus, Gemini and Cancer. This is benefic so the same should be understood for transiting of other planets.

लाभविक्रमखशत्रषु स्थित:
शोभनो निगदितो दिवाकर: ।
खेचरै: सुततपोजलान्त्यगै:
व्यार्किभिर्यदि विद्ध्यते तदा ॥३ ॥

In the above Sloka the houses through which the transit is benefic has been mentioned. There is however an exception to this rule. There is another law which should be applicable according to the conditions of the bye-law, the same law is mentioned in Sloka 3rd to 8th. These are special rules.

Sun has been mentioned as showing benefic results when it is transiting the 3rd house. But if at the same time Moon, Mars, Mercury, Jupiter, Venus, Rahu or Ketu any one of these is also transiting in the 9th house then Sun will not show benefic result. This is called Vedh. Saturn is the son of Sun and Mercury is the son of Moon. When Sun is transiting in the 3rd house then any another planet except Saturn creates Vedh. Saturn being the Son of Sun, there is no Vedh by Saturn. Saturn does not create obstacles in the transit of the father. So among the planets mentioned in the 9th house, when Sun is transiting the 3rd, Saturn's name is not mentioned.

For detailed consideration of Vedh.* please read 'Sugum Jyotish Praveshika by Pt. Gopesh Kumar Ojha. There are two opinion about Vedh. Take for example— Sun is in Cancer in the 3rd house from Taurus. Now from where to count the 9th house? As Moon is in Taurus so the 9th should be counted from Taurus or the transiting Sun is in Cancer so it is to be counted from Cancer? Both the systems are invogue. According to 'Narad' a great scholar, the counting should be done from Taurus and in this book this method has been adopted. The 9th house from Taurus is Capricorn so when Sun is in Cancer, then at that time other planets except Saturn transiting in Capricorn will block Sun and it will not be able to show any benefic result.*

1. See Sugam Jyotish Praveshika by Pandit Gopesh Kumar Ojha.

---

* Similarly if Sun by transit is supposed to show malefic effect then due to Vedh malefic effects is nutralised. This should be applied to other planets also.

2. Astrology and you by the same authors.

As Mercury is only 28 degrees away from Sun on either side and Venus is 48 degrees away from Sun on either side so when Sun will be in Cancer then Mercury and Venus can never be in Capricorn. We have mentioned all the planets except Saturn in order to write what has been written in the original Sloka that except Saturn all the other planets create Vedh.

Now we give below the places of transit and Vedh of Sun—

Benefic Places of Transit	-	3,	6,	10,	11
Place of Vedh	-	9,	12,	4,	5,

Sun in transit shows benefic results in the 11th house. In the horoscope from Taurus, Moon, Pisces is the 11th sign. When Sun will transit Pisces which generally happens every year between 13th March to 13th of April, Sun is always in Pisces in the sidereal Zodiac then it will always give benefic results. However the 5th house from Taurus which is Virgo which has been mentioned as the house creating Vedh at that time if except Saturn any other planet will be transiting it then there will be Veda of Sun and the benefic effects will not be felt.

द्यूनजन्मरिपुलाभखत्रिगाः
चन्द्रमाः शुभफलदः सदा।
स्वात्मजान्त्यमृतिबन्धुधर्मगै
विंध्यते न विबुधैर्यदि ग्रहैः ॥४॥

Moon's benefic Transiting houses	-	1,	3,	6,	7,	10,	11
Vedh houses	-	5,	9,	12,	2,	4,	8

विक्रमायरिपुगः कुजः शुभः
स्यात्तदान्त्यसुतधर्मगैः।
चेन्न विद्ध इनसूनुरप्यसौ
किन्तु घर्मघृणिना न विध्यते ॥५॥

Mars' benefic Transiting houses	-	3,	6,	11
Vedh houses	-	12,	9,	5

The Sloka No. 3 above and in the coming Slokas, the benefic houses has been mentioned when a planet transits them.The Vedh of these are— the 12th is the Vedh of 3rd, 9th is the Vedh of 6th, 5th is the Vedh of 11th, it should be understood in the same way. If Mars is transiting the 3rd house then if a planet is in the 12th from that then Vedh should be understood. If in transit Mars is in the 12th and from the birth Moon, 4th or 5th are transited by a planet then there will be no Vedh for Mars. If Mars is transiting the 6th house and there is any planet in the 9th house (transit) then Vedh should be judged. Here the transit of other planet is mentioned and not the placement at birth. When Mars is in the 11th house and there is any other planet in the 5th in transit from Moon then there will be Vedh of Mars and the benefic results will not ensue- *i.e.* the benefic results will not take place. The benefic houses of Saturn in transit are the same as has been mentioned for Mars *i.e.* the transit of the Saturn in 3, 6, and 11 will give benefic results.

Transit of Saturn	-	3,	6,	11
Vedh houses	-	12,	9,	5

The only difference is that Sun, Moon, Mercury, Jupiter, Venus and Saturn as well as Rahu and Ketu, they obstruct and create Vedh for Mars. But Sun and Saturn have father— son relationship so Saturn does not create Vedh for Sun. Only Moon, Mars, Mercury, Jupiter, Venus, Rahu and Ketu does Vedh for Saturn to make it more clear Sun does not create Vedh for Saturn, and Saturn does not cause Vedh for Sun.

स्वाम्बुशत्रुमृतिखायगः शुभो
ज्ञस्तदा न खलु विध्यते सदा।
स्वात्मजत्रितप आद्यनैधन
प्राप्तिगैर्विबुधुभिर्यदि ग्रहैः ॥५॥

The benefic houses for Mercury in transit are-	2,	4,	6,	8,	10	11
Vedh houses -	5,	3,	9,	1,	8,	12

स्वायधर्मतनयास्तसंस्थितो नाकनायकपुरोहितः शुभः।
रिःफरन्ध्रखजलत्रिगैर्यदा विध्यते गगनचारिभिर्न हि ॥७॥

The benefic houses for Jupiter in transit are-	2,	5,	7,	9,	11
Vedh houses -	12,	4,	3,	10,	8

आसुताष्टमतपोव्ययायगी विद्ध आस्फजिदशोभनः स्मृतः ।
नैधनास्ततनुकर्मधर्मधीलाभवैरिसहजस्थखेचरैः ॥८॥

The benefic houses for the transit of Venus are-	1,	2,	3,	4,	5,	8,	9,	11,	12
Vedh house-	8,	7,	1,	10,	9,	5,	11,	3	6

जन्मन्यायासदाता क्षपयति विभवान् क्रोधरोगाध्वदाता
वित्तभ्रंशं द्वितीये दिशति न सुखदो वञ्चनामाग्रहं च ।
स्थानप्राप्तिं तृतीये धननिचयमुदाकल्यकृच्चारिहन्ता
रोगान् दत्ते जनयति च मुहुःस्रग्धराभोगविघ्नम् ॥९॥

वित्तक्षोभं सुतस्थो वितरति बहुशो रोगमोहादिदाता
षष्ठेऽर्को हन्ति रोगान् क्षपयति च रिपूञ्छोकमोहान्प्रमार्ष्टि ।
अध्वानं सप्तमस्थो जठरगुदभयं दैन्यभावं च तस्मै
रुक्त्रासावष्टमस्थः कलयति कलहं राजभीतिं च तापम् ॥१०॥

Now what is the result of Sun when it transits different houses from the Moon sign? The effect is given below—

For example— In the example horoscope the placement of Moon is in Taurus. So we start from Taurus. When Sun will transit in the same sign where Moon is placed then it will be called in the first house. In Gemini it will be called as transiting the 2nd house and in the same manner we should count— 1, 2, 3, 4, etc.

In different houses what is the effect of Sun? In the 1st house it makes one work very hard expenses increase and anger comes. (When the situation is not according to the mental aptitude then anger comes). It makes one travel and if he doesn't travel then he walks much in and around the place where he lives.

In the 2nd house loss of wealth or wealth is destroyed, no happiness. A person becomes adament. People cheat and use him.

In the 3rd house gain of position or place. Wealth is accumulated and as such happiness comes, good news through communication or certain type of work is accomplished which give joy. Enemies are destroyed and a person is victorious over them.

In the 4th house it causes disease, obstacles in the matters of happiness.

In the 5th house mental anguish, disease, disappointment in love and all these create uneasiness and disturb the mental equilibrium.

In the 6th house a person overcomes disease, success over enemies, the matters which create emotional distress, sorrows etc. are destroyed *i.e.* the mind is healthy.

In the 7th house, it makes one walk on foot. It causes problems in stomach and urinary tracks. A person feels stressed and low, *i.e.* loss of prestige, loss of respect so much so that a person is very unhappy in the mind.

In the 8th house, disease, fears, anguish, quarrels. Fear from kings, rulers, government or from officials and people in power oppose the native.

In the 9th house calamities, stresses, separation from loved ones and he is humiliated and whatever work a person undertakes results in failure.

In the 10th house— the person accomplishes all that he works for even big things are achieved with ease. Support from people in high position.

In the 11th house gain of wealth, prestige, riches, a person overcomes disease, financial security, good health, rise in status or gain of property.

In the 12th house— sorrow, unhappiness, loss of wealth, feverishness etc. even friends become enemies.

आपद्दैन्यं तपसि विरहं चित्तचेष्टानिरोधं
प्राप्नोत्युग्रां दशमगृहगे कर्मसिद्धिं दिनेशे।
स्थानं मानं विभवमपि चैकादशे रोगनाशं
क्लेशं वित्तक्षयमपि सुहृद्वैरमन्त्ये ज्वरं च॥११॥

These are in order the effect of the transit of Sun in 12 different houses. Every year almost around a certain date Sun goes in one sign for a month and then after the month is over it enters into a 2nd sign. In general it is for 30 days in one sign.

The English dates when Sun enters in a sign.

	Sign			Dates
1.	Aries	Enters	On	13/14 April
2.	Taurus	,,	,,	14/15 May
3.	Gemini	,,	,,	15 June
4.	Cancer	,,	,,	16/17 July
5.	Leo	,,	,,	16/17 August
6.	Virgo	,,	,,	17 September
7.	Libra	,,	,,	17 October
8.	Scorpio	,,	,,	15-16 November
9.	Sagittarius	,,	,,	16 December
10.	Capricorn	,,	,,	13/14 January
11.	Aquarius and	,,	,,	12 February
12.	Pisces	,,	,,	14 March.

The dates that we have mentioned above are in a rough manner are the dates when Sun enters into a second sign from the first one. This is called Sankranti. Sometimes there are 28 days in February and at times 29 on a leap year, so it is possible that there will be a difference of 1 day or so in the change of sign by Sun, it can not be more than one day.

Now a person can go back to his earlier and past experiences and he can visualise and make a chart when and in which month eventful happenings or eventful things took place in his life. These months should be counted not from 1st to 30th or 31st but from 15th to 15th, 15th to 16th, like the solar months. It is definite that every year does not go the same and in the same manner every month for every year is not repeated because Sun is only one solar transit. There are other planets and the transit of them also effect. Beside the major and minor periodical influences of planets also keep on changing.

Transit of Sun due to Sankranti of Sun

Now we bring to the notice of readers a new method. This has not been written and elaborated by Mantreshwar but we have taken it from other places. This is the transit of the Sun.

1. The day there is the Surya Sankranti *i.e.* Sun is entering from one sign to another. That should be observed from a correct ephemeris. Observe the time, the hours and minutes when Sun is changing sign or note the Ghatis and Palas when Sun changes sign.
2. Note where moon was at that time.
   (i) Note the constellation occupied by Moon when Sun changes sign.
   (ii) Note the preceding Nakshatra which Moon occupied when Sun is changing Sign.

For example— If there is change of Sun sign and Moon is in Jeshta Nakshatra then Anuradha being the previous Nakshatra before Jeshta we should note it down or suppose Sun is changing and Moon at that time is in Pushya Nakshatra then note Punarvasu which is the preceding Nakshatra before Pushya.

Now start counting from this preceding Nakshatra which we have noted down upto your own Janma Nakshatra *i.e.* the constellation, that Moon occupied when you were born.

For example— If a person has his birth in the constellation of Bharani *i.e* the Moon occupied the constellation of Bharani and we have to consider and take into account how this month is going to be for him? How the transit of Sun will effect him?

Then for example if at the time of the changing of signs of Sun, Moon is in Jeshta then we start to count from the proceeding Nakshatra of Jeshta which is Anuradha. Then we count from Anuradha to Bharani. Anuradha -1, Jestha-2, Mool-3, Purvashad- 4, Uttraashad-5, Sarvan-6, Danishta-7, Satbhisa -8, Purva Bhadrapada -9, Uttra Bhadrapada-10, Revati-11, Ashwini-12, Bharani-13, so the number 13 come. According to this number the effect of the entrance of the

Sun in a different sign will be as follows—

(a) If the number of Nakshatra is 1, 2, or 3 then during that month travelling or walking or movement is indicated.

(b) If the number comes to be 4, 5, 6, 7, 8, 9, then enjoyment is indicated.

(c) If the number is - 10, 11, 12, then sorrow *i.e.* unhappiness and sufferings.

(d) If the number is - 13, 14, 15, 16, 17, 18 then gain of new clothes and dresses.

(e) If the number is - 19, 20, 21, then losses.

(f) If the number is -22, 23, 24, 25, 26, 27 any of them then it indicates tremendous gains of wealth. We repeat again we count from the preceding Nakshtra which the Moon occupies at the time when Sun changes sign to the constellation at birth.

क्रमेण भाग्योदयमर्थहानिं जयं भयं शोकमरोगतां च।
सुखान्यनिष्ठं गदमिष्टसिद्धिं मोदं व्ययं च प्रददाति चन्द्रः ॥१२॥

Moon

Now we consider the transit of Moon (from the sign occupied by Moon by birth) which is called radical Moon. The result of the transit in different houses is as follows—

1. In the 1st house good fortunes and fortunate time
2. Loss of wealth
3. Victory
4. Fear
5. Sorrow
6. Good health
7. Happiness
8. Negative period— hindrance and delays
9. Disease
10. Success in work, attainment of desire
11. Happiness
12. Expenses.

When Moon is in the sign of the radical Moon then good fortunes start to began. In the 2nd house loss of wealth, in the 3rd house victory, in the 4th house from the radical Moon fear and in the same manner the transit should be understood, through various houses.

अन्तः शोकं स्वजनविरहं रक्तपित्तोष्णरोगं
लग्ने वित्ते भयमपि गिरां दोषमर्थक्षयं च।
धैर्ये भौमो जनयति जयं स्वर्णभूषांप्रमोदं
स्थानभ्रंशं रुजमुदरजां बन्धुदुःखं चतुथे ॥१३॥

ज्वरमनुचिताचिन्तां पुत्रहेतुव्यथां वा
कलयति कलहं स्वैः पञ्चमे भूमिपुत्रः।
रिपुकलहनिवृत्तिं रोगशान्तिं च षष्ठे
विजयमथ धनाप्तिं सर्वकार्यानुकूल्यम् ॥१४॥

कलत्रकलहाक्षिरुग्जठररोगकृत्सप्तमे
ज्वरक्षतजरुक्षितो विगतवित्तमानोऽष्टमे।
कुजे नवमसंस्थिते परिभवोऽर्थनाशादिभि-
र्विलम्बितगतिर्भवत्यबलदेहधातुक्षयैः ॥१५॥

दुश्चेष्टा वा कर्गविघ्नः श्रगः खे
द्रव्यारोगयक्षेत्रवृद्धिश्च लाभे।
भौमः खेटो गोचरे द्वादशस्थो
द्रव्यच्छेदस्ताप उष्णामयाद्यैः ॥१६॥

Mars

Now we talk about the transit of Mars from the radical Moon which will be as follows—

1. In the 1st house inner discontentment or worries, loss of relatives, blood disorder or disease connected with biles, high temperature or any other disease which occurs due to heat and dryness.

2. In the 2nd house fear, loss of wealth, sarcastic remarks, quarrels.
3. In the 3rd house victory, success, gain of wealth, happiness.
4. In the 4th house loss of position and or loss of residence or house or loss of job. Disease connected with stomach and unhappiness due to relatives.
5. In the 5th house fever, worries due to no reason, suffering to children, ir-rationale anxiety and mental imbalance, differences with own people.
6. In the 6th house - victory over enemies and opponents or some type of pact with them. Disease subsides victory gain of wealth and success in all work.
7. In the 7th house fight with own wife and business partners. Eye disease, stomach problems.
8. In the 8th house, fever, injury, wounds, loss of wealth, loss of prestige.
9. In the 9th house defeat, loss of prestige, loss of wealth, weakness in the body, slowness in walking due to lack of strength Tuberculosis, loss of semen etc.
10. In the 10th house obstacles in work or failure in work, hard work. The person is engaged in such type of work which he should not undertake (low type of works).
11. In the 11th house, gain of wealth, good health, benefit from lands and properties etc. good results.
12. In the 12th house loss of wealth, heat in the body resulting in disorder of the system, which will cause disease, mental apprehensions, worries.

वित्तक्षयं श्रियमरातिभयं धनाप्तिं
भार्यातनूजकलहं यिजयं विरोधम्।
पुत्रार्थलाभमथ विघ्नमशेषसौख्यं
पुष्टिं पराभवभयं प्रकरोति चान्द्रि: ॥१७॥

Mercury

The transit of Mercury in different houses from the radical Moon will show the following results-

1. In the 1st house loss of wealth.
2. In the 2nd house gain of money.
3. In the 3rd house fear from enemies.
4. In the 4th house realisation of wealth.
5. In the 5th house quarrels with own wife and children.
6. In the 6th house, success, victory.
7. In the 7th house, opposition, quarrels.
8. In the 8th house happiness from son, gain of wealth.
9. In the 9th house obstacles.
10. In the 10th house happiness of various types.
11. In the 11th house increase of prosperity, gains.
12. In the 12th house defeat and loss of face.

जीवे जन्मनि देशानिर्गमनमप्यर्थच्युतिं शत्रुतां
प्राप्नोति द्रविणं कुटुम्बसुखमप्यर्थे स्ववाचां फलम्।
दुश्चिक्ये स्थितिनाशमिष्टवियुतिं कार्यान्तरायं रुजं
दु:खैर्बन्धुजनोद्भवैश्च हिबुके दैन्यं चतुष्पाद्भयम्॥१८॥

पुत्रोत्पत्तिमुपैति सज्जनयुतिं राजानुकूल्यं सुते
षष्ठे मन्त्रिणि पीडयन्ति रिपव: स्वज्ञातयो व्याधय:।
यात्राँ शोभनहेतवे वनितया सौख्यं सुताप्तिं स्मरे
मार्गक्लेशमरिष्टमगते नष्टं धनै: कष्टताम्॥१९॥

भाग्ये जीवे सर्वसौभाग्यसिद्धि:
कर्मण्यर्थस्थानपुत्रदिपीडा।
लाभे पुत्रस्थानमानादिलाभो
रि:फे दु:खं साध्वसं द्रव्यहेतो:॥२०॥

Jupiter

When Jupiter transits the 12 sign as counted from the Moon sign at birth by then the results will be as follows—

1. In the 1st house *i.e.* in the sign occupied by Moon. Travel out of place or country, loss of money in a big way, money is destroyed, enmity etc. bad results.
2. In the 2nd house, gain of wealth, happiness from family, realisation of good speech, whatever one says comes true. People care for his advise or a person earns money from speech.
3. In the 3rd house loss of place, status or position, losses in financial matters or position, separation from relatives and loved ones. Obstacels in work, disease etc. negative results.
4. In the 4th house unhappiness and insults from relatives, danger from four legged animals like— cows, horses, elephants etc.
5. In the 5th house increase in family, birth of a son, happiness from children meeting with learned people, favour from kings etc. are the benefic results.
6. In the 6th house problem created by kinsmen, cousin from the father's side. Also problems due to enemies, disease etc. all negative results.
7. In the 7th house, travelling in connection with some good work, happiness from own wife birth of son- all good results.
8. In the 8th house, difficulties in travelling, efforts go waste due to wandering around for no reason, loss of money and problems in many ways.
9. In the 9th house good fortunes of all types, gains, fortunates times commences, success in work etc. good results.
10. In the 10th house financial tightness, displacement in job, setback in work or status, danger of insults and bad name, unhappiness to children etc., the negative results.
11. In the 11th house gain of son, gain of position, new position, or upliftment or one gets betterment in own place etc.
12. In the 12th house financial disaster, fear, anxiety and imbalance of mind etc. - negative results.

अखिलविषययोगं वित्तसिद्धिं विभतिं
सुखसुहृदभिवृद्धिं पुत्रलब्धिं विपत्तिम्।
दिशति युवतिपीडां सम्पदं वा सुखाप्ति
कलहमभयमर्थप्राप्तिमिन्द्रारिमन्त्री॥२१॥

Venus

The transit of Venus in different houses are as follows-

1. All kinds of enjoyment.
2. Money comes, gain of wealth.
3. Increase of wealth and beautiful things are attained.
4. Happiness, increase in the numbers of friends.
5. Child birth, gain of a son, happiness from children.
6. Problems, sorrow.
7. Problem connected with wife or any other women.
8. Inheritance, property.
9. Happiness.
10. Quarrels.
11. Fear
12. Gain of wealth and other beneficial results.

All these places which has been mentioned above are as counted from the radical Moon *i.e.* the position of Moon in a sign at birth.

For example— If a person was born in radical Moon posited in Cancer and at the time when we want to know whether it is a good time or a bad time, then we look to Venus which we find in Aquarius. Then as counted from Cancer, Aquarius is the 8th sign. We count both Cancer and Aquarius, then the effect of the 8th house which is gain of property or inheritance will happen.

रोगाशौचक्रियाप्तिं धनसुतविहतिं स्थानभृत्यार्थलाभं
स्त्रीबन्ध्वर्थप्रणाशं द्रविणसुतमतिप्रच्युतिं सर्वसौख्यम्।
स्त्रीरोगाध्वावभीतिं स्वसुतपशुसुहृद्वित्तनाशामयातिं
जन्मादेरष्टमान्तं दिशति पदवशेनार्कसूनुः क्रमेण॥२२॥

दारिद्रं धर्मविघ्नं पितृसमविलयं नित्यदु:खं शुभस्थे
दुर्व्यापारप्रवृत्तिं कलयति दशमे मालभङ्गं रुजं वा।
सौख्यन्येकादशस्थो बहुविधविभवप्राप्तिमुत्कृष्टकीर्ति
विश्रान्ति व्यर्थकार्याद्वसुहृतिमरिभि: स्त्रीसुतव्याधिमन्त्ये ॥२३॥

Saturn

1. When Saturn transits the sign where Moon is placed at birth then it causes disease or impurity in the family due to the death of a close relative etc. - negative results.
2. When Saturn is in the 2nd house from the Moon, then problems and worries to children, loss of wealth.
3. In the 3rd house it gives gains, new position or a new job, new business, own commanding position, gain of servants, gain of wealth etc. are the good results.
4. In the 4th house Saturn is a malefic and shows bad results viz. loss of wealth, loss of wife or spouse. Not good relationship with relatives and kinsmen or anxiety and problems caused by them.
5. In the 5th house Saturn gives loss of wealth or financial tightness. Problem to children, mind is confused and a person takes improper decisions. Many types of anxiety, apprehensions which lead to loss of peace.
6. When Saturn goes in the 6th house from the radical Moon then it gives benefic results. All types of happiness, success over rivals etc. are the good effects.
7. Saturn in the 7th house gives sufferings. Causes problems to wife/spouse, or disease to wife, quarrels with her, many types of fears, tiring journies.
8. In the 8th house Saturn is again is very bad. Loss of children, problem to them, loss of animals like— Cow, Buffalo etc. loss of wealth and extreme problems. A person loses his friends or they die, animals die, loss of wealth in particular. A person gets worried on account of his own health due to some type of serious health problem.

9. When Saturn is in the 9th house then it causes poverty. Obstacles in spiritual and religious activities. Person who are equal to father and like him. Viz., Guru, Uncle, Maternal Uncle etc. pass away at that time or certain types of sorrow comes to them.

10. When Saturn is in the 10th house from the radical Moon, then loss of prestige, bad name, some chronic disease or it involves a person in a certain type of work which results in extreme losses and failure in the end. A person is engaged in certain bad activities which results in loss of prestige.

11. In the 11th house Saturn makes a person travel. It gives good effect, all types of happiness and prosperity, big name and fame etc. are realised.

12. In the 12th house a person is engaged in work which are not fruitful. He works hard and doesn't get any results and so it increases worries and sorrows. The enemies cause loss of wealth. Disease to wife and children.

देहक्षयं वित्तविनाशसौख्ये
दुःखार्थनाशौ सुखनाशमृत्यून।
हानिं च लाभं सुभगं व्ययं च
कुर्यात्तमो जन्मगृहात्क्रमेण ॥२४॥

Rahu

The effect of Rahu transiting through different sign as counted from Moon are-

1. In the 1st house *i.e.* in the house where Moon is at birth, sickness, loss of power, physical power in particular.
2. Loss of wealth in the 2nd house.
3. In the 3rd house happiness.
4. In the 4th house unhappiness.
5. In the 5th house loss of wealth.
6. In the 6th house happiness.
7. In the 7th house losses.
8. In the 8th house sorrow and suffering like death.

9. In the 9th house big losses.
10. In the 10th house gains.
11. In the 11th house good fortunes.
12. In the 12th house expenses.

क्षितितनयपतङ्गौ राशिपूर्वत्रिभागे
सुरपतिगुरुशुक्रौ राशिमध्यत्रिभागे।
तुहिनकिरणमन्दौ राशिपाश्चात्यभागे
शशितनयभुजङ्गौ पाकदौ सार्वकालम्॥२५॥

The timings of the special effect of Planets

When Sun and Mars enter into any sign then they start to show their effect as soon as they enter it. In one sign there are 30 degree. The main effect of Sun and Mars are in the first 10 degree *i.e.* in the first decanet. Jupiter and Venus show effect in the 2nd decanet *i.e.* from 10 degree to 20 degree. They show special results and effect. Moon and Saturn show effect in the last decanet *i.e.* from 20 degree to the 30 degree *i.e.* when they are about to move out of the sign, they show more results.

Mercury and Rahu show the same results throughout the sign *i.e.* from the 1st degree to the 30 degree. Rahu always moves backward and Mercury can be direct in motion or retrograde. But Rahu is most of the time retrograde and so is Ketu. We have given the effect of Rahu and as Ketu is always opposite to Rahu so its results should be surmised. *

---

*Comments- In Muhurta Chintamani an authentic Book on Astrology and many other books on Astrology, have put up a question if Vedh should be observed from the radical Moon or from the planet under consideration? An opposite view of Vipreet Vedh is also considered. However in this small book it is not possible to compare the views and opinions of different Rishi's like- Narad, Kashyap and many other learned Astrologers and then to draw a conclusion. The learned people who are more interested can directly study the original Sanskrit Books to get more information about this subject.

Chart showing the transit effects of Vedh of Sun, Moon, Mars etc. –another opinion.

Sun	Moon	Mars	Mercury	Jupiter	Venus	Saturn	Rahu	Ketu
Loss of place Travels	Health and gain of grains	Fears and pains	Imprisonment fears	sad events fears destroyed	happiness enemies are	all is lost fears, pains	Losses sufferings	Losses, fear of disease
Losses and Fears	gain of wealth happiness	wealth loss eye trouble	gain of wealth	money gained money	happiness gain of	sorrow wealth loss	expenses	enmity loss of wealth
Happiness Wealth is Gained	money is received happiness	happiness money	fears of enemies	Fear disease	happiness wealth	gain of wealth happiness	health wealth	happiness prosperity
Fear of disease Insults Lost	Disease wealth is enemies	sufferings fear of wealth	gain of happiness &	loss of wealth	wealth comes enemies increase	sufferings fears	enmity sorrow	fears pains
Poverty Loss of wealth Hampered wealth	happiness work is loss of	fear of disease	sorrows & sufferings	Gains & happiness a son	gains birth of destroyed.	wealth and sons	losses sorrow lost	sorrow wealth loss
Enemies are Destroyed Happiness	gain of money	gains & happiness	No gain no promotions	disease and sorrow	increase of enemies & sufferings	happiness wealth is gained	happiness wealth	happiness wealth
Wealth is lost Travels Happiness	money is received lost	work and wealth is disorganised	fear of sufferings	honour & happiness	sorrow great fears	bad name sufferings	losses quarrels	insults pains

Disease and fears death in sins	fear of sufferings involvement	fears mental etc.	gain of wealth, grains sufferings	fear of death & wealth enemies	calamities loss of increase of	fear of sorrow unhappiness	fear of disease losses	fear of pains &
loss of glamour and sinful attitude	fear of kings loss of presgtige	fear of disease	fear of disease' loss of wealth	happiness honour	happiness gains	sins loss of wealth	involvement in sinful activities	sins & poverty
Happiness Accomplish- ment	good events happiness	happiness sorrow	happiness luxuries	great poverty	loss of religion un- happiness	jealousy enmity	enmity happiness	fears & sorrow
gain of wealth happiness	many types of gains	gains happiness	Expenses in good things wealth	happiness gain of comes	sorrow wealth & wealth	gains of happiness & wealth	gain of happiness health	good name gain of
loss of wealth fear of sufferings wealth	disease loss of	disease sorrow wealth	sorrow & loss of fears	pains in body	wealth is gained big sorrow	mental anguish	losses & pains	sufferings enmity
Benefic 3, 11, 6, 10	7,6,10 1,3,11	3,6,11	2, 4, 6 8,10,11	5, 2, 9 7, 11	1, 2, 3 4, 5, 8 9, 12, 11	6, 11, 3	3, 6, 11,	3, 6, 11
Vedh 9, 5 12, 4 exception Saturn	2,12,4 5, 9, 8, exception Mercury	12,9,5	5,3,9 1, 8, 12 exception Moon	4, 12, 10 3, 8	8, 7, 1 10, 9, 5 11, 6, 3	9, 5, 12 exception Sun	12, 5, 9	12, 9, 5

Chart of the Transit Effects

Sun	Moon	Mars	Mercury	Jupiter	Venus	Saturn Rahu Ketu	Planet
3,6,10, 11	1, 2, 3, 5, 6, 7, 9, 10, 11	3, 6, 10, 11,	2, 6, 10, 11,	2, 5, 7, 9,	1, 2, 3, 9, 11,	3, 6, 10, 11	Excellent
1, 2, 5, 7, 9	+ +	1, 2, 5 7, 9	1, 3, 5 7, 9	1, 3, 6 10	5, 6, 7, 10	1, 2, 5 7, 9	Evil
4, 8, 12	4, 8, 12	4, 8, 12	4, 8, 12	4, 8, 12	4, 8, 12	4, 8, 12	Very bad

Generally the effects of transits which have been mentioned above, the same are advocated by Varahmihir and other well known Acharyas. Therefore these effects have not been analyzed. The Learned persons have expressed the effect of transits and the same has been given above in the format of a chart. In the same context, Mantreshwar has considered Constellation- Transit and when planets show less effect in transit and when they show more effects. This has been given on the next page.

Constellation - Transits

Draw 7 horizontal lines and 7 vertical lines so that they intersect as shown on next page in the diagram. Beginning from the North-East write the numbers of constellations (including Abhijit in clockwise direction).

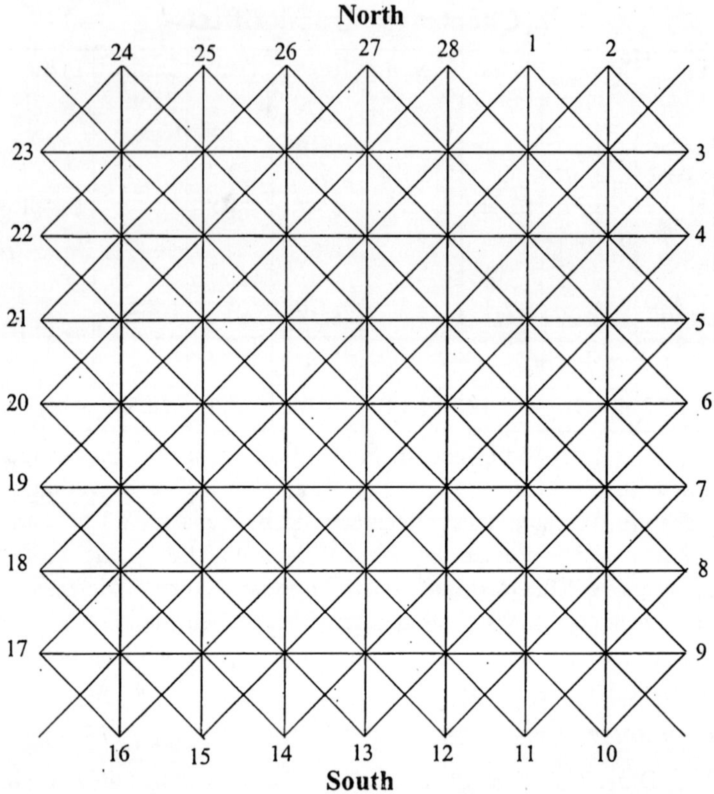

Number Corresponds to various Nakshatras viz., 1 for Aries, 2 for Taurus and so on.

रेखाः सयतसमालिखेदुपरिगास्तिर्यक्तथैव क्रमा-
दीशादग्निभमादितोऽपि गणयेदादित्यभयस्यावधि।
वेधा जन्मदिने मृतिर्भयमथाधानाख्यनक्षत्रके
कर्मण्यर्थविनाशनं खलु रविर्दद्यात्सपापो मृतिम् ॥२३॥

If Sun is transiting the constellation which is getting a Vedh from the constellation occupied by radical Moon, then danger to life can happen.

If Adhana Nakshatra *i.e.* the 19th constellation from the birth star is getting Vedh then fear and anxiety will take shape. If the Karma constellation, which is 10th Nakshatra from the birth constellation, is having Vedh then loss of money should be predicted. If there is a malefic planet with Sun at the time of transit then the negative effect will be more intensified.

एवं विद्धे खचरैः क्ररन्यैर्मरणम्।
सौम्यैर्विद्धे न मृतिर्विद्यादेवं सकलम्॥२७॥

The three constellation which we have mentioned above if they are getting Vedh from other malefic planets then death can happen. If simultaneously benefic planets are also having Vedh then there will be no death. Similarly the transit of other planets in the constellation as/ has been considered for the transit of Sun in constellation should be considered. Malefic will indicate negative things and benefic will show good results and also will be able to ward off the evils.

आधानकर्मर्क्षविपन्निजर्क्षे
वैनाशिके प्रत्यरभे वधाख्ये।
पापग्रहो मृत्युभयं विदध्या
द्वेधेतथा कार्यहरः शुभाख्ये॥२८॥

A. The 19th Nakshatra from the constellation occupied by the Moon, is called a Adhan Nakshatra.

B. The 10th Nakshatra is called the Karma Nakshatra. Karma means works.

C. The 3rd constellation from the Moon's constellation at birth is called 'Vipat' i.e. dangers.

D. The 22nd Nakshatra is called Vainashik it can cause death.

E. The 5th Nakshatra is Pratyari and

F. The 7th Naksharta is called 'Vadha' like being 'assasination'.

In the 6th constellation mentioned above as well as in the birth constellation if any one of them has Vedh from a malefic then fear of death or death takes place. If simultaneously there is Vedh from benefic then only loss of work or loss of fortunes or losses in general etc. will take place.

आदित्यसङ्क्रान्तिदिने ग्रहाणां
प्रवेशने वा ग्रहणे च युद्धे।
उल्कानिपाते च तथाद्भुते च
जन्मत्रयं स्यान्मरणदिदुःखम्॥२९॥

1. The day Sun changes from one sign to the other sign (this is called Sankramana).
2. Or any other planet is changing from one sign to another.
3. There is an Eclipse.
4. There is a war between planets. We have already mentioned that war between planets are— when two planets are in the same sign, degree and minute.
5. Ulka Nipat *i.e.* there are lightening and stars with tale, are visible. Or
6. Any other out of the ordinary happenings happens in the sky. On that day if these events happen in the birth constellation or Anu Janma *i.e.* the 10th Nakshatra from the birth star or Tri Janma *i.e.* the 19th Nakshatra from the birth star then death etc. i.e. sorrowful events take place.

असत्फलः सौम्यनिरीक्षतो यः
शुभप्रदश्चाप्यशुभेक्षितश्च।
द्वौ निष्फलौ द्वावपि खेचरेन्द्रौ
यः शत्रुणा स्वेन विलोकितश्च॥३०॥

In this Sloka, three conditions have been mentioned where planets in transit are unable to show their effect or results—

1. If a malefic planet which is supposed to show negative effects receives the aspect or associates with a benefic, then the malefic effect is mitigated.
2. If there is a benefic planet and during transit it gets aspect from a malefic, then the benefic effect does not take place and is destroyed.
3. If any planet receives the aspects from a planet, which is his

enemy, then the power of the planet to show benefic results are reduced or destroyed.

अनिष्टभावस्थितखेचरेन्द्रः
स्वोच्चस्वगेहोपगतो यदि स्यात्।
न दोषकृच्चोत्तमभावगश्चेत्
पूर्णं फलं यच्छति गोचरेषु ॥३१॥

If a planet in transit is in a negative house, (Negative house means where it can cause harm) but if that sign is its exalted or own sign, then it does not cause bad effects *i.e.* does not cause losses. If the transiting planet is in a benefic house and that house is own sign or exalted sign, then it shows full benefic effect.

ग्रहेश्वरारुते शुभगोचरस्था
नीचारिमोढ्यं समुपाश्रिताश्चेत्।
ते निष्फलाः किन्त्वशुभाङ्कसंस्थाः
कष्टं फलं संविदधत्यनल्पम् ॥३२॥

If the transiting planet is in a benefic place, but that benefic place is its sign of debilitation or the sign owned by an enemy or is very close to the Sun so it is combust then the planet is not able to show its benefic results. If in the same condition viz., debilitated sign or in an enemy sign or combust and the planet is in a bad house, then it causes very bad results.

द्वादशाष्टमजन्मस्थाः शन्यर्काङ्गिरका गुरुः।
कुर्वन्ति प्राणसन्देहं स्थानभ्रंशं धनक्षयम् ॥३३॥

When Sun, Mars, Jupiter and Saturn are in transit passing through the 1st, 8th and 12th sign, from the radical Moon then they cause loss of wealth, loss of place, loss of residence and all types of evil effects. Sometimes there are doubts if the native will survive.

चन्द्राष्टमे च धरणीतनयः कलत्रे
राहुः शुभे कविररौ च गुरुस्तृतीये।

अर्क: सुतऽर्किरुदये च बुधश्चतुर्थे
मानार्थहानिमरणानि वदेद्विशेषात् ॥३४॥

If from the radical Moon, Moon in transit is in the 8th house, Mars is transiting the 7th house, Rahu in the 9th house, Mercury in the 4th house, Jupiter in the 3rd house, Venus in the 6th house and Saturn is in the 1st house and Sun in the 5th house, then they show great negative results like— loss of wealth, loss of prestige, death or sufferings equal to death.

Now we talk about another method of the transit in various constellations.

The transit of Sun in different constellation as counted from the birth star is equated with the different parts of the Kalapurush. The details transit vis-a-vis parts of Kalapurush are given below—

1. In the 1st constellation on the face.
2. In the 2, 3, 4 and 5 on the head.
3. 6, 7, 8 and 9 constellation on the chest.
4. 10, 11, 12, 13 right arm.
5. 14, 15, 16, 17, 18 and 19 constellation both feet.
6. 20, 21, 22, 23 left arms.
7. 24 and 25 constellation both eyes.
8. 26 and 27 constellation in the urinary and private parts.

वक्त्रे क्ष्मा मूर्ध्नि चत्वार्युरसि च चतुरः सव्यहस्ते चतुष्कं
पादे षड्वामहस्ते चतुरथ नयने द्वौ च गुह्ये द्वयं च।
भानुर्नाशं विभूतिं विजयमथ धनं निर्धनं देहपीडां
लाभं मृत्युं च चक्रे जनयति विविधान् जन्मभाद्देहसंस्थ ॥३५॥

The effect of these transits in order are:-

A. Destructions

B. Wealth- Prosperity

C. Victory

D. Wealth

E. Poverty

F. Physical pains and sufferings

G. Gains

H. Death.

शीतांशोर्वदने द्वयोरतिभयं क्षेमं शिरस्यम्बुधौ
पृष्ठे शत्रुजयं द्वयोर्नयनयोर्नेत्रे धनं जन्मभात्।
पञ्चस्वात्मसुखं हृदि त्रिषु करे वामे विरोधं क्रमात्
पादौ षट्सु विदेशतां जनयति त्रिष्वर्थलाभं करे ॥३६॥

As we have indicated the transit of Sun in different constellation in the same way the effect of the transit of Moon in the 27 constellation are given below:-

1. As counted from birth star *i.e* the constellation occupied by Moon at birth.
   - A. 1 and 2 on the face and the result is great fears.
   - B. 3, 4, 5 and 6 on the head, result happiness and well being.
   - C. 7 and 8 on the back, result victory over enemies.
   - D. 9 and 10 both eye - gain of wealth, money is realised.
   - E. 11, 12, 13, 14, 15 on the heart, inner contentment.
   - F. 16, 17, 18 left hand— results- quarrels.
   - G. 19, 20, 21, 22, 23 and 24 - both feet travelling.
   - H. 25, 26, 27 right hand— it means gains.

वक्त्रे द्वे मरणं करोत्यवनिजः षट् पादयोर्विग्रहं
क्रोडे त्रीणि जयं चतुर्विधनतां वामे करे मस्तके।
द्वे लाभं चतुराननेऽधिकभयं क्षेमंकरे दक्षिणे
वार्द्धिर्द्वे नयने विदेशगमनं चक्रे स्वजन्मर्क्षतः ॥३७॥

Now the transit of Mars in different constellation as counted from Moon and it should be understood in the body of Vishal Purush. 'Vishal Purush' stands for the almighty God, the Supreme Power of god head.

Now we give in order

When counted from the constellation occupied by Moon at birth—

A. In the 1 and 2 face - result death.

B. In the 3, 4, 5, 6, 7, 8 both feet results- quarrels and fight.

C. In the 9, 10, 11 in lap result- victory.

D. In the 12, 13, 14, 15 left hand- result poverty.

E. In 16, 17 on the head result- gain.

F. In 18, 19, 20, 21 on the face- result- extreme fear.

G. In 23, 24, 25 in the right hand- result- conferring happiness.

H. In 26, 27 for trips, travelling away from home.

मूर्ध्नि त्रीणि मुखे त्रयं च करयोः षट् पञ्च कुक्षौ तथा
लिङ्गे द्वे द्विचतुष्टयं चरणयोः प्राप्तेऽमरेन्द्रार्चितः ।
शोकं लाभमनर्थमर्थनिचयं नाशं प्रतिष्ठां तथा
दद्यादात्मदिनात्तथैव भृगुजस्तद्वद्बुधोऽपि क्रमात् ॥३८ ॥

Now we speak of the transit and result of Mercury, Jupiter and Venus in the different portion of the constellation Purush. Mercury, Jupiter and Venus all the three of them has the same result in the same order. So they have been plugged together. The counting should be from the birth constellation.

A. 1, 2, 3 i.e. on the head- result- grief, sorrow.

B. 4, 5, 6 on the face- result- gains.

C. 7, 8, 9, 10, 11, 12 in both hands - result- calamities.

D. 13, 14, 15, 16, 17 in the Flanks- result- gain of grains.

E. In the 18, 19 constellation from the birth star, private parts- result- destruction.

F. In the 20, 21, 22, 23, 24, 25, 26 and 27 constellation in both feet- result- honour, high status.

भूवेदवह्निगुणवेदशराग्निनेत्र-
दस्रं च वक्त्रकरपादपदेषु हस्ते ।

कुक्षौ च मूर्ध्नि नयनद्वयपृष्ठभागे
नयस्य क्रमेण शनिसंयुतभान्निजर्क्षात् ॥३९ ॥

दुःखं च सौख्यं गमनं च नाशं
लाभं स्वभोगं सुखसौख्यमृत्यून् ।
वक्त्रक्रमादाह फलानि मन्द-
स्यैवं तमःखेचरयोर्वदन्तु ॥४० ॥

Now we speak of the transit of the Saturn, Rahu and Ketu in different constellations of the Constellation Purush. In all the three, the results of the transit are the same, so they have been clubbed together. The counting is done from the radical Moon. Here one thing should be kept in mind that Saturn moves, forward and Retrograde both, but Rahu and Ketu are most of the times retorgrade in motion.

A. 1st constellation on the face- result- sorrow.

B. 2, 3, 4, 5 constellations- right hand- result- happiness, satisfaction.

C. 6, 7, 8 right feet- result- travelling, changes.

D. 9, 10, 11- left legs- result- destruction.

E. 12, 13, 14, 15 left hand - result- gains.

F. 16, 17,18, 19, 20 constellation flanks- result- enjoyment and satisfaction in relationship.

G. 21, 22, 23 on the head result- happiness, contentment.

H. 24, 25 in the eyes- result- happiness, good thing happens.

I. 26, 27 on the back - result- death.

Now we give a new method of the transit of planets

यत्राष्टवर्गेऽधिकबिन्दवः स्यु-
स्तत्र स्थितो गोचरतो ग्रहेन्द्रः ।
तद्वत्फलं प्राह शुभं व्ययारि-
रन्ध्रस्थितो वाऽपि शुभं विधत्ते ॥४१ ॥

We have elaborately talked about the transit of planets in different constellations. Still we come back to the transit according to the Ashtakvarga theory. We would like to point out that if in any sign of the Ashtakvarga there are more benefic points then a planet even if it is transiting in the trik *i.e.* 6th, 8th or 12th house, still it will show good effects. The purpose of saying is that although the 6th, 8th and 12th houses are not good houses yet as the number of benefic bindus are more, so the result will be always beneficial and never malefic. The bindus that we have referred to are used in the books written in the South of India. The same bindus are called Rekhas like lines in the Sanskrit Books written in North India.

रवेर्द्वादशनक्षत्रं भसुतस्य तृतीयकम्।
गुरोः षट्तारकं चैव शनेरष्टमतारकम्॥४२॥

एतेषां च पुरोलत्ता पृष्ठलत्ताः प्रकीर्त्तिताः।
शुक्रस्य पञ्चमः तारं चन्द्रस्य तु सप्तमम्॥४३॥

राहोस्तु नवमं चैव द्वाविंशं भं हिमद्युतेः।
मरणं जीवलत्तायां जन्मभे व्यथा॥४४॥

रवेः सर्वार्थहानिः स्यात्तमसोर्दुःखमुच्यते।
मरणं जीवलत्तायां बन्धुनाशो भयावहः॥४५॥

शुक्रस्य कलहो भ्रशं अनर्थः शशिजस्यतु।
चन्द्रस्य तु महाहानिर्लत्तामात्रफलं भवेत्॥४६॥

सर्वत्र लत्तासाङ्कर्ये द्विगुणत्रिगुणादिकम्।
वदेद्दोषफलं नृणां ग्रहाल्लत्ताधिकक्रमात्॥४७॥

When we have to consider the transit of a planet as to what results it will show then we should take into account–

A. The 12th constellation from the constellation in which Sun is in transits.

B. The 3rd constellation from the constellation in which Mars is.

C. The 6th constellation from the constellation Jupiter is in transit.

D. The 8th constellation from the constellation which is transited by Saturn.

These are called Purolatta. Now we always count in front of it *i.e.* in order of the Nakshatra.

For example- If Sun is in the constellation of Ashwini then the 12th constellation will be Ultraphalguni. So the Purolatta will be in Uttraphalguni.

E. The constellation in which Venus is we start to count the 5th constellation in reverse order.

F. The constellation in transit occupied by Mercury. We count in the reverse order the 7th constellation from the one occupied by Mercury in transit.

G. We count the 9th Nakshatra in the reverse order from the one occupied by Rahu and Ketu.

H. The 22nd constellation counted in the reverse order from the constellation occupied by Moon. These are the Pristhalatta. The one in front are Purolatta and those we get by counting backward are Pristhalatta.

Illustration - When we count in the reverse order that means if Venus is in the constellation of Ashwini then Satbhisa will be the Pristhalatta of Venus which is the 5th Nakshatra that we get by counting that way.

If the latta is on the birth star i.e. the star occupied by Moon at birth then it causes sorrows, sufferings more like mental anguish.

If the latta is that of the Sun then all types of financial losses.

If it is of Rahu or Ketu then unhappiness.

If it is of Jupiter then death, loss of relatives and fears.

In that of Venus the latta causes quarrels.

In the latta of Mercury loss of place. Calamities.

In the latta of Moon huge losses.

These are the effect of the latta's of different planets. The evil effect that we have talk about if it is that of only one planet, then the negative effect will be ordinary.

If it is of two or more, then the negative effects multiplies because if the latta's are together then it causes more malefic results and may multiply many times.

The more the number of latta's on the birth star, that much more malefic and evil, will be the result.

Sarvatho Bhadra Chakram - Consideration

Now we state another method to see the transits. We have given below a chart called Sarvatho Bhadra Chakram. In this Sarvatho Bhadra Chakram–

1. The Swar- the sound.
2. Constellation.
3. the 1st letter of the name.
4. The sign occupied by Moon.
5. The lunar date, called Tithi and
6. The planets are considered.

The order is as given below–

Chart given in the next page— Where different letters are shown indicating constellation and letters of alphabet which fall under them also the direction are given on the top East, at the bottom West and then other directions. Now we give the chart of the Sarvatho Bhadra Chakram–

Sarvato Bhadra Chakra

East: घ ङ छ

N.E. — S.E.

अ	3	4	5	6	7	8	9	आ
2	उ	अ	व	क	ह	ड	ऊ	10
1	ल	लृ	Taurus	Gemini	Cancer	लृ	म	11
28	च	Aries	ओ	सू नन्दा मं	औ	Leo	ट	12
27	द	Pisces	रिक्ता	Purna	Bhadra	Virgo	प	13
		शु	Saturn	Moon Mercury				ठ
26	श स	Aquirius	अ:	जया Jup.	अं	Libra	र	14
25	ग	ऐ	Capri corn	Sagi ttarius	Scorpio	ए	त	15
24	ऋ	ख	ज	भ	य	न	ॠ	16
ई	23	22	21	20	19	18	17	इ
		Abhijit						

North: थ झ ञ

South: ष ण

N.W. — S.W.

West: ध फढ़

N.B. 1, 2, 3, 4, to 28 are the nos for nakshatras viz. Aries Tauras etc.22nd Abhijit so is all 28 constellation.

For conversion of Hindi/Devnagri Alphabets to English Equivalent, Refer to 'Hindi self Taught' by Ashutosh Ojha.

Sarvato Bhadra Chakra

East

N.E. — gha, ng, chha — S.E.

North: ny, jha tha

a	3	4	5	6	7	8	9	aa
2	u	a	va wa	ka	ha	da	oo	10
1	la	lree	Taurus	Gemini Sun	Cancer	lri	ma	11
28	cha	Aries	o	Nanda Mers	au	Leo	ta	12
27	da	Pisces	Rikta Venus	Purna Saturn	Bhadra Moon Mercury	Virgo	pa	13
26	sha, sa	Aquirius	ah	Jaya Jupiter	an%	Libra	ra	14
25	ga	ai	Capri corn	Sagi ttarius	Scorpio	e	ta	15
24	ri	kha	ja	bha	ya	na	ree	16
ee	23	22 Abhijit	21	20	19	18	17	i

South: sha, na tha

N.W. — dha pha dhna — S.W.

West

N.B.: 1,2, 3, 4 etc. Stand for west the constellation in order 22nd is Abhijit so in all 28 Nakshatras

Hindi: Devanagri Scripts are converted into their English Equivalent. Please refer to Hindi self Taught - by Ashutosh Ojha.

1. Swar *i.e.* the sound in the North East called Eshankoan, then in the clockwise direction. Earnearkoan which is the then Nairityakoan and Vaibhyakoan. And we have placed the Sanskrit alphabet- अ, आ, इ, ई। In the same manner in these Koanas we have placed the other alphabets- उ, ऊ, ऋ, ॠ। After that in the same corners we have placed- लृ, लृह, ए, ऐ। And inside four corner we have written the remaining four letters- आ, औ, अं, अः। This way we have written down the 16 alphabet in order.
2. Constellation are in the 1st line beginning from the Krittika on the four side we have written the 28 Nakshatra's. Why 28 ? There are 27 well known Nakshatra and one which is not visible is called Abhijit. So the 28 Nakshatras are written into the chart it will be clear.
3. Below the constellation we have written - अ, ब, क, अ, ड़। Then म, ट, प, र, त। Then ग, श, द, च, ल। These 20 Varna are here. Above we have written- अ, आ, इ, ई and in the order 'अ' which comes is an indicator of the sound- स्वर called मात्रा and अ, ब, क, ह, ड। In order the 'अ'। which comes here is the indicator of the beginning of the 1st letter of the name. So there are two things one- The Swar- the sound the second- The first letter of name.

   For example- If the name of the one person is - अजय। Then the first letter is- 'अ' So the second one is in the order of - अ, ब, क, ह, ड। will indicate the first letter of the name.

   In the Ephemeris the 27 Nakshatras are divided in 108 quarters. We write 108 letters depicting the beginning of the name if someone is born in those quarters. (The 27×4= 108 and each one of them represents one letter).

   For example- If one person is born in the first quarter of Ashwini Nakshatra *i.e.* constellation of Ashwini. Then the beginning of his name will start from the first letter which is Chu. Generally the system was prevailing for 75 to 100 years ago in most part of India. Now in some parts the system does not exist and although in the birth chart which is made at the time of birth the beginning letter of the name is mentioned still the name by which a person is called is generally different. Generally every constellation has been succeeded by the मात्रा। like the sound which combines the letter the way it is spoken.

For example- Chaa, (चा) adding it to (ई) Che, (ची) adding it to (उ) Chu, (चू) same manner (चे) Chey, (चौ) Cho, (चा) Cha, (खा) Kha, (च) Cha, (छ) Cha. But (खा) Kha and (ज) Ja here has only just two matras. One is- (अ) and other is - (इ) the (खा) Kha letter has four matras- (खी) Khee, (खू) Khoo, (खे) Khey, (खो) Kho.

See Makar Rashi *i.e.* Capricorn sign and the letters which are under it.

The question is what is the reason of this?. The reason is that after the shrawana constellation, there is the Nakshatras Abhijit and Abhijit Nakshatra is also counted.

When Aries rises in the East at that time the top of the earth in the sky which is the 10th house in a horoscope, the Constellation Abhijit is the result. So the Mid - Noon *i.e.* exactly the time of the Noon- 12.00 O 'Clock is called the Abhijit Kaal or Abhijit Muhurata. If this Abhijit Constellation is also included in the letters following under its four quarters, then the letters will be – जू, जे, जो, ख। Similarly - ज and ख will also contain five matras in the constellation.

Now coming back to the matter under discussion. At places only one अक्षर। The letter which has the sound of the just - ए, अ has been given.

For example- घ, ड़, छ, ष, ण, ठ, ध, फ, ढ़, थ, त, झ and ञ।

We do not know why this method has been adopted. Our scriptures expressed and mentioned by the Rishi's has not done any thing in them without certain principles. But we do not know what is the method or how the principles have been selected?

For example– 20 years has been allotted as the periodical

influence of Venus but Sun has been allotted just 6 years. Why is it so anyway?

In this Sarvatho Bhadra Chakra- We have written - अ, ब, क, हृ, ड etc. 20 letters inside and the 12 letter- घ, ङ, छ etc. has been written outside in four directions.

The list of 27 constellation *i.e* Ashwini, Bharani etc. which has been given to indicate the beginning of the letters starting from Krittika Nakshatra first quarters and the letters which comes are in order- अ, ब, क, घ, ङ, छ, हृ, ड, म, ट, प, ष, ण, ठ, र, त, न, य, भ, ध, फ, ढ़, ज, ख, ग, स, द, थ, भ, ञ, च, ल। Here the underlined words should be placed together, then we have- अ, ब, क, ह, ङ, म, ट, प, र, त, न, य, भ, ज, ख, ग, स, द, च, ल।

These 20 alphabets has been placed inside the Sarvatho Badhra Chakra. ब Should also be suppose to include व *i.e.* one whose name start with व।

For example– विद्याभूषण That should also fall under ब। Square श। and स। Both are considered from the same square.

4. Taurus, Gemini, Cancer in order the 12 signs are written inside all around the 4 sides. First the starting used to be from the constellation of Krittika, so the three quarters of Krittika which are the 2nd, 3rd, 4th falls in the sign of Taurus. The signs have been placed, beginning from Taurus.

5. Inside the inside square the lunar dates called Tithis and 'war' which are the week days, have been placed. There are five sections of the lunar dates and these are called- Nanda, Bhadra, Jaya, Rikta and Purna. Now the chart given below-

Name of Tithis

1. Nanda - Parthipada *i.e.* the 1st day of the lunar Moon. 2. Bhadra- द्वितीय- The 2nd day of the lunar Moon. 3. Jaya- तृतीया The 3rd day of the lunar Moon. 4. Rikta- चतुर्थी The 4th day of the Lunar Moon. 5. Poorna- पंचमी। The 5th day of the lunar Moon.	पड़वा। In the Local languages it is called in. द्वितीय is called Doja. तृतीया is called Teej. चतुर्थी - is called Chauth and the rest has the same name.	षष्ठि (छठ) सप्तमी अष्ठमी नवमी दशमी	एकादशी द्वादशी त्रियोदशी चतुर्दशी पूर्णिमा is the full Moon. अमावस्या- is when the Sun and Moon are in the same degree.

6. The seven week days are also entered in the Sarvatho Bhadra Chakra. The Hindi names are - सूर्यवार, रविवार, चन्द्रवार, सोमवार, मंगलवार इत्यादि। In English they are–Sunday, Monday, Tuesday, Wednesday, Thursday, Friday, Saturday. Why do we called it Sarvatho Bhadra Chakra? The reason is that it is made in the same manner from all four sides. The house which is similar from all the four sides is called a square and on all the four sides of the house the East, West, North and South. The main door is in the centre on all the foursides then we call them a house of the type of or the form of the Sarvatho Bhadra Chakra.

In all the four directions we have respectively written - घ ङ छ, ष ण ठ, ध फ ढ, थ झ ञ। The letters घ ङ छ। are the first letters of name for person born in the constellation of Ardra. So these letters are written above Ardhra.

See similarly further the constellation Hasta. The letters- ष ण ठ।

Similarly below Purvaasada constellation ध फ ढ। and under Uttra Bhadra constellation थ झ ञ। Swastik or Sarvatho Bhadra Chakra is similar from all the four sides.

Now we speak about how to decide from the Sarvatho Bhadra Chakra the good and the evil.

Rule No. 1

a. Saturn, Sun, Rahu, Ketu are malefic - All the reamaing planets are benefic.

b. If Mercury is with malefic then it is considered a malefic.

c. The waining Moon is a malefic.

Rule No. 2

First decide as to which planet you want to consider, if it is good or bad in transit.

For example– Suppose we have to consider the transit of Saturn. Then during the time of the transit *i.e* when Saturn is transiting we should observe as to which constellation it is placed in. In any Nakshtra the planet does Vedh in three manners–

a. With the aspect from the left.

b. Aspect from the right.

c. Aspect from the front.

   (i) When the planet is retrograde then it's aspect is right.

   (ii) When a planet is moving faster then its average motion then the aspect it throws is left.

   (iii) When a planet is in normal motion (average) then it is supposed to have aspect from the front.

Rule No. 3

a. The placement of a planet in any constellation and when this planet does Vedh from the left then it does the Vedh of the constellation, Swar- Varna *i.e.* of the मात्रा and Consonants, etc.

b. When in a constellation a planet is placed and it does the Vedh with the right aspect then it also does the Vedh of the constellation, Swar and Varna *i.e.* the मात्रा etc.

c. When a planet in a constellation does the Vedh with the front aspect at that time it does not do the Vedh for Swar, Varna etc. but does the Vedh of the Constellation (only).

Rule No. 4

For example-

(i) Suppose Saturn is transiting the Rohini constellation then the letter ब। the sign Gemini. The स्वर और मात्रा- औ, Virgo sign the letter- र। The constellation Swati then it does Vedh of all these. Look into the Sarvatho Bhadra Chakra. All this is when it is doing it with Vamadristhi left aspect.

(ii) In the right aspect it does Vedh of – उ। and the Ashwini constellation.

(iii) When it is average in motion then it will do the Vedh from the front aspect, and so here will be only the Abhijit constellation which will get the Vedh.

Second Example- If a planet (the planet whose transit is under consideration) is in the constellation Krittika then..........

(i) By left aspect it is Vedh of the letter- अ। Taurus, sign lunar date, Nanda (1st, 6th and 11th days) planets Sun and Mars, (Bhadra- 2nd, 7th and 12th lunar dates). Libra sign, the letter- त। Constellation Vishakha.

(ii) By right aspect it does Vedh of the Bharani constellation.

(iii) With the front aspect it does Vedh of the constellation Sravana.

Rule No. 5

(i) Sun and Moon always have left aspect.

(ii) Rahu and Ketu always have right aspect.

(iii) The remaining five planets viz. Mars, Mercury, Jupiter, Venus and Saturn have front, left, right at different times. Out of these three one of them is at any time. This has been mentioned in Rule— above.

Some learned persons are of the opinion that Sun, Moon, Rahu and Ketu, the four of them always have all the three types of aspect i.e. left, right and front. But our view is that Sun and Moon have left aspect and Rahu and Ketu always have right aspect.

Rule No. 6

(i) When malefic planets in transit are retrograde then they give more malefic results.

(ii) When benefic planets are retrograde then they show extraordinary benefic results.

(iii) When benefic planets are retrograde then they are capable of conferring kingdom and happiness and good things equal to that.

(iv) When malefic are retrograde then the native (the one whose horoscope is under consideration) enters into many calamities and dangers. He wanders from one place to another with no success. He does hard work but there are no gains, success totally avoids him.

Rule No. 7

(i) When the letter क। is having Vedh then simultaneously the letters- घ ङ छ। also are in Vedh.

(ii) When the letter प is under Vedh then the letters- ष ण ठ। also are in Vedh.

(iii) When the letter भ। is under Vedh then the letters- ध फ ढ। Consonants also get Vedh.

(iv) When the letter द। is having Veda then the letters— थ झ ञ। also get Vedh.

Rule No. 8

(i) When व। is having Vedh then ब। should be taken in Vedh or *vice-versa* when ब as the Vedh व should be under Vedh.

(ii) When स। has Vedh then श also has Vedh and in the reverse way श having Vedh then स is also considered to be in Vedh.

(iii) When ख। has Vedh then ष also has Vedh and *vice-versa*.

(iv) When य has Vedh then ज also is considered to having Vedh and when ज has Vedh then य is considered to in Vedh.

(v) When न has Vedh then ण also has Vedh when ण has Vedh then न is considered in Vedh.

Rule No. 9

(i) अ, आ- Is any of them has Vedh then the 2nd one is also considered to in Vedh.

(ii) इ, ई- When one is in Vedh then the 2nd one is also in Vedh.

(iii) उ, ऊ- When one is in Vedh then the 2nd one is also in Vedh.

(iv) ऋ, ॠ- When one is in Vedh then 2nd one is also in Vedh.

(v) ऌ, ॡ- When one is in Vedh then 2nd one is automatically in Vedh.

(vi) ए, ऐ- Is any one is in Vedh then the 2nd one is automatically in Vedh.

(vii) ओ, औ- When one has Vedh, the second one also has Vedh.

(viii) अ- in the Vedh then अं, अ: both of them are in Vedh.

Rule No. 10

(i) When a planet is in the fourth quarter of the constellation Bharani or in the 1st quarter of Krittika constellation then it does Veda of the letters - आ, ऊ, ॡ, औ।

(ii) When any planet is in the last quarter of Ashlesha (आश्लेषा) or in the first quarter of Magha (मघा) then it does the Vedh of आ, ऊ, ॡ, औ।

(iii) When any planet is in the fourth quarter of Vishakha or in the first quarter of Anuradha then it does Veda of ई, ऋ, ए, अं। These four Vowels are in Vedh.

(iv) When a planet is in the last quarter of the Sarvana, then the Vowels in Veda are- ई, ऋ, ऐ, and अ: ।

(v) Out of the above four conditions if any one exists then the Lunar date which have Vedh are Purna Tithi i.e. (5th, 10th day, full Moon Amavasya).

Rule No. 11

Now whoever is the person whose good and bad has to be considered or analysed from the Sarvotho Bhadra Chakra then note on a paper his -

(i) Name. The first letter of the name by which he is known to other people.

(ii) The Swar- the Vowels.

(iii) His birth star *i.e* the constellation occupied by Moon at birth.

(iv) The lunar date when he was born

(v) The Moon sign.

The readers are familiar with the following which has been recommended to be noted down viz. The first letter of the name, the birth star, the lunar date of birth, and the Moon sign. So it is not necessary to explain it to them. But what about the Vowels? It needs to be explained in details. How to decipher the Vowels that will be applicable.

Look into the table given below-

Varna- Swar Chakra- It has Seven Columns

1	2	3	4	5	6	7
क	छ	ड	ध	भ	व	The Vowel of these is - ा
ख	ज	ढ़	न	म	श	The Vowel of these is - ा
ग	झ	त	प	य	ष	The Vowel of these is - ा
घ	ट	थ	फ	र	स	The Vowel of these is - ा
च	ठ	द	ब	ल	ह	The Vowel of these is - ा

1. ब and व।

2. श and स।

3. ष and ख।

All these Vowels are mentioned in separate places but when one of them for example- ब and व । gets the Vedh then the second one is also supposed to be in Vedh. Vedh means- Pricked.

From- क to ह are- 33 Consonants. But (in the Chakra) in the table above only 30 has been given. We have not given - ङ, ञ, ण । Because in general no names start from these letters. But if the Vowels have to be decided about then these have to be taken into the account viz., - ङ, ञ, ण । for - ङ it will be- उ; for ञ, इ; for ण, अ । These will be the vowels for ङ and ण ।

Rule No. 12

(i) Now we explain the effect of the Vedh. We have given above the birth star, the moon sign, the lunar date of birth, the first letter with which the name starts and the Vowel of first letter with which the name starts. Out of these if one has Vedh then there will be uneasiness, mental apprehensions, worries, anxieties.

(ii) If two of them have Vedh then the result is fears.

(iii) If three of them has Vedh it means losses. Loss of wealth, property, position.

(iv) If four of them has Vedh then there will be sickness, disease.

(v) If all the five mentioned above have Vedh, then the conclusion is death or sufferings equivalent to death.

If the radical Moon or the Moon sign has Vedh from Saturn, Mars, Rahu, Ketu and Sun, then also death or sufferings equal to death.

2. The way the result of the Vedh of malefic have been given above as evil in the same manner when there is Vedh from benefic planets, then the results is beneficial. The number of benefic planet giving Vedh to birth star, Moon sign etc. so much better will be the good effect. The benefic planets are– Jupiter, Venus, Moon (of the Shukla pakshas), Mercury etc. We repeat if the Vedh is from many malefic the result is extremely bad and if it is with benefic (more the number of the benefic) doing Vedh then the result will be so much more benefic.

3. If malefic and benefic both type of planets cause Vedh then logical conclusion should be drawn.

VEDH OF MALEFIC

Rule No. 13

(i) Generally when the birth star has Vedh then the mind is confused (wondering- I should this or I should do that and so many impractical ideas come to the brain, which are not feasable) when the first letter by which the name starts has Vedh then losses. When the Swar- *i.e.* the Vowels have Vedh then losses. When the lunar date has Vedh then calamities and big obstacles; If all the five have Vedh then the native does not survive.

(ii) Now if a person is engaged in a war (*i.e.* we want to know the good and bad about a person who is fighting with weapons in the battle field), then- (One) the birth name, the birth star etc. The Vedh of any one can create fears in the native. If two of them have Vedh then losses of wealth and if he is involved in legal dispute then loss in dispute.

If three of them has Vedh then there is a possibility of fracture in the hands or feet or serious injuries to some portions of the body.

If the four of them has Vedh then it can give death.

Rule No. 14

(i) When Sun has Vedh then the result is— worries, anxieties, mental anguish.

(ii) Mars having Vedh creates loss of wealth.

(iii) When Saturn has Vedh *i.e.* the planet Saturn himself is in Vedh then disease and pains.

(iv) When Rahu or Ketu has Vedh then the conclusion is obstacles, hindrances, calamities.

(v) When Moon has Vedh then the effect is mixed. If the Moon is waning and very weak then great negative effects. If the Moon is very strong and powerful then the Vedh of the Moon gives benefic results.

(vi) When Venus is in the Vedh then in the horoscope of male persons it indicates indulgence and association of women. Intimate relationships. In the horoscope of women good times—and men come in their life and general results are gain of clothes, ornaments, luxurious items and other beautiful objects.

(vii) When Mercury has Vedh then the mind becomes penetrating and good, new ideas come, shortcut method of efficiency, increase of knowledge, success in debates and good news through correspondence or communication.

(viii) When Jupiter has Vedh then all type of benefic results should be concluded.

Rule No.15

(i) When the planet who is having the Vedh is retrograde then the effect doubles up. When it is a malefic then the negativity becomes double too. Benefic planets create and give two times more gains and happiness.

(ii) When the planet having Vedh is exalted then the results are three times more.

(iii) If it is in ordinary sign which is - neither a friend nor an enemy, nor own sign, nor exalted then the result is ordinary.

(iv) In the sign of debilitation the Vedh creates only half the effect.

Look for Vedh at the time of Muhurta - (Time for starting a new work)

Rule No. 16

(i) The lunar dates, the signs, the Navansha, or the constellation having Vedh with malefic should not be selected to start a good work. For example—Ashtami, the lunar date is receiving a Vedh from a malefic, then no new work should be started on that Ashtami.

(ii) One who falls sick at this time when there is a Vedh takes a long time to recover. If one is married at this time then there is no conjugal happiness. If travelling is commenced at that time then travels are not beneficial and does not bring in good results.

(iii) If the day of week is having Vedh see Sarvatho Bhadra Chakra, then in the squares of lunar date, the small letter meaning Sun,

Moon, Mars etc. have been written from them their week day should be understood *i.e.* the Sun- means- Sunday, Moon-means- Monday, Mars- means- Tuesday and so on then that week day when it is having the Vedh then there is no inner contentment rather worries occur.

Rule No. 17

The Combust Direction

The combust direction in the Sarvatho Bhadra Chakra

(i) Taurus, Gemini and Cancer represents East. When Sun in transit is passing through any of these sign then it should be concluded that the East is combust. The letters written in the North East direction viz. अ, ऊ, लृ and ओ should also be taken to be combust.

(ii) In the South– Leo, Virgo and Libra are the signs– when Sun is transiting in any of these signs then the South direction should be supposed to be combust- आ, उ, ऊ, लहृ and औ। These four Vowels are also combust when Sun is in Leo, Virgo and Libra.

(iii) In the West– Scorpio Sagittarius and Capricorn are the signs. The transit of Sun in any of the three will make the West combust. In the South West the Vowels- इ, ऋ, ए अं। are also written and so they are also combust.

(iv) In the North Aquarius, Pisces and Aries are the signs and when Sun is in these signs then the North is combust. Side-by-side the North-West which has the

Vowels- ई, ॠ, ऐ, अः। will also be taken as combust whenever Sun in transit passes in any of the three sign of Aquarius, Pisces and Aries.

(v) The signs which are combust then at the same time the constellation the Vowels, the Consonants, the lunar date, all of them in that direction will be combust.

(vi) Page- 665- When the first letter of the name the Swar- which is the Vowel, birth star, Moon sign, lunar date all of them are combust then what is the different results. If birth star is combust then the result is sickness, If the first letter of the name is combust then losses should be understood. In case the Vowels is combust then sorrow. If Moon sign is combust then obstacles. If the lunar date is combust then fear should be concluded.

(vii) One should not travel in the direction which is combust. One should not keep the main door of the house in that direction.

(viii) When the first letter of the name is combust then generally success does not come in work.

(ix) If the birth star rises *i.e.* when the combust effect is over then Pusthi- vigour; if the first letter of the name rises then gains. When the Vowels rise then happiness, when the birth sign rises *i.e* comes out of the combust effect then victory. If the lunar date rises then luster on the face and fame increases. If all the five are rising like none of them is combust then a person attains a height like— a new position or status.

The Logic in the Sarvatho Bhadra vis-a-vis the satellites.

Rule No. 18

Look to the constellation Sun is transiting, then from it,

(i) The 5th constellation is called- 'Vidyun Mukh'.

(ii) The 8th Nakshatra is called 'Shool'.

(iii) The 14th Nakshatra is 'Sannipat'.

(iv) The 18th Nakshatra is 'Ketu'.

(v) The 21st Nakshatra is 'Ulka'.

(vi) The 22nd Nakshatra is 'Kump'.

(vii) The 23rd Nakshatra is 'Vajrak'.

(viii) The 24th Nakshatra is called 'Nirdhat'.

If out of these 8 constellations mentioned above any planet is present in one or more constellation then they create obstacles in work.

Consideration of the transit of Moon

The constellation occupied by Moon at birth is called the birth star.

The 10th constellation from the birth star is 'Karma'.

The 16th constellation is the 'Sanghatik'.

The 18th is 'Samudayik'.

The 19th is 'Aadhan'.

The 23rd is 'Vinashi'.

The 26th is 'Jaati'

The 27th is 'Desha' and

The 28th Nakshtra is Abhishek.

If malefic planet in transit are passing through the birth star, karma constellation, aadhan or in vinasha constellation then the result is suffering, quarrels, sorrow, mental anguish etc. In the Samudayik Nakshtra, a malefic causes unforeseen calamities. In the Jaati Nakshtra Vedh creates family - sorrow. In the Abhishek a Vedh with a malefic creates, sufferings like- imprisonment, hospitalization etc. In the 'Desha' Nakshtra malefic cause- one to leave one's country on account of the law.

If benefic planets create Vedh then benefic result should be understood.

सर्वतो भद्र चक्रोक्त शुभवेधाः शुभावहाः ।
पापवेधा दुःखतरा गोचरेताश्च चित्तयेत् ॥४८ ॥

Malefic creating Vedh are givers of suffering and sorrow. Benefic if they are the Vedh planet then they give and endow one with benefic results. Therefore whatever results good and bad that have been described in the 'Sarvatho Bhadra Chakra' about Vedh should also be considered.

दशापहाराष्टक वर्गगोचरे
ग्रहेषु नृणां विषमस्थितेष्वपि ।
जपेच्च तत्प्रीतिकरैः सुकर्मभिः
करोति शान्तिं व्रतदानवन्दनैः ॥४९ ॥

If a planet in transit is malefic or the major and minor periods of malefic planets are running then good deeds to pacify the planet viz.- fasting, donations, worshipping, Japa and Shantipaath should be performed to mitigate the evil effect of the planet.

अहिंसकस्य दान्तस्य धर्मार्जितधनस्य च।
सर्वदा नियमस्थस्य सदा सानुग्रहा ग्रहा: ॥५० ॥

The planets are always kind to that person, who does not desire the ill of others, doesn't want to kill others, has control on his mind and emotions, and one who is engaged in earning money on the path of religion in the righteous manner and always follows the principles laid down in scriptures.

27

Sanyas Yoga

In this chapter different combinations for Ascetic life (Sanyas) has been dealt with.

ग्रहैश्चतुर्भिः सहिते खनाथे
त्रिकोणगैः केन्द्रगतैस्तु मुक्तः ।
लग्ने गृहान्ते सति सौम्यभागे
केन्द्रे गुरौ कोणगते च मुक्तः ॥१ ॥

If the lord of the 10th house occupies 1st, 4th, 7th, 10th, 5th or 9th house together with four other planets then the native attains liberation after this life *i.e.*, he will overcome the wheel of life and death.

एकर्क्षसंस्थैश्चतुरादिकैस्तु
ग्रहैर्वदेतत्र बलान्वितेन ।
प्रव्रज्यकां तत्र वदन्ति केचित्
कर्मेशतुल्यां सहिते खनाथे ॥२ ॥

Four planets in one house constitute Sanyas. The type of Sanyas will depend upon the strongest planet out of the four *i.e.*, the Sanyas will be as indicated by the nature of the strongest planet. If the lord of 10th house is one of the four planets constituting Sanyas then it will have priority over other planets and the native's Ascetic life will be according to the lord of the 10th house. This is the opinion of a few.

शशी दृगाणे रविजस्य संस्थितः
कुजार्किदृष्टः प्रकरोति तापसम् ।

कुजांशके वा रविजेन दृष्टो
नवांशतुल्यां कथयन्ति तां पुनः ॥३ ॥

If Moon occupies the Dreshkana (Decanet) owned by Saturn, and Mars and Saturn simultaneous aspect Moon, then the native will be a 'Tapaswi' and a Sanyasi. This is one yoga. Now we state the second one. If Moon is in the Navansha of Mars, and Saturn aspects it then the native will take Sanyas according to the Navansha of Moon *i.e.* as indicated by Mars.

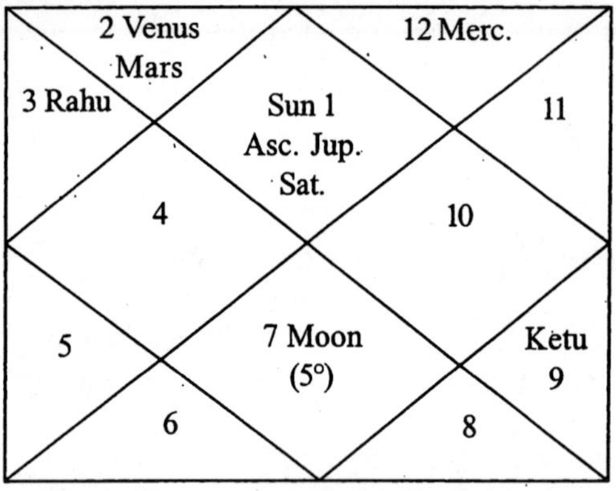

In the example horoscope Moon is in the Navansha of Mars and is aspected by Saturn. This person took sanyas and founded places of worship all over the world. He has already constructed temples of lord Hanuman in many countries. (The worshipping of Lord Hanuman in this case is due to Moon being in the Navansha of Mars. Hanuman is the presiding diety of Mars).

जन्माधिपः सूर्यसुतेन दृष्टः
शेषैरदृष्ट पुरुषस्य सूतौ।
आत्मीयदीक्षां कुरुते ह्यवश्यं
पूर्वोक्तमत्रापि विचारणीयम् ॥४ ॥

If only Saturn (and no other planet) aspect the lord of the sign occupied by the Moon then the native definitely gets initiated. The type of Sanyas should be considered by the lord of the sign, occupied by the Moon.

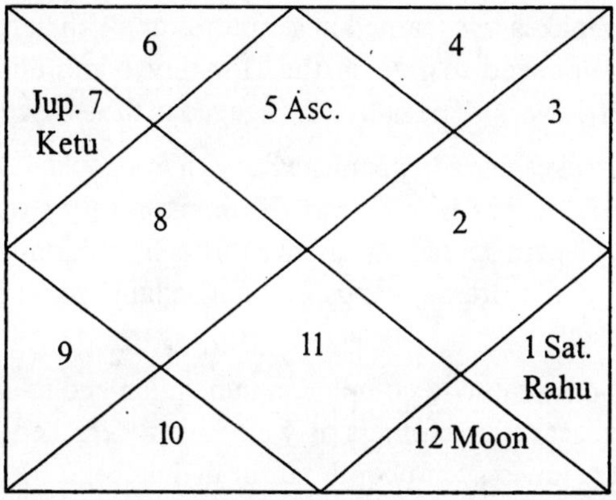

In the horoscope given above Moon occupies the sign of Jupiter, which is aspected by Saturn. There is no other aspect on Jupiter. The association of South Node of Moon (Ketu) did not allow him to take Sanyas. The native is however religious and expert in Tantra - Shastra.

योगीशं दीक्षितं वा कलयति तरणिस्तीर्थपान्थं हिमांशु-
दुर्मन्त्रज्ञ च बौधाश्रयमवनिसुतो ज्ञो मतान्यप्रविष्टम् ।
वेदान्तज्ञानिनं वा यतिवरममरेड्यो भृगर्लिङ्गवृत्ति
व्रात्यं शैलूषवृतिं शनिरिह वाऽथ पाषण्डिनं वा ॥५ ॥

Sun makes one engage in yoga and meditation. The native worships Sun and Gayatri Mantras. Moon makes one a pilgrim. He visits holy places of worship and moves on from one holy place to the other. (He worships lord Shiva).

अतिशयबलयुक्तः शीतगुः शुक्लपक्षे
बलविरहितमेनं प्रेक्षते लग्ननाथः ।
यदि भवति तपस्वी दुःखितः शोकतप्तो
धनजनपरिहीनः कृच्छ्रलब्धान्नपन्नः ॥६ ॥

Mars draws one to a rigorous life. The native will be engaged in strong and forceful attainment of difficult Mantras [can be a Vam a margi] (He worships Lord Hanuman). At times he renounces and becomes Buddhist Monk. Mercury makes one change his religion. (It also draws one to the worship of lord Vishnu) and Krishna.

Jupiter makes one learned in scriptures or a Yati (a religious sect which are supposed to live in the Himalayas and endowed with supernatural powers). The native is engaged in the service of Brahma.

Venus makes one a hypocrat - a Sanyasi from outside but attached to the material things in his heart. If Venus is very strong then the native is engaged in spreading Krishna through Sankirtan, through the medium of music drama, songs etc. and attains proximity to God through music.

Saturn draws one to complete renunciation and at one stage the native will discard his clothers as well (live a detached life in deep forests). Sometimes such people fall in their ascetic life and turn to cheating. (this is so if Saturn is afflicted).

Moon is very strong during the bright half. If Moon is weak in the nativity and is aspected by the lord of the Ascendant then the native will be devoid of wealth, relatives, unhappy and sorrowful if he takes to Sanyas. Moon during the dark half is devoid of strength, directional strength etc. and is considered weak. Such a person gets even food and milk with difficulty.

प्रकथितमुनियोगे राजयोगो यदि स्या-
दशुभफलविपाकं सर्वमुन्मूल्य पश्चात्।
जनयति पृथिवीशं दीक्षितं साधुशीलं।
प्रणतनृपशिरोभिः स्पृष्टपादाब्जयुग्मम्॥७॥

If in the yoga for 'Muni' mentioned above, the nativity also has raja yoga then the bad effects mentioned therein will subside of some extent. If the Raja Yoga is very powerful then the native will be a Sanyasi who will be like a King. He will own lands; will be gentle and endowed with good qualities. He will be worshipped and praised by others.

चत्वारो द्युचराः खनाथसहिताः केन्द्रे त्रिकोणेऽथवा
सुस्थाने बलिनस्त्र यदि तदा सन्याससिद्धिर्भवेत्।
सब्द्बाहुल्यवशाच्च तत्र सुशुभस्थानस्थितैस्तैर्वदेत्
प्रव्रज्यां महितां सतामभिमतां चेदन्यथा निन्दिताम्॥८॥

If four planets (out of which one should be lord of the 10th house) occupy an angular position (1, 4, 7, 10th) or a trine (5, 9), or if three strong planets occupy good houses in a nativity the native desires to attain Sanyas and becomes powerful after he turns to Sanyas. He is satisfied and he is a Sanyasi in its true senses. If in the above case benefic planets are more and occupy good houses then the native gets honour and respect from Good people. If malefic are posited in such a manner the native does not receive praise from others.

28

Upsanharadhdyaya

संज्ञाध्यायः कारको वर्गसंज्ञो
वीर्याध्यायः कर्मजोवोऽथ योगः।
योगो राज्ञां राशिलीलो ग्रहाणां
मेषादीनां लग्नसम्प्राप्तशीलः ॥१॥

भार्याभावो जातकं कामिनीनां
सूनुर्बालारिष्टयोगोऽथ रोगः।
भावस्तस्माद्द्वादशावाप्तभावा
निर्याणं स्यादू द्विग्रहाद्याश्च तस्मात् ॥२॥

सूर्यादीनां यत्फलं तद्दशाप्तं
भावादीनामीश्वराङ्का दशा च।
सूर्यादीनामन्तराख्या दशाऽथ
सव्यासव्या कालचक्रोऽष्टवर्गः ॥३॥

होरासारावाप्तयद्यष्टवर्गो
मान्द्यध्यायो गोचर स्यात्प्रव्रज्यः।
अध्यायानां विंशतिः सप्तयुक्तान्
जन्मन्येतद्गोलजं संवदामि ॥४॥

श्रीशालिवाटिजातेन मया मन्त्रेश्वरेण वै।
दैवज्ञेन द्विजाग्रेण सतां ज्योतिर्विदां मुदे ॥५॥

सकुन्तलाम्बां सम्पूज्य सर्वाभीष्टप्रदायिनीम्।
तत्कटाक्षविशेषेण कृता या फलदीपिका॥६॥

I, the resident of SHALI VATI (Samprati Tinnevalley) am a Superior Astrologer among the Brahmins. After worshipping and seeking the grace of the Giver of all blessings, Sukantala Mata, I have constructed the present Phaldeepika for the happiness of Astrologers. My name is Mantreshwar. In the preceding 27 Chapters, I have analysed the following subject.

1. Introduction of signs and what they signify (Definition).
2. Planets and their meanings.
3. Divisions, Hora, Decanate etc.
4. Strength and Weakness of Planets.
5. Career - the method of livelihood.
6. Yoga- combination of planets and their interpretations.
7. Raj Yoga- Yoga for attaining - Kingdom, high position.
8. The effect of different planets in different signs.
9. The interpretation of Aries, Taurus etc. in the Ascendant.
10. The Seventh House (Wife).
11. Special consideration in Female Horoscopes.
12. The House of Children (V- house).
13. Intimately death in childhood (Bala rishta).
14. Disease (Sickness)
15. Analysis of the effect of Different houses.
16. The twelve houses– Interpretation.
17. The ending - timing of Death.
18. The effect of the combination of two or more planets.
19. Ududasha (Vimshottari Dasha)- Major Periods of Planets.
20. Interpretation of Planets due to their lordship.
21. Antardasha (minor periods) and Pratyantara Dasha (small periods)
22. Kal Chakra Dasha.

23. Ashtak Vargas.
24. Ashtak Varga Process as is mentioned in 'Horasara'.
25. Mandi and other Satellites of Planets.
26. Transits
27. Sanyas Yoga (combination for Ascetic life).

Which planet is called a defeated planet?

The answer to this question is that–

a. When two planets are in the same sign, degree, minutes– then they are side to be engaged in war with each other.

b. The three balas viz. (i) Sthanbala (ii) Dikbala (iii) Kalabala should be calculated out of the Shadbalas (six type of strength) which includes the above mentioned 3 balas and also (iv) Ayanbala (v) Chestabala (vi) Naisargikbalas.

c. Add the first 3 balas only in order to arrive at the 'Yudhbala'.

d. Subtract the one with lesser strength (bala) from the one which has more strength.

e. The remainder should be divided by the Bimba Parimana (the area inside the circumstances) of the two planets.

f. Add the quotient to the (Yudhbala) (three balas) of the planet in the North direction and subtract the quotient from the planet in the South direction.

g. The planet in the North is the victorious one and the after one in the South is the defeated one. The planetary Bimba Parimana are as follows-

---

If the sign, decanate, Navansha, all the three of a planet are in their own or exalted divisions, then it is said to be in the 'Uttam Varga'. Some astrologers are of the view that if a planet is in any three, out of the ten Vargas, in own or exalted divisions it is in the 'Uttam Varga'. This opinion is considered to be a weak opinion.

Planet	Bimba Parimana
Mars	9.4 Seconds
Mercury	6.6 Seconds
Jupiter	190.4 Seconds
Venus	16.6 Seconds
Saturn	158.0 Seconds

APPENDIX-1

PREFACE

'अं', 'ऊ', 'म' - Alphabets 'ह', 'ँ' One of the five elements - 'Ether'. Vata - Vayu, Wind - one of the three doshas. Shwas - Prashaws - inhaling - exhaling of breath. Maya - The luxuries, the world matters. Chakras - Centres, Wheel. Kundalini - The Sepentine (Power). Moksha - Liberation. Saguna - Nirguna (with formation and visible - not visible).

Dakshin Murti and Jantrasara - Well known books of Tantra. Inhaling - Exhaling - Kumbhik all three are related with breath - in take - outlet and stopping it in between. Kalpa Vriksha - The tree which fulfills all desires - supposed to be located in Haven. Shrividya - Mother Divine. Shiva - The Supreme Power. Ardha Narishwar - Shiva (Half Woman - Half Man). Pran - Life. Hansa - Soul. Atma - Soul. Shri Ramanuja, Mantreshwar, Maharishi Parashar, Gemini Yavanacharya, Narada etc. were great astrologers of their times. karma - Deeds in life/Previous - Present. Ravana - King of Lanka (Ceylon). For details see 'Ramayan'. Sita, Ram, Lakshman - See 'Ramayan'. Duryodhan - See the Epic 'Mahabharat'. 'Helen' - Read 'Helen of Troy'.

INTRODUCTION

Tamil, Telgu, Kannada, Malyalam, Gujrati, etc. are some of the language in India (different parts of India). Saravali - A great treatise on predictive astrology.

DIFFERENT

Chapter - I

Dhruva Loka

The abode named after Dhruva who was the Son of a King and

worshipper of 'Vishnu'. Ganesh - The lord who removes all obstacles - One of the five schools whose worship is done - viz. Ganesh, Vishnu, Shiva, Surya and Shakti.

Maharshi Atri - Rishi

Ghatis - Palas - Vipalas - The method of time measurement indication. The time like Hours - Minutes - Seconds and Ghati has 60 Palas and one Pala has 60 Vipalas - One Ghati = 24 minutes. Kala Purush - The Supreme Power; God. Rashi Sandhi - Where 2 signs meet. The end of one sign and the beginning of the other sign.

Moola Trikona

Certain degrees in a sign are allotted to planets which is called its Mool Trikona. This portion is more powerful then the own sign but has less strength then a planet's sign of exaltation. SeeTable of Moola Trikona (Chapter - I). Urdha. Adha. Sama. Vakra. Bhava - House. Hawana (Yogya) - fire sacrifice/religious rites. Satwa - (strength - physical and mental). Brahmins - Priestly caste in India - Four exists-Brahmins-Shatriya-Vaisya-Shudras. Shruti Smirity-Holy books. Tapasya-Rigorous penance.

Shastha - Goddess. Brahma - God who created the Universe due to the desire of Vishnu. He was born out of the naval of Lord Vishnu. Sheshnag - The Serpent God also holds this earth on his head. The king of Snakes. The one on whose lap lord Vishu takes rest.

Chapter - III

Shadvargas - Six Divisions. Saptavargas - Seven Divisions. Har - Name of Shiva. Parijatansha, Uttamansha, Gopuransha, Singhasansha, Parvatansha, Devlokansha, Surlokansha, Aairavatansha - These are the natives given to indicate the strength of a planet if it is in 2,3,4,5,6,7,8, or 9 divisions endowed with strength due to being in own, sign, exaltation etc. Ansha - Means certains divisions. Avasthas - Bal (very young like 4 years); (Kumar - teenage); Yuga (young - like 21 to 36 years); Prodha (like 45-50-55); Vridhdha - (67 onwards).

Chapter - IV

Graha Bala - Planetary Strength. Roopa - One unit of 60 points. Saptavarga - Seven Divisions. Keshavi Jataka - Book of Astrology. Ayan - Northern or Southern portion of Equator. Cheshtabala - Strength due to the motion . Surya Siddhanta - Book which gives the Astronomical Calculations. Vikram Samvat - The calendar prevailing on India. It starts from the year King Vikramaditya Ascended the throne. Pinda - The total.. Bhavesh - Lord of the house. Shubha - Benefic. Keet - Insects.

Abda

Parivesh, Indrachap, Gullik, Mandi etc. are names. Dhoom, Vyatipate etc. names.

Chapter - V - VI

Names of Yogas

A. Panch Mahapurush viz. Ruchak, Bhadra, Hansa, Malavya, Sasa - Created by Mars, Mercury, Jupiter, Venus and Saturn respectively.

B. Anpha, Sunpha, Durdhara, and Kemudrum.

C. Subhavesi, Subhavasi, Ubahyachari - Papavasi, Papaubahya Chari, Papakartari, Subhakartari.

D. Amla, Mahabhagya Yoga.

E. Kesari Yoga or Gaja - Kesari Yoga, Sakat, Adham, Sama, Varishta.

F. Vasuman Yoga, Pushkal.

G. Subhamala, Asubhamala or Asubhamalika Lakshmi and Gauri, Saraswati.

H. Shrikantha, Srinath, Viranch Yoga.

'Rudraksha' - name of tree which bears small fruits and the kernel (seeds) are used to weave neckless for Japa. These trees are mostly located in Nepal and some parts of North-East of India. Rudraksha - beads are also known in short as 'Rudraksha'. Narayan - name of Lord Vishnu. Maha Yoga - Dainya Yoga, Khala Yoga, Harsha, Saral, Vimal. Uttarakalamrit - Book of Astrology by Kalidas. Kahal

Yoga - Parvat, Shankha, Vallaki, Vina, Dama, Pasha, Kedar, Shool, Yuga, Gola, Adhi, Chamar, Dhenu, Shorya, Amudhi or Jaladhi, Chatra, Astra, Kama, Asur, Bhagya, Khyati, Suparijatu, Masal Avayoga, Niswas, Vimal, Daridra, Mriti, Kuhu, Pamar, Harsh, Dushkriti, Nirbhagya.

Chapter - VII - VIII

Rajyoga - Combination of Planets which endows them due to the ownership of house to the powers equal to that of a king. Ashwini - First constellation. The others are Bharani etc. (see Appendix 2) names of Nakshatas, Karan and Yogas, Tithis etc. Subramanian Shastri - A writer of many Astrological works. The translation and commentaries. His works promoted astrologers and made it available to the English knowing people. Varga - Division. Varahmihir - Famous Astrologer. Neechabhanga-Cancellation of the debilitated effect. Kamadev - The Cupid.

Chapter - IX - X - XI - XII

Santan - Children. Dosha - Negative factors. Parihar-Counteracting - nullifying a negative factor. Chidra Thithis - 4-6-8-9-12-14 days after full Moon or Amavasya is Chidra Thithis. Karan - See name of Karan (Appendix). Purushsukta - Certain Vedic Mantras welded together for and about the Supreme Power of God heed. Nagraj - Head of Snakes. Sharvana - Name of month (in the Hindu calendar) see Appendix. Kartikswami - Name of God - Son of Lord Shiva and Commander of the army of Gods. Ganesh is also the son of Shiva. Garuda - The big Eagle - used by Lord Vishnu for his travels. Yakshini - The female part of Yaksha - The entities living in the 4th dimension and they control treasure. Kubera or Kuvera - God and treasurer of wealth of Gods half brother of Ravana. Yamaraja - God ruler of Hell. Sankirtan - Devotional songs sung by Groups. Shrimad - Bhagvatam/Religious Book Gita-Spiritual Book of philosophical knowledge. Ekadashi - 11th day of Moon (in the bright half and dark half). Shraddha - Rituals performed for the departed forefathers.

Yamakanta

Upanayan-Sacred thread. Ceremony in the upper caste Hindus and also in Zionist.

Chapter - XIII - XIV

Balarishta - danger in a very young (tender) age. 'Sugam Jyotish Praveshika' - An Astrological book in Hindi for learning Astrology by Pandit Gopesh Kumar Ojha. "Astrology and You" in English or "Predictive Astrology of the Hindus" by Pandit Gopesh Kumar Ojha. Marak - which kills (Fatal). Punya Karma - Good deeds. Sripati - Astrologer. Vidyadharas, Yaksha, Kinnars, Gods - Matrikas Entities living in the 4th dimensions. Urdhawasya. Urdhagati. Ubhayodaya. Vaikuntha - The abode of Lord Vishnu.

Chapter - XV

Trik - The 6th, 8th and 12th house are called Trik.

Chapter - XVI - XVII - XVIII

Kalapurusha - God - The Supreme Power. Dushthan- 6th, 8th and 12th houses. Veda, Scriptures - Spiritual Books. Saumya - Soft, benefic, mild. Siddhakaal - Timing of fruitfulness.

Chapter - XIX

Divyagyan - Celestial knowledge. Yogini dasha has - One of the type of dashas Astottari, Kalchakra etc. are various type of Dashas (Periods). Dakshina - donations after rituals - Yagya (fire sacrifice) etc. Acharya Siddhi - Gains a Guru or himself becomes a Guru. Ratnakar - Samudra - Sea. Tarang - Waves. Ganga - Ganges - The holy river in India - Bathing in if removes all sins and helps in liberation after death. Hindi/Sanskrit names of signs. Hindi/Sanskrit names of Planets and Lagna. Paapi - Malefic. Names of houses - Viz. Tanu, Dhano, Sahaj, Sukh, Putra, Riku, Bharya, Mrityu, Bhagya, Karma, Labha, Vyaya, Jataka Deshmarg. Saravali.

Chapter - XX

Antardasha - The minor period of Planet Arohi - Moving towards the exaltation degree. Avrohi - Moving towards the debilitation degree. Brihat Jatak - Book of Astrology of Kalyan Vermic. Udoo Dasha. Udai Pradeep (Nakshatradasha).

Chapter - XXI - XXII

Pratyantar dasha - Sub Periods of Planets. Yoga Karak- when a planet owns an angle and a trine at the same time then it is called a Yoga Karaka. Jataka Parijata - Brihat Parashar Horashastra. Raphael's Ephemeris - Printed in England for each year. Lahiri's Ephemeris - from Kolkata. Deha - Body. Jeeva - Living Entity/soul. Jeevadhip - Lord of Jeeva sign. Dehadhip - Lord of the Deha sign. Utpanna Mahadasha - The Mahadasha which starts from the 5th Constellation from the birth star - is the Utpunna Mahadasha. Adhan Mahadasha - The Dasha which starts from the 8th Constellation from the birth star. Shema Dasha - The Persian Master - great Astrologer. Ansha Dasha - Based in the longitudes of the Planet and its strength. Satyacharya. Maya. Jeevasharma. Pindayur Dasha - Best way to measure the longevity. But many other Masters do not agree with this Manithya. Chankya. Shruti. Nisargayu- Natural periods. Gurujan - Older and respected person.

Chapter - XXIII

Ashtakvarga - Eight Divisions. Seven for the Sun, Moon, Mars, Mercury, Jupiter, Venus and Saturn. The eight is for the Ascendant. Bindus - Benefic Points - These are shown in the chart as 'O'.

Chapter - XXIV

Horsar. Shodhya Pind. Trikona Shodhan - The signs are grouped in 4 Trines (1-5-9) and then correction is done in the number of the benefic points. Prasnamarg. Bhagwat Gita. Sanyas. Niskam Karma. Bhakti. Sayankya. Yoga. Ekadhipatya Shodhan. Mandan - Cycle. Shambhu Hora Prakash. Haran - Reduction in Dasha.

Chapter -XXV - XXVI - XXVII - XXVIII

Gullika etc. Uppagrahas - Sattelite. Upketu- Dhoom, etc. Tyajakala - Times to be discarded. (No auspicious work should be done in these). Visghatis. Ashtak - Eight. Mana - The emotions - The desires. Varahmihir. Brihat Jatak. W.J. Tucker - Author of "Fixed Stars and Your Horoscope". Vedh - Obstruction - Piercing - Muhurata Chintami. Narad. Kashyap (Rishis). Vipreet Vedh - Adhan - The 19th Constellation from the Moon. Vipat - The 3rd Constellation from the Moon. Vainashik - 22nd Constellation from the Moon. Pratyari - The 5th Constellation from the Moon. Vadha - The 7th Constellation from the Moon. Sankaramara - Change of sign by Sun. Ulka Nipat - Comets.

Anujanma - The 10th from birth. Tri Janma - The 19th Nakshtra.

Name of Thithis

Page 616

Days of Week (Page 645 see App.-2)

'Prasana Marg' is a rare book of Prasna (Horary) and Predictive Part of Astrology. It was earlier available in the local language in Kerala (Malayam). It has 32 Chapters and then it was printed in 2 parts of 16 chapters each.

'Laghu Prashari' is an abridged version of Parashar Horashastra. It is a book which is good in a manner but it is like trying to till the entire sea in a pot. For basics it is fine.

Brihat Jataka was written by Varah Mihir. Many people have written commentary and notes in it.

'Hora Sar' is an authoritative book of predictive Astrology and Mantreshwar in his 'Phaldeepika has mentioned it.

APPENDIX - 2

Some more words which occur in the book

म ह स Alphabets १ २ ३ ४ ५ ६ ७ ८ ९ १० ११ १२ १३ १४ १५ १६ १७ १८ १९ २० Akash tatwa - one of the five elements viz., Ether

Vata - vayu, wind one of the three Doshas in Ayurvada

Shawas - Prashwas - Inhaling and exhaling of breath

Maya - The luxuries of life, the wordly matters vis a vis spiritualism

Chakras - Centres, wheel.

Moksha - Liberation

Saguna - Nirguna (with formation and visible and - not visible)

Dakshini Murti Samhita - and Tantrasara Books of Mantra and Tantra

Inhaling-exhaling-Kumbhak - all related to breathing - intake, outlet, and stopping of breathe in between.

Kalpavrishka- The tree which fulfills all desires, located in Heaven

Sri Vidya - The Mother Divine

Shiva - The Supreme Power.

Weekdays

Sunday

Monday

Tuesday

Wednesday

Thursday

Friday

Saturday

Ardha-Narishwar - Lord Shiva in the form of half woman and half male.

Pran Life

Hansa Soul

Ama soul

Names of Astrologers : Shri Ramanuja, Mantreshwar, Maharishi Parashar, Gemini, Yavanacharya, Narada, Kalyan Varma.

Karma (Deeds in Life)

Ravana - King of Lanka (Ceylon), for details read Ramayan Sita, Rama, Lakshaman, read Ramayan 'the Epic'

Duryodhan - The eldest son of Dhritrashtra for details read 'The Epic Mahabharat'

Helen - read "Helen of Troy'

Introduction

What is the meaning of the words used in the decanet table? We mention them now.

Ayudh	-	Weapon or one who bears them
Chatushpada	-	Four Legged
Kolanan	-	Pig faced.
Gridhasya	-	Vulture faced
Pash	-	Net
Pakshi	-	Bird
Sarpa	-	Snake
Nigad	-	One who is chained.

Nakshatra Dasha	Nakshatras	Nakshatras	Planets	Years of (these are fixed yrs.)
1 Krittika	Uttra Phalguni	Uttrashada	- Sun	6
2. Rohini	Hasta	Shravana	- Moon	10
3. Mrigsiras	Chitra	Dhanishta	- Mars	7
4. Ardra	Swati	Shatbhisa	- Rahu	18
5. Punarvasu	Vishakha	Porva-Bhadrapada	-Jupiter	16
6. Pusya	Anuradha	Uttara-Bhadrapada	- Saturn	19
7. Aslesa	Jyestha	Revati	- Mercury	17
8. Magha	Moola	Ashwini	- Ketu	7
9. Poorva Phalguni	Porvashada	Bharani	- Venus	20

Introduction

Tamil, Telgu, Kannada, Malyalum, Gujarati, Hindi etc. are some of the languages in India (These are spoken in different parts of the country)

Saravali - a great treatise on predictive astrology by Kalyan Varma

Contents

Ch I, II, III

Manushya, Chatushpada, Jalachar, etc are the names used to decipher characteristics of Constellation.

Vargas - Divisions

Uttamansha, Parijatansha, etc. to indicate the strength of Planets.

Pradipta, Sukhit etc. indicate the class of Moon

Hora - Two equal Divisions of a house/sign

Dreshkan - Decanet - three divisions of a sign

Dasha vargas - Ten Divisions.

APPENDIX - 3

Table of the balance of the Kaal Chakra dasha from the Longitudes of Moon 100 years

	1	2	3	4	5	6	6	8	9	10
Nakshatra	Pada	lon of moon	lon of moon	lon of moon	lon of moon	lon of moon	lon of moon	lon of moon	lon of moon	lon of moon
		S-DE-MIN								
Ashwini	1	0-0-0	0-0-54	0-0-50	0-1-15	0-1-40	0-2-5	0-2-30	0-2-55	0-3-20
Bharani	1	0-13-20	0-13-45	0-14-10	0-14-35	0-15-00	0-15-25	0-15-50	0-16-25	0-16-40
Krittika	1	0-26-40	0-27-5	0-27-30	0-27-55	0-28-20	0-28-45	0-29-10	0-29-35	1-0-0
Rohini	4	1-20-0	1-20-25	1-20-50	1-21-15	1-21-40	1-22-5	1-22-30	1-22-55	1-23-20
Mrigsiras	4	2-3-20	2-3-45	2-4-10	2-4-35	2-5-00	2-5-25	2-5-50	2-6-15	2-6-40
Ardra	4	2-16-40	2-17-5	2-17-30	2-17-55	2-18-20	2-18-45	2-19-10	2-19-35	2-20-0
Punarvasu	1	2-20-0	2-20-25	2-20-50	2-21-15	2-21-40	2-22-5	2-22-30	2-22-55	2-23-20
Pusya	1	3-3-20	3-3-45	3-4-10	3-4-25	3-4-50	3-5-15	3-5-40	3-6-5	3-6-40
Aslesa	1	3-16-40	3-17-5	3-17-30	3-17-55	3-18-20	3-18-45	3-19-10	3-19-34	3-20-0
Magha	4	4-10-0	4-10-25	4-10-50	4-11-15	4-11-40	4-12-5	4-12-30	4-12-55	4-13-20
Purva Phalguni	4	4-23-20	4-23-45	4-24-10	4-24-35	4-25-0	4-25-25	4-25-50	4-26-15	4-26-40
Uttara Phalguni	4	5-6-40	5-7-5	5-7-30	5-7-55	5-7-20	5-7-45	5-9-10	5-9-35	5-10-0
Hasta	1	5-10-0	5-10-25	5-10-50	5-11-15	5-11-40	5-12-5	5-12-30	5-12-55	5-13-20
Chitra	1	5-23-20	5-23-45	5-24-10	5-24-35	5-25-0	5-25-25	5-25-50	5-26-15	5-26-40
Swati	1	6-6-40	6-7-5	6-7-30	6-7-55	6-8-20	6-8-45	6-9-10	6-9-35	6-10-0
Vishakha	4	7-0-0	7-0-25	7-0-50	7-1-15	7-1-40	7-2-5	7-2-30	7-2-55	7-3-20
Anuradha	4	7-13-20	7-13-45	7-14-10	7-14-35	7-15-0	7-15-25	7-15-50	7-16-15	7-16-40
Jeshtha	4	7-26-40	7-27-5	7-27-30	7-27-55	7-28-20	7-28-45	7-29-10	7-29-35	8-0-0
Mool	1	8-0-0	8-0-25	8-0-50	8-1-15	8-1-40	8-2-5	8-2-30	8-2-55	8-3-20

Prvashada	1	8-13-20	8-13-45	8-14-10	8-14-35	8-15-0	8-15-25	8-15-50	8-16-25	8-16-40
Uttarashada	1	8-26-40	8-27-5	8-27-30	8-27-55	8-27-20	8-28-45	8-29-10	8-29-35	9-0-0
Shravana	4	9-20-0	9-20-25	9-20-50	9-21-15	9-21-40	9-22-5	9-22-30	9-22-55	9-23-20
Dhanishtha	4	10-3-20	10-3-45	10-4-10	10-4-35	10-5-0	10-5-25	10-5-50	10-6-15	10-6-40
Shatbhisha	4	10-16-40	10-17-5	10-17-30	10-17-55	10-18-20	10-18-45	10-19-10	10-19-35	10-20-0
Purva bhadrapada	1	10-20-0	10-20-25	10-20-50	10-21-15	10-21-40	10-22-5	10-22-30	10-22-55	10-23-20
Uttara bhadrapada	1	1-3-20	11-3-45	11-4-10	11-4-25	11-4-50	11-5-15	11-5-40	11-6-5	11-6-40
Revati	1	11-16-40	11-17-5	11-17-30	11-17-55	11-18-20	11-18-45	11-19-10	11-19-35	11-20-0
Balance of dasha		100 yrs.	87 yrs 6 mn	75 yrs	62 yrs 6 mn	50 yrs	37 yrs 6 mn	25 yrs	12 yrs 6 mn	nill

Table of the balance of the Kaal Chakra dasha from the Longitudes of Moon 85 years

	1	2	3	4	5	6	6	8	9	10
Nakshatra	Pada	lon of moon	lon of moon	lon of moon	lon of moon	lon of moon	lon of moon	lon of moon	lon of moon	lon of moon
		S-DE-MIN								
Ashwini	2	0-3-20	0-3-45	0-4-10	0-4-35	0-5-0	0-5-25	0-5-50	0-6-15	0-6-40
Bharani	2	0-16-40	0-17-5	0-17-30	0-17-55	0-18-20	0-18-45	0-19-10	0-19-35	0-20-0
Krittika	2	1-0-0	1-0-25	1-0-50	1-1-15	1-1-40	1-2-50	1-2-30	1-2-55	1-3-20
Rohini	3	1-16-40	1-17-5	1-17-30	1-17-55	1-18-20	1-18-45	1-19-10	1-19-35	1-20-0
Mrigsiras	3	2-0-0	2-0-25	2-0-50	2-1-15	2-1-40	2-2-5	2-2-30	2-2-55	2-3-20
Ardra	3	2-13-20	2-13-45	2-14-10	2-14-35	2-15-0	2-15-25	2-15-50	2-16-15	2-16-40
Punarvasu	2	2-23-20	2-23-45	2-24-10	2-24-35	2-25-0	2-25-25	2-25-50	2-26-15	2-26-40

Pusya	2	3-6-40	3-7-5	3-7-30	3-7-55	3-8-20	3-8-45	3-9-10	3-9-35	3-10-0
Aslesa	2	3-20-0	3-20-25	3-20-50	3-21-15	3-21-40	3-22-5	3-22-30	3-22-55	3-23-20
Magha	3	4-6-40	4-7-5	4-7-30	4-7-55	4-8-20	4-8-45	4-9-10	4-9-35	4-10-0
Purva Phalguni	3	4-20-0	4-20-25	4-20-50	4-21-15	4-21-40	4-22-5	4-22-30	4-22-55	4-23-20
Uttara Phalguni	3	5-3-20	5-3-45	5-4-10	5-4-35	5-5-0	5-5-25	5-5-50	5-6-15	5-6-40
Hasta	2	5-13-20	5-13-45	5-14-10	5-24-35	5-15-0	5-15-25	5-15-50	5-16-15	5-16-40
Chitra	2	5-26-40	5-27-5	5-27-30	5-27-55	5-28-20	5-28-45	5-29-10	5-29-35	6-0-0
Swati	2	6-10-0	6-10-25	6-10-50	6-11-15	6-11-40	6-12-5	6-12-30	6-12-55	6-13-20
Vishakha	3	6-26-40	6-27-5	6-27-30	6-27-55	6-28-20	6-28-45	6-29-10	6-29-25	7-0-0
Anuradha	3	7-10-0	7-10-25	7-10-50	7-11-15	7-11-40	7-12-5	7-12-30	7-12-55	7-13-30
Jeshtha	3	7-23-20	7-23-45	7-24-10	7-24-35	7-25-0	7-25-25	7-25-50	7-26-15	7-26-40
Mool	2	8-3-20	8-3-45	8-4-10	8-4-35	8-5-0	8-5-25	8-5-50	8-6-15	8-6-40
Prvashada	2	8-16-40	8-17-5	8-17-30	8-17-55	8-18-20	8-18-45	8-19-10	8-19-35	8-20-0
Uttarashada	2	9-0-0	9-0-25	9-0-50	9-1-15	9-1-40	9-2-5	9-2-30	9-2-55	9-3-20
Shravana	3	9-16-40	9-17-5	9-17-30	9-17-55	9-18-20	9-18-45	9-11-20	9-11-35	9-20-0
Dhanishtha	3	10-0-0	10-0-25	10-0-50	10-1-15	10-1-40	10-2-5	10-2-30	10-2-55	10-3-20
Shatbhisha	3	10-13-20	10-13-45	10-14-10	10-14-35	10-15-0	10-15-25	10-15-50	10-16-15	10-16-40
Purva bhadrapada	2	10-23-20	10-23-45	10-24-10	10-24-35	10-25-0	10-25-25	10-25-50	10-26-1	10-26-40
Uttara bhadrapada	2	11-6-40	11-7-5	11-7-30	11-7-55	11-8-20	11-8-45	11-9-10	11-9-35	11-10-0
Revati	2	11-20-0	11-20-25	11-20-50	11-21-15	11-21-60	11-22-5	11-22-30	11-22-55	11-23-20
Balance of dasha		85 yrs.	74 yr 4 mn 15d	63 yr 9 mn	43 yr 1 mn 15 d	42 yr 6 mn	31 yr 10 mn 15d	21 ys 3 mn	10 yr 7 mn 15 d	nill

Table of the balance of the Kaal Chakra dasha from the Longitudes of Moon 83 years

	1	2	3	4	5	6	6	8	9	10
Nakshatra	Pada	lon of moon	lon of moon	lon of moon	lon of moon	lon of moon	lon of moon	lon of moon	lon of moon	lon of moon
		S-DE-MIN								
Ashwini	3	0-6-40	0-7-5	0-7-30	0-7-55	0-8-20	0-8-45	0-9-10	0-9-35	0-10-0
Bharani	3	0-20-0	0-20-25	0-20-50	0-21-15	0-21-40	0-22-5	0-22-30	0-22-55	0-23-20
Krittika	3	1-3-20	1-3-45	1-4-10	1-4-35	1-5-0	1-5-25	1-15-50	1-16-15	1-16-40
Rohini	2	1-13-20	1-13-45	1-14-10	1-14-35	1-15-0	1-15-25	1-15-50	1-16-15	1-16-40
Mrigsiras	2	1-26-40	1-27-5	1-27-30	1-27-55	1-28-20	1-28-45	1-29-10	1-29-35	2-0-0
Ardra	2	2-10-0	2-10-25	2-10-50	2-11-35	2-11-40	2-12-5	2-12-30	2-12-55	2-13-20
Punarvasu	3	2-26-40	2-27-5	2-27-30	2-27-55	2-28-20	2-28-45	2-29-10	2-29-35	3-0-0
Pusya	3	3-10-0	3-10-25	3-10-50	3-11-15	3-11-40	3-12-5	3-12-30	3-12-55	3-13-20
Aslesa	3	3-23-20	3-23-45	3-24-10	3-24-35	3-25-0	3-25-25	3-25-50	3-26-15	3-26-40
Magha	2	4-3-20	4-3-45	4-4-10	4-4-35	4-5-0	4-5-25	4-19-10	4-19-35	4-20-0
Purva Phalguni	2	4-16-40	4-17-5	4-17-30	4-17-55	4-18-20	4-18-45	4-19-10	4-19-35	4-20-0
Uttara Phalguni	2	5-0-0	5-0-25	5-0-50	5-1-15	5-1-40	5-2-5	5-2-30	5-2-55	5-3-20
Hasta	3	5-16-40	5-17-5	5-17-30	5-17-55	5-18-20	5-18-45	5-19-10	5-19-35	5-20-0
Chitra	3	6-0-0	6-0-25	6-0-50	6-1-15	6-1-40	6-2-5	6-2-30	6-2-55	6-3-20
Swati	3	6-13-20	6-13-45	6-14-10	6-14-35	6-15-0	6-15-25	6-15-50	6-16-15	6-16-40
Vishakha	2	6-23-20	6-23-45	6-24-10	6-24-35	6-25-0	6-25-25	6-25-50	6-26-5	6-26-40
Anuradha	2	7-6-40	7-7-5	7-7-30	7-7-55	7-8-20	7-8-45	7-9-10	7-9-35	7-10-0
Jeshtha	2	7-20-0	7-20-25	7-20-50	7-21-15	7-21-40	7-22-5	7-22-30	7-22-55	7-23-20
Mool	3	8-6-40	8-7-5	8-7-30	8-7-55	8-8-20	8-8-45	8-9-10	8-9-35	8-10-0

Prvashada	3	8-20-0	8-20-25	8-20-50	8-21-15	8-21-40	8-22-5	8-22-30	8-22-55	8-23-20
Uttarashada	3	9-3-20	9-3-45	9-4-10	9-4-35	9-4-0	9-5-25	9-5-50	9-6-15	9-6-40
Shravana	2	9-13-20	9-13-45	9-14-10	9-14-35	9-15-0	9-15-25	9-15-50	9-16-15	9-16-40
Dhanishtha	2	9-26-40	9-27-5	9-27-30	9-27-55	9-28-20	9-28-45	9-29-10	9-29-35	10-0-0
Shatbhisha	2	10-10-0	10-10-25	10-10-50	10-11-15	10-11-40	10-12-5	10-12-30	10-12-55	10-13-20
Purva bhadrapada	3	10-26-40	10-47-5	10-27-30	10-27-55	10-28-55	10-28-45	10-29-10	10-29-35	11-0-0
Uttara bhadrapada	3	11-10-0	11-10-25	11-10-50	11-11-15	11-11-40	11-12-5	11-12-30	11-12-55	11-13-20
Revati	3	11-23-20	11-23-45	11-24-10	11-24-35	11-25-0	11-25-25	11-25-50	11-26-15	11-26-40
Balance of dasha		83 yr	72 yrs 7 mn 15d	62 yr 3 mn	41 yr 10 mn 15d	41 yr 6mn	31 yr 1 mn 15d	20 yr 9 mn	10 yr 4 mn 15 d	nill

Table of the balance of the Kaal Chakra dasha from the Longitudes of Moon 86 years

	1	2	3	4	5	6	6	8	9	10
Nakshatra	Pada	lon of moon	lon of moon	lon of moon	lon of moon	lon of moon	lon of moon	lon of moon	lon of moon	lon of moon
		S-DE-MIN								
Ashwini	4	0-10-0	0-10-25	0-10-50	0-11-15	0-11-40	0-12-5	0-12-30	0-12-55	0-13-20
Bharani	4	0-23-20	0-23-45	0-24-10	0-24-35	0-25-0	0-25-25	0-25-50	0-26-15	0-26-40
Krittika	4	1-6-40	1-7-5	1-7-30	1-7-5	1-8-20	1-8-45	1-9-10	1-9-35	1-10-0
Rohini	1	1-10-0	1-10-25	1-10-50	1-11-15	1-11-40	1-12-5	1-12-30	1-12-55	1-13-20
Mrigsiras	1	1-23-20	1-23-45	1-24-10	1-24-35	1-25-0	1-25-25	1-25-30	1-26-5	1-26-40
Ardra	1	2-6-40	2-7-5	2-7-30	2-7-55	2-8-20	2-8-45	2-9-10	2-9-35	2-10-0
Punarvasu	4	3-0-0	3-0-25	3-0-50	3-1-15	3-1-40	3-2-5	3-2-30	3-2-55	3-3-20

Pusya	4	3-13-20	3-13-45	3-14-10	3-14-35	3-15-0	3-15-25	3-15-50	3-16-15	3-16-40
Aslesa	4	3-26-40	3-27-5	3-27-30	3-27-55	3-28-20	3-28-45	3-29-10	3-29-35	4-0-0
Magha	1	4-0-0	4-0-25	4-0-50	4-1-15	4-1-40	4-2-5	4-2-30	4-2-55	4-3-20
Purva Phalguni	1	4-13-20	4-13-45	4-14-10	4-14-35	4-15-0	4-15-25	4-15-50	4-16-15	4-16-40
Uttara Phalguni	1	4-26-40	4-27-5	5-5-27-30	4-27-55	4-28-20	4-28-45	4-29-10	4-29-35	5-0-0
Hasta	4	5-20-0	5-20-25	5-20-50	5-21-15	5-21-40	5-22-5	5-22-30	5-22-45	5-23-20
Chitra	4	6-3-20	6-3-45	6-4-10	6-4-35	6-5-0	6-5-25	5-5-50	6-6-15	6-6-40
Swati	4	6-16-40	6-17-5	6-17-30	6-17-55	6-18-20	6-18-45	6-19-10	6-19-35	6-20-0
Vishakha	1	6-20-0	6-20-25	6-20-50	6-21-15	6-21-40	6-22-5	6-23-30	6-22-55	6-33-20
Anuradha	1	7-3-20	7-3-45	7-4-10	7-4-35	7-5-0	7-5-25	7-5-50	7-6-15	7-6-40
Jeshtha	1	7-16-40	7-17-5	7-17-30	7-17-55	7-18-20	7-18-45	7-19-10	7-19-35	7-20-0
Mool	4	8-10-0	8-10-25	8-10-50	8-11-15	8-11-40	8-12-5	8-12-30	8-12-55	8-13-20
Prvashada	4	8-23-20	8-23-45	8-24-10	8-24-35	8-25-0	8-25-25	8-25-50	8-26-15	8-26-40
Uttarashada	4	9-6-40	9-7-5	9-7-30	9-7-55	9-8-20	9-8-45	9-9-10	9-9-35	9-10-0
Shravana	1	9-10-0	9-10-25	9-10-50	9-11-15	9-11-40	9-12-5	9-12-30	9-12-55	9-13-20
Dhanishtha	1	9-23-20	9-23-45	9-24-10	9-24-35	9-25-0	9-25-25	9-25-50	9-26-15	9-26-40
Shatbhisha	1	10-6-40	10-7-5	10-7-30	10-7-55	10-8-20	10-8-45	10-9-10	10-9-35	10-10-0
Purva bhadrapada	4	11-0-0	11-0-25	11-0-50	11-1-15	11-1-40	11-2-5	11-2-30	11-2-55	11-3-20
Uttara bhadrapada	4	11-13-20	11-13-45	11-14-10	11-14-35	11-15-0	11-15-25	11-15-50	11-16-15	11-16-40
Revati	4	11-26-40	11-27-5	11-27-30	11-27-55	11-28-20	11-28-45	11-29-10	11-29-35	12-0-0
Balance of dasha		86 yr	75 yrs 3 mn	64 yr 6 mn	53 yr 9 mn	43 yr	32 yr 3 mn	21 yr 6 mn	10 yr 9 mn	nill

APPENDIX-4

Minor periods in the Major Periods of Kalchakra

(i) As far as minor periods in the major periods are concerned, whether we call them as Leo in Aries, or Sun in Mars – this minor period will come only once in the full duration of the Dasha. If we give all the minor periods in the **12 signs**, then the Table of minor periods would be too lengthy to cope up with. Therefore we have given the minor period of **Planets** in the major periods of Planets.

The second thing to be noted is that the minor period of *Mars in Sun is the same as the minor period of Sun in Mars*. We have therefore written Sun x Mars only one time.

(ii) The minor periods of Capricorn or Aquarius (signs) do not come when the

Birth is in the constellation where the longevity is of 100 years duration. Therefore in the section of 100 years longevity, the minor periods of Saturn (or Capricorn – Aquarius) is not given in the Major Periods of signs.

(iii) The Major Periods of Sun (Leo) and Moon (Cancer) do not come in when the

Longevity is of 83 years duration. Therefore the minor periods of these two also do not come. This is the reason why the minor periods of Sun and Moon are not given in the major periods of other planets and *vice-versa*.

(iv) If we calculate the minor periods in the major periods by the method of

Proportions then the minor periods of planets comes in Years, Months, Days, Hours and Minutes. But for practical purposes the Hours and Minutes are omitted. If the sum total in the minor period is more by a day or two then from the bigger minor periods, we should reduce a day or two to bring it exactly to the duration of the dasha. Similarly if the total duration comes to be less by a day or two then a day or two should be added to the bigger periods to bring the total at par.

Table of Minor Periods in the Major Periods of Kalchakra

Planet (Signs)	Long. 100 yrs. Yrs Mn Days	Long. 86 yrs. Yrs Mn Days	Long. 85 yrs. Yrs Mn Days	Long. 83 yrs. Yrs Mn Days
Sun x Sun	0-3-00	0-3-15	0-3-15	
Sun x Moon	1–0-18	1-2-20	1-2-25	
Sun x Mars	0–4-06	0-4-27	0-4-28	
Sun x Merc.	0–5-12	0-6-08	0-6-10	
Sun x Jup.	0-6-00	0-6-29	0-7-01	
Sun x Venus	0-9-18	0-11-05	0-11-09	
Sun x Sat.		0-2-24	0-2-25	
Moon x Moon	4–4-28	5-1-16	5-2-08	
Moon x Mars	1-5-20	1-8-15	1-8-23	
Moon x Merc.	1-10-20	2-2-11	2-2-21	
Moon x Jup.	0-10-24	2-5-09	2-5-20	
Moon x Venus	3-4-10	3-10-26	3-11-13	
Moon x Sat.		0-11-12	0-11-26	
Mars x Mars	0-5-26	0-6-25	0-6-27	0-7-02
Mars x Merc.	0–7-17	0-8-24	0-8-27	0-9-04
Mars x Jup.	0–8-12	0-9-23	0-9-27	0-10-04
Mars x Venus.	1–1-13	1-3-19	1-3-24	1-4-06
Mars x Sat.		0-3-27	0-3-29	0-4-01
Merc. x Merc.	0–9-22	0-11-09	0-11-13	0-11-21

Merc. x Jup.	0 – 10 - 24	1-0-17	1-0-21	1-01 -00
Merc. x Venus	1 – 5 - 08	1-08-03	1-8-10	1 - 8- 24
Merc. x Sat.		0-05-00	0-5-02	0 - 5-06
Jup. x Jup.	1 - 00 - 00	1-01-29	1-2-03	1 -2-14
Jup.x Venus	1 - 07 - 06	1-10-10	1-10-17	1-11-04
Jup. x Sat.		0-05-17	0-5-19	0-5-23
Venus x Venus	2 – 06 - 22	2-11-12	3-0-04	3-1-00
Venus x Sat.		0-8-27	0-9-01	0-9-08
Sat. x Sat.		0-2-07	0-2-08	0-2-09

APPENDIX - 5

The following Table is adopted from the Lahiri's Ephemeris. It gives an easy method to work out the balance of the Mahadasha from the longitude of the Moon. In the first column, longitude of Moon is given. In the rows above, the names of the Zodiacal Signs to which the column below pertains to, are indicated. By combining the two we shall get the balance of Dasha at birth. For example if Moon is in Cancer at 3°–40' and then we look to the first column at 3°–40' and then we look to the 5th column under Cancer, and it gives us the balance of Saturn as 18 years 6 months 9 days at birth. In subsequent pages (3rd to 9th page) the Antardashas of Planets are given in Tabular form.

Table of Balance of Vimshottari Dasha and Antar-dasha

Balance of Vimshottari Dasha by Longitude of Moon

Long. of Moon		Moon in Aries Leo, Sagittarius				Moon in Taurus Virgo, Cap.				Moon in Gemini Libra, Aquarius				Moon in Cancer Scorpio, Pisces			
°	'		Y	M	D		Y	M	D		Y	M	D		Y	M	D
0	0	Ketu	7	0	0	Sun	4	6	0	Mars	3	6	0	Jup.	4	0	0
0	20		6	9	27		4	4	6		3	3	27		3	7	6
0	40		6	7	24		4	2	12		3	1	24		3	2	12
1	0		6	5	21		4	0	18		2	11	21		2	9	18
1	20		6	3	18		3	10	24		2	9	18		2	4	24
1	40		6	1	15		3	9	0		2	7	15		2	0	0
2	0		5	11	12		3	7	6		2	5	12		1	7	6
2	20		5	9	9		3	5	12		2	3	9		1	2	12
2	40		5	7	6		3	3	18		2	1	6		0	9	18
3	0		5	5	3		3	1	24		1	11	3		0	4	24
3	20		5	3	0		3	0	0		1	9	0	Satn.	19	0	0
3	40		5	0	27		2	10	6		1	6	27		18	6	9
4	0		4	10	24		2	8	12		1	4	24		18	0	18
4	20		4	8	21		2	6	18		1	2	21		17	6	27
4	40		4	6	18		2	4	24		1	0	18		17	1	6
5	0		4	4	15		2	3	0		0	10	15		16	7	15
5	20		4	2	12		2	1	6		0	8	12		16	1	24

Long. of Moon		Moon in Aries Leo, Sagittarius			Moon in Taurus Virgo, Cap.			Moon in Gemini Libra, Aquarius			Moon in Cancer Scorpio, Pisces		
°	'	Y	M	D	Y	M	D	Y	M	D	Y	M	D
5	40	4	0	9	1	11	12	0	6	9	15	8	3
6	0	3	10	6	1	9	18	0	4	6	15	2	12
6	20	3	8	3	1	7	24	0	2	3	14	8	21
6	40	3	6	0	1	6	0	Rahu 18	0	0	14	3	0
7	0	3	3	27	1	4	6	17	6	18	13	9	9
7	20	3	1	24	1	2	12	17	1	6	13	3	18
7	40	2	11	21	1	0	18	16	7	24	12	9	27
8	0	2	9	18	0	10	24	16	2	12	12	4	6
8	20	2	7	15	0	9	0	15	9	0	11	10	15
8	40	2	5	12	0	7	6	15	3	18	11	4	24
9	0	2	3	9	0	5	12	14	10	6	10	11	3
9	20	2	1	6	0	3	18	14	4	24	10	5	12
9	40	1	11	3	0	1	24	13	11	12	9	11	21
10	0	1	9	0	Moon 10	0	0	13	6	0	9	6	0
10	20	1	6	27	9	9	0	13	0	18	9	0	9
10	40	1	4	24	9	6	0	12	7	6	8	6	18
11	0	1	2	21	9	3	0	12	1	24	8	0	27
11	20	1	0	18	9	0	0	11	8	12	7	7	6
11	40	0	10	15	8	9	0	11	3	0	7	1	15
12	0	0	8	12	8	6	0	10	9	18	6	7	24
12	20	0	6	9	8	3	0	10	4	6	6	2	3
12	40	0	4	6	8	0	0	9	10	24	5	8	12
13	0	0	2	3	7	9	0	9	5	12	5	2	21
13	20	Venus 20	0	0	7	6	0	9	0	0	4	9	0
13	40	19	6	0	7	3	0	8	6	18	4	3	9
14	0	19	0	0	7	0	0	8	1	6	3	9	18
14	20	18	6	0	6	9	0	7	7	24	3	3	27
14	40	18	0	0	6	6	0	7	2	12	2	10	6
15	0	17	6	0	6	3	0	6	9	0	2	4	15
15	20	17	0	0	6	0	0	6	3	18	1	10	24
15	40	16	6	0	5	9	0	5	10	6	1	5	3
16	0	16	0	0	5	6	0	5	4	24	0	11	12
16	20	15	6	0	5	3	0	4	11	12	0	5	21
16	40	15	0	0	5	0	0	4	6	0	Merc. 17	0	0
17	0	14	6	0	4	9	0	4	0	18	16	6	27
17	20	14	0	0	4	6	0	3	7	6	16	1	24
17	40	13	6	0	4	3	0	3	1	24	15	8	21

Long. of Moon		Moon in Aries Leo, Sagittarius				Moon in Taurus Virgo, Cap.				Moon in Gemini Libra, Aquarius				Moon in Cancer Scorpio, Pisces			
°	'		Y	M	D		Y	M	D		Y	M	D		Y	M	D
18	0		13	0	0		4	0	0		2	8	12		15	3	18
18	20		12	6	0		3	9	0		2	3	0		14	10	15
18	40		12	0	0		3	6	0		1	9	18		14	5	12
19	0		11	6	0		3	3	0		1	4	6		14	0	9
19	0	Venus	11	6	0	Moon	3	3	0	Rahu	1	4	6	Merc.	14	0	9
19	20		11	0	0		3	0	0		0	10	24		13	7	6
19	40		10	6	0		2	9	0		0	5	12		13	2	3
20	0		10	0	0		2	6	0	Jup.	16	0	0		12	9	0
20	20		9	6	0		2	3	0		15	7	6		12	3	27
20	40		9	0	0		2	0	0		15	2	12		11	10	24
21	0		8	6	0		1	9	0		14	9	18		11	5	21
21	20		8	0	0		1	6	0		14	4	24		11	0	18
21	40		7	6	0		1	3	0		14	0	0		10	7	15
22	0		7	0	0		1	0	0		13	7	6		10	2	12
22	20		6	6	0		0	9	0		13	2	12		9	9	9
22	40		6	0	0		0	6	0		12	9	18		9	4	6
23	0		5	6	0		0	3	0		12	4	24		8	11	3
23	20		5	0	0	Mars	7	0	0		12	0	0		8	6	0
23	40		4	6	0		6	9	27		11	7	6		8	0	27
24	0		4	0	0		6	7	24		11	2	12		7	7	24
24	20		3	6	0		6	5	21		10	9	18		7	2	21
24	40		3	0	0		6	3	18		10	4	24		6	9	18
25	0		2	6	0		6	1	15		10	0	0		6	4	15
25	20		2	0	0		5	11	12		9	7	6		5	11	12
25	40		1	6	0		5	9	9		9	2	12		5	6	9
26	0		1	0	0		5	7	6		8	9	18		5	1	6
26	20		0	6	0		5	5	3		8	4	24		4	8	3
26	40	Sun	6	0	0		5	3	0		8	0	0		4	3	0
27	0		5	10	6		5	0	27		7	7	6		3	9	27
27	20		5	8	12		4	10	24		7	2	12		3	4	24
27	40		5	6	18		4	8	21		6	9	18		2	11	21
28	0		5	4	24		4	6	18		6	4	24		2	6	18
28	20		5	3	0		4	4	15		6	0	0		2	1	15
28	40		5	1	6		4	2	12		5	7	6		1	8	12
29	0		4	11	12		4	0	9		5	2	12		1	3	9
29	20		4	9	18		3	10	6		4	9	18		0	10	6
29	40		4	7	24		3	8	3		4	4	24		0	5	3
30	0		4	6	0		3	6	0		4	0	0		0	0	0

Proportional Parts for Dasha of Planets

(To be subtracted from the balance of *dasha* for increase by minutes of the longitude of Moon)

	Ketu (7y)		Venus (20y)		Sun (6y)		Moon (10y)		Mars (7y)		Rahu (18y)		Jup. (16y)		Saturn (19y)		Merc. (17y)		
	m	d	m	d	m	d	m	d	m	d	m	d	m	d	m	d	m	d	
1	0	3	0	9	0	3	0	5	0	3	0	8	0	7	0	9	0	8	1
2	0	6	0	18	0	5	0	9	0	6	0	16	0	14	0	17	0	15	2
3	0	9	0	27	0	8	0	14	0	9	0	24	0	22	0	26	0	23	3
4	0	13	1	6	0	11	0	18	0	13	1	2	0	29	1	4	1	1	4
5	0	16	1	15	0	14	0	23	0	16	1	11	1	6	1	13	1	8	5
6	0	19	1	24	0	16	0	27	0	19	1	19	1	13	1	21	1	16	6
7	0	22	2	3	0	19	1	2	0	22	1	27	1	20	2	0	1	24	7
8	0	25	2	12	0	22	1	6	0	25	2	5	1	28	2	8	2	1	8
9	0	28	2	21	0	24	1	11	0	28	2	13	2	5	2	17	2	9	9
10	1	1	3	0	0	27	1	15	1	1	2	21	2	12	2	26	2	17	10
15	1	17	4	15	1	11	2	8	1	17	4	2	3	18	4	8	3	25	15
20	2	3	6	0	1	24	3	0	2	3	5	12	4	24	5	21	5	3	20

VIMSHOTTARI DASHA SUB PERIODS

Sun—Sub-Periods—6 Years

Sun—Inter-Periods

SUN-Sun				SUN-Moon				SUN-Mars			
	m	d	h		m	d	h		m	d	h
Sun	0	5	10	Moon	0	15	0	Mars	0	7	8
Moon	0	9	0	Mars	0	10	12	Rahu	0	18	22
Mars	0	6	7	Rahu	0	27	0	Jupiter	0	16	19
Rahu	0	16	5	Jupiter	0	24	0	Saturn	0	19	23
Jupiter	0	14	10	Saturn	0	28	12	Mercury	0	17	21
Saturn	0	17	2	Mercury	0	25	12	Ketu	0	7	8
Mercury	0	15	7	Ketu	0	10	12	Venus	0	21	0
Ketu	0	6	7	Venus	1	0	0	Sun	0	6	7
Venus	0	18	0	Sun	0	9	0	Moon	0	10	12
Total 3		**18**	**0**	**Total**	**6**	**0**	**0**	**Total**	**4**	**6**	**0**

SUN-Rahu				SUN-Jupiter				SUN-Saturn			
	m	**d**	**h**		**m**	**d**	**h**		**m**	**d**	**h**
Rahu	1	18	14	Jupiter	1	8	10	Saturn	1	24	3
Jupiter	1	13	5	Saturn	1	15	14	Mercury	1	18	11
Saturn	1	21	7	Mercury	1	10	19	Ketu	0	19	23
Mercury	1	15	22	Ketu	0	16	19	Venus	1	27	0
Ketu	0	18	21	Venus	1	18	0	Sun	0	17	2
Venus	1	24	0	Sun	0	14	10	Moon	0	28	12
Sun	0	16	5	Moon	0	24	0	Mars	0	19	23
Moon	0	27	0	Mars	0	16	19	Rahu	1	21	7
Mars	0	18	22	Rahu	1	13	5	Jupiter	1	15	15
Total	**10**	**24**	**0**	**Total**	**9**	**18**	**0**	**Total**	**11**	**12**	**0**

SUN-Mercury				SUN-Ketu				SUN-Venus			
	m	**d**	**h**		**m**	**d**	**h**		**m**	**d**	**h**
Mercury	1	13	8	Ketu	0	7	8	Venus	2	0	0
Ketu	0	17	20	Venus	0	21	0	Sun	0	18	0
Venus	1	21	0	Sun	0	6	7	Moon	1	0	0
Sun	0	15	7	Moon	0	10	12	Mars	0	21	0
Moon	0	25	12	Mars	0	7	8	Rahu	1	24	0
Mars	0	17	21	Rahu	0	18	22	Jupiter	1	18	0
Rahu	1	15	22	Jupiter	0	16	20	Saturn	1	27	0
Jupiter	1	10	19	Saturn	0	19	23	Mercury	1	21	0
Saturn	1	18	11	Mercury	0	17	20	Ketu	0	21	0
Total	**10**	**6**	**0**	**Total**	**4**	**6**	**0**	**Total**	**12**	**0**	**0**

Moon—Sub-Periods—10 Years

Moon—Inter-Periods

MOON-Moon				MOON-Mars				MOON-Rahu			
	m	d	h		m	d	h		m	d	h
Moon	0	25	0	Mars	0	12	6	Rahu	2	21	0
Mars	0	17	12	Rahu	1	1	12	Jupiter	2	12	0
Rahu	1	15	0	Jupiter	0	28	0	Saturn	2	25	12
Jupiter	1	10	0	Saturn	1	3	6	Mercury	2	16	12
Saturn	1	17	12	Mercury	0	29	18	Ketu	1	1	12
Mercury	1	12	12	Keru	0	12	6	Venus	3	0	12
Ketu	0	17	12	Venus	1	5	0	Sun	0	27	0
Venus	1	20	0	Sun	0	10	12	Moon	1	15	0
Sun	0	15	0	Moon	0	17	12	Mars	1	1	0
Total	**10**	**0**	**0**	**Total**	**7**	**0**	**0**	**Total**	**18**	**0**	**0**

MOON-Jupiter				Moon-Saturn				Moon-Mercury			
	m	d	h		m	d	h		m	d	h
Jupiter	2	4	0	Saturn	3	0	6	Mercury	2	12	18
Saturn	2	16	0	Mercury	2	20	18	Ketu	0	29	18
Mercury	2	8	0	Ketu	1	3	6	Venus	2	25	0
Ketu	0	28	0	Venus	3	5	0	Sun	0	25	0
Venus	2	20	0	Sun	0	28	12	Moon	1	12	12
Sun	0	24	0	Moon	1	17	12	Mars	0	29	18
Moon	1	10	0	Mars	1	3	6	Rahu	2	16	12
Mars	0	28	0	Rahu	2	25	12	Jupiter	2	8	0
Rahu	2	12	0	Jupiter	2	16	0	Saturn	2	20	18
Total	**16**	**0**	**0**	**Total**	**19**	**0**	**0**	**Total**	**17**	**0**	**0**

MOON-Ketu				MOON-Venus				MOON-Sun			
	m	d	h		m	d	h		m	d	h
Ketu	0	12	6	Venus	3	10	10	Sun	0	9	0
Venus	1	5	0	Sun	1	0	0	Moon	0	15	0
Sun	0	10	12	Moon	1	20	0	Mars	0	10	12
Moon	0	17	12	Mars	1	5	0	Rahu	0	27	0
Mars	0	12	6	Rahu	3	0	0	Jupiter	0	24	0
Rahu	1	1	12	Jupiter	2	20	0	Saturn	0	28	12
Jupiter	0	28	0	Saturn	3	5	0	Mercury	0	25	12
Saturn	1	3	6	Mercury	2	25	0	Ketu	0	10	12
Mercury	0	29	18	Ketu	1	5	0	Venus	1	0	0
Total	**7**	**0**	**0**	**Total**	**20**	**0**	**0**	**Total**	**6**	**0**	**0**

Mars—Sub-Periods—7 Years

Mars—Inter-Periods

MARS-Mars				MARS-Rahu				MARS-Jupiter			
	m	d	h		m	d	h		m	d	h
Mars	0	8	13.8	Rahu	1	26	16.8	Jupiter	1	14	19.2
Rahu	0	22	1.2	Jupiter	1	20	9.6	Saturn	1	23	4.8
Jupiter	0	19	14.4	Saturn	1	29	20.4	Mercury	1	17	14.4
Saturn	0	23	6.6	Mercury	1	23	13.2	Ketu	0	19	14.4
Mercury	0	20	19.8	Ketu	0	22	1.2	Venus	1	26	0.0
Ketu	0	8	13.8	Venus	2	3	0.0	Sun	0	16	19.2
Venus	0	24	12.0	Sun	0	18	21.6	Moon	0	28	0.0
Sun	0	7	8.4	Moon	1	1	12.0	Mars	0	19	14.4
Moon	0	12	6.0	Mars	0	22	1.2	Rahu	1	20	9.6
Total	**4**	**27**	**0.0**	**Total**	**12**	**18**	**0.0**	**Total**	**11**	**6**	**0.0**

MARS-Saturn				MARS-Mercury				MARS-Ketu			
	m	d	h		m	d	h		m	d	h
Saturn	2	3	4.2	Mercury	1	20	13.8	Ketu	0	8	13.8
Mercury	1	26	12.6	Ketu	0	20	19.8	Venus	0	24	12.0
Ketu	0	23	6.6	Venus	1	29	12.0	Sun	0	7	8.4
Venus	2	6	12.0	Sun	0	17	20.4	Moon	0	12	6.0
Sun	0	19	22.8	Moon	0	29	18.0	Mars	0	8	13.8
Moon	1	3	6.0	Mars	0	20	19.8	Rahu	0	22	1.2
Mars	0	23	6.6	Rahu	1	23	13.2	Jupiter	0	19	14.4
Rahu	1	29	20.4	Jupiter	1	17	14.4	Saturn	0	23	6.6
Jupiter	1	23	4.8	Saturn	1	26	12.6	Mercury	0	20	19.8
Total	**13**	**9**	**0.0**	**Total**	**11**	**17**	**0.0**	**Total**	**4**	**27**	**0.0**

MARS-Venus				MARS-Sun				MARS-Moon			
	m	d	h		m	d	h		m	d	h
Venus	2	10	0	Sun	0	6	7.2	Moon	0	17	12
Sun	0	21	0	Moon	0	10	12.0	Mars	0	12	6
Moon	1	5	0	Mars	0	7	8.4	Rahu	1	1	12
Mars	0	24	12	Rahu	0	18	21.6	Jupiter	0	28	0
Rahu	2	3	0	Jupiter	0	16	19.2	Saturn	1	3	6
Jupiter	1	26	0	Saturn	0	19	22.8	Mercury	0	29	18
Saturn	2	6	12	Mercury	0	17	20.4	Ketu	0	12	6
Mercury	1	29	12	Ketu	0	7	8.4	Venus	1	5	0
Ketu	0	24	12	Venus	0	21	0.0	Sun	0	10	12
Total	**14**	**0**	**0**	**Total**	**4**	**6**	**0.0**	**Total**	**7**	**0**	**0**

Rahu—Sub-Periods—18 Years

Rahu—Inter-Periods

RAHU-Rahu				RAHU-Jupiter				RAHU-Saturn			
	m	d	h		m	d	h		m	d	h
Rahu	4	25	19.2	Jupiter	3	25	4.8	Saturn	5	12	10.8
Jupiter	4	9	14.4	Saturn	4	16	19.2	Mercury	4	25	8.4
Saturn	5	3	21.6	Mercury	4	2	9.6	Ketu	1	29	20.4
Mercury	4	17	16.8	Ketu	1	20	9.6	Venus	5	21	0.0
Ketu	1	26	16.8	Venus	4	24	0.0	Sun	1	21	7.2
Venus	5	12	0.0	Sun	1	13	4.0	Moon	2	25	12.0
Sun	1	18	14.4	Moon	2	12	0.8	Mars	1	29	20.4
Moon	2	21	0.0	Mars	1	20	9.6	Rahu	5	3	21.6
Mars	1	26	16.8	Rahu	4	9	14.4	Jupiter	4	16	19.2
Total	**32**	**12**	**0.0**	**Total**	**28**	**24**	**0.0**	**Total**	**34**	**6**	**0.0**

RAHU-Sun				RAHU-Moon				RAHU-Venus			
	m	d	h		m	d	h		m	d	h
Mercury	4	10	1.2	Ketu	0	22	1.2	Venus	6	0	0
Ketu	1	23	13.2	Venus	2	3	0.0	Sun	1	24	0
Venus	5	3	0.0	Sun	0	18	21.6	Moon	3	0	0
Sun	1	15	21.6	Moon	1	1	12.0	Mars	2	3	0
Moon	2	16	12.0	Mars	0	22	1.2	Rahu	5	12	0
Mars	1	23	13.2	Rahu	1	26	16.8	Jupiter	4	24	0
Rahu	4	17	16.8	Jupiter	1	20	9.6	Saturn	5	21	0
Jupiter	4	2	9.6	Saturn	1	29	20.4	Mercury	5	3	0
Saturn	4	25	8.4	Mercury	1	23	13.2	Ketu	2	3	0
Total	**30**	**18**	**0.0**	**Total**	**12**	**18**	**0.0**	**Total**	**36**	**0**	**0**

RAHU-Sun				RAHU-Moon				RAHU-Mars			
	m	d	h		m	d	h		m	d	h
Sun	0	16	4.8	Moon	1	15	0	Mars	0	22	1.2
Moon	0	27	0.0	Mars	1	1	12	Rahu	1	26	16.8
Mars	0	18	21.6	Rahu	2	21	0	Jupiter	1	20	9.6
Rahu	1	18	14.4	Jupiter	2	12	0	Saturn	1	29	20.4
Jupiter	1	13	4.8	Saturn	2	25	12	Mercury	1	23	13.2
Saturn	1	21	7.2	Mercury	2	16	12	Ketu	0	22	1.2
Mercury	1	15	21.6	Ketu	1	1	12	Venus	2	3	0.0
Ketu	0	18	21.6	Venus	3	0	0	Sun	0	18	21.6
Venus	1	24	0.0	Sun	0	27	0	Moon	1	1	12.0
Total	**10**	**24**	**0.0**	**Total**	**18**	**0**	**0**	**Total**	**12**	**18**	**0.0**

Jupiter—Sub-Periods—16 Years

Jupiter—Inter-Periods

JUPITER-Jupiter				JUPITER-Saturn				JUPITER-Mercury			
	m	d	h		m	d	h		m	d	h
Jupiter	3	12	9.6	Saturn	4	24	9.6	Mercury	3	25	14.4
Saturn	4	1	14.4	Mercury	4	9	4.8	ketu	1	17	14.4
Mercury	3	18	19.2	Ketu	1	23	4.8	Venus	4	16	0.0
Ketu	1	14	19.2	Venus	5	2	0.0	Sun	1	10	19.2
Venus	4	8	0.0	Sun	1	15	14.4	Moon	2	8	0.0
Sun	1	8	9.6	Moon	2	16	0.0	Mars	1	17	14.4
Moon	2	4	0.0	Mars	1	23	4.8	Rahu	4	2	9.6
Mars	1	14	19.2	Rahu	4	16	19.2	Jupiter	3	18	19.2
Rahu	3	25	4.8	Jupiter	4	1	14.4	Saturn	4	9	4.8
Total	**25**	**18**	**0.0**	**Total**	**30**	**12**	**0.0**	**Total**	**27**	**6**	**0.0**

JUPITER-Ketu				JUPITER-Venus				JUPITER-Sun			
	m	d	h		m	d	h		m	d	h
Ketu	0	19	14.4	Venus	5	10	0	Sun	0	14	9.6
Venus	1	26	0.0	Sun	1	18	0	Moon	0	24	0.0
Sun	0	16	19.2	Moon	2	20	0	Mars	0	16	19.2
Moon	0	28	0.0	Mars	1	26	0	Rahu	1	13	4.8
Mars	0	19	14.4	Rahu	4	24	0	Jupiter	1	8	9.6
Rahu	1	20	9.6	Jupiter	4	8	0	Saturn	1	15	14.4
Jupiter	1	14	19.2	Saturn	5	2	0	Mercury	1	10	19.2
Saturn	1	23	4.8	Mercury	4	16	0	Ketu	0	16	19.2
Mercury	1	17	14.4	ketu	1	26	0	Venus	1	18	0.0
Total	**11**	**6**	**0.0**	**Total**	**32**	**0**	**0**	**Total**	**9**	**18**	**0.0**

JUPITER-Moon				JUPITER-Mars				JUPITER-Rahu			
	m	d	h		m	d	h		m	d	h
Moon	1	10	0	Mars	0	19	14.4	Rahu	4	9	14.4
Mars	0	28	0	Rahu	1	20	9.6	Jupiter	3	25	4.8
Rahu	2	12	0	Jupiter	1	14	19.2	Saturn	4	16	19.2
Jupiter	2	4	0	Saturn	1	23	4.8	Mercury	4	2	9.6
Saturn	2	16	0	Mercury	1	17	14.4	Ketu	1	20	9.6
Mercury	2	8	0	Ketu	0	19	14.4	Venus	4	24	0.0
Ketu	0	28	0	Venus	1	26	0.0	Sun	1	13	4.8
Venus	2	20	0	Sun	0	16	19.2	Moon	2	12	0.0
Sun	0	24	0	Moon	0	28	0.0	Mars	1	20	9.6
Total	**16**	**0**	**0**	**Total**	**11**	**6**	**0.0**	**Total**	**28**	**24**	**0.0**

Saturn—SubPeriods—19 Years

Saturn—Inter-Periods

SATURN-Saturn				SATURN-Mercury				SATURN-Ketu			
	m	d	h		m	d	h		m	d	h
Saturn	5	21	11.4	Mercury	4	17	6.6	Ketu	0	23	6.6
Mercury	5	3	10.2	Ketu	1	26	12.6	Venus	2	6	12.0
Ketu	2	3	4.4	Venus	5	11	41.0	Sun	0	19	22.8
Venus	6	0	12.0	Sun	1	18	10.8	Moon	1	3	6.0
Sun	1	24	3.6	Moon	1	20	18.0	Mars	0	23	6.6
Moon	3	0	6.0	Mars	1	26	12.6	Rahu	1	29	20.6
Mars	2	3	4.2	Rahu	4	25	8.4	Jupiter	1	23	4.8
Rahu	5	12	10.8	Jupiter	4	9	4.8	Saturn	2	3	4.1
Jupiter	4	24	9.6	Saturn	5	3	10.2	Mercury	1	26	12.5
Total	**36**	**3**	**0.0**	**Total**	**32**	**9**	**0.0**	**Total**	**13**	**9**	**0.0**

SATURN-Venus				SATURN-Sun				SATURN-Moon			
	m	d	h		m	d	h		m	d	h
Venus	6	10	0	Sun	0	17	2.4	Moon	1	17	12
Sun	1	27	0	Moon	0	18	12.0	Mars	1	3	6
Moon	3	5	0	Mars	0	19	22.8	Rahu	2	25	12
Mars	2	6	12	Rahu	1	21	7.2	Jupiter	2	16	0
Rahu	5	21	0	Jupiter	1	15	14.4	Saturn	3	0	6
Jupiter	5	2	0	Saturn	1	14	3.6	Mercury	2	20	18
Saturn	6	0	12	Mercury	1	18	10.8	Ketu	1	3	6
Mercury	5	11	12	Ketu	0	19	22.8	Venus	3	5	0
Ketu	2	6	12	Venus	1	27	0.0	Sun	0	28	12
Total	**38**	**0**	**0**	**Total**	**11**	**12**	**0.0**	**Total**	**19**	**0**	0

SATURN-Mars				SATURN-Rahu				SATURN-Jupiter			
	m	d	h		m	d	h		m	d	h
Mars	0	23	6.6	Rahu	5	3	21.6		4	1	14.4
Rahu	1	29	20.4	Jupiter	4	16	19.2		4	24	9.6
Jupiter	1	23	4.8	Saturn	5	12	10.8		4	9	4.8
Saturn	2	3	4.2	Mercury	4	25	8.4		1	23	4.8
Mercury	1	26	12.6	Ketu	1	29	20.4		5	2	0.0
Ketu	0	23	6.6	Venus	5	21	0.0		1	15	14.4
Venus	2	6	12.0	Sun	1	21	7.2		2	16	0.0
Sun	0	19	22.8	Moon	2	25	12.4		1	23	4.8
Moon	1	3	6.0	Mars	1	29	20.4		4	16	19.2
Total	**13**	**9**	**0.0**	**Total**	**34**	**6**	**0.0**		**30**	**12**	**0.0**

Mercury-sub-Periods—17 Years

Mercury—Inter-Periods

MERCURY-Mercury				MERCURY-Ketu				MERCURY-Venus			
	m	d	h		m	d	h		m	d	h
Mercury	4	2	19.8	Ketu	0	20	19.8	Venus	5	20	0
Ketu	1	20	13.8	Venus	1	29	12.0	Sun	1	21	0
Venus	4	24	12.0	Sun	0	17	20.4	Moon	2	25	0
Sun	1	13	8.4	Moon	0	29	18.0	Mars	1	29	12
Moon	2	12	6.0	Mars	0	20	19.8	Rahu	5	3	0
Mars	1	20	13.8	Rahu	1	23	13.2	Jupiter	4	16	0
Rahu	4	10	1.2	Jupiter	1	17	14.4	Saturn	5	11	12
Jupiter	3	25	14.4	Saturn	1	26	12.6	Mercury	4	24	12
Saturn	4	17	6.6	Mercury	1	20	13.8	Ketu	1	29	12
Total	**28**	**27**	**0.0**		**11**	**27**	**0.0**		**34**	**0**	**0**

MERCURY-Sun				MERCURY-Moon				MERCURY-Mars			
	m	d	h		m	d	h		m	d	h
Sun	0	15	7.2	Moon	1	12	12	Mars	0	20	19.8
Moon	0	25	12.0	Mars	0	29	18	Rahu	1	23	13.2
Mars	0	17	20.4	Rahu	2	16	12	Jupiter	1	17	14.4
Rahu	1	15	21.6	Jupiter	2	8	0	Saturn	1	26	12.6
Jupiter	1	10	19.2	Saturn	2	20	18	Mercury	1	20	13.8
Seturn	1	18	10.8	Mercury	2	12	6	Ketu	0	20	19.8
Mercury	1	13	8.4	Ketu	0	29	18	Venus	1	29	12.0
Ketu	0	17	20.4	Venus	2	25	0	Sun	0	17	20.4
Venus	1	21	0.0	Sun	0	25	12	Moon	0	29	18.0
Total	**10**	**6**	**0.0**	**Total**	**17**	**0**	**0**	**Total**	**11**	**27**	**0.0**

MERCURY-Rahu				MERCURY-Jupiter				MERCURY-Saturn			
	m	d	h		m	d	h		m	d	h
Rahu	4	17	16.8	Jupiter	3	18	19.2	Saturn	5	3	10.2
Jupiter	4	2	9.6	Saturn	4	9	4.8	Mercury	4	17	6.6
Saturn	4	25	8.4	Mercury	3	25	14.4	Ketu	1	26	12.6
Mercury	4	10	1.2	Ketu	1	17	14.4	Venus	5	11	12.0
Ketu	1	23	13.2	Venus	4	16	0.0	Sun	1	18	10.8
Venus	5	3	0.0	Sun	1	10	19.2	Moon	2	20	18.8
Sun	1	15	21.6	Moon	2	8	0.0	Mars	1	26	12.6
Moon	2	16	12.0	Mars	1	17	14.4	Rahu	4	25	8.4
Mars	1	23	13.2	Rahu	4	2	9.6	Jupiter	4	9	4.8
Total	**30**	**18**	**0.0**	**Total**	**27**	**6**	**0.0**	**Total**	**32**	**9**	**0.0**

Ketu—Sub-Periods—7 Years

Ketu—Inter-Periods

KETU-Ketu				KETU-Venus				KETU-Sun			
	m	**d**	**h**		**m**	**d**	**h**		**m**	**d**	**h**
Ketu	0	8	13.8	Venus	2	10	0	Sun	0	6	7.2
Venus	0	24	12.0	Sun	0	21	0	Moon	0	10	12.0
Sun	0	7	8.4	Moon	1	5	0	Mars	0	7	8.4
Moon	0	12	6.0	Mars	0	24	12	Rahu	0	18	21.6
Mars	0	8	13.8	Rahu	2	3	0	Jupiter	0	16	19.2
Rahu	0	22	1.2	Jupiter	1	26	0	Saturn	0	19	22.8
Jupiter	0	19	14.4	Saturn	2	6	12	Mercury	0	17	20.4
Saturn	0	23	6.6	Mercury	1	29	12	Ketu	0	7	8.4
Mercury	0	20	19.8	Ketu	0	24	12	Venus	0	21	0.0
Total	**4**	**27**	**0.0**	**Total**	**14**	**0**	**0**	**Total**	**4**	**6**	0.0

KETU-Moon				KETU-Mars				KETU-Rahu			
	m	**d**	**h**		**m**	**d**	**h**		**m**	**d**	**h**
Moon	0	17	12.0	Mars	0	8	13.8	Rahu	1	26	16.8
Mars	0	12	6.0	Rahu	0	22	1.2	Jupiter	1	20	9.6
Rahu	1	1	12.0	Jupiter	0	19	14.4	Saturn	1	29	20.4
Jupiter	0	28	0.0	Saturn	0	23	6.6	Mercury	1	23	13.2
Saturn	1	3	6.0	Mercury	0	20	19.8	Ketu	0	22	1.2
Mercury	0	29	18.8	Ketu	0	8	13.8	Venus	2	3	0.0
Ketu	0	12	6.0	Venus	2	24	12.0	Sun	0	18	21.6
Venus	1	5	0.0	Sun	0	7	8.4	Moon	1	1	12.0
Sun	0	10	12.0	Moon	0	12	6.0	Mars	0	22	1.2
Total	**7**	**0**	**0.0**	**Total**	**4**	**27**	**0.0**	**Total**	**12**	**18**	0.0

KETU-Jupiter				KETU-Saturn				KETU-Mercury			
	m	**d**	**h**		**m**	**d**	**h**		**m**	**d**	**h**
Jupiter	1	14	19.2	Saturn	2	3	4.2	Mercury	1	20	13.8
Saturn	1	23	4.8	Mercury	1	26	12.6	Ketu	0	20	19.8
Mercury	1	17	14.4	Ketu	0	23	6.6	Venus	1	29	12.0
Ketu	0	19	14.4	Venus	2	6	12.0	Sun	0	17	20.4
Venus	1	26	0.0	Sun	0	19	22.8	Moon	0	29	18.0
Sun	0	16	19.2	Moon	1	3	6.0	Mars	0	20	19.8
Moon	0	28	0.0	Mars	0	23	6.6	Rahu	1	23	13.2
Mars	0	19	14.4	Rahu	1	29	20.4	Jupiter	1	17	14.4
Rahu	1	20	9.6	Jupiter	1	23	4.8	Saturn	1	26	12.6
Total	**11**	**6**	**0.0**	**Total**	**13**	**9**	**0.0**	**Total**	**11**	**27**	**0.0**

Venus-Sub-Periods-20 Years

Venus-Inter-Periods

VENUS-Venus				VENUS-Sun				VENUS-Moon			
	m	**d**	**h**		**m**	**d**	**h**		**m**	**d**	**h**
Venus	6	20	0	Sun	0	18	0	Moon	1	20	0
Sun	2	0	0	Moon	1	0	0	Mars	1	5	0
Moon	3	10	0	Mars	0	21	0	Rahu	3	0	0
Mars	2	10	0	Rahu	1	24	0	Jupiter	2	20	0
Rahu	6	0	0	Jupiter	1	18	0	Saturn	3	5	0
Jupiter	5	10	0	Saturn	1	27	0	Mercury	2	25	0
Saturn	6	10	0	Mercury	1	21	0	ketu	1	5	0
Mercury	5	20	0	Ketu	0	21	0	Venus	3	10	0
Ketu	2	10	0	Venus	2	0	0	Sun	1	0	0
Total	**40**	**0**	**0**	**Total**	**12**	**0**	**0**	**Total**	**20**	**0**	**0**

VENUS-Mars				VENUS-Rahu				VENUS-Jupiter			
	m	d	h		m	d	h		m	d	h
Mars	0	24	12	Rahu	5	12	0	Jupiter	4	8	0
Rahu	2	3	0	Jupiter	4	24	0	Saturn	5	2	0
Jupiter	1	26	0	Saturn	5	21	0	Mercury	4	16	0
Saturn	2	6	12	Mercury	5	3	0	Ketu	1	26	0
Mercury	1	29	12	Ketu	2	3	0	Venus	5	10	0
Ketu	0	24	12	Venus	6	0	0	Sun	1	18	0
Venus	2	10	0	Sun	1	24	0	Moon	2	20	0
Sun	0	21	0	Moon	3	0	0	Mars	1	26	0
Moon	1	5	0	Mars	2	3	0	Rahu	4	24	0
Total	**14**	**0**	**0**	**Total**	**36**	**0**	**0**	**Total**	**32**	**0**	**0**

VENUS-Saturn				VENUS-Mercury				VENUS-Ketu			
	m	d	h		m	d	h		m	d	h
Saturn	6	0	12	Mercury	4	24	12	Ketu	0	24	12
Mercury	5	11	12	Ketu	1	29	12	Venus	2	10	0
Ketu	2	6	12	Venus	5	20	0	Sun	0	21	0
Venus	6	10	0	Sun	1	21	0	Moon	1	5	0
Sun	1	27	0	Moon	2	25	0	Mars	0	24	12
Moon	3	5	0	Mars	1	29	12	Rahu	2	3	0
Mars	2	6	12	Rahu	5	3	0	Jupiter	1	26	0
Rahu	5	21	0	Jupiter	4	16	0	Saturn	2	6	12
Jupiter	5	2	0	Saturn	5	11	12	Mercury	1	29	12
Total	**38**	**0**	**0**	**Total**	**34**	**0**	**0**	**Total**	**14**	**0**	**0**